MW01419674

BOOK COVER DESIGN AND ILLUSTRATIONS (OTHER THAN FROM SPECIFIC STUDIES) BY EASHWARRAN KOHILATHAS.

WWW.CALLINGOUTTHESHOTS.XYZ

WWW.DRKOHILATHAS.CO.UK

TO HUMANITY,
MAY WE CONTINUE TO QUESTION,
TO SEEK JUSTICE,
AND HEAL TOGETHER.

CONTENTS

DISCLAIMER

THE INFORMATION PROVIDED IN THIS BOOK AND RELATED WEBSITE IS FOR EDUCATIONAL AND RESEARCH PURPOSES ONLY. IT IS NOT INTENDED TO BE A GUIDE FOR SELF-DIAGNOSIS OR SELF-MEDICATION. I ACCEPT NEITHER LIABILITY NOR RESPONSIBILITY TO ANY PERSON WITH RESPECT TO LOSS, INJURY OR DAMAGED CAUSED, OR ALLEGED TO BE CAUSED DIRECTLY OR INDIRECTLY BY THE INFORMATION CONTAINED IN THIS BOOK AND/OR RELATED WEBSITE.

"FIRST DO NO HARM"

HIPPOCRATIC OATH

"PATIENTS NEED GOOD DOCTORS. GOOD DOCTORS MAKE THE CARE OF THEIR PATIENTS THEIR FIRST CONCERN: THEY ARE COMPETENT, KEEP THEIR KNOWLEDGE AND SKILLS UP TO DATE, ESTABLISH AND MAINTAIN GOOD RELATIONSHIPS WITH PATIENTS AND COLLEAGUES, ARE HONEST AND TRUSTWORTHY, AND ACT WITH INTEGRITY AND WITHIN THE LAW.

GOOD DOCTORS WORK IN PARTNERSHIP WITH PATIENTS AND RESPECT THEIR RIGHTS TO PRIVACY AND DIGNITY. THEY TREAT EACH PATIENT AS AN INDIVIDUAL. THEY DO THEIR BEST TO MAKE SURE ALL PATIENTS RECEIVE GOOD CARE AND TREATMENT THAT WILL SUPPORT THEM TO LIVE AS WELL AS POSSIBLE, WHATEVER THEIR ILLNESS OR DISABILITY."

GENERAL MEDICAL COUNCIL

“THE INTERESTS AND WELFARE OF THE INDIVIDUAL SHOULD HAVE PRIORITY OVER THE SOLE INTEREST OF SCIENCE OR SOCIETY.”

UNIVERSAL DECLARATION ON BIOETHICS AND HUMAN RIGHTS

"ALL TRUTH PASSES THROUGH THREE STAGES. FIRST, IT IS RIDICULED. SECOND, IT IS VIOLENTLY OPPOSED. THIRD, IT IS ACCEPTED AS BEING SELF-EVIDENT."

ARTHUR SCHOPENHAUER

"WHY OF COURSE THE PEOPLE DON'T WANT WAR. WHY SHOULD SOME POOR SLOB ON A FARM WANT TO RISK HIS LIFE IN A WAR WHEN THE BEST HE CAN GET OUT OF IT IS TO COME BACK TO HIS FARM IN ONE PIECE? NATURALLY THE COMMON PEOPLE DON'T WANT WAR NEITHER IN RUSSIA, NOR IN ENGLAND, NOR FOR THAT MATTER IN GERMANY. THAT IS UNDERSTOOD. BUT, AFTER ALL, IT IS THE LEADERS OF THE COUNTRY WHO DETERMINE THE POLICY AND IT IS ALWAYS A SIMPLE MATTER TO DRAG THE PEOPLE ALONG, WHETHER IT IS A DEMOCRACY, OR A FASCIST DICTATORSHIP, OR A PARLIAMENT, OR A COMMUNIST DICTATORSHIP.

VOICE OR NO VOICE, THE PEOPLE CAN ALWAYS BE BROUGHT TO THE BIDDING OF THE LEADERS. THAT IS EASY. ALL YOU HAVE TO DO IS TELL THEM THEY ARE BEING ATTACKED, AND DENOUNCE THE PEACEMAKERS FOR LACK OF PATRIOTISM AND EXPOSING THE COUNTRY TO DANGER. IT WORKS THE SAME IN ANY COUNTRY."

HERMANN GOERIN, HIGH-RANKING NAZI, AT THE NUREMBERG TRIALS

FOREWORD
BY ALEX MITCHELL

My own personal journey over the past two years has been one of many paths on the road to here in late October 2023.

My journey began in late March 21 when I thought I was doing the right thing and got the first Astrazeneca vaccine, little did I know then of the horrific consequences that awaited me.

I am now a medically certified and UK government acknowledged VITT (Vaccine induced thrombotic thrombocytopenia).

I am now an amputee, I lost my left leg from above the knee and I have other issues.

Since April 21 I have been contacted by many who reached out to me and said that they were going to do something and very rarely did they do so, which does nothing for my trust and faith and continues to do so to today, but Eash wasn't one of them.

Eash said from the very first contact that he was going to write a book to try to help the vaccine injured out there and that's exactly what he has done. Eash has been in regular contact sometimes just asking if I was ok.

That is the true measure of the man.

I have to say that not only is Eash a man of his words and convictions but he is also a very nice decent person and I have enjoyed our conversations along the way and look forward to many more my friend.

On a very personal note I am truly humbled and honoured to be asked to write the foreword thank you.

Alex Mitchell VITT

"You don't know how strong you are until strong is all you've got."

SURVIVORS GUILT

I am one of the lucky ones. I was at the right place at the right time. Lucky to have the ability to see situations from both sides. Aware of the disease and the "cure". Lucky to know our natural ability to ward off infections. Lucky to be aware of the wonders of modern medicine. And lucky to understand the limitations of both.

I am one of the lucky ones. Lucky to have the ability to read, understand, and analyse scientific papers. Lucky to know the limitations of peer-reviewing and reductionist science. Lucky to understand the inner workings of healthcare institutions. Lucky to know how decisions are made on the ward to how policies are made in government. Lucky to understand micro and macro politics. Lucky to have read the works of those like Yevgeny Zamyatin, Haing S. Ngor and Malcolm X. Lucky to have a family who fled genocide. Lucky to understand tyranny and fear.

I am one of the lucky ones. Lucky to have worked in emergency departments, general practices, mental health wards, paediatrics, neonatology, geriatrics, and in intensive care units. Lucky to have been in positions where I have helped to save lives and in other situations where I have made it possible for people to go peacefully. Lucky to have helped introduce new life into this world and lucky to have held the hands of those who breathed their final breath. I am lucky to have seen it all.

I am one of the lucky ones. Lucky to have a wonderful family. Lucky to be brought up with a sense of love and purpose. Lucky to question things if they don't make sense. Lucky to have the patience to sit with a problem until it is solved. Lucky to stand up and speak out if I see wrongdoing. Lucky to want better for humanity and the world as a whole. Lucky enough to understand the preciousness of life and freedom.

I am one of the lucky ones. Lucky to have been at an age and a position in my life where I could say "no". Lucky to have the strength to endure the feeling of loneliness. Lucky to have ignored the ostracisation and unfair treatment at work and society.

Lucky to have the ability to understand the importance of medical ethics and evidence-based science. Lucky to have not gotten swayed by the opinions of those who did not have my best interest at heart.

I am one of the lucky ones. Luckier than the members of my family and friends who have recently been diagnosed with cancer. Lucky to have the courage to stand up to the matron who called security on me and my grieving family for visiting my dying grandmother. Luckier than my friend who collapsed whilst playing football and never woke up.

I am one of the lucky ones. Luckier than those who have been tricked into giving their health away for 'freedom'. Luckier than those buried and cremated without proper autopsy. Luckier than those who could not be with their loved ones to say their final goodbyes. Luckier than those turned into a statistic for political gain. Luckier than those who have damaged their heart. Luckier than those who have lost limbs. Luckier than those who have ruined their immune system. Luckier than those who have been murdered.

I am one of the lucky ones. I do not have brain fog. I can breathe deeply. I do not suffer from debilitating anxiety. I do not feel a deep betrayal as the truth reveals itself day after day. I do not live in fear not knowing when I will die. I do not constantly worry about my fertility or the health of my family. I am luckier than parents who are grieving their deceased children. I am luckier than children who lost out on education and their childhood.

But though lucky, I wish I had done more.

HOW TO READ THIS BOOK?

The information in this book comes from 15 years of my medical knowledge, real-life events, my experience working on the COVID-19 frontline and in different medical specialties, and many more years of research spent looking for answers.

Even though I've done my best to explain complicated ideas in simple terms, I can't hide the fact that some parts of this work may be hard to understand. I will not only reveal scientific theories and words that many of you may have never heard of, but by understanding these concepts, you will realise that what has occurred in recent years is the greatest government-sponsored miscarriage of science and harm to population health that humanity has ever faced.

The reasons for the recent atrocities are based on a multitude of geopolitical reasons, but ultimately, we are living through what happens when science is politicised and used as a tool for power, control, and Big corporate greed.

The subsequent attempted power grab by and the greatest transfer of wealth to the world's corrupt 1% were only possible via two factors: the induction of population-wide fear and a lack of understanding of one's health and sovereignty. Both fear and freedom are intimately tied together. They are both negatively correlated; as one increases, the other goes down.

My aim is to not only shed light on what has been going on in the scientific realm and uncover what the studies *actually* say, but also to help educate you on ways you may be able to strengthen your immune system and highlight research that may be useful for those with jab-related side effects.

And so I have split this book into three main parts. In part one, I will be going through common questions about the jab, what studies that have been kept hidden have noted, and how our immune system actually works. There has been a global narrative to only provide government-vetted answers to common questions about the shot and our health, labelling anything that goes against this as "misinformation" and even censoring those who have other opinions.

By highlighting what the evidence *really* says, I hope you will appreciate that what has been injected into the arms of millions was done ultimately through cohesion, false promises, and scientific fraud. No one has been properly informed with regards to the shots since their introduction.

Part one is my attempt to openly show you, without the threat of being "cancelled", the hidden facts and figures that have been kept from you by the mainstream media. Only once the scene has been set can the story unfold, and so part two will use the evidence gathered in part one, as well as other scientific research, to look at what we may be able to do now to help humanity in the future.

In part two, you'll be shown ways to naturally improve your immune system so we're better prepared for another pandemic. We'll also look into how to help people with long-term effects from the virus and/or injuries from the shot. Part two is dedicated to rebuilding humanity's strength.

And finally, in part three, we will take a collective deep breath and explore what is needed to prevent another pandemic from happening again in the future, what we need to do now to rebuild society, and ways justice can be served to those who have done us wrong.

I understand that there is a lot to take in throughout this book, but I encourage you to try very hard to take in the information and absorb it. Your individual understanding, and thus ownership of your own health, is what stands between humankind and medical tyranny. I also think it is paramount that we move away from the culture of needing to simplify everything. We lose the meaning of concepts through oversimplification, and the appreciation for the interconnectedness of life goes with it too.

Though I have put pen to paper, I have tried my very hardest to write this book without bias or ulterior motives other than to give you clear-cut information. And so, in that sense, the information contained within this book is not mine; it is all of ours.

Take your time, take notes, read the studies, and question the assumptions and theories made in this book. Make up your own mind. Think and come to your own conclusions.

Let's practise actual science again.

Let's aim to evolve.

Let's aim to work together.

Let's become free.

UNDERSTANDING THE PRODUCT, YOURSELF AND THE SITUATION YOU'RE IN.

SO YOU'VE TAKEN THE SHOT, NOW WHAT?

You might have taken three and are awaiting your fourth. You might have only had one. And some of you might have had none. But judging by the fact that you're reading this, you're probably looking for some answers or even some help now.

If you did get the shot, I'm not here to pass judgement with regards to whether or not your initial choice to get it (or your fourth one) was correct. You did what you thought was right. *And in fact, how would you have known any better?* There's been a purposeful, politically-backed narrative forcing people to take it. The UK government alone spent more than one hundred million pounds on COVID-19 communications in 2020.[1] And the US Department of Health and Human Services (HHS) and the Centers For Disease Control and Prevention (CDC) supposedly paid stand-up comedians, screenwriters, production companies, and tech companies to promote COVID-19 jabs to the masses, while ridiculing and shaming those who refused the jab. This was all part of the COVID-19 stimulus push, estimated to be around $1 billion.[2]

In my personal life, I know of university students who were warned that they had to show evidence of vaccination if they wanted to continue to study. I know caregivers and other health professionals who had to get jabbed to keep their jobs. I know of others who felt violated as the needle was driven into their skin. And we all know what happened to some professional athletes who refused to take it, as well as what is happening to and has happened to some of them who did. When push comes to shove and it's your family you've got to feed, risks seem like they have to be taken. And most of us trusted our governments and doctors. I get it.

It's not your fault, but I will urge you to now at least pause, think, and ask for more scientific evidence before injecting yourself with unknown agents. If you're unsure, don't do it. It's your health we're talking about here and an irreversible medical procedure.

Regardless of jab status, I must ask that we begin to question and speak up whenever we see wrongdoing so that we do not end up in this mess again. There were people who were unethically refused medical treatments, like organ transplants,[3] solely because of their vaccine status. Others injured after being inoculated are continuing to be dismissed and gaslighted into thinking that what they are suffering from is all in their heads. *Why don't more people stand up for their fellow man?*

From the start, it was us who allowed this circus act to continue by following idiotic rules like wearing masks when standing and removing them when sitting at restaurants. When people were refused the chance to hug and say goodbye to their loved ones in hospitals or at funerals, no one said a word. When they came for our children. Silence. Fear gripped us all.

If something doesn't sit right or is obviously wrong and/or idiotic, we *must* speak up. Society is shaped by every single citizen it houses. As a result, we must each take individual responsibility for the group. More of us would have been protected if more of us had spoken up at the start.

But anyway, you've already rolled up your sleeve and have had the procedure, or you may know of someone who has. The deed is done, and we all know that it can't be reversed. We must now move on. And move on as one.

There is no "us versus them," "blue versus red," or "vaccinated versus unvaccinated." The fueling of division is what politicians want. Our strength is greater in numbers, and so I also urge you to work with one another, especially as there has been a targeted objective to cause intersocietal conflict by reducing others to disease vectors and various inhuman slurs. We've been divided, and so we must come and work together.

I get it if some of you are angry, especially if you or someone you know has been negatively impacted by these shots. I am angry too. To you, I say direct that energy into learning and thus preventing a situation like this from happening again. Direct that energy toward acquiring justice. Direct that anger progressively. Build, do not destroy. Do not be mad at each other, but at those who tricked us.

In the sections below, once the introductions and formalities have taken place, I will go through an overview of our immune system, what exactly mRNA technology is, the various injuries these vaccines have caused, and what you *may* be able to do to mitigate these. I cannot promise success, and please do not take anything in this book as medical advice. I must also state that, due to the novelty of the virus and mRNA technology, data around this subject matter is still sparse. We are currently at the stage of scientific discovery. No one, including myself, knows what will happen to those who have had the jab in the future. There are many unknowns and even more unknown unknowns.

What makes the whole situation worse is that much of the scientific data surrounding the jabs and virus may be compromised. A lot of science is controlled by major pharmaceutical companies and influenced by politics, rendering it no longer science. This is no better highlighted than when the world's most politically powerful man declared, "You're not going to get COVID if you have these vaccinations."[4] We are waking up to this lie now.

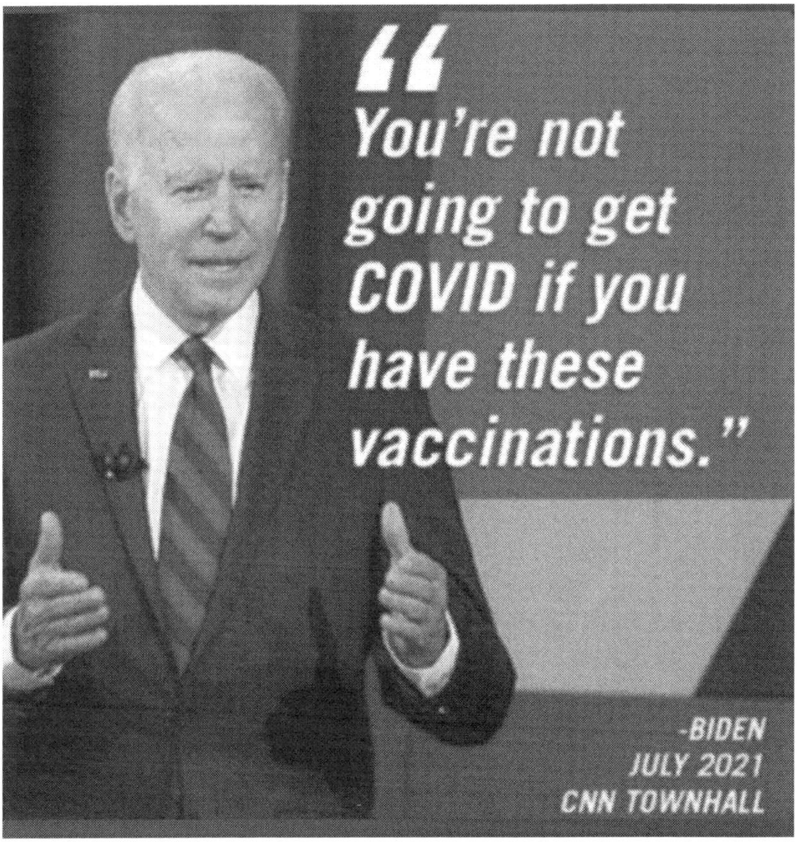

President Joe Biden spreading misinformation, from: https://twitter.com/business/status/1553464129012252673

Other prominent figures who led the COVID-19 response have also made unscientific statements in efforts to promote the product. See this. Understand this. Come with an open mind.

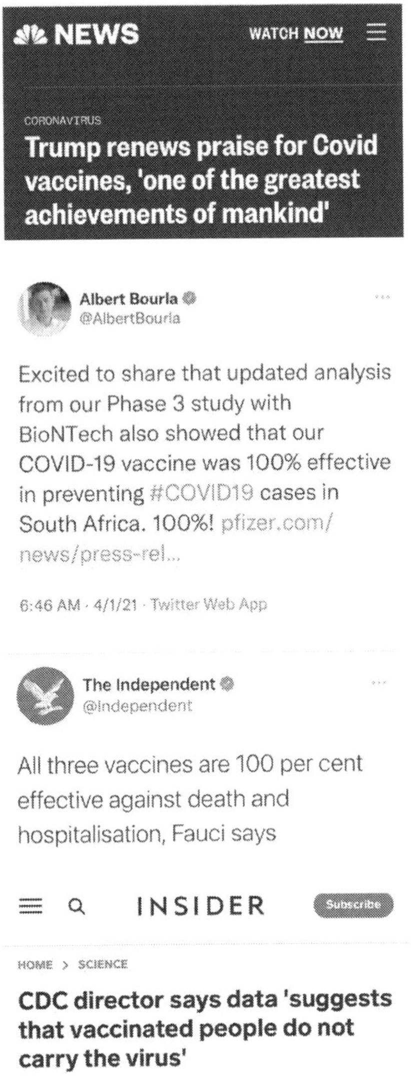

NEWS WATCH NOW

CORONAVIRUS

Trump renews praise for Covid vaccines, 'one of the greatest achievements of mankind'

Albert Bourla
@AlbertBourla

Excited to share that updated analysis from our Phase 3 study with BioNTech also showed that our COVID-19 vaccine was 100% effective in preventing #COVID19 cases in South Africa. 100%! pfizer.com/news/press-rel...

6:46 AM · 4/1/21 · Twitter Web App

The Independent
@Independent

All three vaccines are 100 per cent effective against death and hospitalisation, Fauci says

INSIDER Subscribe

HOME > SCIENCE

CDC director says data 'suggests that vaccinated people do not carry the virus'

Other prominent figures spreading misinformation, from: https://www.nbcnews.com/politics/donald-trump/trump-renews-praise-covid-vaccines-one-greatest-achievements-mankind-n1286551 https://twitter.com/albertbourla/status/1377618480527257606?lang=en https://twitter.com/independent/status/1366125427144732672?lang=en-GB https://www.businessinsider.com/cdc-director-data-vaccinated-people-do-not-carry-covid-19-2021-3?r=US&IR=T

Please understand that I'm not here to change your mind one way or the other.

I'm just looking for the truth. I'm also not here to make you feel bad or worried. My purpose is to highlight certain scientific journals that weren't circulated in the mainstream and to question the science behind these shots. I am learning about this whole scenario as time goes on too.

All in all I'd like to help you become more informed and, therefore, more in control of your health. You've heard one side of the story; I'm here to give you the other.

I have written this book to help you understand the science behind the virus, the shot, and your immune system. Only through understanding can we begin to think about what we might be able to do to mitigate the side effects post-vaccination. Don't be alarmed if the answer is nothing. And don't be alarmed if I release "version two" later down the line that contradicts everything I say here. That is how science works. And remember, take nothing in this book as medical advice.

WHAT IS MY STORY?

My name is Eashwarran Kohilathas. I am a medical doctor and, to some, an annoyingly curious questioner. In 2020, I was working on the front lines of an emergency department during the first wave of the pandemic, and probably one of only a few doctors to encounter the first COVID-19 cases in hospital in the UK.

As you can guess, it was stressful. Not only were we dealing with a nasty virus and the introduction to things like personal protective equipment (PPE) and respirators (now unfortunately embedded in common language), but none of us really knew what we were doing. When I say "we," I mean the scientific community as a whole. *And how could we?* This was a new virus; we had no idea how to deal with it. People were getting seriously ill from it, and others were dying from it.

I spent many long shifts diagnosing and treating people with COVID-19, and I used this time to learn about the disease and how it affected me and others. I tested the basic idea of natural immunity on myself by breathing in virus-filled air on several occasions. I did this on the foundation of natural pharmaceuticals and changes to my own physiology that I had begun prior to the virus's official arrival to the UK. I understood the uselessness of all types of masks very early on and was willing to work maskless with patients coughing on me if need be.

During this time, I read up on immunology and learned as much as I could about the virus. To me, it was a once-in-a lifetime event, and we had this wonderful thing called the internet. *How could one not take this opportunity to learn?* But the more I understood what was going on, the more holes and errors I noted in my workplace. My colleagues were following the rules, but a lot of the rules did not hold up to scientific or logical scrutiny.

We were sending the elderly back to care homes too soon. Windows were closed in many parts of the emergency department, reducing air circulation. We were counting anyone who had died *with* COVID-19 as dying *from* it. Family members were denied the chance to see their loved ones, and death certification and post-mortems seemed to happen very rarely now. The rules were so backward that I felt like they were actually *helping* to spread disease and cover up mistakes. Regardless, I continued, assuming that those enforcing the rules must have had a better understanding of pandemic than I did. I hoped it would all make sense soon. Whatever I learned, I shared on Twitter and on my website. It was well received.

After eight months of working in the emergency department, I worked with children and babies in paediatrics and neonatology; this was during the second wave. To give you some context of how busy it was, there was only *one* child admitted due to COVID-19 in my four months working there. This child was not in a serious state and was quickly discharged. The wards were largely empty.

As time passed, I became increasingly aware of discrepancies between what I saw and what we were supposed to believe. Unfortunately, the majority of my colleagues seemed blind to real-life data. Worryingly, I noticed that the people I worked with, regardless of their specialty or qualifications, had a serious lack of scientific knowledge about the pandemic and the virus during conversations. When I probed them to explain their reasoning behind unscientific rules, like needing to wear a mask on the ward but not in the staff room, for example, they reeled out pre-prepared statements. It was like speaking to parrots.

I worked in a psychiatric hospital after leaving paediatrics. As I worked, I continued to observe, read journals, research, and write. I knew that lockdowns had taken a toll on people's mental health, but I was horrified to find out just how much. I predominantly worked on the young people's ward, and I saw firsthand just *how much* the pandemic had taken from them.

I encountered children as young as 13 who tried to kill themselves. Others were there with eating disorders and signs of psychosis, both conditions worsened by stress and a lack of routine. Many stayed for up to a year, not improving, their education and future ruined. The nurses and psychiatrists agreed that they were seeing record numbers of young people being admitted. There was a growing admissions waiting list for this particular hospital.

Working in mental health was emotionally draining, but to make matters worse, I felt that the rules placed by the infection control department were harming the children. Upon admission, many children were placed in rooms alone, with only sporadic interactions with staff members who were masked and gowned up and sat outside their doors. This appeared to be done in an effort to limit viral spread. Children were placed in this room alone until two polymerase chain reaction (PCR) tests were taken and confirmed negative before letting them enter the main ward.

In my four months working there, not one child was symptomatic with COVID-19; not one child had a positive test, and yet these children, with serious underlying mental health issues like psychosis and severe depression, were placed in solitary confinement on admission, sometimes for up to four days in a row.

To get to those rooms in the first place, these children had to traverse the ward, so if they were hypothetically infectious, they'd be spreading the virus everywhere anyway. And yet we had people from outside the hospital visiting the ward who did not need to be tested before entering. Staff members were free to interact and go shopping after work and on the weekends, then come back to work without being tested or placed in confinement. Many of the staff had taken the shot, so in theory they were protected too. *What was the concern?* I did not get any of it.

What I saw was that we were jeopardising these young people's mental health and recovery due to personal ignorance and fear. When I brought these rules up with senior colleagues, they told me it was just the way things were. The case of admissions confinement is only one example of stupidity bordering on a breach of human rights out of many.

My final placement was in general practice, but things were heating up as there were talks of bringing in mandatory vaccinations for healthcare staff. During this time, I was also seeing at least two patients per day who were experiencing vaccine-related side effects. What was astonishing was that most of these patients and other general practitioners (GPs) simply denied or turned a blind eye to the fact that these vaccines were causing all this chaos.

After work, I'd go home and continue to read multiple scientific papers per day. Things were beginning to get serious as children were advised to get vaccinated too. I knew from firsthand experience that children very rarely fell ill with COVID-19 and were even less likely to die from it. And statistically, I knew children were more likely to die from getting struck by lightning than from the virus. So in rebuttal and a plea for help, I wrote to the General Medical Council (GMC), the organisation supposedly in charge of protecting patients, to re-evaluate the government's decision. I posted this letter online along with an online petition. The petition was taken down. The GMC replied back with a generic, unhelpful response.

Things were getting personal at work as my vaccine status was requested. After my answer, things changed. I felt my working environment had become colder and that a few of my colleagues were more distant. I wasn't allowed to see patients face-to-face anymore. I initially took these changes in stride, possibly secretly hoping my colleagues would magically begin to read scientific journals and, in doing so, see the errors of their ways.

I have never been sick with COVID-19. I was one of the youngest people working at the surgery and possibly one with the greatest real-life and scientific knowledge about the subject. In other words, I was low-risk and knew it. Not being able to see patients made no sense whatsoever. Whenever I brought this up, I was given reasons based on emotions and politics. Under scientific scrutiny, what I was subjected to did not hold up.

Every day that went by became less and less bearable. During general conversation, I was exposed to the ignorance of scientific data and the snobbery that some of my colleagues had. I would be astonished that they did not know about basic concepts like T cell (an immune cell) immunity and the importance of vitamin D in immunity. These were people whose whole job was supposed to revolve around looking after people to the best of their ability using up-to-date scientific knowledge. It was concerning, to say the least.

With the decision of mandatory healthcare vaccines looming closer, I felt more alone. The people I worked with didn't really care about this verdict. Again, this is astounding, given that informed consent and the right to refuse treatment are the supposed foundations of medical ethics.

I realised that I was becoming stupider at work and more unhappy. I realised that I was different, too informed, and needed to get out. During my time working in the pandemic, I discovered that I knew far too much to continue working in healthcare while remaining willfully ignorant. I also couldn't bear hearing the cries of children getting jabbed next door.

I quit my job voluntarily less than a year before I could become a GP, and a few months before it was decided whether or not health care workers would have to get the vaccine to keep their jobs. I could no longer work for a corrupt and anti-scientific organisation. I knew too much to stay. I chose freedom and the truth.

The decision placed me in a difficult position financially. The flat my girlfriend and I were intending to buy fell through. We had to continue to live with my parents. I began receiving welfare from the government. Everything I had worked so hard for felt like it had been taken from me. But I knew I was doing the right thing. There are certain things in life that are a lot more important than a career.

I am grateful to have worked in various areas of healthcare during the pandemic. I also count myself lucky to have the ability to understand scientific literature as well as the curiosity and open-mindedness to piece it all together. And, because I am neither paid nor affiliated with any organisation, I have examined and will continue to examine data free of vested interests. I know everyone has their biases, but I try to be as unattached to information as I can.

Because of this, though I am no PhD-holding "expert" in this matter, I can confidently say that I have a deep and personal understanding of the virus, vaccines, masks, and what lockdowns and other pandemic measures did and continue to do to people. I've seen it all.

In fact, though they provide useful contributions, I am wary of so-called "experts" and our blind reliance on them. I would even go to the extent of saying that their blinkered approach to solving real-life matters can be life-threatening. And so, I'd like to say that I am no expert. I'm just a person interested in learning and sharing. I'm also an advocate of listening to those with lived experience.

Plus, if you were wondering about my knowledge around immunology, what's more "skin in the game" than the fact that, since the start of the pandemic and to this very day, I have not taken one day off sick nor been symptomatically unwell with any respiratory illness, COVID-19 included?

And finally, I am not an "anti-vaxxer." I disdain that derogatory term. But I am certainly anti-mRNA and DNA technology.

WHAT HAVE YOU INJECTED INSIDE OF YOURSELF?

If you've been paying attention, you'd have known that the definition of vaccines changed overnight in 2021 to something more, let's say, forgiving of these new agents.

One day, the CDC's definition of vaccines changed from "a product that stimulates a person's immune system to produce immunity to a specific disease" to "a preparation that is used to stimulate the body's immune response against diseases."[1]

As you can see, "to produce immunity" was removed. Making it okay to not be immune after vaccination The change also made those with an up-to-date Merriam-Webster dictionary unbearable during scientific debates.

Well, I'm sticking with the traditional definition of vaccines because I understand that if definitions of words become malleable, then their meaning disintegrates. And when meaning disintegrates, words become useless, and we become lost. No one knows what the other is talking about. Progressive discussion stops. Confusion ensues.

I'm also sticking to the former definition because these agents don't produce total immunity to COVID-19; they also likely do the reverse, *reducing* the body's immune response against disease. We'll get to that later. But firstly, *what did you have injected inside yourself exactly*?

Conventional vaccines, which I will call just "vaccines," try to act like an infection to get the body's immune system to react without actually making someone sick. This is done by injecting the individual with a weakened or inactivated virus or a piece of viral protein, called an antigen. mRNA shots like Pfizer-BioNTech and Moderna work differently.

Ribonucleic acid (RNA) is a molecule similar to DNA; they both hold genetic information. But unlike DNA, RNA is single-stranded. DNA encodes all genetic information and serves as a repository for it to be passed down from generation to generation. RNA functions as the reader that decodes this genetic material.

mRNA stands for messenger ribonucleic acid and is one type of RNA. mRNA copies portions of the genetic code and transports these copies to ribosomes, which are the cellular factories that facilitate the production of proteins from this code.

If you didn't already know, SARS-CoV-2 stands for "severe acute respiratory syndrome coronavirus 2," the name of the virus that causes COVID-19 (coronavirus disease 2019). The spike protein is part of this virus.

Instead of a protein antigen, mRNA agents contain mRNA, and it is these mRNA strands that have the information for making the SARS-CoV-2 spike protein. Once injected into your upper arm, the content of the injection ends up in your muscle cells. Here the mRNA is translated into spike proteins and is then displayed on the cell surface, where it is recognised by the immune system. From here, the sequence of events is said to be similar to that of conventional vaccines. The immune system is activated, antibodies are produced, the spike protein is recognised and the spike-protein-producing cell killed.[2] The body is trained to recognise the spike protein as a threat and remembers this via the activation of memory immune cells.

But that's not it; for mRNA agents to work, the mRNA must be packaged within lipid nanoparticles (LNPs). LNPs are more or less spherical structures containing different types of fat and cholesterol. More specifically, LNPs are made of ionisable lipids, phospholipids, cholesterol, and polyethylene glycol (PEG)-lipids. All together, the LNP is essential to package, protect, and deliver mRNA inside cells.

Other shots, such as those from Johnson & Johnson and Oxford-AstraZeneca,[3,4] store instructions to make spike proteins in double-stranded DNA rather than mRNA. The DNA here is added to and carried by another virus called an adenovirus.

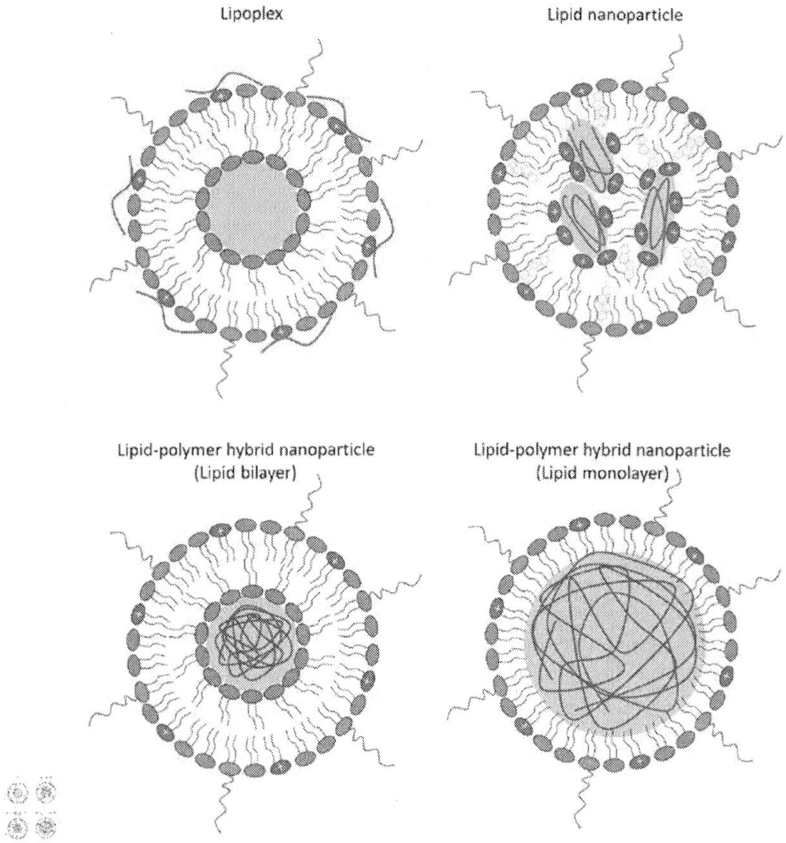

Lipid nanoparticles, from: https://www.frontiersin.org/files/Articles/589959/fchem-08-589959-HTML/image_m/fchem-08-589959-g001.jpg

I have simplified this scientific process down significantly, but to move forward, you've got to understand this process well. Traditional vaccines do not induce human cells to produce viral proteins, and thus don't flag themselves up to be targeted by our immune system. On the contrary, mRNA and DNA shots induce human cells to make spike proteins and then rely on an autoimmune reaction to take place on all cells that have taken in the genetic strand.

This mechanism of action, along with the fact that the contents of the shots do not only stay in the arm, is how they primarily cause system-wide damage. Imagine if our immune system killed heart, brain, or sperm cells that had been trained to make spike proteins. *What would happen then? What if they interfered with our own genetics?*

Note: Since these genetic shots came out, most of the scientific work has been on mRNA technology, so that's where I'll be focusing most of my attention for the rest of this book.

ARE THESE 'GENE THERAPIES'?

The FDA states that "human gene therapy seeks to modify or manipulate the expression of a gene or to alter the biological properties of living cells for therapeutic use."[1] Going by this definition, these shots *aren't* gene therapies. So as far as we know, no, our DNA isn't involved. This is because a multiple-step process is needed to convert the mRNA into DNA, enter the nucleus, and integrate into the cell's DNA.

Well, that's what they have been telling us, but these claims of safety are not backed up by scientific evidence in the literature.[2] As one review of this topic notes, ***"many studies simply state that vaccine mRNA cannot integrate into the host genome without explaining why this is not possible."***[2]

In genetics, the process of putting a piece of RNA into a DNA genome is called "retroposition." mRNA *can* be reintegrated into the genome via a process called reverse-transcription. In fact, retroposition is a natural process that makes a lot of functional genes and about 10,000 copies of genes in the human genome.[3]

One way in which reverse transcription takes place is via a molecule called long interspersed element-1 (LINE-1 or L1) retrotransposons.[4] And so various mRNAs in humans could be reverse-transcribed and integrated into the genome via L1 retroelements, which would have negative health consequences.

It is important to note that the vaccine mRNA was genetically modified to reduce our immune response to it and enhance translation and stability.[5,6] And the information we have about how vaccine mRNA was made shows that vaccine mRNAs were not made to avoid being taken by the L1 retroposition machinery. Also, it has been thought that the length of the Pfizer BioNTech (BNT162b2) mRNA sequence probably won't stop retroposition because it is very close to the average length of the mRNA from the parental genes.[2]

In a single 30 mcg dose of the shot, there are an estimated 1.3×10^{13} synthetic mRNA molecules.[7] To put that into perspective, that's enough to give every nucleated cell in your body about 26 copies of mRNA. People don't get one dose of stable, immune-evading mRNA, but several doses. This makes it more likely that vaccine mRNA will run into L1 machinery in many different types of cells in the body.

Also, it's important to remember that several papers have said that when viruses, like SARS-CoV-2, infect human cells, the activity of cellular endogenous L1 retroelements goes up.[8,9] So, this means that getting an mRNA vaccine during an active viral infection or after the infection has gone away may increase the chance that the vaccine mRNA will become part of the genome.

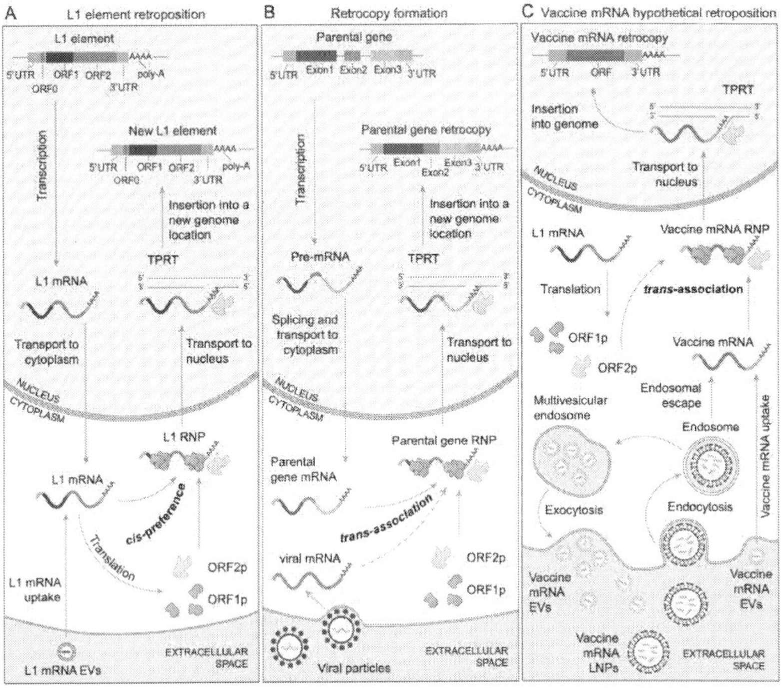

Vaccine mRNA hypothetical retroposition, from: https://www.ncbi.nlm.nih.gov/pmc/articles/PMC9141755/figure/genes-13-00719-f001/

So far, these are all speculations and have not been noted to occur in real life. Not because it does not happen, but because there is an extreme paucity of data. The absence of evidence, however, is not proof of absence.

In a study of host cells in culture, it was found that reverse-transcribed SARS-CoV-2 RNA could integrate into the genome of cultured human cells and could be expressed in patient-derived tissues.[10] And another lab (*in vitro*) study showed the uptake of mRNA material from these novel "vaccines" into human liver cell lines.[11]

If more evidence amounts to the fact that DNA integration is possible via these vaccines, then we're in big trouble. It means that a large part of the population could naturally make spike proteins, and that some people could pass this trait on to their children forever. More evidence of better quality is needed before we open that can of worms.

Hopefully you can see why I wince at calling these mRNA agents "vaccines," simply because they are not. So, for the remainder of the book, I will refer to these agents as anything other than "vaccines."

Pedantic? No, just scientifically correct.

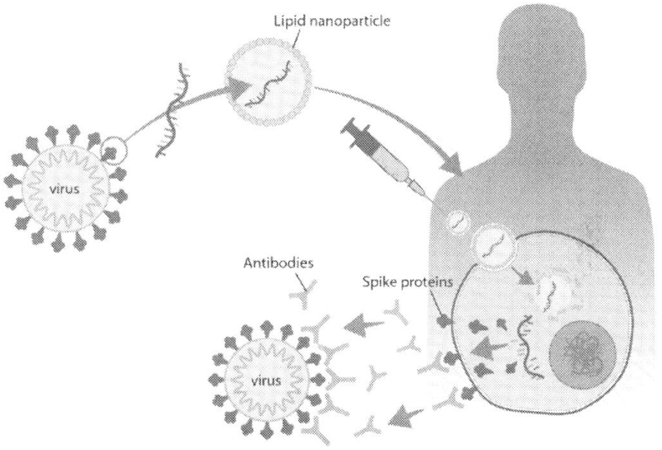

Genetic agent mechanism of action, from: https://healthfeedback.org/how-were-mrna-vaccines-developed-for-covid-19/

HOW RELIABLE IS THE ORIGINAL STUDY DATA?

Thank your lucky stars that you're still able to read this book; there are many thousands who haven't been so fortunate. If you don't believe me, at least believe the data.

From the very start, the original jab trials indicated something wasn't right, even though we were made to believe that these new therapeutic agents were some sort of scientific miracle.

If we were to look at the data from the early period in Pfizer's trial, then yes, there were fewer cases of symptomatic and severe COVID in the jabbed group than in the non-jabbed group.[1] However, if we were to look at *all* adverse events, not just COVID-19, the jabbed group outperforms (i.e., has more adverse events) than the non-vaccine group. More importantly, there were 15 total deaths in the jabbed group and 14 deaths in the control group.

What's even more worrying is that these trials, yes, the same ones that were later used to justify the mass jabbing of millions around the world, may have been produced using poor data and at the cost of patient safety.

Brook Jackson was a former regional director employed at the research organisation Ventavia Research Group, a subcontractor on Pfizer's COVID-19 vaccine trial. She spoke to the British Medical Journal (BMJ) in 2021, explaining that the company she worked for ***"falsified data, unblinded patients, employed inadequately trained vaccinators, and was slow to follow up on adverse events reported in Pfizer's pivotal phase III trial. Staff who conducted quality control checks were overwhelmed by the volume of problems they were finding."***[2]

After repeatedly notifying Ventavia of these issues, Brook Jackson emailed a complaint to the US Food and Drug Administration (FDA). Jackson was fired by Ventavia later the same day.

Jackson is a trained clinical trial auditor with more than 15 years' experience in clinical research coordination and management, and reading through what she had noted in her two weeks working in Pfizer's phase III trial makes my stomach turn.

Blinding is the process of keeping information from the participants and sometimes the experimenters until the experiment is over. This is done to prevent experimental biases from happening. For example, if you knew you were taking paracetamol in a study to see how it affected pain, your perception of pain might change, which would make the study useless. The only way to study an experimental agent properly is if you and the experimenter don't know the changing variable.

Even though the first part of Pfizer's trial was supposed to be blinded, Jackson pointed out that it may have been accidentally unblinded early on because drug assignment confirmation printouts were left in the charts of participants, where blinded staff could see them. So the data from the original trial was likely compromised.

The BMJ article[2] is a must-read and highlights other concerns that Jackson noted, including:

- Participants placed in a hallway after injection and not being monitored by clinical staff.
- Lack of timely follow-up of patients who experienced adverse events.
- Protocol deviations not being reported.
- mRNA agents not being stored at proper temperatures.
- Mislabelled laboratory specimens.
- Targeting of Ventavia staff for reporting these types of problems.

And remember, for notifying this, she was fired. This is not how scientific studies should ever be conducted, and yet plans went ahead and billions received the jab.

You must question why someone like Jackson would speak out against a multi-billion-dollar company and willingly risk jeopardising her career in the process. She certainly wasn't getting paid to do so.

Jackson spoke up most likely because she thought it was the right thing to do, and analysis of court-ordered Pfizer documents released in May 2022 indicates that she was rightfully concerned.[3]

The Pfizer document is riddled with inconsistencies and questionable data. One thing noted was a possible lack of patient files. This would mean that Pfizer wasn't running trials with 44,000 patients, but with a lot fewer, and that 97% of the data from the patients might have been made up using "synthesised" numbers. This would be a very strong sign of fraud, which would make the trial data useless and unreliable. Patient safety data would have also likely been downplayed.

We will see if Pfizer is able to explain these concerning findings. And, if proven to be a forgery, we'll see what happens when people realise the entire government-created approach to fighting the virus was based on false data.

It doesn't get better. Real-life data that has subsequently emerged confirms the worst. Professor Norman Elliott Fenton, a Professor of Risk Information Management at Queen Mary London University, and colleagues released what I think is the most important scientific study to date.

The study is titled, "*Official mortality data for England suggest systematic miscategorisation of vaccine status and uncertain effectiveness of Covid-19 vaccination.*"[4] and uses data from the Office for National Statistics (ONS), which, at first glance, seems to show that all-cause mortality is lower in each of the older age groups among those who had been jabbed than among those who have not. But don't get your hopes up yet, because on closer inspection, the data showed a range of fundamental inconsistencies and flaws.

One of these flaws was the fact that people were still classified as "unvaccinated" up to fourteen days after having the shot. And so if they died in those two weeks, it would have been noted as an "unvaccinated death". In fact, this is what was shown. **In each age group, there was a spike in non-Covid mortality in the unjabbed at exactly the same time as the shot roll-out peaked for that age group.**

This is another example of why we must be stringent with definitions. I've always identified people as vaccinated the second they get inoculated, not two weeks later. *"Yeah, but the vaccine manufacturers claim that they are only effective when the recipient is fully vaccinated, which they define as being more than 14 days after the second dose."* Well, too bad, that's not how definitions work, and if that were the case, then the ONS should have specifically highlighted it.

When changes were made to the data to make it clearer, the numbers showed that the jabs did not lower all-cause mortality. Instead, they showed spikes in all-cause mortality right after inoculation. All-cause mortality, which is death from any cause, correlated with genetic agent roll-outs. Simply put, deaths from any cause went up around the same time as jab rollouts.

A horrifying finding, and yet bigger medical journals have systematically rejected this paper without review. That's probably why you haven't heard about it.

One journal that *has* alluded to a worrying problem is The Wall Street Journal. In their piece titled "Rise in Non-Covid-19 Deaths Hits Life Insurers", they write that U.S. life insurers are seeing a jump in non-COVID-19-related death claims.[5] The article goes on to say that experts believe that many of these fatalities are tied to delays in medical care and the effects of lockdown.

There's no mention of jabs however, maybe because they're 95% effective, remember?

ARE THESE SHOTS "95% EFFECTIVE"?

In November 2020, Pfizer and BioNTech announced that the efficacy portion of their COVID-19 jab trial had been completed, showing the shots were able to prevent 95% of cases of the disease.[1]

"Hooray!" Many of us shouted on hearing this news and proceeded to pick up the phone and book a doctor's appointment to receive a jab. In fact, I believe there is a large subset of the population that still believes this to be true.

With so many of those inoculated still becoming ill with COVID-19, it should now be clear that this shouldn't have been popularised at all. This is another example of why it is important to search for data yourself and not rely on new sources wholeheartedly. The "95% effective" claim was a marketing tactic, and a sneaky one at that.

Why sneaky? Well, vaccine efficacy is generally reported as a "relative risk reduction" (RRR). RRR is the relative decrease in the risk of an adverse event in the exposed group compared to the unexposed group, i.e., the ratio of those with COVID with and without a vaccine. Ranking by reported efficacy gives relative risk reductions[2] of:

- 95% for the Pfizer–BioNTech
- 94% for the Moderna–NIH
- 91% for the Gamaleya
- 67% for the J&J
- 67% for the AstraZeneca–Oxford vaccines.

Looks impressive right? Well, using the RRR is a trick that drug companies use when talking to the press about how well their drug works. While it sounds impressive, the benefit really depends on how common the condition is. In our case, RRR should be seen against the background risk of being infected and becoming ill with COVID-19, which varies between populations and over time.

There is another way to calculate risk: absolute risk reduction (ARR). The absolute risk of disease is your chance of contracting the disease over time. The ARR is a reduction of this risk after the individuals are treated.

RRR only looks at people who might benefit from the shot, while ARR looks at the whole population. ARR is the difference between the number of positive COVID-19 cases with and without being inoculated.

Still confused? Well, for example, let's say women have a 4 in 100 risk of developing a certain disease by the time they reach the age of 60. Then, say that research shows that a new treatment reduces the relative risk of getting this disease by 50%. The 50% is the RRR and is referring to the effect on the 4 (in 100). 50% of 4 is 2. But this means that the absolute risk is reduced from 4 in 100 to 2 in 100. Or 0.04 - 0.02 = 0.02 or 2%.

ARRs tend to be ignored because they are much less impressive when read out loud. For example, the ARRs[2] for the vaccines are:

- 1·3% for the AstraZeneca–Oxford
- 1·2% for the Moderna–NIH
- 1·2% for the J&J
- 0·93% for the Gamaleya
- 0·84% for the Pfizer–BioNTech vaccines.

"1% effective" vaccines sound a *lot* less impressive than "95% effective." As we dig deeper and uncover the truth, keep in mind that **people have died or continue to suffer as a result of a medical "therapy" that is only at best "1.3% effective."** This form of reporting bias skews the public's perception of therapeutic efficiency. And it also brings into question why these pharmaceutical companies had to modify the way they promoted their shots in the first place.

When methodologies used in scientific trials become questionable, the end data becomes null. In this case, Pfizer told us that their vaccine was "95% effective," but the FDA's briefing document for the Vaccines and Related Biological Products Advisory Committee (VRBPAC) meeting on December 10, 2020, for the Pfizer-BioNTech COVID-19 shots tells another story.[3] Sonia Elijahm, a former BBC researcher and investigative journalist, has carefully looked at these documents and found that Pfizer's widely publicised vaccine efficacy rate of 95% may be closer to 12%.

The 95% efficacy rate came from polymerase chain reaction (PCR) test results from a central lab. Dr. Kary Mullis invented the PCR test in 1993, originally to detect genetic mutations in order to identify genetic diseases such as sickle cell anaemia.[4]

PCR tests work by replicating strands of DNA or RNA in order for them to become large enough to be identified. The number of cycles it takes to do this is called the "cycle threshold value (CT)." The problem with it is that at a high enough cycle, tests may be positive even though the person is not symptomatic with the given disease.

Dr. Mullis has even said this about PCR tests: *"It's just a process that is used to make a whole lot of something out of something. It doesn't tell you that you are sick and it doesn't tell you that the thing you ended up with was going to hurt you or anything like that."* [5]

According to one study, when PCR tests were run with 35 cycles or more, the accuracy of the PCR dropped to 3%, meaning up to 97% of positive results could be false positives.[6] Sometimes I wonder if this is why the flu seemingly disappeared in 2021.[7]

Returning to Pfizer, the CT used at one of their central laboratories is unknown. But it's not completely crazy to think that the PCR-CTs in the jabbed and unjabbed groups could have been changed separately to make it more likely that the placebo group would get a positive result. I'm not saying this happened, but with everything going on so far, I have a hard time ruling it out. Unfortunately, I don't think we'll get to the bottom of the central lab CT number.

Anyway, separate from the dataset that was used by Pfizer to show the world that their vaccine was a success, on page 42,[3] what Sonia Elijahm did find was this paragraph:

"Among 3410 total cases of suspected but unconfirmed COVID-19 in the overall study population, 1594 occurred in the vaccine group vs. 1816 in the placebo group. Suspected COVID-19 cases that occurred within 7 days after any vaccination were 409 in the vaccine group vs. 287 in the placebo group."

These are the numbers of suspected cases of symptomatic COVID-19 that were not confirmed by PCR and thus were not subject to possible manipulation. And if you crunch the data, shot effectiveness is shown to be 12 percent.

What is also interesting is that there were more suspected COVID-19 cases in the vaccine group too. *More*, not less. By the way, all of this data was known to the FDA back in 2020, raising questions about potential collusion. Though seemingly kept undercover, it has not all gone unnoticed.

One journal that has been fairly unbiased throughout the last few years is the BMJ. This could be because Peter Doshi, who is a senior editor at The BMJ, has publicly questioned the endpoints of the trials.

In his BMJ feature titled "Will covid-19 vaccines save lives? Current trials aren't designed to tell us",[8] Doshi states that the **phase III trials are not designed to detect a reduction in any serious outcome, such as hospital admissions, use of intensive care, or deaths. Nor were the jabs studied to determine whether they could interrupt transmission of the virus.**

In a separate BMJ blog,[9] Doshi questions why over **3,400 "suspected COVID-19 cases" were not included in the interim analysis of the Pfizer vaccine data submitted to the FDA**. Plus, **individuals with a known history of SARS-CoV-2 infection or a previous diagnosis of COVID-19 were excluded from Moderna's and Pfizer's trials**. But still, 1125 and 675 of the participants in Pfizer's and Moderna's trials, respectively, were deemed to be positive for SARS-CoV-2 at baseline. For these and other reasons, the interim efficacy estimate of around 95% for both vaccines is suspect.

All that maths aside, these vaccines were never going to be 95% effective anyway, which is maybe why the CDC's definition of vaccines changed. This is because viruses mutate. Mutation is usually a good thing; it is when viruses change ever so slightly in relation to selection pressures, usually becoming more spreadable but less dangerous in the process. We'll get to the science behind this later on.

At the time this was written, the COVID-19 shots and boosters that are on the market were made for the original alpha variant, not for the vast majority of other variants that are now in circulation. *So when told about effectiveness in the future, it is important to ask "for how long" and "effective against what exactly"?*

Another question to ask is, *"Will it make me live longer?"* Ask that question first, actually. Whether it's statins or these shots, the end goal for therapeutics claiming to save lives, as you will agree, is whether they will help you live longer than if you didn't take them.

Unfortunately for us, there is no clear data around this. The UK doesn't have the data of those who have been harmed or have suffered illness from a COVID-19 shot, as this is not recorded on the death certificate.[10] But by using Professor Fenton's study, we cannot rule out the very likely fact that these jabs do the opposite of increasing lifespan.

So are these shots 95% effective at reducing infection?

Certainly not.

DOES IT REDUCE SYMPTOM SEVERITY?

In the beginning, I believed, and the evidence suggested, that the shots seemingly worked, in the sense that they were shown to be effective in reducing SARS-CoV-2 infections and COVID-19-related hospitalisations, severe disease, and death.[1] However, as time went on, this belief of mine became less and less optimistic.

"Reducing the severity" was the last go-to reason for getting the jab for many, as the prevention of disease and spread did not work out as expected. And for a lot of people who have only had a mild case of COVID-19 post-jab, the shots seem to have done the job. But this conclusion, though reasonable to draw, may be incorrect, all thanks to "survivorship bias."

Survivorship bias is a flawed way of thinking where the individual believes that something works for them because they weren't affected negatively after the intervention was made. What they appear to overlook are the many other people who *were* adversely affected by the intervention but were unable to express their concerns due to the negative outcome.

Struggling to understand? Well, one good example of survivorship bias includes a study performed on cats. This 1987 study reported that cats who fell from *less* than six stories and were still alive had *greater* injuries than cats who fell from higher heights.[2] They hypothesised that this was the case due to cats being able to reach terminal velocity at greater heights, which allowed them to right themselves and relax themselves, leading to fewer severe injuries. In 1996, The Straight Dope newspaper column proposed another possible explanation. They said this phenomenon would be due to survivorship bias. The cats that die in falls are less likely to be brought to the vets, and thus many of the cats killed in falls from higher buildings were not reported in studies of the subject, skewing the data.[3]

Keep in mind that thousands of people are likely to have developed severe disease after receiving the shot. And you've got to ask yourself, "*How do you know that they wouldn't have contracted the disease without the therapy?*" Just because the stars were aligned for one person doesn't make the procedure foolproof.

As time goes on, I'm beginning to question my views regarding symptom severity from a scientific standpoint. *Why?* Well, one outbreak in an Israeli hospital led to the deaths of five fully jabbed hospital patients.[4] Another study found that COVID-19 killed 34/152 (22%) of fully jabbed patients in 17 Israeli hospitals.[5] If the jab proved to be effective, fully jabbed people shouldn't be dying of COVID-19.

And even if the shots do reduce symptom severity, we must ask ourselves, *"at what cost"?*

WHAT IS IMMUNITY?

For the last three years or so, the concept and inner workings of the human immune system have been underappreciated, misunderstood, and greatly ignored.

Whether or not natural immunity, a biological fact in all living organisms, was purposefully ignored by the mainstream media and international governments in efforts to maximise vaccine take-up is another issue, an issue I will explore later in this book. But for now, the only thing I know for certain is that if more people really understood the immune system, then better personal health decisions would have been made.

Immunity is not a shield, nor is it an invisible force field that is found covering the body. It also certainly cannot be “boosted” or "recharged" since you are not a smartphone. All these dehumanising metaphors may help conceptually, as well as look cool in ads trying to sell antibacterial sprays and genetic shots, but it’s a lot more complicated than that.

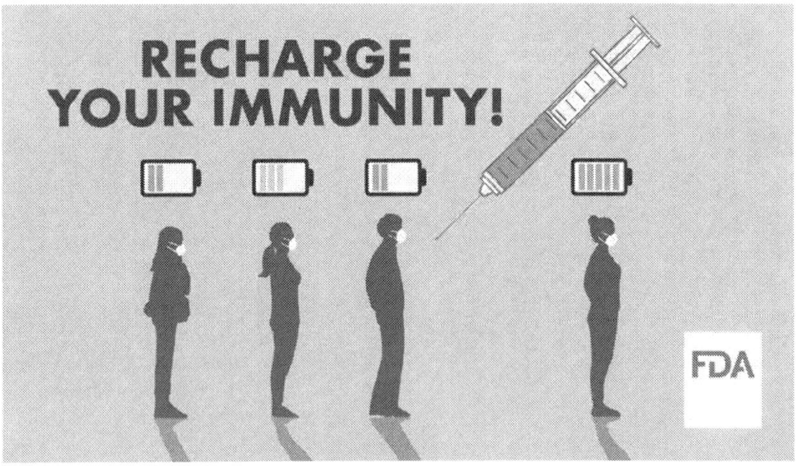

"Recharge Your Immunity" by the FDA, from:
https://twitter.com/US_FDA/status/1568264993921015809?ref_src=twsrc%5Etfw

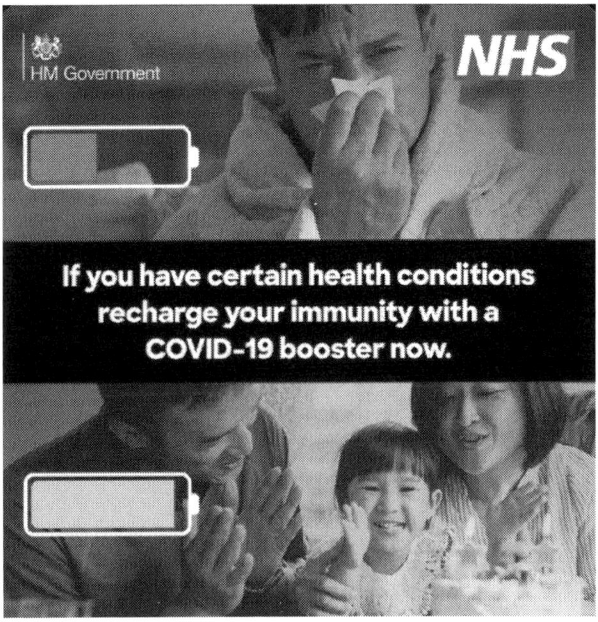
HM Government
NHS
If you have certain health conditions
recharge your immunity with a
COVID-19 booster now.

A recent NHS advert, from:
https://twitter.com/NHSuk/status/1600823702693855232

The immune system is an extraordinarily complex, interconnected universe of various cell types and communicating molecules that exists in a state of flux.

It has been described as "the second-most complicated system in your body after your brain"[1] consisting of hundreds of cell types and signalling molecules controlled by some 8000 genes, which all teeter like a gymnast on a tightrope, *relying* on balance for proper functioning.

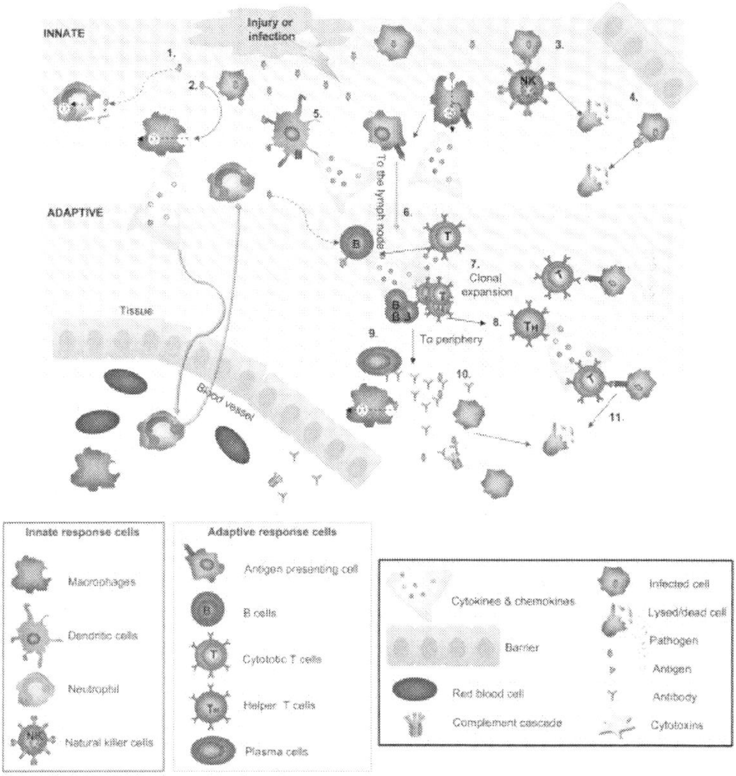

A simplified schematic of the two branches of the immune system, from: https://www.researchgate.net/figure/Innate-and-adaptive-immunity-A-simplified-schematic-of-the-two-branches-of-the-immune_fig1_50597034

When the immune system is overstimulated and out of control, it attacks its own cells, which leads to autoimmune diseases and makes it more likely to overreact. An under-stimulated and unprepared immune system is one that is prone to infection and associated ill health.

It's also important to remember that your immune system not only protects you from infections, but it also plays an important role in controlling inflammation and cancer growth and spread. And thus, immune dysfunction can lead to various forms of cancer, increased inflammation, and sepsis. To *really* understand the immune system we've got to dive a little deeper.

WHAT IS THE INNATE IMMUNE SYSTEM?

The immune system can be grouped into two groups: the innate and adaptive systems. This is extremely important to understand, so pay attention.

The innate system is an evolutionary ancient defence strategy and the dominant one found in plants, fungi, and insects. It is the reason why the trees in your local park have continued to stand strong and rot-free for hundreds of years.

In humans, it is the first line of defence and is constantly working to keep us safe and healthy. But because it has been ignored by others for three years now, I'm going to purposely shine the spotlight a little brighter on the innate immune system in this book. Here are some of the important (though extremely simplified) things it does:

It acts as a physical barrier to the outside world. Physical barriers include parts of the body like your skin, gastrointestinal tract, respiratory tract, nose, eyes and blood-brain barrier. These physical barriers do not only work like a stand-alone wall but are home to additional defence mechanisms. For example the gastrointestinal tract has gastric acid, molecules called thiocyanates and defensins and is home to our gut microflora. All of these play an important role in our immunity.

It triggers inflammation. *Know that red and painful sensation around a fresh wound or burn?* Thank the innate immune system for that. Inflammation is stimulated by chemical factors released by injured cells and this helps to stop the spread of infection, promotes healing and clears damaged tissue once the pathogen has been cleared.

It recruits other immune cells to sites of infection by producing various chemical factors, one of them being a group of chemicals called cytokines. Cytokines are small secreted proteins released by cells that have a specific effect on the interactions and communications between cells.[1] Examples include tumour necrosis factor alpha (TNF-α), interleukin-2 (IL-2) and macrophage inflammatory protein-1 alpha (MIP-1α). Cytokines also trigger other white cells to perform anti-pathogenic activities such as causing cell death.

It activates molecules called complements. These "complement" antibodies to clear pathogens trigger the recruitment of other inflammatory cells, tag pathogens for destruction by other cells, clear antigen-antibody complexes and form holes on the outside of pathogens causing them to die. The complement system also has the capacity to discriminate our own cells from non-self cells, as well as identify microorganisms that have no "intent" to do harm vs harmful pathogens. For example, the bacteria that are part of the commensal flora—i.e. non-self but with no "intent" to do harm—that are abundant in our body, including in our digestive tract, are not normally targeted by the complement system, but infective microorganisms that enter our body to do harm are.[2]

It activates the adaptive immune system through complement cascade and a process called antigen presentation. An antigen is a molecule that can bind to a specific antibody or T cell receptor. In layman's terms, an antigen is any substance that causes the body to make an immune response against that substance. Antigen presenting cells include dendritic cells, macrophages, Langerhans cells and B cells. All these cells apart from B cells are part of the innate immune system.

It is composed of various forms of white cells called natural killer cells, mast cells, eosinophils, basophils, macrophages, neutrophils, and dendritic cells. They all have various roles and reside in different locations of the body. For example, mast cells reside in connective tissue and mucous membranes and are often associated with allergy and anaphylaxis. Natural killer cells destroy our own cells that are compromised, such as tumour cells or virus-infected cells.

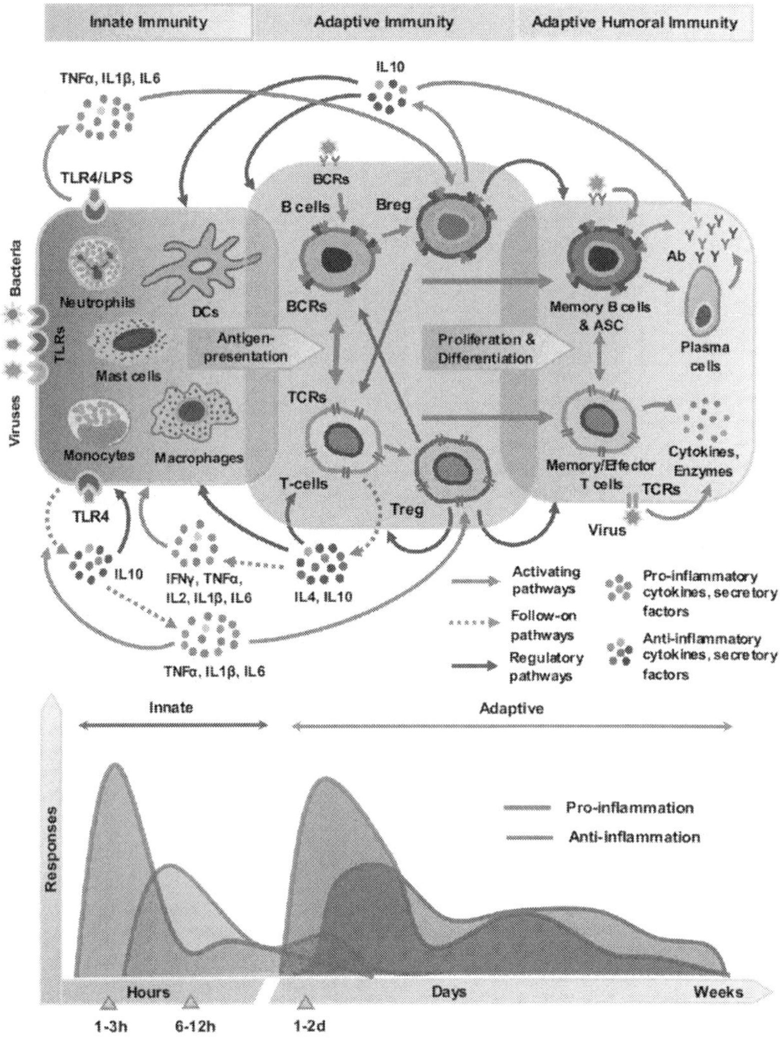

A simplified schematic of the two branches of the immune system, from: https://www.researchgate.net/figure/A-simplified-schematic-diagram-of-the-innate-and-adaptive-immune-response-activating-and_fig1_342490143

WHAT IS THE ADAPTIVE IMMUNE SYSTEM?

The innate immune system uses pattern recognition receptors (PRRs), which recognise molecules that are broadly shared by pathogens but differ from molecules found in the body naturally. These receptors and the system as a whole are pre-programmed to react to broad categories of common pathogens. Think of it like a big magnet in a scrap yard—great at what it does, but not so specific.

The adaptive immune system makes up the rest of our immune system, and though it is slower to act than the innate immune system, it is highly specific to each particular pathogen it encounters. It can be so specific because of the body's amazing ability to create new, specially designed antibodies in response to novel antigens. The white cells that make up the adaptive immune system are B cells and T cells, and there are a handful of differences between the two.

T cells live longer, they move to the site of infection, they can act against tumour cells, they have an inhibitory effect on the immune system, and they can destroy cells infected with pathogens within. B cells have a shorter half-life and produce antibodies, but they cannot do the other things mentioned that T cells can do. Both are important and work closely together. As well as forming and working with antibodies, adaptive immunity also creates immunological memory through memory B and memory T cells. This is the underlying mechanism for why conventional vaccines work.

The adaptive immune system is also called the "acquired immune system" because pathogen-specific receptors are "acquired" over the course of an organism's life, while the innate immune system is written into our DNA.

As time goes by and we are exposed to more pathogens, the adaptive immune system is able to create specific antibodies to antigens and remember these for future use.

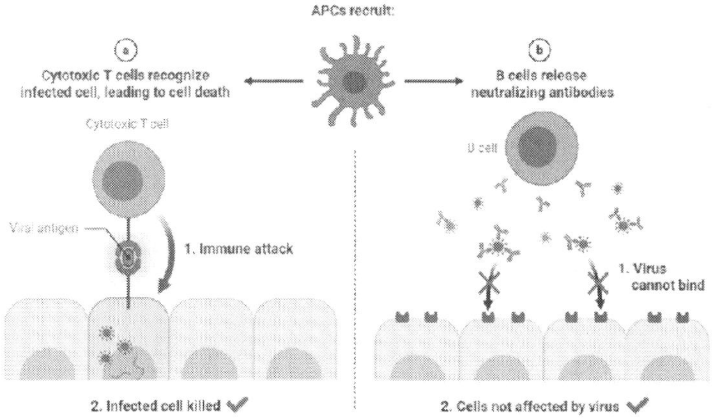

T and B cells, from: https://www.the-scientist.com/news-opinion/the-search-for-immune-responses-that-stop-covid-19-67769

Out of all the things mentioned, antibodies were the only immunological factor that kept coming up in the news. *Tell me, how many of you knew about the comple-*

ment system? T cells? or what role the gut microbiome plays in the severity and risk of COVID-19? I see very few hands raised.

All I want you to do now is appreciate the complexity of your immune system. And though science divides it into two groups, please begin to see the immune system as a whole. The innate and adaptive immune systems *need* each other to work properly, and a compromise in one can cause issues in the other.

CHARLIE'S STORY

I am Charlie. I am 45 years old. I thought I was fit and healthy before I had my COVID vaccine but looking back at my timeline I wasn't. I should never have had a COVID vaccination as I think I've had something since I was very young, maybe I was even born with it. By the age of 2, I had been diagnosed with severe gluten intolerance and was put on a gluten free diet, I was also sensitive to MSG and white sugar so my mum ensured I didn't eat anything with those foods in.

Fast forward, to the age of 45, a week after having my one and only Pfizer vaccination I had hives, skin peeling off my face and neck and oedema in my face. My head also felt like it was going to explode and I had a raging thirst. This turned into a histamine intolerance and severe food intolerances that gave me GI issues and really whacked out my nervous system. My worst symptoms were the head issues, brain fog, burning stomach and throat along with my throat feeling like it was swelling up.

I was constantly at the hospital on IV drips with steroids and fluids to flush my system out. At one point all I could eat was chicken, rice and broccoli, I couldn't drive or work due to the symptoms I was having, especially the brain fog and the feeling like my head was going to explode.

The doctors in Spain were and are adamant that the

vaccine hasn't caused this, they have said it just happens sometimes, they even put pressure on me to have my second vaccination and boosters, which I declined.

I've had to be my own detective and find out how to help myself, treat my symptoms and recover. I've discovered a syndrome that I may have (mast cell activation syndrome) and histamine intolerance. I think I've had this from a very early age, most of the symptoms were mild and I could ignore them , and never joined the dots together until the symptoms were extremely debilitating after my Covid vaccination.

I am now 18 months after my vaccination and I am feeling much better. I still have a very limited diet and have to be very careful what I eat. In the last month I have started working 30 hours a week and I feel like I'm finally getting back to be me again.

I started seeing a Homoeopath 6 months ago and this has really helped me and my recovery. I have also started fasting 2 days a week and this has been a game changer, in the last month since starting the fasting I'm trying foods that used to cause a reaction and not having a reaction.

I'm also off all my medications that the doctor prescribed for me and just take homoeopathic remedies now.

WHAT WERE MY ANTIBODY RESULTS?

After six months of working with COVID-19-positive patients, adhering poorly to social distancing rules, and breathing in SARS-CoV-2-infested air, work asked me (along with other employees) to have an antibody test.

I had not, and I have not to this day, had symptoms of COVID-19. And so back then, I was certain my antibody test would come back positive, explaining my immunity. But surprisingly, my IgM and IgG antibody blood tests came back negative. *Why?*

Antibodies, also known as immunoglobulins, are "Y"-shaped proteins made by B cells that are used by the immune system to neutralise pathogens.[1] The ends of the antibody recognise a unique molecule on the pathogen called the antigen. Antibodies can attach to pathogens and highlight their presence for other immune cells. They can also neutralise the target directly.

Antibodies come in different varieties called isotypes; there are five: IgA, IgD, IgE, IgG, and IgM. Each isotype has distinctive roles, differs in functional locations, and has the ability to deal with different antigens.[2]

For the purpose of SARS-CoV-2 infections, let's focus on IgA, IgG, and IgM.

IgA

- IgA is the first line of defence in the resistance against infection especially at mucosal surfaces like the gastrointestinal, respiratory and urogenital tracts.[3]
- It is the most common type of antibody found in the sweat, saliva, and tears of people.[3]

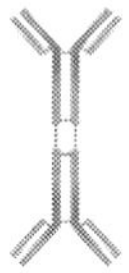

IgA

IgG

- IgG is the most abundant antibody in the blood, making up nearly 75% of human antibodies.[4]
- IgG binds onto the antigen and can signal other immune cells to react.[4]
- IgG can also be transferred to the foetus through the placenta, protecting the infant.[4]
- IgG is largely responsible for long-term immunity.[4]

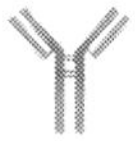

IgG

IgM

- IgM usually circulates in the blood, accounting for about 10% of human antibodies.[5]
- B cells produce IgM first in response to an infection, therefore IgM is detected and developed during acute infection.[5]

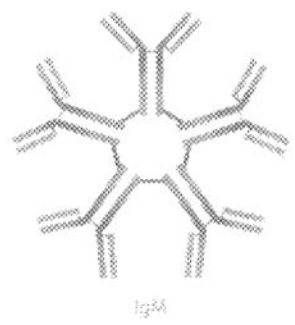

https://logicalbiological.com/sars-cov-2-iga/

Also crucial to know is that there are two main categories into which all antibodies fall: neutralising antibodies and non-neutralising antibodies.

A neutralising antibody is one that protects a cell from a pathogen or infectious particle by neutralising any biological effects that the particle may have, making it no longer infectious or pathogenic.[6]

Non-neutralizing antibodies, also known as "binding antibodies," bind firmly to the pathogen but have no effect on its capacity to infect. That could be a result of them not binding to the proper region of the antigen. Non-neutralising antibodies may be crucial for alerting immune cells to the target status of the particle, which allows them to process and subsequently eliminate the particle.[7]

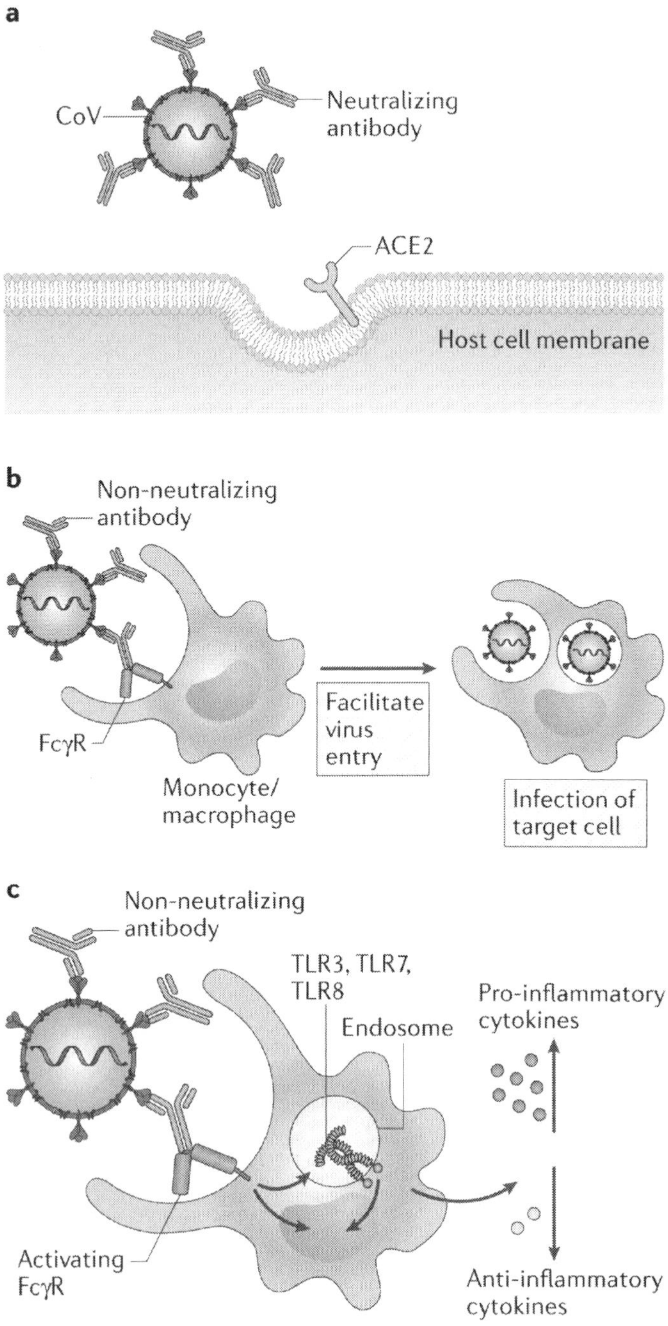

Differences between neutralising and non-neutralising antibodies, from: https://www.nature.com/articles/s41577-020-0321-6

When I first glanced at the words "negative antibody test" on the medical document that was sent to me, my initial reflex was to make sure that these results were in fact mine. Name checked. I was confused, but research revealed that I was not alone.

You can, in fact, have a negative antibody test and yet have no symptoms (remain asymptomatic). Here are the five occurrences where this might happen:

1. You have not had the infection yet.
2. You have been very recently infected, but have not produced antibodies yet.
3. You've had an infection a long time ago, and not been exposed recently, and so your antibody levels have now waned (and the test isn't sensitive enough to pick this up)
4. The test is inaccurate and shows false-negatives.
5. You've had an independent T cell response.

I knew I was constantly breathing in virus-filled air, which ruled out options 1, 2, and 3. I had no control over option 4. So all that was left was option 5, and a study at that time seemed to indicate I might have been onto something.

CAN YOU BE IMMUNE WITH A NEGATIVE ANTIBODY TEST?

"SARS-CoV-2 induces robust memory T cell responses in antibody-seronegative and antibody-seropositive individuals with asymptomatic or mild COVID-19." I was reassured by reading this sentence from the 2020 paper by Karolinska University Hospital.[1]

In other words, they found memory T cell activation in people with mild or no symptoms of COVID-19 who had no antibodies against the virus.

The researchers made a map of SARS-CoV-2-specific T cell responses in 203 people, including people who had never been exposed to the virus, family members who had been exposed, and people with acute COVID-19 or who were getting better from it. They found that different clinical markers of disease severity turned on different SARS-CoV-2-specific T cells.

The paper optimistically concludes by saying, *"Our collective dataset shows that SARS-CoV-2 elicits robust memory T cell responses akin to those observed in the context of successful vaccines, suggesting that natural exposure or infection may prevent recurrent episodes of severe COVID-19 also in seronegative individuals."*[1] In other words, natural infections are as good as vaccines and may prevent future infections from happening, even in those with negative antibody responses.

This fact was repeated again:

"The observation that most individuals with asymptomatic or mild COVID-19 generated highly functional durable memory T cell responses, not uncommonly in the relative absence of corresponding humoral responses, further suggested that natural exposure or infection could prevent recurrent episodes of severe COVID-19."

A humoral response is basically an antibody response. And so, in other words, most people with asymptomatic or mild COVID-19 maintained highly functional permanent memory T cell responses, often in the absence of comparable humoral responses, showing that natural exposure or infection could prevent recurring bouts of severe COVID-19.

I vividly remember reading this scientific paper on my break in the emergency department staff room. As I read the above paragraph, the background noises of people talking, machines beeping, and alarms seemed to stop. I thought I had struck gold. This study found that natural exposure to the virus could prevent severe COVID-19 from happening in the future. If this were the case, then the pandemic could be over fairly quickly through natural exposure. It also showed that checking antibody responses without also checking T cell responses was a waste of time when trying to figure out one's natural immunity status.

But instead of celebrating, a great feeling of confusion enveloped me. *If natural exposure worked, why did institutions ignore it as a way to prevent disease and insist only on using mRNA and DNA shots? And why were the studies assessing shot effectiveness only focusing on antibodies?*

WHY WAS NATURAL IMMUNITY IGNORED?

Since then, nothing has really changed. The CDC Director Rochelle Walensky, for example, was deceptive in her October 2020 published LANCET statement that "there is no evidence for lasting protective immunity to SARS-CoV-2 following natural infection" and that "the consequence of waning immunity would present a risk to vulnerable populations for the indefinite future." [1]

"No evidence for lasting protective immunity to SARS-CoV-2 following a natural infection?" Explain that to the many millions of individuals who aren't dead even though they didn't get the shot. Explain that to those who were inoculated but still became ill, spreading disease. Explain that to groups of individuals like me who have continued to live COVID-19-free for three years so far, all naturally.

Explain that to the growing body of scientific evidence demonstrating that natural immunity outperforms genetic jab immunity. By October 2021, there would be more than 150 studies affirming naturally acquired immunity to COVID-19, yet we were told the shots were the only way out.[2]

Some people *still* believe that these jabs confer better immunity than the natural virus, and I don't get why. The whole underlying concept of vaccine success is dependent on natural immunity. If natural immunity didn't exist, then vaccines wouldn't work. The only way these shots would have proven more effective than the real thing is if they contained a *more* dangerous strain than the original one.

Denying natural immunity is a heinous crime. With one drop of a hat, many centuries of biological research were thrown into the trash. The marvellously complex, interconnected network of cells and all the communicating molecules and receptors keeping you alive right now were ignored. And anyone even daring to bring up this biological fact was labelled a conspiracy theorist. The scary part was that scientific institutions like medical schools, universities, and research labs all went along with this circus act too.

I have been racking my brain trying to find some sort of scientific explanation for it all, but I can't. And so I have concluded that papers on natural immunity and T cell immunity like the one mentioned in the previous chapter were purposefully ignored by the mainstream media and medical institutions for reasons other than ones pertaining to science.

I wish the world followed science properly, but I know this is wishful thinking. Greed and ulterior motives always want a piece of the pie too. In this case, I have a strong suspicion that economic and political needs were placed above scientific facts. I think natural immunity was pushed aside for two reasons: one, to drive Big Pharma profits, and two, to help with the dehumanisation of the individual. Both strategies helped increase the individual's dependency on the government and placed the genetic jabs as the only key to freedom.

Why dehumanisation? Well, being told to ignore our natural capability to fend off infections unconsciously translates to "you are not enough," when in fact this is far from the truth. Our natural protective defences, like our lung microflora, nasal air filtration system, and antibody-abundant mucus membranes, continue to be viewed as second-best compared to masks and genetic shots. For the vast majority of the population, being human was and is currently seen as being prone to sickness and thus incomplete without the help of lab-manufactured pharmaceuticals.

Accepting natural immunity obliterates the need for population-wide inoculation; it empowers the individual and reinstates sovereignty. Natural immunity is anti-pharma.

Natural immunity is pro-freedom.

WHY IS NATURAL IMMUNITY THE ONLY WAY OUT?

I think the *greatest* reason for the international denial of natural immunity was because it was our only way to end the pandemic. It always has been. Prior infection provides approximately 85% protection against reinfection and a further 90% protection against severe illness if reinfected.[1]

Immunity to the natural virus is broader than jab immunity alone. We saw this with Omicron, where those with existing anti-SARS-CoV-2 T cell responses were safe from the Omicron strain.[2] And we're also seeing it in the lower numbers of cases among the previously infected compared to those inoculated.

There are also emerging studies now pointing towards jab-induced immunodeficiencies.[3] Combine this with jab-produced jab-resistance variants,[4] and you get a never-ending loop of infection and reinfection within the population. The pandemic would have theoretically gone on forever if people continued to take boosters. Only a non-genetic agent infection or exposure is capable of stopping this cycle, increasing the breadth of immunity while simultaneously not causing the individual to become immunocompromised. *No genetic shots, no dragged out pandemic.*

Lucky for us, scientific truths always find a way to rise to the surface. An April 2022 study of 124,500 people showed that ***"Naturally acquired immunity confers stronger protection against infection and symptomatic disease caused by the Delta variant of SARS-CoV-2, compared to the BNT162b2 two-dose vaccine-induced immunity."*** [5]

Furthermore, *"it was highlighted that the vast majority of the individuals after suffering from COVID-19 develop a natural immunity both of cell-mediated and humoral type, which is effective over time and provides protection against both reinfection and serious illness.* ***Vaccine-induced immunity was shown to decay faster than natural immunity."*** according to a comprehensive review of 900 studies and 246 scientific articles, published in October 2022.[6]

The review goes on to note, *"..**natural immunity after COVID-19, which seems comparable or superior to the one induced by anti-SARS-CoV-2 vaccination. Consequently, vaccination of the unvaccinated COVID-19-recovered subjects may not be indicated.**"*

Jabbing those already exposed should never have had taken place.

Natural immunity will always be superior.

WHO ARE THE UNSUNG HEROES?

Antibodies are great, but their popularity has overshadowed other equally important components of our immune system, like T cells. And I'd go so far as to say that solely focusing on antibodies is neither scientifically sound nor helpful, as this study concludes:

"Circulating antibody titers were not predictive of T cell memory. ***Thus, simple serological tests for SARS-CoV-2 antibodies do not reflect the richness and durability of immune memory to SARS-CoV-2.****"* [1]

T cells develop in the thymus, hence the "T." They can be distinguished from other white cells by the presence of a T receptor on the cell surface. There are two main types of T cells: CD4+ "helper T cells" and CD8+ "killer (or cytotoxic) T cells."

Killer T cells directly kill the virus-infected cells and also use signalling proteins called cytokines to mount an immune response. They are important for clearing an infection that has already started; their response can reduce the severity of the infection, and they are known to restrict the number of circulating viruses in an infected individual.

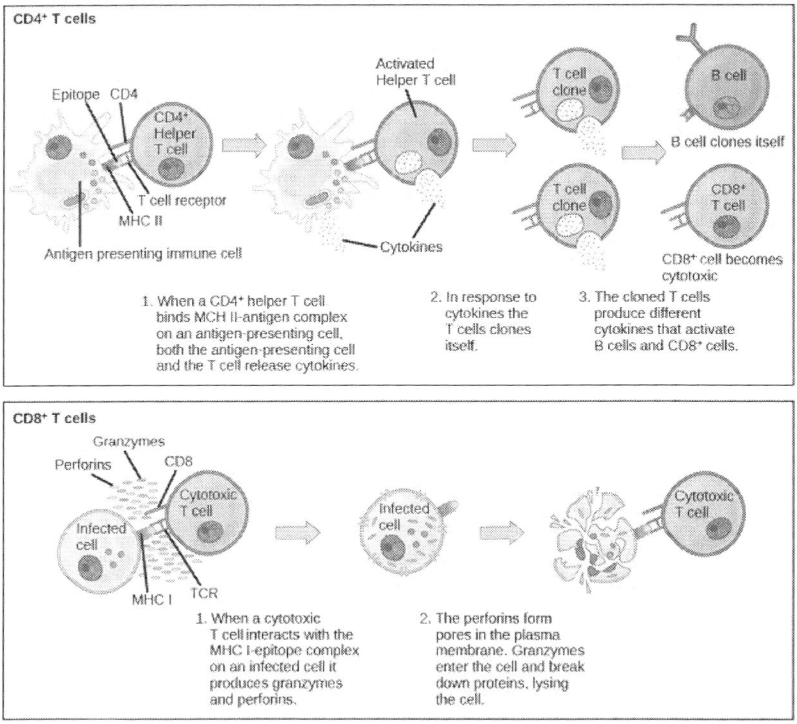

CD4+ and CD8+ T cells, from: https://pediaa.com/what-is-the-difference-between-cd4-and-cd8-t-cells/

Helper T cells may be the most important cells in adaptive immunity, as they are required for almost all adaptive immune responses. They not only help activate B cells to secrete antibodies and macrophages (a type of white cell that can phagocytose, or "eat and digest," pathogens) to destroy ingested microbes, but they also help activate killer T cells to kill infected target cells.

T cells work widely. When the body comes into contact with the natural SARS-CoV-2 virus, it is exposed to the virus's proteins, such as the membrane (M), nucleocapsid (N), envelope (E), and spike (S) proteins. And it has been demonstrated that this elicits a stronger and broader killer T cell response than spike-protein-only-producing mRNA jabs.[2] As one study puts it, "*Natural infection induced expansion of larger CD8 T cell clones occupied distinct clusters, likely due to the recognition of a broader set of viral epitopes presented by the virus not seen in the mRNA vaccine.*" [3]

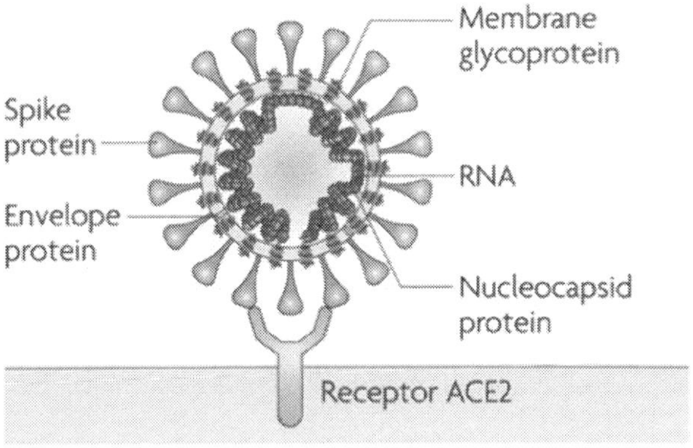

SARS-CoV-2 proteins, from:
https://pubs.acs.org/doi/10.1021/acscentsci.0c00272

T cells work quietly and sometimes independently. As previously discussed, many of us had killer T cell responses to SARS-CoV-2 prior to the shot rollout, even if we had negative antibodies. This evidence has been repeated in another study of patients and their families that showed that six out of eight family members who caught SARS-CoV-2 at home had T cell responses but no detectable antibodies.[4] Thus further highlighting, **"T cell responses may be more sensitive indicators of SARS-CoV-2 exposure than antibodies."** [4]

T cells don't forget. Unlike antibodies, which detect and attach to proteins that decorate the outside of the cell, T cells target the stable viral proteins expressed inside infected cells,[5] and therefore their existence may mean long-term immunity to COVID-19 and its many strains. One study suggested that those exposed naturally to the virus are likely immune to 23 different variants of it.[6]

T cell memory for those infected with SARS-CoV-1 is at 17 years and running.[7] There is now emerging data indicating that T cell immunity for those infected with SARS-CoV-2 is long-lasting in individuals too.[8] Longitudinal analysis has shown durable and broad immune memory after SARS-CoV-2 infection, with persisting antibody responses and memory B and T cells. [9]

Another study of over a thousand participants a year after infection found that SARS-CoV-2-specific neutralising antibodies and T cell responses were still present 12 months later.[10] And though antibody levels waned, as they do, memory T cell responses to the original strain were not disrupted by new variants. Another study found that T-cell immunity to SARS-CoV-2 can last for up to a year too.[11]

And this memory isn't static; as another paper noted, *"Following a typical case of mild Covid-19, SARSCoV2–specific* ***CD8+ T cells not only persist but continuously differentiate in a coordinated fashion well into convalescence into a state characteristic of long-lived, self-renewing memory****".*[12] It is not far-fetched to assume that T cell memory to SARS-CoV-2 is lifelong.

All in all, T cells have an excellent memory; I can't find studies suggesting otherwise. Unlike T cells, antibody levels wane over time, but this is a normal physiological response too. *So I have to ask, were T cells ignored, yet antibodies were not, to justify using boosters?*

Here's the best bit. Before the introduction of COVID-19 shots, it was estimated that **40–60% of unexposed individuals already had SARS-CoV-2-reactive CD4+ T cells,**[13] suggesting cross-reactive T cell recognition between circulating "common cold" coronaviruses and SARS-CoV-2.[14] Another study, in the Lancet (a highly respected scientific journal), notes, "*In summary,* ***we demonstrate the existence of naïve and memory SARS-CoV-2-reactive CD8 T cells in peripheral blood of unexposed healthy subjects***".[15]

In layman's terms, a lot of us were already protected from COVID-19 before the pandemic thanks to previous exposure to viruses like the one that causes the common cold.[16] It may also answer why some, like me, continue to live COVID-19-free. This isn't "new science" or a "ground-breaking" immunological discovery, however hard the Telegraph tries to portray it as such with posts like this[17]:

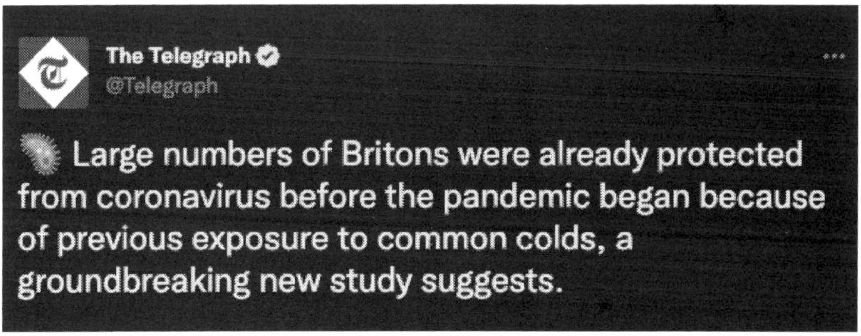

The Telegraph
@Telegraph
Large numbers of Britons were already protected from coronavirus before the pandemic began because of previous exposure to common colds, a groundbreaking new study suggests.

A headline from The Telegraph on Twitter, from: https://twitter.com/Telegraph/status/1480496590049755141

All of this information should make you wonder why genetic shots, lockdowns, and masks were and continue to be pushed so hard. The National Health Service (NHS) text message service is one example of this. I just wish the NHS texted us actionable weight loss advice rather than going on and on about booking a jab appointment.

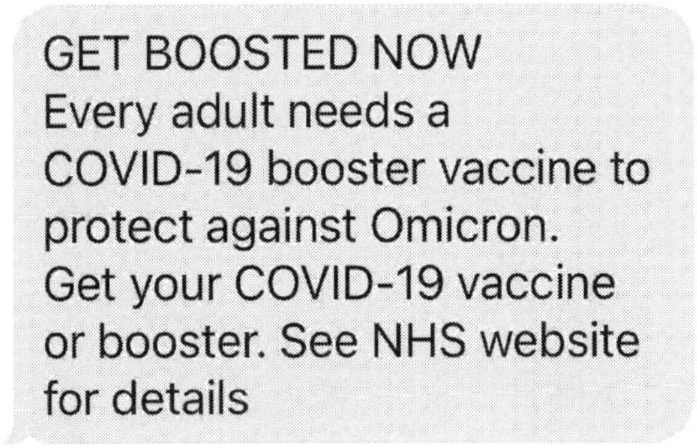

GET BOOSTED NOW
Every adult needs a
COVID-19 booster vaccine to
protect against Omicron.
Get your COVID-19 vaccine
or booster. See NHS website
for details

A text message sent to my phone.

This is what happens when immunological science is twisted. Many were already protected before the pandemic, and so they didn't need any sort of jab at all. Boosters are also ineffective, making each shot exponentially more dangerous. This is no better highlighted than in one recent study published in the BMJ, which shows that in those aged 18 to 29 years old, ***"per COVID-19 hospitalisation prevented, we anticipate at least 18.5 serious adverse events from mRNA vaccines"***. And "***To prevent one COVID-19 hospitalisation over a 6-month period, we estimate that 31207–42836 young adults aged 18–29 years must receive a third mRNA vaccine***."[18]

But we are told another narrative.

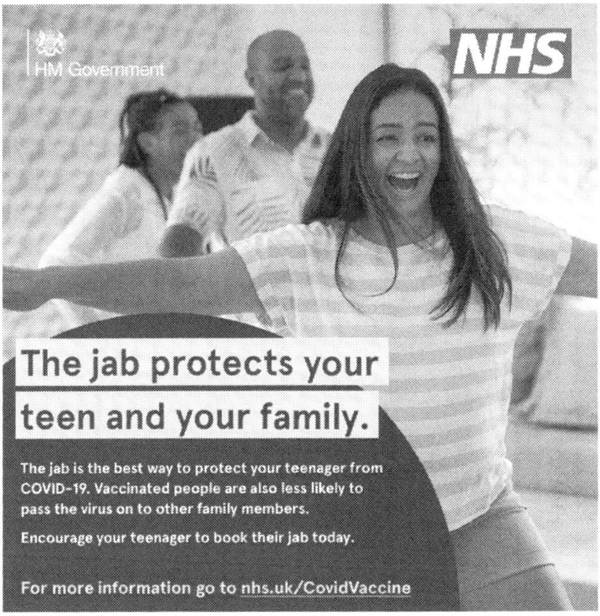

NHS advert, from: https://notts.icb.nhs.uk/your-health/covid-19-and-flu/covid-19/childrens-vaccinations/

Jabs don't protect us; T cells do.

Thanks to our T cells, you can be immune with a negative antibody test; I am a living example of this. *Forget antibodies*. And don't just take it from me. In a June 28 FDA meeting, Pfizer Vice President for Viral Vaccines Kena Swanson even acknowledged that ***"there is no established correlate' between antibody levels and protection from disease."*** [19]

We should have always focused on T cells. They remain the cornerstone of natural immunity. Differences in T cell immunity are also why some people are affected by COVID-19 worse than others, and may also point towards why others are affected badly by the jabs too.

It's time we give them the attention they deserve.

WHAT IS THE KEY TO A WELL FUNCTIONING IMMUNE SYSTEM?

Looking back, I was lucky to have a blood test showing negative antibody results and even luckier to have the curiosity and knowledge to read and understand scientific literature. We're all different and react to pathogens differently. It is our differences that should be studied; that is where the answers lie.

Fortunately for us, there have been studies that have looked into these differences and specifically into why there is a wide difference in symptom severity between different people.

It appears that how severe one suffers with COVID-19 is a good indicator of one's health and, thus, the balance of one's immune system. People who are healthy and asymptomatic respond only through cellular (antibody-independent) immunity,[1] whereas those who have symptoms respond through antibody formation.[2] In rare cases, individuals who suffer very severe and long-lasting symptoms show highly imbalanced cellular *and* humoral (antibody-dependent) immune responses, whereby the levels of SARS-CoV-2-specific T cells or antibody immunity are very low.[3]

Death due to SARS-CoV-2 has been postulated to be due to lung injury and/or clotting issues due to an excessive release of cytokines, termed "a cytokine storm."[4] We must understand that, though the virus acts as the finger pushing the first domino, disease progression is ultimately down to how the body reacts afterwards. Imbalances cause massive inflammation and disease. Immunological balance can lead to no symptoms whatsoever.

Find balance.

WHY ARE SOME PEOPLE AFFECTED WORSE BY THE VIRUS?

You may know someone in their 80s who has never had symptomatic COVID-19 (I add the word "symptomatic" there because, as you now know, you can mount an immune response to this virus without becoming ill from it). And you might know a "fit and healthy" 20-year-old who has been sick with COVID-19 on multiple occasions. It may not make sense at first glance, but deeper inquiry may reveal potential answers.

To begin, keep in mind that your observations of those who are still alive and well should not skew your perception of the pandemic as a whole. Older people *are* more prone to severe illness and death,[1] and so the older folk you are seeing now are the luckier ones who survived it all. Don't forget survivorship bias.

I say luckier, but I think it is important to step back, unplug from the fear-mongering narrative, and assess the actual severity of SARS-CoV-2.

Let's take Peru as the worst-case example. Peru, at the time of writing this, has the worst case-fatality rates of all nations at 6.0%, with 645.60 deaths per 100,000 people due to COVID-19.[2] Dividing the number of deaths by the total population of Peru gives us 0.0065% of the population who have died with COVID-19, or, in other words, 99.35% of Peru (the worst-hit nation in terms of concentration of COVID-19 deaths) were not killed because of COVID-19.

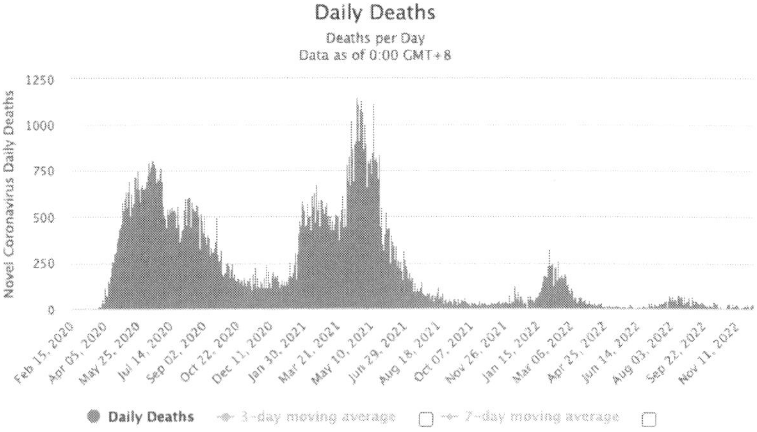

Daily deaths during the pandemic in Peru, from:
https://www.worldometers.info/coronavirus/country/peru/

Please don't take this as me being callous or disregarding the millions of people who have suffered or died as a result of COVID-19 worldwide. *Trust me, I've seen what this virus can do.* I'm just trying to put it all into perspective for you.

If you're from the UK, then the figures are 258.60 deaths per 100,000 people due to COVID-19, which means 99.7% of the population hasn't been killed by COVID-19.[2] This is disregarding the somewhat questionable methods (COVID-19 deaths within 28 days of a positive test and no postmortems) from which these figures have been calculated. And sticking with the UK, the average age of death due to COVID-19 is 80.4 years.[3] To put that into perspective, the average life expectancy in the UK is 79.4 years for males and 83.1 years for females.[4]

The overwhelming majority of people were not badly affected by the virus. But it does pose a question: *why did some die? And why are others seemingly fine?*

We now know that many factors like age, gender, existing medical conditions, blood type, and even body weight all play a part in whether or not someone suffers from symptomatic COVID-19. Furthermore, your day-to-day lifestyle also affects your risk of infection. Circulating blood sugar levels, the amount of sunlight you had last summer, previous infections, stress, alcohol consumption, exercising too much, the food you eat, and lack of sleep all play a massive part in one's immunity.

Actually, let's make a list of the various risk factors that increase one's likelihood of having a symptomatic COVID-19 infection. In no particular order:

- Increased age[5]
- Male gender[6]
- Obesity[7]
- Metabolic diseases[8] (diabetes, blood pressure, obesity)
- High circulating blood sugar levels (independent of diabetes)[9]

- Lack of sleep[10]
- Alcohol consumption[11]
- Mineral deficiencies (e.g. selenium and zinc)[12,13,14]
- Unfavourable gut microbiome[15]
- Vitamin D deficiency[16]
- Over-exercising[17]
- Physical inactivity[18]
- Increased stress and anxiety[19]
- Blood group A, B, and Rh+[20]
- Immunocompromisation[21]
- Reduced amount of previous general coronavirus (common cold) infections[22]
- Reduced repeated exposure to SARS-CoV-2[23]
- Exposure to newer, more spreadable strains of SARS-CoV-2[24]
- Having the COVID-19 shot (we'll get to this later on don't worry)[25]

If you look at that list, a lot of it, apart from your age, sex, and blood type, are all modifiable and thus controllable. This is why I am a big proponent of the phrase I made up: **"One does not *give* the virus, one accepts it."** It's easy to go to a BBQ, drink heavily, sleep badly, and become unwell with COVID-19 the next day and blame one of your friends or the cashier working at Tesco's for making you unwell with COVID-19. It's easy, but it's wrong.

Yes, the amount of virus in the air increases if someone is coughing and sputtering everywhere in a closed environment, but it's ultimately up to your immune system to mount an effective response to it or not. And in fact, viruses are everywhere; it's their world, and they were here first. Even deer have been shown to carry SARS-CoV-2.[26] *Does that mean you're going to stop going for walks in the forest?* I didn't think so. This is also why the "Zero COVID policy" is an utterly stupid idea.

Whether asymptomatically or not, we must assume that getting infected is (and has been in many cases) a definite eventuality. This is because SARS-CoV-2 is extremely transmissible and will always be under selection to become more transmissible. The ability to infect more hosts is key to the evolutionary success of viruses. Any proposed man-made external intervention is destined to fail.

You will be infected and have most likely already been infected by the virus. And here's the kicker: You *will* very likely get infected by SARS-CoV-2 and its variants in the future too. There is no hiding. Ever.

But not all infections lead to illness. If you get sick, you are solely responsible. And no mask or plastic screen will help you. So, the only thing you can do to reduce your chances of getting sick from pathogens is to stay healthy. It's time to stop blaming others and focus on your own health. *Don't fret if you don't know how; I'll explain various things you might be able to do to improve your immunity later on in this book.*

See, the immune system is extraordinarily complicated, and though its primary aim is to keep you free from pathogen-causing diseases, it moulds your life and biology in unimaginably numerous ways from the moment you are born to the day you die.[27] This is why seemingly unrelated factors like anxiety and blood sugar levels all play a part in your immunity.

As a side note, this is also why I disdain the term "fit and healthy." It is a term tossed around too easily. If one were actually fit and healthy, then one wouldn't have been so sick with the virus. If you have been very unwell with COVID-19, especially if you are young, then take this as a sign to explore why.

Going back to that list, some of you may have noticed that I included two seemingly opposing risk factors one after the other.

- Reduced repeated exposure to SARS-CoV-2
- Being exposure to newer, more transmissible strains of SARS-CoV-2

"How can a reduced exposure to the virus and being exposed to newer, more transmissible strains of the virus both increase the chances of symptomatic infection?" I hear you asking.

I think the answer to this question could be key to figuring out why some people are more likely to get a severe COVID-19 infection than others.

WHY MAY AN INCREASED EXPOSURE TO SARS-COV-2 IMPROVE IMMUNITY?

In July 2021, I published a blog on my website titled "The vaccinated getting infected marks the end of the pandemic."[1] In it, I wrote that we were seeing a rise in COVID-19 cases, particularly among those who have been double-jabbed because those who have been inoculated have antibodies **only** to the vaccine-coded spike proteins;[2] something we have discussed earlier in this book.

"Viruses have a tendency to mutate and preferentially at the spike though, rendering vaccines somewhat useless against newer more mutated forms of the virus, e.g. delta.", I wrote.[1]

And I continued, *"If natural immunity is far superior at reducing re-infection and if circulating strains of the virus are less harmful than before, then it would make the most sense now to allow everyone to restart life back as usual. Everyone should be exposed to the virus naturally so we can all build long-lasting robust immunity to it. We must aim to naturally improve people's immune systems through diet and lifestyle[3] (something we should have been doing for the last two years). No need for boosters, no need for lockdowns,[4] no need for masks,[5] for which the evidence for effectiveness is poor anyway."*.

Nothing changed after writing that.

People queued up for their boosters.

I wasn't surprised, just saddened.

More than a year later, my sentiment still stands, and the evidence that these shots are more useless than natural infection against newer strains holds up to scientific scrutiny too. Here, one paper notes,[6]

"Together, our results indicate that Omicron can evolve mutations to specifically evade humoral immunity elicited by BA.1 infection. The continuous evolution of Omicron poses great challenges to SARS-CoV-2 herd immunity and suggests that

BA.1-derived vaccine boosters may not be ideal for achieving broad-spectrum protection."[6]

It seems like the best approach to protecting yourself against rapidly mutating respiratory viruses is repeated mucosal exposure in one's respiratory tract.

The mucosa, which is also called the mucous membrane, is the thin layer of tissue that lines body cavities and covers the outside of organs. It is made up of epithelial cells and the substances they secrete.[7] Basically, it's the surface layer that covers our eyes, mouth, throat, tongue, and the rest of our insides that separates us from the outside world.

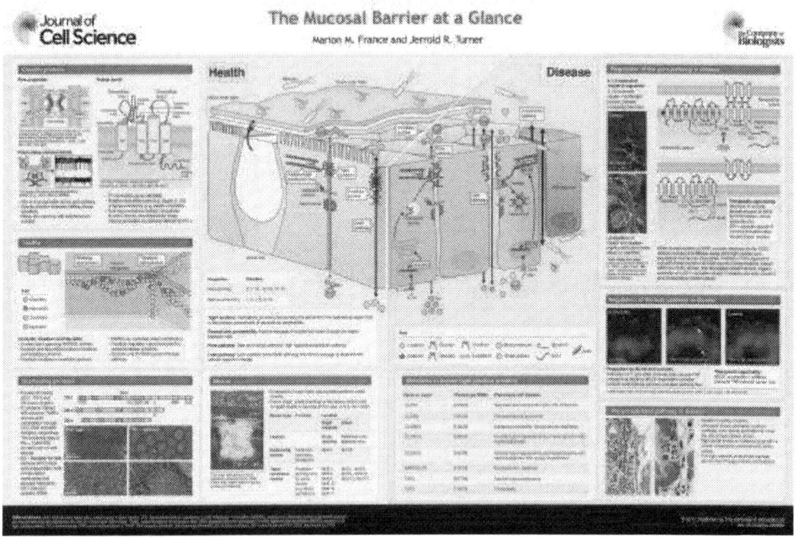

The mucosal barrier at a glance, from:
https://www.ncbi.nlm.nih.gov/pmc/articles/PMC5278669

Those surfaces are our main sites of infectious threat since various microorganisms and allergens in our environment invade through the nose, mouth, eyes, and gut all the time. To keep these dangerous buggers out, we have evolved the mucosal immune system, the largest component of the entire immune system.[8]

The mucosal immune system consists of innate and adaptive immunity components that are found in circulating blood, but what (among other things) makes the mucosal immune system unique are secretory IgA (SIgA) antibodies and a special set of T cells called resident memory T (TRM) cells.

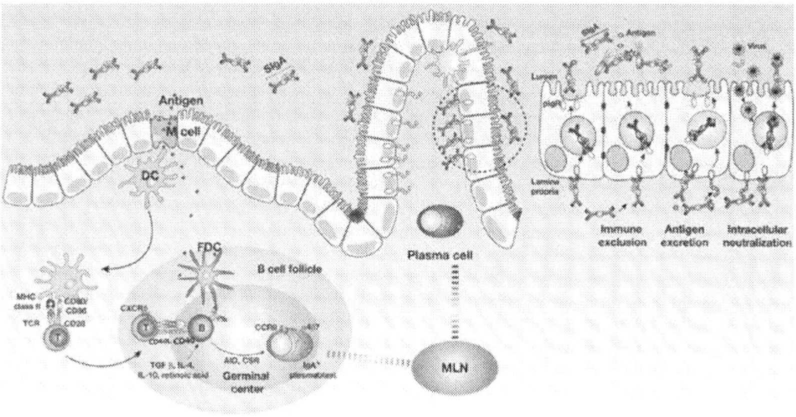

The mucosal immune system, from: https://www.researchgate.net/figure/Schematic-diagram-of-mucosal-immune-induction-to-generate-T-cell-dependent-IgA_fig1_260809430

SIgA is the major antibody in mucosal secretions. SIgA in the mucosa cannot kill pathogens or activate the complement system. It works by attaching to the microorganisms and then eliminating them from the upper respiratory tract through coughing up phlegm (mucociliary transport). And though it is an antibody, SIgA is considered a component of the innate immune system. It is vital to note that **these shots do *not* activate SIgA**.[8]

TRM cells are a special type of T cell that stays in mucosal tissues for a long time and doesn't move around in the blood. They can kill infected cells, make cytokines, and have innate-like "sensing and alarming" properties that can recruit other immune cells to fight antimicrobial infections.[9] Overall, TRM cells give us immediate and long-lasting frontline immunity, which protects us from getting sick again and again.

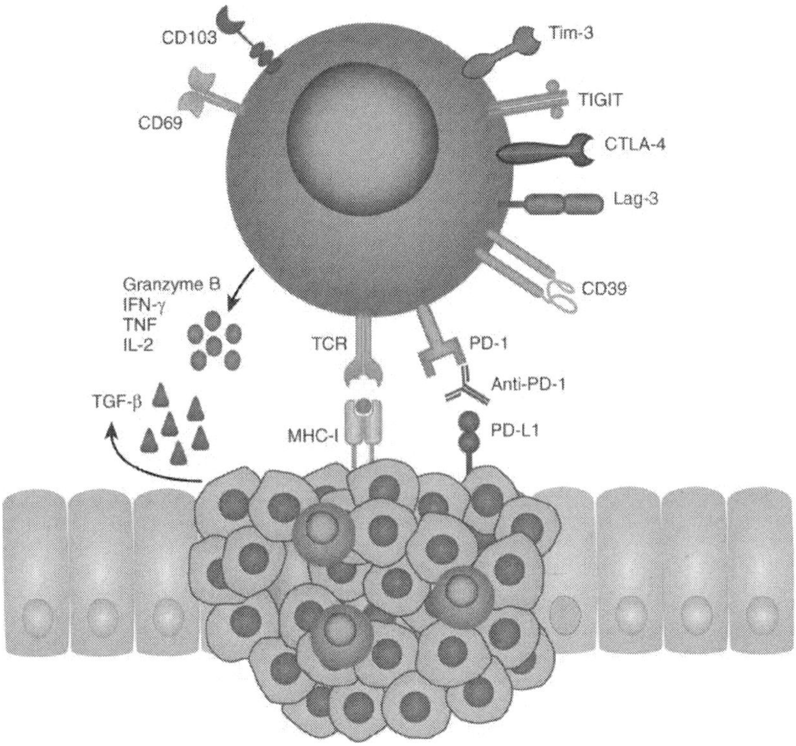

Tissue-resident memory T cells, from: https://www.nature.com/articles/s41385-021-00467-7

However, not all TRM cells are created equal. In the skin, TRMs remain in the tissue long after infection and antigen clearance. In contrast, lung TRM are lost 4-5 months after an acute infection, resulting in a loss of protection from reexposure.[8]

As a result, I believe that repeated mucosal exposure in the respiratory tract is the best way to protect yourself against rapidly mutating respiratory viruses. As this paper notes,

"Not only is antigen required for TRM formation as previously documented, but unlike the situation in most other organ sites, ***persistent antigen is essential for the continual replenishment and long-term maintenance of TRM population in the lungs****."*[10]

In other words, theoretically (as studies specifically on SARS-CoV-2 haven't been performed yet), if you encountered SARS-CoV-2 once, formed TRM cells to the virus, and then locked yourself away at home for 5 months alone, you'd lose your TRM cells and become as susceptible to SARS-CoV-2 reinfection as you were at the start. *Who still thinks that lockdowns are a good idea?*

Continuous exposure to SARS-CoV-2 and other coronaviruses may help TRM cells to retain memory and prevent reinfection.[11] Don't take it from me, look at the first line of this study ***"Resident memory T cells positioned within the respiratory tract are probably required to limit SARS-CoV-2 spread and COVID-19".*** [12]

And like SIgA, I must note that **shots injected into the blood *cannot* induce TRM cell formation.**[10]

Repeatedly being exposed to respiratory pathogens in short amounts of time, either naturally or through a vaccination, helps to stop people from getting sick again and again. But the trick is not to become ill from the virus every time you are exposed to it.

I think that the key to making this work is to always have a very strong innate immune system and T cell responses.

See, viruses are trying to infect us at all times; it is the only way they can replicate. And we are surrounded by them. It has been estimated that there are 380 trillion viruses living on and inside your body right now.[13] That is 10 times the number of cells that make up our body.

During a respiratory virus infection, a person who is sick can make 10^{12} infectious viral particles.[14] *That's 10 with 12 zeros after it, or 1 000 000 000 000 viral particles.*

It has been estimated that we encounter 6 million virus-like particles in the air every day.[15] A teaspoon of seawater typically contains about fifty million viruses.[16] And even in supposedly pristine environments,[17] like way up in the sky above the atmospheric boundary layer, the concentrations of viruses have been found to range from 0.26×10^9 to more than $7\times10^9 m^2$ per day.

It is a viral world, and we are simply living in it. Trying to "control" viruses is a futile affair. *Laughable really.*

Not only that, but remember that viruses are always changing, and the ones that stick around are the ones that our immune systems fail to stop. And so, in turn, viruses become *more* transmissible over time. They also become *less* deadly, we think, due to a proposed theory that was formed more than 30 years ago called the "virulence-transmissibility evolutionary trade-off." [18]

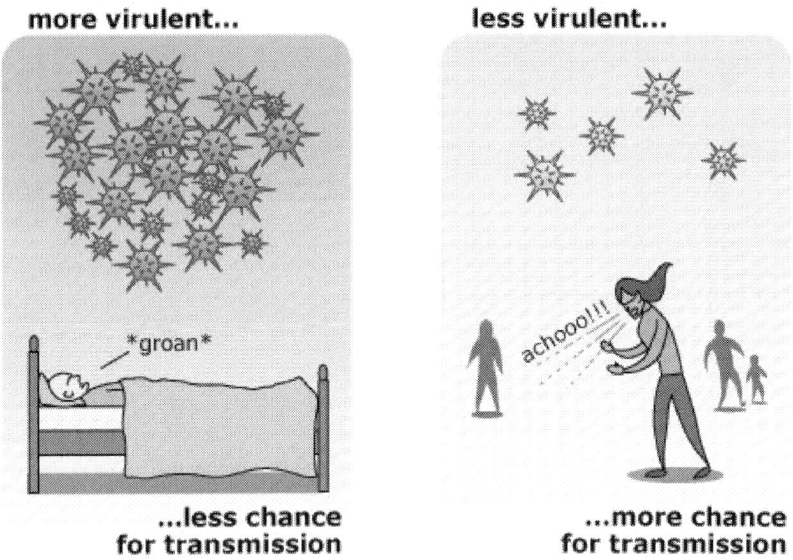
more virulent...
groan
...less chance for transmission
less virulent...
achooo!!!
...more chance for transmission

Virulence-transmissibility evolutionary trade-off, from: https://evolution.berkeley.edu/evo-news/evolution-from-a-viruss-view/

In short, the trade-off hypothesis says that virulence, which is when a pathogen hurts its host by making the host unwell, is an unavoidable cost that the virus has to pay for using the host's resources to make more copies of itself. And thus, the greater the harm the virus imposes, the greater the chance its host (us, in this case) will die and no longer be able to spread to other people and survive. So for transmission to be maximised, intermediate levels of virulence are needed. And though this theory is continuously debated, it seems to hold true for COVID-19. [19]

I say "hold true" tentatively, as it seems like the natural progression of the virus has been tampered with. Scientists noted in one paper that vaccines that do not prevent transmission (like the COVID-19 ones) can **create conditions that promote the emergence of pathogen strains that cause more severe disease in unvaccinated hosts.**[20]

And authors of another paper evaluating the Omicron variant noted that unnatural changes to its **spike protein were highly likely a product of artificial genetic modification**.[21]

When large groups of people are treated with imperfect vaccines to treat modified viruses, the trade-off hypothesis may fall apart, but this is a reflection of manipulated public health measures and not natural viral progression. If more studies show that pathogens are being changed genetically and then released to the general population, we could be moving toward a future where new variants are made in labs to promote cultural and social changes. *We'll get into this later.*

For now, it looks like less people are getting sick from the current versions of SARS-CoV-2, which is a good sign. Soon SARS-CoV-2 will morph into a form of the common cold, we hope. The subtype H1N1 of influenza is a good example of this; it is still deadly and circulating now, but less so than when it caused the 1918 influenza pandemic, also known as the Spanish flu.[22]

Because the risk of getting sick from SARS-CoV-2 (and related viruses) is always there and getting worse, I'd say we should always be on guard to prevent this from happening. Remember, the immune system is in flux, and through negative external factors, one can be "immune" one day and not so "immune" the next.

It seems like the key to overall respiratory immunity is a strong and well-balanced innate and mucosal T cell response because these are our first-line defences. Only after this level is breached do people begin to experience symptoms and the formation of antibodies.

The thing is, it's not like the scientific community didn't know about mucosal immunity. This article, titled - "Mucosal Immunity in COVID-19: A Neglected but Critical Aspect of SARS-CoV-2 Infection" was published in November 2020.[23]

And more recently, I was brought to the attention of this May 2022 study on hamsters titled "A live attenuated vaccine confers superior mucosal and systemic immunity to SARS-CoV-2 variants."[24] In this study, hamsters were either given a weakened SARS-CoV-2 virus through their nose or an mRNA vaccine through an injection. They found that the intranasal vaccine did better on all fronts. They conclude, ***"Our results demonstrate that use of live-attenuated 10 vaccines may offer advantages over available COVID-19 vaccines, specifically when applied as booster, and may provide a solution for containment of the COVID-19 pandemic."***[24]

At the start, those who were only injected without natural exposure lacked mucosal immunity, which may be one reason why jabbed people still became infected and transmitted the virus. A natural infection (or nasal vaccine) is paramount for mucosal immunity stimulation, as one paper puts it, ***"We also speculate that the extraordinarily high antibody titers observed in vaccinated individuals who develop breakthrough infections may lead to subsequent long-term protection in those individuals."*** [25]

In other words, becoming naturally infected is the only way for a jabbed person to gain long-lasting and sterilising immunity that prevents further infection and transmission.

If mucosal live attenuated vaccines are better than injected mRNA agents, you must ask yourself why so-called "experts" dismissed the former? And, once again, why was natural immunity so demonised?

While you think about that, let's look at the science behind T cell balance and why some people fare worse than others when infected.

WHAT IS THE DIFFERENCE BETWEEN A TH1 AND TH2 RESPONSE?

I am aware that I may come across as being unhealthily obsessed with T cells. I may be. I am not ashamed; it's all for a good reason. I just think that the media doesn't give them nearly enough credit for how important they are to our overall biological function. Not only that, but a proper understanding of them and their role may help you reduce your risk of infections in the future.

There are a few different types of T cells. Naive T helper (Th) cells are T cells that have no role; they are like children with so much potential but no job or university degree. Th are activated by the recognition of a peptide antigen–class II major histo-compatibility complex (MHC) presented on antigen-presenting cells (APCs) through the interaction with the T cell receptor (TCR).

That may have sounded like gibberish, so simply put, when pathogenic material is presented on a special receptor (MHC) by certain cells like dendritic cells, macrophages, Langerhans cells, and B cells (also known as a group as APCs); Th cells interact with this receptor and with another receptor (TCR) to turn them into effector Th cells, also known as CD4+ cells.

See it as a business deal. APCs eat pathogenic material and show it to naive T helper cells. The naive T helper cells see this, interact with the APCs through a TCR, and now have a job to do.

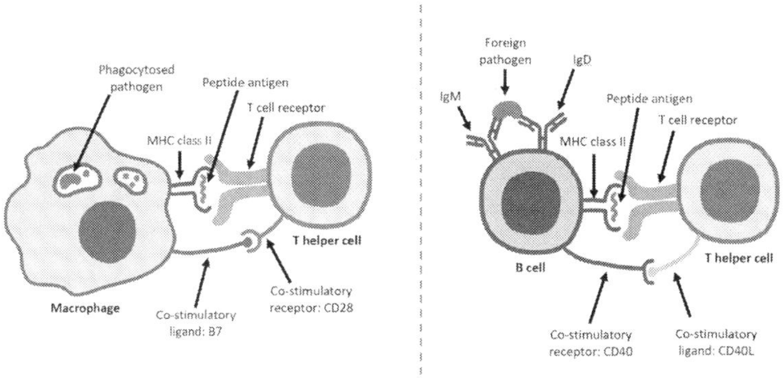

Activation of T and B cells, from:
https://en.wikipedia.org/wiki/T_helper_cell#/media/File:Activation_of_T_and_B_cells.png

These effector Th cells are further divided into three main types, identified by the cytokines they secrete. If you've forgotten (and I understand; it can feel like a lot), cytokines are small secreted proteins released by cells that have a specific effect on cell interactions and communication. *Remember now?*

The three effector Th cells are referred to as Th type-1 (Th1), Th type-2 (Th2), or Th type-17 (Th17) cells.

Th1 cells secrete the cytokines interferon (IFN)-γ, and tumour necrosis factor (TNF)-β. This makes it easier for these cells to fight infections caused by viruses, bacteria, and other microorganisms that grow inside macrophages. They are also effective in eliminating cancer cells.[1]

Th2 cells secrete another type of cytokine called interleukins, specifically IL-4, IL-5, IL-10, and IL-13, which up-regulate antibody production and target parasitic organisms and allergens. Th2 cells activate B cells, which are adapted for defence against parasites. Th2 cells are predominantly responsible for the development of asthma.[1]

Th17 was later discovered and shown to secrete IL-17, IL-17F, IL-6, IL-22, and TNF-α, and it appears to play an important role in tissue inflammation as well as neutrophil activation to combat bacteria existing outside cells.[1]

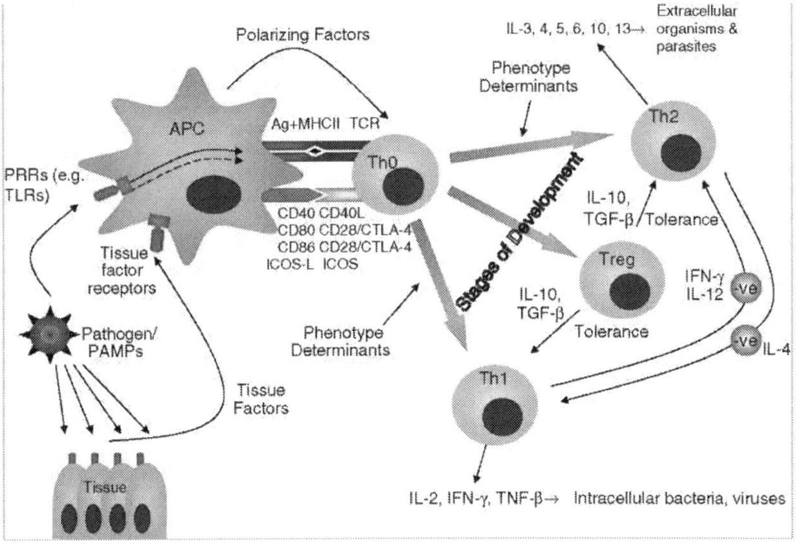

Various effector Th cells, from: https://www.ncbi.nlm.nih.gov/pmc/articles/PMC2433332/

In broad terms, Th1 cells work best against viral infections, Th2 cells work best against parasites, and Th17 cells work best against bacterial and fungal infections. Th1, Th2, and Th17 populations and the cytokines they release are antagonistic to each other, meaning that they work in opposition. And so during an infection, one predominant type of effector Th takes control, depending on the pathogen.

There is another form of T cell that can be formed around this time called regulatory T (Treg) cells.[1] They were formerly known as suppressor T cells, and act like mediators. They secrete IL-10 and transforming growth factor (TGF)-β, which modulates helper T cell activity and suppresses some of their functions. They are thought to maintain tolerance to self-antigens, and help prevent autoimmune disease.[1]

I hope you can appreciate that the immune system relies on certain cells doing their job properly and communicating with other cells in the correct way. The immune system is a sensory system of sorts, constantly on alert, detecting external and internal environments and making sure the ship runs smoothly. It has its own intelligence.

However, like any finely tuned system, asynchronicity causes chaos. And with regards to the immune system, this chaos causes downstream detriment, and, for some, death.

A small number of studies have found some differences in the immune systems of people who had mild COVID-19 and those who had severe COVID-19 or died from SARS-CoV-2. I have summarised the findings of these studies in the following table.

Mild/non-hospitalised COVID-19	Severe COVID-19
Those who were non-hospitalised showed a greater T helper and T killer cell response secreting IL-10.[2]	Hospitalised patients show a bias towards an T killer cell response characterised by IFN-γ and IL-4 secretion - which is in response to the S peptides on the virus.[2]
The only cytokine that was higher in non-hospitalised compared to hospitalised groups was IL-12p70.[2]	The one deceased patient studied had the second lowest level of IL-12p70 of the severe group.[2]
M and N-specific responses dominated in nonhospitalized and mild-hospitalised cases.[2]	
A broader Th profile in CD8+T cells induced by the nonspike viral proteins was associated with a less severe infection[2]	Spike responses dominated by IL-4+ T killer cells represented a hallmark of disease severity, being the sole response in the fatal

	case.[2]
An N-specific effector memory Th1 profile has been associated with non-hospitalization during symptomatic COVID-19.[2]	
T-bet expression is associated with patients with a better prognosis.[3]	
CXCR3 (a chemokine receptor) is also found on a subset of CD4+Foxp3+T cells, and the control of inflammatory responses at mucosal surfaces requires IL-10 producing Treg cells.[2]	Reduced frequencies of Treg cells have been noted in severe COVID-19 cases. [4,5]
	"elevated fraction of HLA-DR+CD38hi rather than HLA-DR+CD38+ CD8+ T cells were persistently accumulated in COVID-19 patients, especially in severe and

	critical cases."[6]
	Increased inflammatory markers, low white cell levels (lymphopenia), pro-inflammatory cytokines, and high anti-receptor binding domain (RBD) antibody levels.[7]
"Asymptomatic SARS-CoV-2 infected individuals showed a potent and robust Th1 immunity, with a lower Th17 and less activated T-cells at the time of sample acquisition compared not only with symptomatic patients, but also with healthy controls."[8]	"COVID-19 patients who eventually died had established a potent Th2 response as a compensatory mechanism for an impaired Th1 response"[8]
Asymptomatic patients have shown higher median total lymphocyte	"Hospitalised patients presented global lymphopenia, this being in

(white cell) counts.[8]	line with previous studies where lymphocyte count had been proposed as a predictor of severity"[8]
A higher proportion of IFNy-producing T helper 1 (Th1)- like cells in patients with moderate disease than in patients with severe disease has been noted.[9]	"The stu dy has shown that increased levels of IL-15 and a high Th2 response are associated with a fatal outcome of the disease."[10]
	"a significant reduction of %Th1 and %Th17 cells with higher activated %Th2 cells in the COVID-19 patients compared with reference population."[10]
	"Senescent (the process of growing old) Th2 cell percentage was an independent risk factor for death accompanied by the numbers of total

	lymphocytes"[10]
	"Patients who did not survive presented significantly higher levels of IL-15 than those who recovered"[10]
	"we also observed a higher Th17/Th1 cytokine imbalance in all deceased patients compared to those that survived"[11]

Okay, there is a lot to unpack here. First of all, I want to say that I left some boxes blank on purpose because, even though opposites could be inferred, these were not mentioned in studies. Secondly, I'd only take the study results as correlations with regard to disease severity. Immunology lies on a spectrum. Remember too that the table above is far from being fully complete.

If I had to sum it all up, **people with severe COVID-19 were more likely to make antibodies, react more strongly to spike proteins, have lower levels of lymphocytes (T and B cells) overall, and have less Th1 than Th2 and Th17. T reg cells tended to be lower in those with severe COVID-19 too.**

Those who had mild or non-hospitalised COVID-19 tended to have responses predominantly to the M and N proteins of the virus, had greater Th1 and better T reg activation.

Interestingly too, M peptides induced the strongest IFNγ secretion in CD4+ T cells, N peptides enhanced cytotoxicity (cell killing) in CD8+ T cells and S peptides had an overall predominant Th2 profile.[2]

T bet, also called T-box transcription factor TBx21, is a protein that was originally thought to be the master regulator of Th1 development,[12] although it is now recognised to have a role in both the adaptive and innate immune systems.[13] And so it makes sense why its expression was found higher in those who only suffered with mild COVID-19.

Overall, it looks like the bodies of people who had severe COVID-19 responded to the virus as if it were a parasite instead of a virus. And because the predominance of one Th cell reduces the evolution of others, their disease took off like a runaway train. This train only got faster and more out of control due to a lack of or dysfunction of its braking system: T reg cells.

Unfortunately, in those who died, their immune system became so exhausted that it ceased to work at all, as noted here: *"Senescent Th2 cell percentage was an independent risk factor for death accompanied by the numbers of total lymphocytes".*[10] Senescence is the process by which a cell ages, stops dividing for good, but doesn't die. It's kind of like the cell just gives up.

This information brings up more questions than answers, like, why do some people have lower circulating levels of lymphocytes than others? Was this caused by the infection, or did it occur prior to it? Why did they develop and then administer a vaccine that is only able to produce SARS-CoV-2 spike proteins? What are some risk factors for Th1/Th2 disruption?

One study found that men, asthmatics, people over 40, smokers, and people with high ACE2 (Angiotensin-Converting Enzyme 2) expression in their sputum all had Th1/Th2 dysfunction.[11] This could explain why their risk of severe COVID-19 was higher than others'. ACE2 is the receptor responsible for the SARS-CoV-2 viral entry.[14]

This image, shown below, from another study shows beautifully the range of COVID-19 severity and how well the immune system works.[2] When infections were very bad, both T helper cells and T killer cells made more IL-4 which is a sign of Th2 activation. Whereas in mild or non-hospitalised patients, T cells produce less IL-4 and more IL-10.

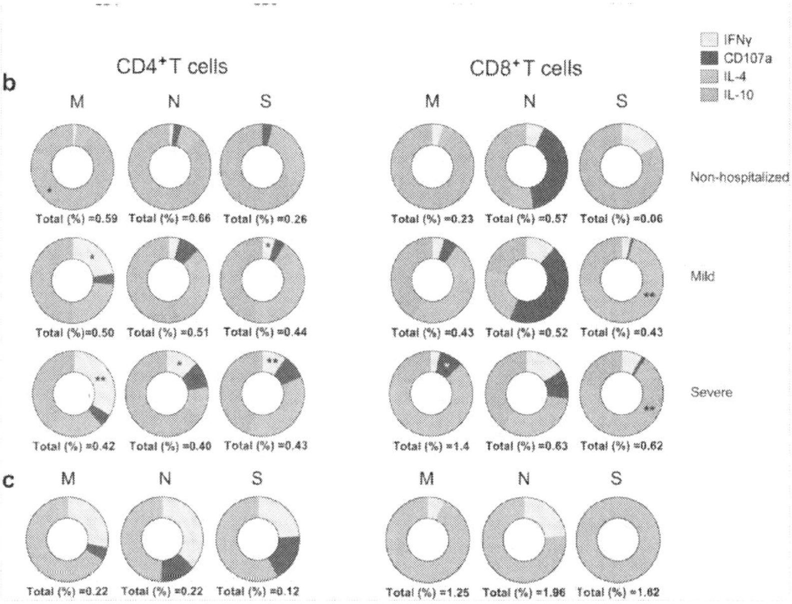

CD4+ and CD8+ T cell ratios in non-hospitalised, mild and severe COVID-19 patients, from: https://www.ncbi.nlm.nih.gov/pmc/articles/PMC8140108/

IL-10 was originally thought to be a Th2 cytokine; its identity as such originated from its association with Th2 clones in mice.[15] In humans though, both Th1, Th2 and regulatory T cells secrete IL-10. And now IL-10 is emerging as more of an anti-inflammatory cytokine.[15] This idea was backed up by the discovery of regulatory T cells, which have suppressor functions and are helped by molecules like IL-10.

The immune system is a sensing system that requires balance for proper functioning. When this is disrupted, we get fulminant disease. By the way, I'm not talking only about COVID-19; it has long been known that patients infected with HIV who show a Th1 response are seronegative (antibody negative) and do not develop acquired immunodeficiency syndrome (AIDS), whereas Th2 patients become seropositive and evolve to AIDS.[16]

Balance needs to be kept for the immune system to work well, and there is more and more evidence that these mRNA agents greatly upset this balance.

DO THE JABS INCREASE OUR RISK OF INFECTION?

In the process of leaving my profession, I had many meetings, and during a lot of them, I was encouraged to take the shot to protect myself against the virus. To my coworkers at the time, I was being selfish by willingly allowing myself to remain vulnerable to infection and thus a walking threat to them and my patients. They were scared of the virus and wanted me to get the shot to protect them. That's what it really all boiled down to. Fear and flawed thinking.

In all of history, these agents were the first known pharmaceutical products whose effectiveness was measured by how much they affected others. It's the same as getting a rabies vaccine to protect your mother or taking paracetamol to relieve your partner's headache. It makes no sense.

Abhorrently orchestrated studies, which were then popularised in mainstream media, did not help either.

Unvaccinated disproportionately risk safety of those vaccinated against COVID-19, study shows

https://www.theglobeandmail.com/canada/article-unvaccinated-covid-risk-for-vaccinated-canada/?utm_source=dlvr.it&utm_medium=twitter

Luckily, I understood the importance of natural immunity and keeping healthy.

And as my colleagues tried to convince me, I stared blankly and confidently, reassured by the various high quality medical studies that circulated in my mind. I knew the scientific facts, and I also knew that a lot of my then colleagues had to take time off work due to COVID-19 very soon after having their shot.

"If you've taken it and are masked, what are you worrying about?" I'd ask during meetings. No answer. "And why am I the only one here who has never had COVID, while a lot of you have been unwell after the jab?" Again, no answer.

If jabs were effective, we would have seen fewer cases and daily new confirmed COVID-19 deaths in countries with the highest vaccine uptake rates. Two shots, no more COVID-19, the end of the pandemic, the return to normal life, the end. But this hasn't happened. In fact, the opposite did.

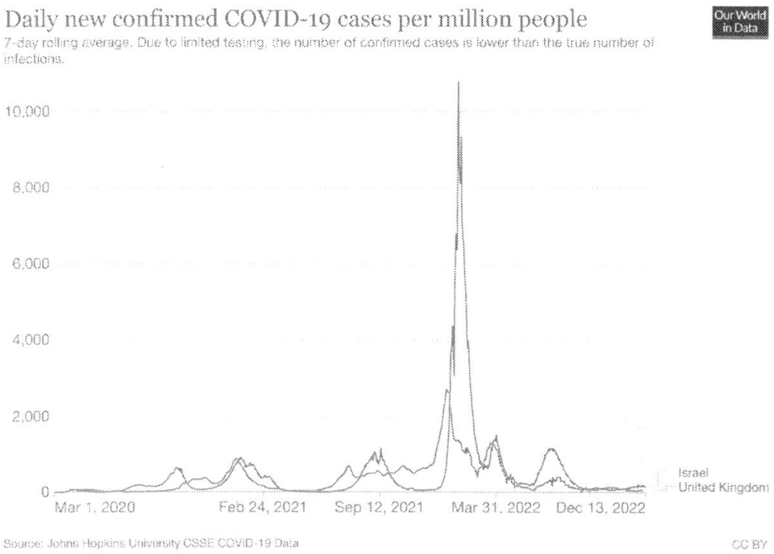

Daily new confirmed COVID-19 cases per million, *Israel and the United Kingdom, March 2020 to December 2022- https://ourworldindata.org/*

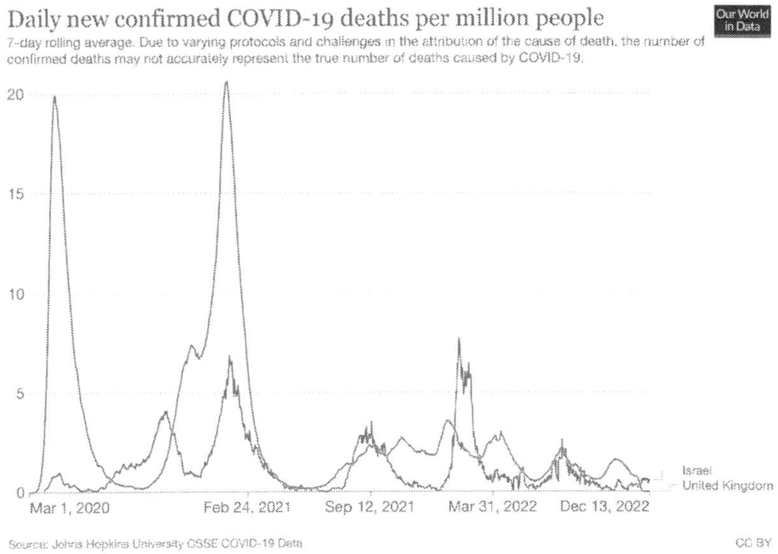

Daily new confirmed COVID-19 deaths per million, Israel and the United Kingdom, March 2020 to December 2022- https://ourworldindata.org/

As you can see from the graphs above, cases and deaths in the United Kingdom and Israel, two nations with extremely high levels of shot administration and documentation, went *up* as shots were administered. The UK was first introduced to the jabs in December 2020 and the first booster in September 2021.[1,2] While 80% of the eligible population in Israel have received two doses plus a booster jab,[3] and yet they had their biggest spike in cases in 2022. I am using these graphs because the UK does not collect figures for those who may have been harmed or suffered illness from a COVID-19 shot, as this is not recorded on death certificates.[4]

And emerging evidence continues to pile up pointing to the fact that the jabbed are *more* likely to have COVID-19 than the unjabbed. For example, New Zealand Government data shows that the jabbed have up to six times the infection rate of the unvaccinated.[5]

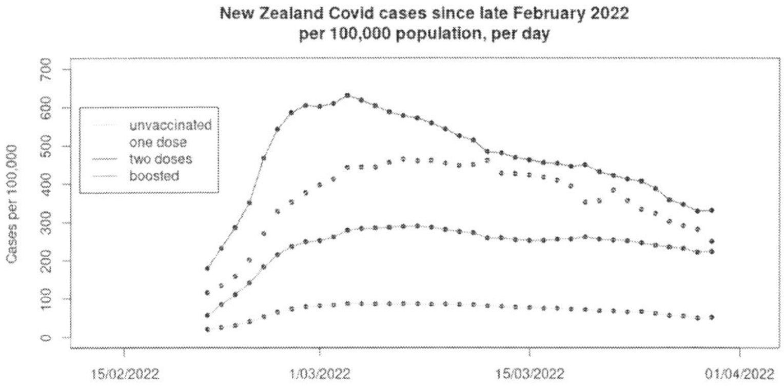

New Zealand COVID-19 cases since late Feb 2022 per 100,000 population, per day, from: https://dailysceptic.org/2022/04/09/vaccinated-have-up-to-six-times-the-infection-rate-of-unvaccinated-new-zealand-government-data-show/

Other than being totally counterproductive, when I noticed this, it worried me a lot. Because if people were more likely to get COVID-19 after the vaccine, it could mean that their immune systems were being compromised. So I went out looking for answers.

There are now various theories and potential mechanisms by which these agents may indeed cause immunocompromisation in recipients. Let's explore them.

Firstly, **the shot is known to cause an immunosuppressive state in individuals during the first three days post-first jab**.[6] Note the drop in white cells during days 1–3 post-shot in the graph on the next page.

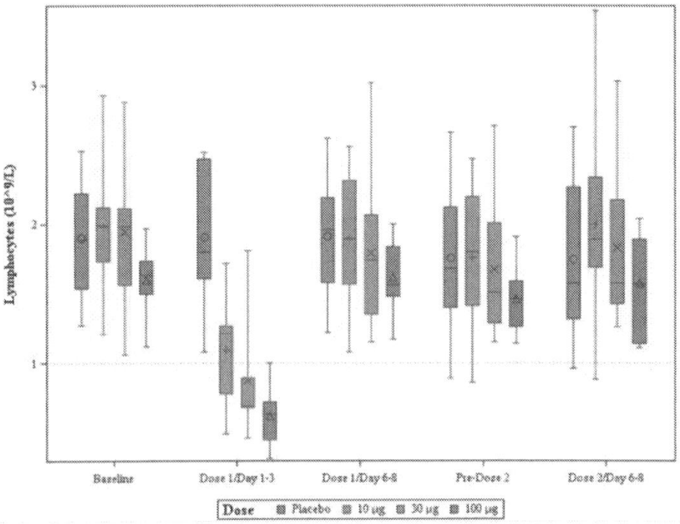

A reduction in lymphocytes during day 1-3, from: https://www.researchgate.net/publication/343607804_Phase_12_study_of_COVID-19_RNA_vaccine_BNT162b1_in_adults

People appear to become more susceptible to SARS-CoV-2 a few days after vaccination, as seen with Yellow Fever vaccination. [7]

Pfizer has also confirmed that after the first dose, white blood cells drop for a short time in people of all ages. From the horse's mouth: *"Clinical laboratory evaluations showed a* ***transient decrease in lymphocytes that was observed in all age and dose groups after Dose 1****, which resolved within approximately 1 week, were not associated with any other clinical sequelae, and were not considered clinically relevant.*

Ribonucleic acid (RNA) vaccines are known to induce type I interferon, and type I interferons regulate lymphocyte recirculation and are associated with transient migration and/or redistribution of lymphocytes. This rapid rebound of lymphocytes supports that the lymphocytes are not depleted, but temporarily migrated out of the peripheral blood, and subsequently re-entered the bloodstream by the time of the next assessment."[8]

In plain English, they agree that white cells drop temporarily after the first dose, but they say it's because these white cells move away from the blood and toward sites of infection (injection site), likely because type I interferon (IFN) is triggered.

This explanation is all well and good after dose one, but why are those who have more than one dose even *more* likely to get infected than the unvaccinated? We need better answers.

Another idea is that viruses from the gut become active again when the immune system is weak after a vaccine. Some viruses have a tendency to hide in various parts of the body and reemerge when the body's defences are weakened. This may not be so different for SARS-CoV-2. Case reports suggest that SARS-CoV-2 may be hiding in the gut even after the chest infection is resolved, further perpetuating the patient's hospital stay.[9]

Is this also why shingles reactivation is being noted after people have been jabbed? Varicella zoster, the virus causing shingles, usually lays hidden and dormant in the nerve cells near the spinal cord and brain after infection. In some, it has been noted to become reactivated after the mRNA jab.[10]

Remember, too, that respiratory vaccines injected into the arm cannot elicit mucosal immunity. Secretory IgA antibodies and resident memory T cells are not activated. This could be another reason why those who have been injected are likely to become ill after the shot. As this study notes *"**The increasing numbers of breakthrough infections in fully vaccinated individuals with waning immunity suggest that current SARS-CoV-2 vaccines do not provide durable sterilizing immunity, particularly against viral variants with enhanced transmissibility and reduced neutralization sensitivity.**"*[11]

The study found that the levels of mucosal IgA and IgG were lower in people who had not been infected but had been injected. Therefore concluding the only way a jabbed person can gain long lasting and sterilising immunity is by becoming naturally infected. Or in other words, the jab only provides partial protection, and you need to get naturally infected for full immunity.

So far, I believe that reactivation and mucosal immunity non-activation are only partial answers to the question of immunocompromisation, simply because previously naturally immune people must have had the jab and had COVID-19 again. There are also others who have also supposedly had COVID-19 multiple times after the jab. And the risk of reinfection seems to coincide with the number of jabs one has had.

This all begs the question: *Are jabs causing longer-term dysregulation of our immune systems?*

Raw data points towards this being the case in some instances. A preprint study looking at Israeli data found that **those who were injected had a nearly six-fold increased risk for breakthrough infection and a seven-fold increased risk for symptomatic disease compared to those who were naturally infected**.[12] The study also noted that those who were jabbed were also at a greater risk of COVID-19-related-hospitalisations compared to those who were previously infected. Becoming unwell post-jab occurred regardless of when the individual was naturally exposed to the virus.

To summarise and answer the original chapter question, I present to you a graph from a recent preprint study noting that the more doses of genetic shots one has, the more likely they are to have COVID-19.[13] *More.*

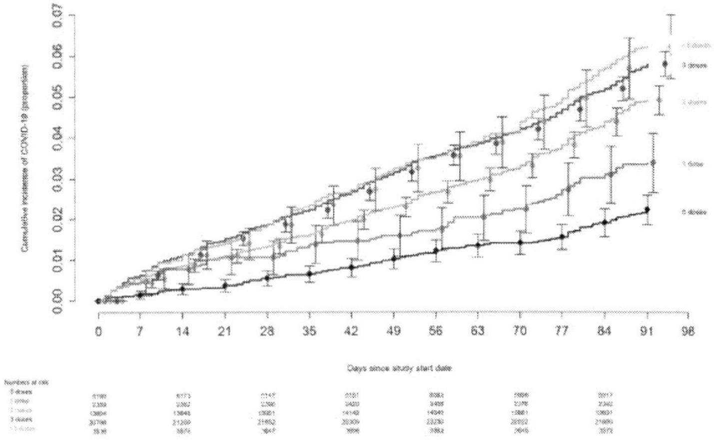

A plot comparing the cumulative incidence of COVID-19 for subjects stratified by the number of COVID-19 vaccine doses previously received, from: https://www.medrxiv.org/content/10.1101/2022.12.17.22283625v1.full.pdf

The idea of immunosuppression becomes more plausible when one truly understands how these shots affect our immune system on a cellular level.

WHAT MAY BE SOME LONGER TERM IMMUNOLOGICAL IMPLICATIONS OF TAKING THE SHOT?

The reason why I spent so much time going over our immune system was firstly to educate you about the extraordinary importance of this network of cells and, secondly, to help you understand what may happen if this system were to be damaged. And as you can guess, things aren't looking too good.

Numbers and charts aside, there are lab-based biochemical findings that indicate vaccine-induced immune dysregulation.

CAN THESE AGENTS DOWNREGULATE INNATE SYSTEMS?

The prize for the 2022 study packing the most bad news goes to one titled "Innate immune suppression by SARS-CoV-2 mRNA vaccinations: The role of G-quadruplexes, exosomes, and MicroRNAs".[1] (I hope there won't be a new contender.)

Here are the study highlights:

Highlights

- mRNA vaccines promote sustained synthesis of the SARS-CoV-2 spike protein.
- The spike protein is neurotoxic, and it impairs DNA repair mechanisms.
- Suppression of type I interferon responses results in impaired innate immunity.
- The mRNA vaccines potentially cause increased risk to infectious diseases and cancer.
- Codon optimization results in G-rich mRNA that has unpredictable complex effects.

https://www.sciencedirect.com/science/article/pii/S027869152200206X#bib119

- *mRNA vaccines promote sustained synthesis of the SARS-CoV-2 spike protein.*
- *The spike protein is neurotoxic, and it impairs DNA repair mechanisms.*
- *Suppression of type I interferon responses results in impaired innate immunity.*
- *The mRNA vaccines potentially cause increased risk to infectious diseases and cancer.*
- *Codon optimization results in G-rich mRNA that has unpredictable complex effects.*

Told you it wasn't looking good.

In it the authors explain the various ways the mRNA agents differ from the natural virus and how lab-made alterations in the jab causes differences in our immune response to it compared to the real life virus. They go on to predict, and back claims with biochemical evidence, that the various biological disturbances caused by these mRNA agents may lead to conditions like cancer, neurodegenerative disease, myocarditis, immune thrombocytopenia, Bell's palsy, liver disease, impaired adaptive immunity and an impaired DNA damage response. They end by showing evidence from the Vaccine Adverse Event Reporting System (VAERS) database supporting their hypothesis.

The main takeaway is that the mRNA agents and the natural virus are not similar, the differences are due to manmade alterations and these alterations are overall harmful. I have summarised the differences between a natural infection and mRNA jab noted in the study on the next page.[1]

mRNA vaccination	Natural infection
Impairs type I IFN signalling.[1]	Upregulation of both type I and type II IFNs.[1]
IgG is the principal antibody class that is raised against the SARS-CoV-2 spike glycoprotein, not IgA.[2]	IgA dominates the early neutralising antibody response to SARS-CoV-2.[3]
"Those vaccinated with BNT162b2 mRNA vaccines developed a robust adaptive immune response which was restricted only to memory cells."[4]	
mRNA in the COVID-19 vaccines is present in germinal centres in secondary lymphoid tissue long after the vaccine is administered, and that it continues to synthesise spike glycoprotein up to at least	

sixty days post-vaccination.[5]	
Vaccine mRNAs contain GC enrichment and increases the risk for potential G-quadruplex (pG4) formations in these structures.[6]	No GC enrichment.
Contains lipid nanoparticles	No lipid nanoparticles
microRNA (miR) - miR148a and miR-590 and their inflammatory effects are unique to vaccination-induced SARS-CoV-2 spike glycoprotein production.[7]	miR-148a nor miR-590 are excessive or deficient.[7]
Suppresses both Interferon regulatory factor 7 (IRF7) and Signal transducer and activator of transcription 2 (STAT2).[8]	
No expansion of	Expansion of circulating

circulating hematopoietic stem and progenitor cells (HSPCs).[9]	HSPCs in COVID-19 patients.[9]
No expansion of circulating plasmablasts.[9]	Expansion of circulating plasmablasts.[9]
Substantial loss of neutralising antibodies induced by the BNT162b2 mRNA vaccine due to mutating spike protein.[10]	
Spike glycoprotein mRNA is further "humanized" with the addition of a guanine-methylated cap, 3′ and 5′ untranslated regions (UTRs)[11]	
A synthetic cationic lipid has been added, since it has been shown experimentally to work as an adjuvant to draw immune cells to the	

injection site and to facilitate endosomal escape.[12]	
Those jabbed acquired circulating exosomes containing the SARS-CoV-2 spike glycoprotein by day 14 following first vaccination and number of circulating spike-glycoprotein-containing exosomes increased by up to a factor of 12 after second.[13]	
Injecting the contents of the vaccine into the deltoid muscle, bypasses the mucosal and vascular barriers.[1]	

Going through the study, the first thing I noticed was an incongruence between what this paper notes and what Pfizer has said about their agents. Pfizer specifically agreed that there was a transient decrease in white cells after the first jab and attributes this to the induction of type I IFN.

In their words, *"Ribonucleic acid (RNA) vaccines are known to induce type I interferon, and type I interferons regulate lymphocyte recirculation and are associated with transient migration and/or redistribution of lymphocytes."*[14]

However, this study found that type I IFN signalling is impaired after mRNA inoculation rather than with the natural virus.[1] *Something isn't adding up.*

IFN, or interferon (a type of cytokine), was discovered in 1957 after scientists recognised that cells challenged by a weakened influenza A virus created a substance that "interfered with" a subsequent infection by a live virus.[15]

There are three main types of IFN, each with numerous subtypes. Type I IFNs have diverse effects on innate and adaptive immune cells during infection. Type I IFNs also slow down tumour growth and inhibit the production of blood vessel growth in tumours.[16]

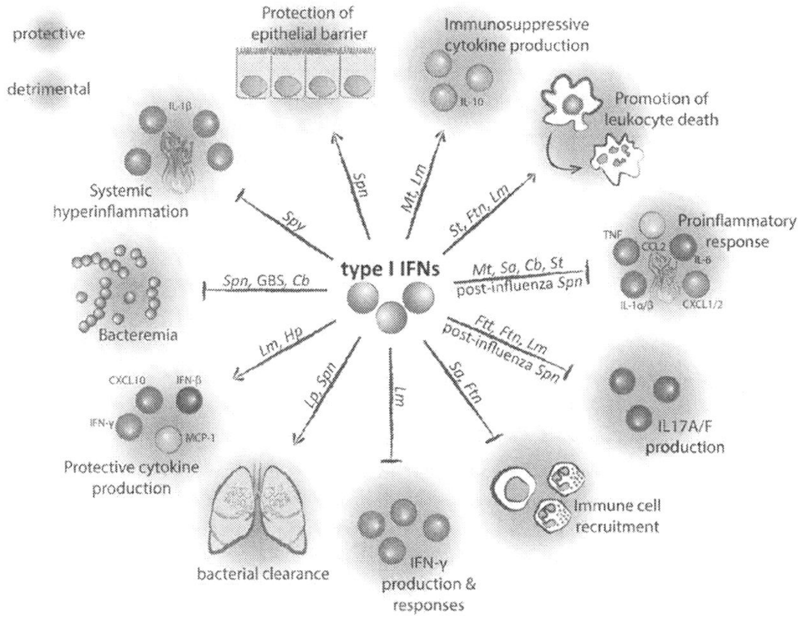

Various roles of type I IFNs, protective with regards to protection of epithelial barrier, systemic hyperinflammation, bacteremia, protective cytokine production and bacterial clearance. Detrimental with regards to other areas on the diagram, from: https://www.frontiersin.org/articles/10.3389/fimmu.2016.00652/full

IFNs play a vital role in the immune response to multiple stressors, and we've even harnessed it as a therapeutic agent for a variety of conditions, including viral infections, solid tumours, bone marrow disorders, blood-related cancers, and autoimmune diseases such as multiple sclerosis.[17,18]

The coordination of IFN is regulated through the activity of the family of IFN regulatory factors, or IRFs.[19] IRFs, IRF9 in particular, is directly involved in antiviral as well as anti-tumor immunity and genetic regulation.[1]

Impaired type I IFN signalling is linked to many disease risks, most notably cancer and infections. This is also similarly true when IRFs are blocked. And, yes, the shots have also been demonstrated to suppress the IRF subtype IRF7.[8]

What does the suppression of IRFs mean? Well, the study goes on to explain, ***"This can be expected to interfere with the cancer-protective effects of BRCA1 as described above. Cancers associated with impaired BRCA1 activity include breast, uterine, and ovarian cancer in women; prostate and breast cancer in men; and a modest increase in pancreatic cancer for both men and women. Reduced BRCA1 expression is linked to both cancer and neurodegeneration.*** *"*[1]

BRCA1, or Breast cancer type 1 susceptibility protein, is a protein related to breast and ovarian cancer that is involved in DNA repair and tumour suppression. People with changes in the BRCA gene are more likely to get breast cancer and ovarian cancer at any age.[20]

Through IRF suppression, these mRNA jabs not only make people more likely to get sick, but they may also make them more likely to get a number of cancers.

Also noting that type I IFN is suppressed after mRNA shots, another study states, ***"together, these data suggested that after vaccination, at least by day 28, other than generation of neutralizing antibodies, people's immune systems, including those of lymphocytes and monocytes, were perhaps in a more vulnerable state.*** *"*[8]

The rest of the table is a little complicated, so I will go through some of the more pertinent points in layman's terms so you can appreciate the significance of it all.

CAN THESE JABS WIPE IMMUNE MEMORY?

The third row on the table above notes,

"Those vaccinated with BNT162b2 mRNA vaccines developed a robust adaptive immune response which was restricted only to memory cells."[4]

The jabbed have been shown to develop a robust immune response, but only in memory cells.

Now, I must say that the significance of this is currently unknown. But I have nonetheless added it to the table as a potential mechanism that may drive "T cell exhaustion." It's unlikely, but it could happen.

T cell exhaustion is a broad term that has been used to describe the unfavourable response of T cells to long-term antigen stimulation.[21] This phenomenon has been noted in the setting of chronic viral infections as well as in response to tumours. Basically, it's when T cells stop working if exposed to a pathogen for too long.

It has been found that if T cells are exposed to a persistent antigen for 2–4 weeks, T cell exhaustion sets in. These cells don't turn back into normal memory T cells, even if they are no longer exposed to the antigen.[22]

At the start of 2022, the European Union's drug regulator warned that too many doses of COVID-19 vaccines could eventually weaken the body's immune system, rendering the extra shots ineffective.[23] Repeated shots at short intervals were warned may overload people's immune systems and lead to immunological fatigue in the population.[24]

We do know that T cells specific to SARS-CoV-2 can become exhausted, worsening disease states in some.[25] The scientific community has also speculated that there may be an increased risk of T cell exhaustion if one jabs a person who has already had COVID-19.[26] And this in turn may impede the shot-induced development of T cell memory.

So a link between jabs, COVID-19 and T cell exhaustion exists. Thinking out loud, if the jabs *only* produced a robust immune response to memory cells, then there may be an increased risk of memory-wiping through T cell exhaustion of memory T cells.

But the term "exhaustion" is used mainly to refer to effector T cells, not memory T cells.[27] As a result, this thought may have to be put on hold until more evidence is gathered.

But never say never, as one 2011 study states,

"Our model shows that ***immunization against persistent viral infections can, under some circumstances, lead to an increase in pathology following infection****. This increased pathology is greatest for noncytopathic viruses and occurs at intermediate levels of T cell memory."*[28]

WHAT IS GC ENRICHMENT?

The spike protein naturally expressed in SARS-CoV-2 is *not* the same as the spike protein made by mRNA jabs.

They are *not* bioequivalent.

This is paramount to understand, as I bet most of the general public think otherwise. This often leads one to assume that the pathologies that arise from genetic agent-expressed spike protein should be a subset of those you might experience with the full-length live virus. Think again.

mRNA spike has been genetically modified. One way this has been done is by increasing the guanine (G) and cytosine (C) content of the mRNA.[6] G and C are two bases (also known as nucleotides) that help form DNA or RNA.

DNA and RNA hold the instruction manual for specific proteins to be made. A sequence of three consecutive nucleotides is called a codon, and GC enrichment (the addition of G and C) is a process called "codon optimisation."

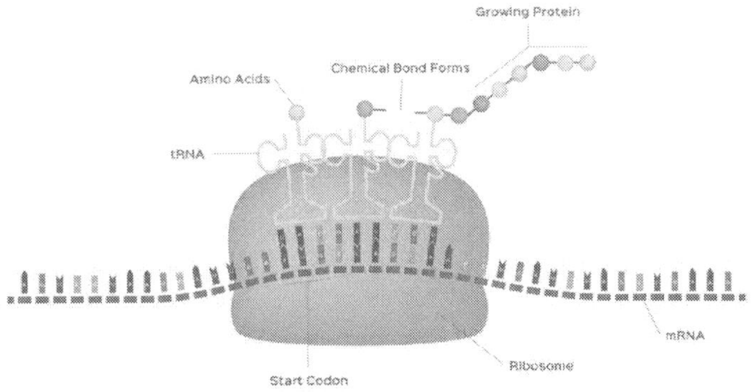

Codon optimisation, from: https://peakproteins.com/the-two-sides-of-codon-optimisation/

All these additional GCs alter the structure of mRNA. See next.[6]

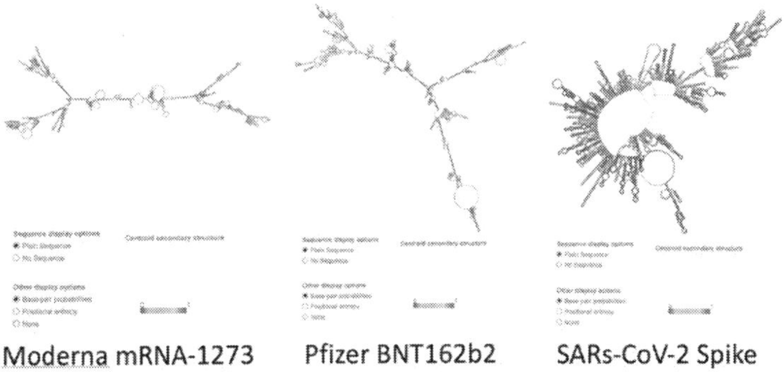

The three different Spike Protein Sequences (Moderna (left), Pfizer (middle), SARs-CoV-2(right)) analysed with RNAfold, from: https://osf.io/bcsa6/

If you look at the image above, you can appreciate that the spike protein naturally expressed in SARs-CoV-2 will not be the same as the spike protein made by mRNA jabs.

You're probably asking what the reason for codon optimising a viral mRNA that is already adapted to its host is. Well, the most likely answer is that the mRNA was changed to change or improve the way the protein was made. That is the only reason genetic material is ever modified.

As one paper puts it, *"Codon-optimization describes gene engineering approaches that use synonymous codon changes to increase protein production."*[29]

The spike protein in our case.

It goes on to note however, *"codon-optimization may not provide the optimal strategy for increasing protein production and* ***may decrease the safety and efficacy of biotech therapeutics. We suggest that the use of this approach is reconsidered, particularly for in vivo applications****."*[29]

As noted, codon optimisation doesn't come risk free and can result in immune and genetic dysregulation, leading to disease progression.[6]

Furthermore, GC enrichment can form structures called "G quadruplexes" which have a complicated relationship with conditions like cancer and dementia.[30,31]

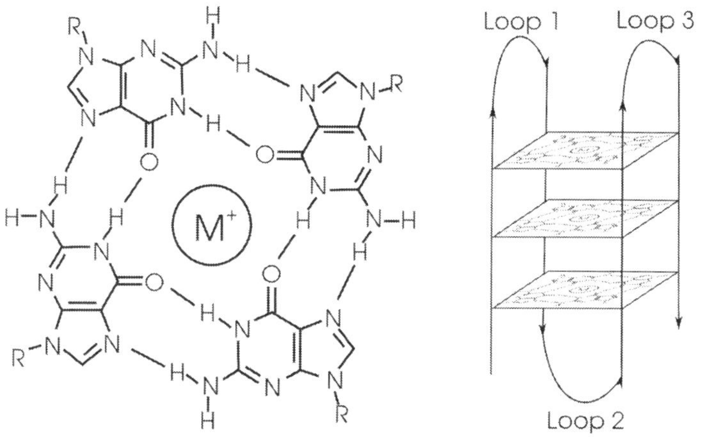

An example of a G-quadruplex, from: https://en.wikipedia.org/wiki/G-quadruplex

Another paper notes, ***"the enrichment of GC content in vaccine mRNA will inevitably lead ... to dysregulation of the G4-RNA-protein binding system and a wide range of potential disease-associated cellular pathologies including suppression of innate immunity, neurodegeneration, and malignant transformation****."*[1]

If the only point of codon optimisation was to maximise spike protein production, then it seems to have worked.

It has been predicted that each jab equates to 13 Trillion to 40 Trillion mRNA molecules injected in a few seconds with each injection. Each of these mRNAs can produce 10-100 spike proteins. And you have 30-40 Trillion cells.[6]

Do the maths.

WHAT ARE MICRORNAS?

microRNAs (abbreviated miRNA or miR) are small, single-stranded types of non-coding RNAs that play important roles in regulating gene expression.[32]

They are well conserved in both plants and animals, are thought to be a vital and evolutionarily ancient component of gene regulation, and have the potential to be used as biomarkers in a number of diseases.[33,34]

miRs regulate many other aspects of human physiology, from T cell exhaustion to sleep.[35,36] MiR profiles change with disease status and have even been shown to improve COVID-19 detection accuracy. [37]

Other than being formed naturally, it has been noted that immune cells that have taken up the jab nanoparticles release large numbers of exosomes containing spike protein along with critical miRs that induce a signalling response in recipient cells in other areas of the body.[1]

Two microRNAs, **miR148a** and **miR-590** have been postulated to be unique to vaccination-induced SARS-CoV-2 spike protein production.[1]

On immune brain cells grown in a lab, both of these have been shown to cause acute inflammatory responses.[38] And in further exploration, the authors of the same study proposed a specific mechanism by which these two microRNAs could specifically disrupt type I INF signalling.[38] The same component of the immune system that has been shown to be impaired by the jabs.

miR-148a is found in cancers at an abnormally high level,[39] and miR-590 has been shown to play a key role in cellular growth, differentiation, death, and ageing, as well as in the development and progression of many diseases, including cancer.[40]

WHAT ARE GUANINE-METHYLATED CAPS?

Concerns have been raised with regards to mRNA caps, which are molecules that are found at the ends of mRNA and help with mRNA stability, export, and protein translation.[41]

Caps are found naturally; they are not the issue per se. The speculated issue is the synthetic caps on the mRNA in these agents. The caps in the jabs contribute to increased protein production; they help deceive our bodies into thinking they are from our own cells and increase their binding capacity to certain proteins.[41] This was done all in an effort to optimise vaccine performance.

This is all well and good under normal bodily conditions. But it has been thought that in the future, when the body is under stress, like when it is sick with an infection, **it may be forced to make spike proteins** from synthetic mRNAs because they are capped.

These synthetic mRNA caps may also increase the likelihood of cancer formation, immune deregulation, neurodegeneration, and ageing in recipients.[41]

Or as Dr. McCullough, the renowned cardiologist and highly published medical scientist, put it on Twitter:

"Normal human "message" is ephemeral and dissolved by RNA-ases after the peptide is synthesized. Mandated novel products have synthetic caps and do not breakdown allowing them to stay in the body for months. Caps may themselves be the cause of disease, particularly cancer." [42]

WHY THE SPIKE PROTEIN?

The SARS-CoV-2 virus uses proteins on its outer surface, called spike (S) proteins, to enter the cells of the body and cause disease. It is also what these genetics shots encode for too.

But *why did all the scientists around the world pick the spike protein out of all the viral proteins to replicate using DNA/mRNA technology?"*

Some scientists have said that the spike was chosen because it is the protein that binds to host cells, and thus it is the only part of the virus that can elicit neutralising antibodies that help prevent infection.

Yes, the spike protein *is* capable of eliciting neutralising antibodies, and though I have researched this thoroughly, I could not find evidence of other parts of the virus having the ability to do the same thing. *Remember that this doesn't rule out the possibility that they can't, however. It just hasn't been tested.*

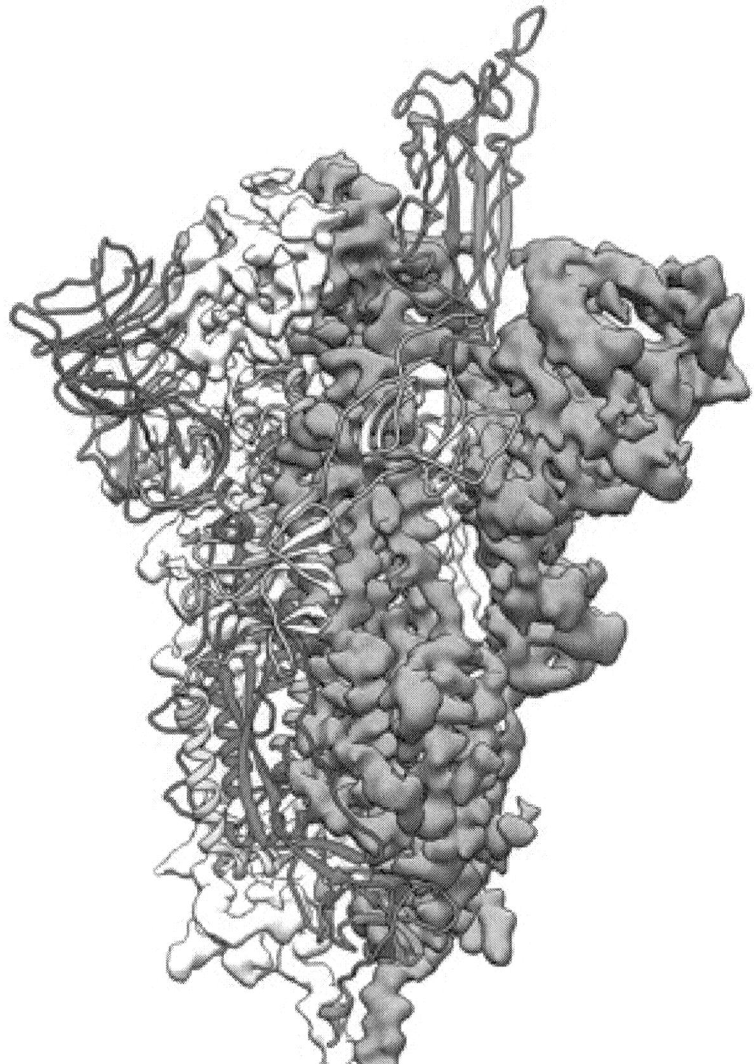

A 3D modelling of the spike protein, from: https://www.eurekalert.org/news-releases/775813

So spike was chosen to elicit neutralisation, okay, or as one paper puts it, "*S glycoprotein is responsible for the entry of the virus into host cells, where it begins to spread, but it can also be recognized by the immune system triggering a protective response, the main objective of vaccines. Several types of new vaccines currently in use are selected based on their ability to generate neutralizing antibodies upon immunization."*[1]

This would be all well and good, but we now know that mRNA-jab-induced neutralising antibodies are highly variable among individuals.[2] In other words, useless.

The spike protein is also rapidly mutating and evades vaccine-induced antibodies with high efficiency.[3] So, once again, useless.

And what makes this all so potentially sinister is that the spike protein is extremely toxic, regardless of what certain "fact checkers" continue to say.[4]

No sign that the COVID-19 vaccines' spike protein is toxic or 'cytotoxic'

IF YOUR TIME IS SHORT

- U.S. public health authorities and vaccine experts say there is no evidence that the vaccines' spike protein is toxic or "cytotoxic," which means toxic to cells.

See the sources for this fact-check

Misinformation spread by "fact-checkers," from: https://www.politifact.com/factchecks/2021/jun/16/youtube-videos/no-sign-covid-19-vaccines-spike-protein-toxic-or-c/

The spike protein is definitely toxic. We know it can cross the blood-brain barrier in mice and cause nerve damage.[5,6] **We know it can cause cardiac damage.**[7] **We know it can cause lung inflammation.**[8] **We know it can cause endothelial cell damage.**[9] **We know it can significantly inhibit DNA damage repair.**[10]

You get the point.

It also may be worth remembering that the COVID-19 lab-leak hypothesis, the hypothesis regarding whether or not SARS-CoV-2 coronavirus emerged from a laboratory and was subsequently leaked, has not been disproven as of yet.[11] Plus other bats haven't been shown to carry relatives of SARS-CoV-2.[12]

I bring this up because it has been found that the SARS-CoV-2 spike protein (both the natural and mRNA kind) have GP120 HIV-1 and Staphylococcus Enterotoxin B (SEB) gene inserts.[13,14]

That's the human immunodeficiency virus, HIV. According to one study, which has since been withdrawn, the GP120 inserts "***suggest unconventional evolution of 2019-nCoV that warrants further investigation.***"[13]

It is noted that the gp120 molecule of HIV-1 can induce cell death and severely alter the immune response to HIV by dampening the antiviral CD8+ T cell response, thus impeding the clearance of HIV.[15]

SEB is one of several harmful substances produced by the bacterium *Staphylococcus aureus*. The symptoms of SEB intoxication, is noted in one review titled "Staphylococcal Enterotoxin B as a Biological Weapon: Recognition, Management, and Surveillance of Staphylococcal Enterotoxin",[16] as the following,

"sudden onset of fever (40-41C), chills, headache, myalgia, non-productive cough. Some patients may develop shortness of breath and chest pain. Fever may last for 2-5 days and cough may continue for up to one month. Patients also present with nausea, vomiting, and diarrhea when the toxin is swallowed."[16]

Now what does that sound like?

In one *in vitro* study, researchers noted that Multisystem inflammatory syndrome in children (MIS-C) was strikingly similar to toxic shock syndrome (TSS).[17] MIS-C is an inflammatory condition that can happen weeks after a child's first SARS-CoV-2 infection or exposure. It involves systemic hyperinflammation and multiorgan involvement, and children have symptoms of fever, rashes, bloodshot eyes, diarrhoea, and vomiting.

TSS is a condition caused by bacterial toxins, specifically *Staphylococcus aureus* superantigens. Superantigens are a class of antigens that can cause excessive immune activation (and harm) due to the way they bind to various receptors in our immune system. TSS can result in fever, low blood pressure, rash, vomiting, diarrhoea, and other serious systemic symptoms. Those affected by TSS usually need to go to the hospital.

The remarkable similarities between MIS-C and TSS prompted researchers to look for superantigen-like sections on the spike protein.[17] And what did they find? You guessed it: *the SEB fragment in the SARS-CoV-2 spike 1 glycoprotein*.

On further analysis, they also noted the spike protein also had neurotoxin-like motifs, which they speculate may contribute to neurological symptoms in COVID-19 and MIS-C patients.

They end their abstract with, *"Accordingly, we hypothesize that* ***continuous and prolonged exposure to the viral SAg-like and neurotoxin-like motifs in SARS-CoV-2 spike may promote autoimmunity leading to the development of post-acute COVID-19 syndromes, including MIS-C and long COVID, as well as the neurological complications resulting from SARS-CoV-2 infection****."*[17]

So I ask again: *Why the spike protein? Why didn't they use a weaker spike, or a live attenuated virus?*[18] *Why not the N-protein?*

The N-protein is highly immunogenic and is the most abundant viral protein during coronavirus infections.[19,20] It is also a major target for antibody and T cell responses.[21]

We shouldn't completely disregard non-neutralising antibodies either. We need them. Non-neutralizing antibodies against N-protein have been shown to protect mice against some other viruses, such as the mouse hepatitis virus and the influenza A virus.[22]

So again, I ask, why the spike protein?
And secondly, how long does it stay in the body?

HOW LONG DO SPIKE PROTEINS STAY IN THE BODY?

This is an important question, and honestly, we don't really know. And it's not just us, Pfizer, Biointech, Moderna, and the rest also seem to have no clue either. We have no published scientific data about this from them whatsoever.

In fact, both Moderna and Pfizer are said to have not looked at the proteins made by their synthetic mRNA shots in cell culture for more than 48 hours after transfection.[1] *I wish I was making this up.*

You'd hope that the manufacturers would have known a little more about their novel pharmacological product *before* millions of people rolled up their sleeves. But no. This is just another example of gross regulatory dereliction by these companies.

What we do know is that these jabs are injected into the deltoid muscle, and in *most people*, drains primarily to the lateral axillary lymph nodes.

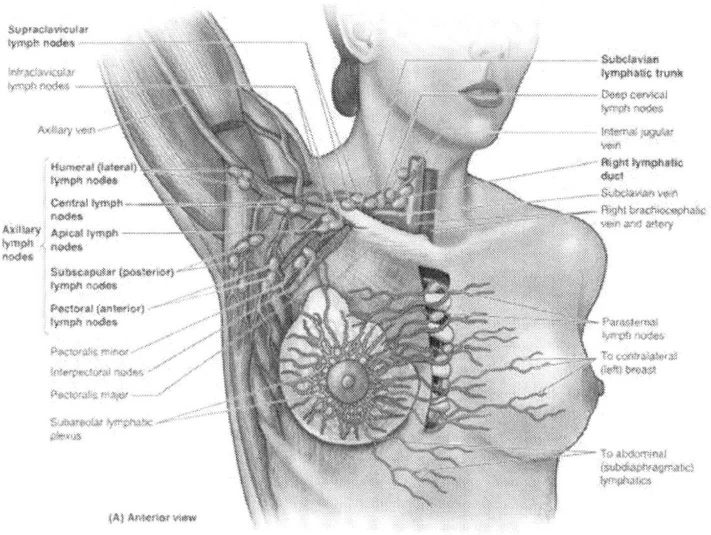

Axillary lymph nodes, from: https://anatomy-medicine.com/immune-and-lymphatic-systems/140-the-axillary-nodes.html

Here they activate areas of lymph nodes and transiently form structures called germinal centres. Germinal centres, which form as the result of natural infection or vaccination, are like boot camps for B cells where antibodies are formed and further developed to better attack the enemy.

As shown in the table above, mRNA from the COVID-19 vaccines was found in germinal centres in secondary lymphoid tissue long after the shot was administered, and it continued to synthesise spike glycoprotein for at least **sixty days** after inoculation.[2]

In a different study of COVID-19 infection, the spike protein lasted up to **15 months** in an individual with long COVID, but jab-status was not noted.[3]

Another study discovered a persistent antigen-specific germinal centre B cell response that remained at or near peak frequencies for at least **12 weeks** after secondary immunisation with these mRNA agents.[4]

To put that into context, and because human studies on the subject are lacking, immunising mice with conventional vaccines containing aluminium adjuvants has been shown to result in germinal centre responses peaking 1-2 weeks after immunisation.[4] Conventional vaccines that use other adjuvants tend to reach their peak about 2–4 weeks after vaccination, and the peak can last for several months at a low frequency.

When these mRNA jabs were first introduced to the market, they were hailed as a remarkable technological advancement that gave the recipient a "really robust immune response"[5] because they induced a B cell response that is maintained at or near peak frequencies for at least 12 weeks and continues to synthesise spike glycoprotein up to at least sixty days post-vaccination.

More isn't always better, though.

As we know now and continue to find out, many who were vaccinated still went on to become ill with COVID-19, and sometimes more than once. In fact, one study published in June 2022 showed not only that natural immunity provided a greater protection than jabs against future infection, but it called into question the very idea of "hybrid immunity" - *a recently coined term to describe those who have had a combination of shots and a prior protection* - as those who had "hybrid immunity" did not do so much better than those only naturally infected.[6]

More spike in our lymph nodes thanks to these jabs does not cause a "really robust immune response".

Well what about circulating blood then?

Most of the jab contents administered is supposed to drain to local lymph nodes, but we now know that at least some contents of these jabs become distributed into the blood.

With regards to mRNA, one study noted that synthetic mRNA persisted in circulation in human participants for at least **2 weeks** following the jab.[7] **This was more than double the time provided by Pfizer-BioNTech, who showed that RNA in ionisable lipids were cleared in the plasma of *rats* after a maximum of 6 days.**[7]

There is an increase in spike protein antigen in the circulating blood after the first dose, and it is still detectable in the plasma of 63% of recipients one week later.[8]

After the second dose, however, it is very hard to find spike antigen. This is likely because anti-spike antibodies join with spike proteins to form immune complexes that are too big for lab machines that can only find spike proteins.[8]

Another study, which also found similar results, put the reduced circulating spike in blood after the second dose down to the production of IgG and IgA. However the study also notes, *"We hypothesise that the cellular immune responses triggered by T-cell activation, which would occur days after the vaccination, lead to direct killing of cells presenting spike protein and an additional release of spike into the blood stream."*[9]

In other words, a few days after getting the shot, T-cell activation causes cellular immune responses that kill spike-presenting cells directly and release more spike into the bloodstream.

With no traditional pharmacokinetic or biodistribution studies having been performed on these genetic shots, it's hard to know what's really going on.[10] I think there is likely a combination of T cell clearance and circulating immune complexes that explains the lower levels of pure spike protein in the blood after the second dose of the jab. But this should have been looked at in studies before genetic technology was made available to people.

I must also point out that the studies mentioned in this section are small and have abrupt end points. As a result, we don't know if other people have prolonged B cell responses and spike glycoprotein synthesis in lymphatic tissue for longer than the ones mentioned. Some people may be producing protein spikes right now, many months after inoculation, for all we know.

There are also other mechanisms that can transport spike protein around the body. For example, another paper has noted that spike protein was released from cells via the induction of small biological transport bubbles called exosomes for up to **four months**.[11]

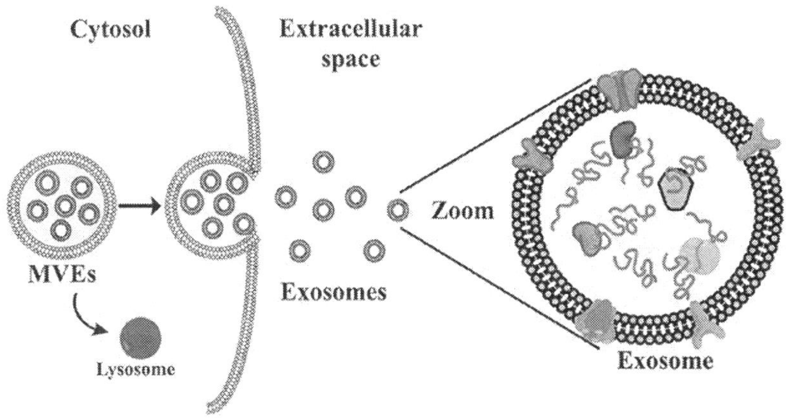

Exosomes, from: https://www.frontiersin.org/articles/10.3389/fgene.2018.00092/full

What's more concerning is that we know exosomes can be exhaled.[12] So naturally, one may ask, *"Do these exosomes contain any jab-derived mRNA?"* and *"Can they be exhaled like other exosomes?"*

With COVID-19 mRNA now being detected in human breast milk,[13] we must also ask whether this will affect newborn babies too.

This is what we know so far, it's still more than what these pharmaceutical companies let on at the beginning though.

WHAT IS THE "HOOK EFFECT"?

This may be a good place to remind everyone that too much of anything is never a good thing, and that this may be especially true with regards to neutralising antibodies.

To cut to the chase, having more neutralising antibodies can in fact *impede* viral clearance. *Yes, you heard that right.*

This phenomenon is called the "Hook" or "prozone" effect and describes a drop in antibody protection efficacy seen at very high antibody concentrations.

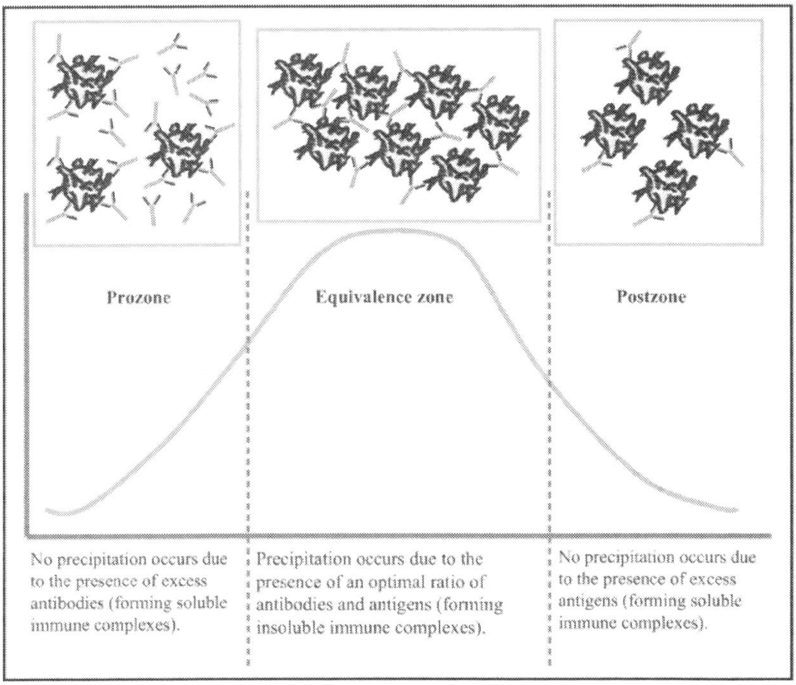
Prozone
Equivalence zone
Postzone
No precipitation occurs due to the presence of excess antibodies (forming soluble immune complexes).
Precipitation occurs due to the presence of an optimal ratio of antibodies and antigens (forming insoluble immune complexes).
No precipitation occurs due to the presence of excess antigens (forming soluble immune complexes).

The hook effect (far right), from: https://link.springer.com/chapter/10.1007/978-3-319-77694-1_3

One way viruses are cleared in our body is through a process called phagocytosis, where certain white blood cells effectively eat the virus. However, for this to happen, antibodies need to bind to parts of the virus (spike protein in our case) and let the virus-eating white cells know that dinner is here and ready.

Only a small number of antibodies are needed to flag these viruses. In fact, a small number of high quality antibodies is all you need for proper immune function, which is what you see in those with mild cases. It may be why children do better, along with better T cell responses and stronger innate immune systems.

Asymptomatic and Mild SARS-CoV-2 Infections Elicit Lower Immune Activation and Higher Specific Neutralizing Antibodies in Children Than in Adults

https://pubmed.ncbi.nlm.nih.gov/34659235/

SARS-CoV-2 specific T cell responses are lower in children and increase with age and time after infection

https://pubmed.ncbi.nlm.nih.gov/33564773/

Robust innate responses to SARS-CoV-2 in children resolve faster than in adults without compromising adaptive immunity

https://pubmed.ncbi.nlm.nih.gov/33564773/

Problems seem to occur in phagocytic systems when there are too many neutralising antibodies. Firstly, too many antibodies create competition within themselves to bind to certain areas of the virus, favouring other forms of binding and reducing the signal for phagocytosis.

Also, when there are a lot of antibodies, they cover the spike in a way that isn't right. This makes it hard for the receptor on the phagocytic cell and the antigen to work together.

In effect, **high concentrations of neutralising antibodies coat the very thing we are trying to get rid of and help it evade our immune system**.

Don't take all of this from me but from a 2022 study titled "Spike-Dependent Opsonization Indicates Both Dose-Dependent Inhibition of Phagocytosis and That Non-Neutralizing Antibodies Can Confer Protection to SARS-CoV-2"[2]

The researchers note using animal data that "**too high doses of neutralizing antibodies are not beneficial in a treatment model and that non-neutralizing antibodies can offer protection to SARS-CoV-2 infection.**"[2]

Yep, the long-ignored non-neutralising antibodies play a major role in controlling infection. *Don't let anyone else say otherwise.*

I hope the study mentioned above gets more coverage because it highlights the important point of not always going for the highest titres of neutralising antibodies as a proxy for immunological success. It also emphasises the significance of the balance between non-neutralizing and neutralising antibodies.

We know that those who are most unwell with COVID-19 have higher antibody titres and poorer antibody quality.[3,4] This may have contributed to the persistence of disease states. Remember: *quality over quantity*.

Importantly, too, solely focusing on high antibody titres post-shot is how researchers and policymakers justified mass inoculation and boosters. And the spike protein was chosen for mRNA replication as it was touted as the only protein on the virus to sufficiently elicit neutralising antibodies.

Now that we can see that more neutralising antibodies may actually be detrimental to our health, we have to question why boosters are still encouraged.

WHAT HAPPENED TO ANTIBODY-DEPENDENT ENHANCEMENT?

A person who has antibodies against one virus (from infection or vaccination) may experience worse disease when infected by a second, closely related virus. This is a phenomenon known as antibody-dependent enhancement (ADE),[1] and it occurs when the antibodies have a special and uncommon reaction with proteins on the surface of the second virus.

ADE is not an uncommon or new phenomenon. The enhancement of disease by antibody-dependent mechanisms has been described clinically in children given formalin-inactivated respiratory syncytial virus (RSV) or measles vaccines in the 1960s;[2,3] in dengue haemorrhagic fever due to secondary infection with another dengue serotype;[4] and in feline infectious peritonitis virus (FIPV) upon re-infection with an identical serotype of the virus.[5]

There are two main ADE mechanisms in viral diseases, and both of them rely on non-neutralising or sub-neutralising antibodies.[6]

- **FcγRIIa-mediated endocytosis:** For viruses that infect primary cultures of macrophages such as dengue virus and FIPV, non-neutralizing or sub-neutralizing antibodies cause increased viral infection of monocytes or macrophages via receptor mediated cell ingestion (FcγRIIa is a receptor), resulting in more severe disease.
- **Immune complexes:** Non-neutralizing antibodies can create immune complexes with viral antigens inside airway tissues for non-macrophage-tropic respiratory viruses like RSV and measles. These immune complexes cause the release of pro-inflammatory cytokines, the recruitment of immune cells, and the activation of the complement cascade within lung tissue. In severe circumstances, the following

inflammation might result in airway blockage and acute respiratory distress syndrome.

These two processes are demonstrated by the diagram below.[6]

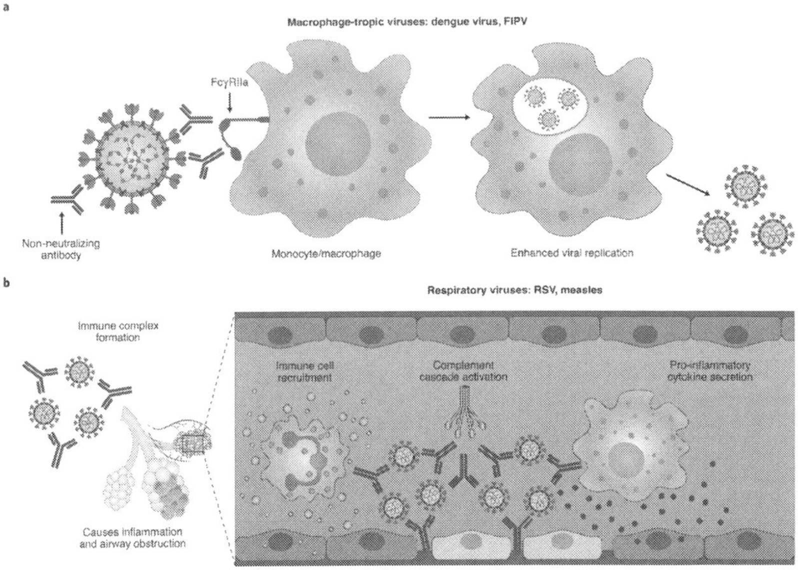

Two main ADE mechanisms, from: https://www.nature.com/articles/s41564-020-00789-5/figures/1

The extent to which ADE plays a role in coronavirus infections is unclear. Reports confirming the existence of ADE in coronavirus infections are based on experiments using cell cultures or animal models.[7,8]

Existing evidence suggests that immune complex formation, complement deposition,[6] and local immune activation present the most likely ADE mechanisms in COVID-19 immunopathology, as SARS-CoV-2 has not been shown to productively infect macrophages.[7]

Currently, though feared by many before these jabs were widely introduced, we have no evidence indicating that ADE is a relevant mechanism counteracting the role of anti-spike protein antibodies generated by vaccines in humans.

A receptor-binding domain (RBD) is a short piece of a virus that is immunogenic and binds to a specific endogenous receptor sequence. This allows the virus to get into the host cell. The RBD for SARS-CoV-2 is located on its "spike" domain, which allows it to dock to body receptors to gain entry into cells and lead to infection.

I note this because one study *did* find that ADE was more likely to develop in patients with high titers of SARS-CoV-2 RBD and S1-specific antibodies and more likely to develop in elderly patients with severe and critical conditions, longer hospital stays, and longer disease duration.[10] However, this was an *in vitro* study.

ADE was also predicted to cause more problems with the emergence of previously unknown strains such as Delta.[11] But again, we've got no real-life evidence so far.

Reassuringly, one very large study of 20,000 people receiving blood from people who've recovered from COVID-19 reported no safety concerns with regard to ADE.[12]

The closest thing so far to ADE that I have found is one autopsy study that did note that viral dissemination within organ systems was higher in jabbed cases versus unjabbed cases.[13] The authors state that one reason for their finding could be ADE. But they also note that the other reason may be that those affected worse after inoculation were more likely to have underlying immunosuppressive conditions and tended to be older.

Currently, we lack real-life evidence of ADE caused by mRNA jabs; this may be due to a handful of reasons. Firstly, there are currently no assays or biomarkers established to prove ADE *in vivo*.[13] Secondly, many people may have already died via ADE mechanisms, but due to the lack of autopsies, we have no way of proving this. And thirdly, maybe ADE isn't as much of a threat as once feared.

Only time will tell.

WHAT IS ORIGINAL ANTIGENIC SIN?

When one is exposed to a new pathogen, memory B cells respond and form antibodies against this pathogen. So when the same pathogen comes around again, the body is adequately ready and produces antibodies quickly to keep us safe. *Great stuff.*

However, not all pathogens remain the same.

Viruses, as we know, have a tendency to mutate. More specifically, viruses may undergo a process called "antigenic drift," in which the proteins on their surface become altered enough to escape the immune system.

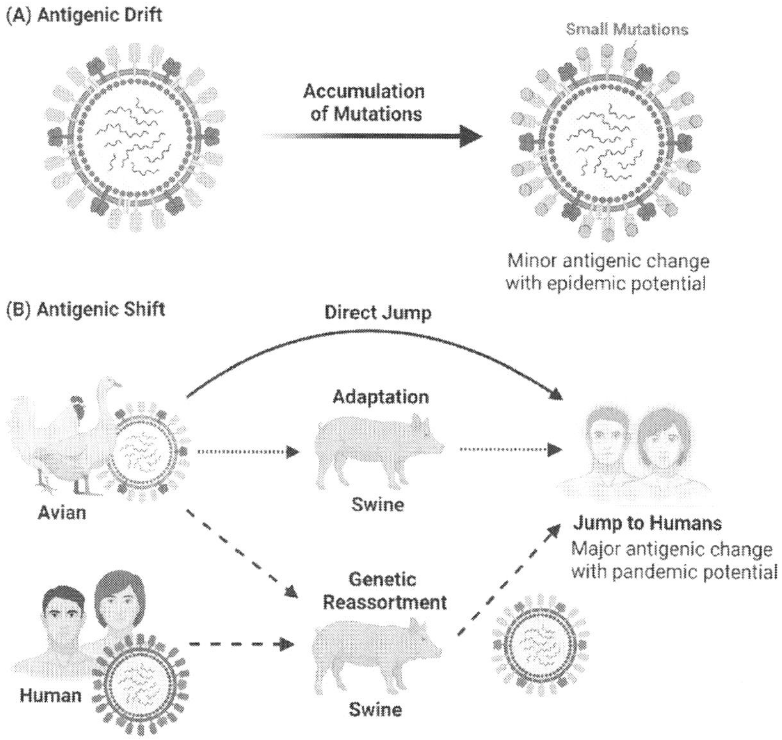

Antigenic drift (A) and antigenic shift (B), from: https://www.researchgate.net/figure/Antigenic-Drift-and-Shift-in-Influenza-A-viruses-A-Antigenic-Drift-results-in-minor_fig2_356263159

When we encounter this "virus 2.0," the body, instead of forming fresh antibodies, may respond by reactivating previously formed antibodies to the first version of the virus. If this happens, then problems may occur, as these antibodies aren't able to neutralise this pathogen, and this process may also diminish the effectiveness of naive B cells' capability of producing neutralising antibodies.

This process is called "original antigenic sin" (OAS) and was first used in the 1960s to describe how one's first exposure to influenza virus shapes the outcome of subsequent exposures to antigenically related strains.[1]

OAS is also known as "antigenic imprinting" or "the Hoskins effect", and is of particular importance in the application of vaccines.

As one study concerning the influenza vaccines states, *"In the present study, we studied the immune responses to the 2009 H1N1 vaccine in subjects who either received the seasonal influenza virus vaccination within the prior 3 months or did not.* ***Following 2009 H1N1 vaccination, subjects previously given a seasonal influenza virus vaccination exhibited significantly lower antibody responses, as determined by hemagglutination inhibition assay, than subjects who had not received***

the seasonal influenza virus vaccination*. This result is compatible with the phenomenon of* ***"original antigenic sin," by which previous influenza virus vaccination hampers induction of immunity against a new variant.****"*[2]

Other than influenza vaccines, a similar scenario has recently played out following the release of the human papillomavirus (HPV) vaccine, Gardasil 9, which contains four antigens present in the original Gardasil vaccine plus an additional five new antigens. It was found that individuals previously immunised with Gardasil who were later vaccinated with Gardasil 9 mounted poor responses to the five new antigens present in the Gardasil 9 vaccine compared to individuals vaccinated with Gardasil 9 who had no prior exposure to Gardasil.[3]

In the 1960s, the first generation of vaccines against Respiratory Syncytial Virus (RSV) were produced; however, when these vaccines were given to children who hadn't encountered RSV, a large proportion of those who later became naturally infected with RSV developed enhanced respiratory disease, in some cases with a fatal outcome.[4]

OAS has also been described for dengue, feline coronaviruses, HIV, and several other viruses too.[5]

What about SARS-CoV-2?

Well, we now know that OAS can be elicited naturally by previous common cold coronaviruses and that this likely plays a role in severe COVID-19.[6] But like anything, it gets slightly more complicated as OAS here may also depend on which region of the common cold coronavirus spike your body has dominant antibody responses to.[7]

When it comes to the mRNA shots, one study noted that memory B cells in those who were never infected with SARS-CoV-2 were similar 5 months after inoculation to those that dominate the initial response.[8] They also found that the antibodies made by these shots were not as strong or as wide-ranging as the antibodies made by natural infection. And so combining those two may mean that those who have received the shots and continue to get jabbed with boosters may be at a higher risk of developing OAS.

Surveillance data from the UK Health Security Agency (UKHSA) showed that people who get sick after two doses of these mRNA agents seem to have lower levels of N antibodies.[9] One reason for this has been hypothesised as being due to a stronger response to the spike than nucleocapsid protein, through OAS-like mechanisms.

In a way, you could see OAS as a form of trauma: certain vaccines may "scare" the immune system so badly during the first round that it responds to all similar pathogens the same way. Rooted in immunological memory, this becomes learned behaviour and "traps" the immune response in the first ineffective response it makes to the pathogen. Similar things have been said about cytotoxic T cells, which may explain why HIV vaccines haven't worked so far.[10]

When the immune system is turned into a one-trick pony against a rapidly mutating virus, bad things happen. Not only are mutations of viruses more likely to happen, but it is also less likely that future vaccines will be able to stop them, even if they are changed to deal with new types.[11] In fact, we might already be seeing this with evidence of certain Omicron subvariants being 4.2 times more resistant than variants in those who have had the jabs.[12]

OAS is a problem rooted in immunological memory, and thus, by toying with it, one can also possibly prevent optimal naturally occurring immunity from occurring later down the line. That's a life of repeated infections and subsequent bodily damage. A life of repeated illness until death.

So what might be the answer?

OAS is a phenomenon affecting the adaptive immune response (mainly primarily B cells, but also cytotoxic T cells),[13] and so those with a higher risk of OAS (but also everyone) may need to optimise their first-line defences, including mucosal secretory antibodies and tissue-resident memory T cells, to prevent both infection and OAS. *The innate and mucosal immune systems again. It's funny how we always come back to the same thing.*

CAN THESE SHOTS CAUSE AUTOIMMUNE DISEASES?

Autoimmunity is an immune response in an organism against its own healthy cells, and any disease resulting from this type of immune response is called an "autoimmune disease."

To make myself more clear, autoimmunity isn't all "bad" per se and, in fact, occurs in all individuals. Low levels of autoimmunity help with the selection of white blood cells, help balance and prepare the immune system, and also help protect the body against organ damage.[1,2]

Even though all healthy people have autoimmune immune cells, only a small percentage of the population gets autoimmune diseases. This is because the immune system is no longer as tightly controlled as it used to be, and because of other things like differences in genetics and exposure to pathogens.

In those with autoimmune disease, immunological tolerance—the ability to ignore "self" while reacting to "non-self" antigens—becomes broken. This breakage leads to an unending attack on one's own body by one's own immune system.

One mediator of immunological tolerance is regulatory T (Treg) cells. Treg cells help modulate helper T-cell activity and restrict fulminant autoimmunity. So, as you might have guessed, problems with the number or function of Tregs are linked to autoimmunity.[3]

Another way autoimmunity may be triggered is via a mechanism called "molecular mimicry." Here, antigens that aren't made in the body share structural similarities with antigens found naturally within the body. And thus antibodies formed to bind to the former and also bind to the latter. It is thought that molecular mimicry is a pervasive strategy employed by viruses to harness or disrupt host cellular functions.[4]

One of the first experiments to identify molecular mimicry was carried out in 1983, and it found that murine antibodies to the measles virus and herpes simplex virus (HSV) reacted against human cells.[5]

Since then, many other studies have cemented the link between molecular mimicry and autoimmunity. Vaccines, too, haven't gotten off scot-free.

The influenza A vaccine has been linked to narcolepsy and Guillain-Barré syndrome (a neurological condition causing muscle weakness and paralysis);[6,7] the hepatitis B vaccine to a 5-fold increased risk of multiple sclerosis;[8,9] and the human papillomavirus (HPV) vaccines to postural orthostatic tachycardia syndromes (POTS, a disorder of the autonomic nervous system characterised by heart rate changes linked to changes in posture).[10] All of this has been postulated to be due to molecular mimicry.

Those prone to autoimmune diseases also commonly show a dysfunction with their CD8+ "killer" (cytotoxic) T cells. In a normal infection, a productive CD8+ T cell response is generated, the pathogen is cleared, and immunological memory is formed.[11] Job done.

By comparison, when there is *chronic antigen stimulation*—in the context of conditions like cancer, long-term infections, and autoimmunity—CD8+ T cells either become "exhausted" or exhibit excessive and inappropriate autoimmunity, causing self-damage. This dysfunction, in turn, contributes to viral persistence and continued tumour growth.[12]

Fig. 1: 'Opposite ends of the spectrum' framework of $CD8^+$ T cells in autoimmunity versus chronic viral infection and cancer.

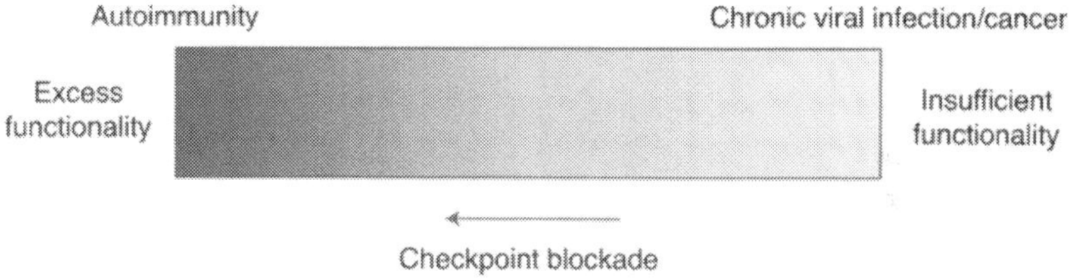

$CD8^+$ T cells in autoimmunity (left) overcome numerous tolerance mechanisms to exhibit excessive and inappropriate effector functionality, causing damage of self-tissue. By contrast, $CD8^+$ T cells in chronic viral infection and cancer (right) become 'exhausted' and exhibit lower effector functionality than that elicited by acute infection. This dysfunction contributes to viral persistence and continued tumor growth. Blockade of immune checkpoints such as the co-inhibitory receptors PD-1 and CTLA-4 can augment the effector functionality of $CD8^+$ T cells in both contexts, leading to better control of chronic viral infection/cancer and exacerbated autoimmunity.

CD8+ T cells in autoimmunity versus chronic viral infection and cancer, from: https://www.nature.com/articles/s41590-021-00949-7#Fig1

We now know that certain traditional vaccines can increase one's risk of certain autoimmune diseases. *But what about mRNA shots?* To understand the risk of developing autoimmune disease after the shots, we've got to first really understand the mechanism by which they work.

As a refresher, traditional vaccines consist of inactivated or weakened viruses, which in turn allows the immune system to mount a response and form immunological memory without causing infection.

mRNA jabs, on the other hand, train regular human cells to make and then present SARS-CoV-2 spike proteins on their surfaces. These cells are identified by the immune system and destroyed.[12] *An autoimmune reaction takes place.*

The whole immunological basis of these mRNA shots relies on autoimmune reactions. This comes as no surprise, as one must remember that mRNA technology was originally made to stimulate T cells to destroy tumour cells.[13]

With regard to molecular mimicry, it isn't looking hopeful either. One study noted that ***"SARS-CoV-2 antibodies had reactions with 28 out of 55 tissue antigens,*** *representing a diversity of tissue groups that included barrier proteins, gastrointestinal, thyroid and neural tissues."*[14]

Another study noted cross-reactivity between an antibody with affinity for spike protein and a human protein and noted that *"consideration of cross-reactivity for SARS-CoV-2 is important for therapeutic intervention and when designing the next generation of COVID-19 vaccines to avoid potential autoimmune interference."*[15]

And the evidence of molecular mimicry between SARS-CoV-2 proteins and our own proteins continues to mount. Here are some excerpts from recent studies on this topic:

- ***"20 novel human peptides mimicked by SARS-CoV-2*** *have not been observed in any previous coronavirus strains"*[16]
- *"We report that SARS-CoV-2 has evolved a unique S1/S2 cleavage site, absent in any previous coronavirus sequenced, resulting in the* ***striking mimicry of an identical FURIN-cleavable peptide on the human epithelial sodium channel α-subunit*** *(ENaC-α)"*[17]
- *"we find that, relative to their proteome size, single-stranded RNA (ssRNA) viruses, including coronaviruses (CoVs), have circumvented the limitations of their small genomes by* ***mimicking human proteins to a greater extent than their large dsDNA counterparts*** *like Pox and Herpes viruses"*[18]
- *"COVID-19 induces a marked humoral response against the major protein of high-density lipoproteins. As a correlate of poorer prognosis in other clinical settings, such* ***autoimmunity signatures may relate to long-term COVID-19 prognosis assessment and warrant further scrutiny in the current COVID-19 pandemic.****"*[19]
- *".. identified previously known autoreactivities, and also* ***detected undescribed neutralizing interferon lambda 3 (IFN-λ3) autoantibodies.****"*[20]
- *"It would be expected that the COVID-19 pandemic and the vaccination against this pathogen could significantly increase the ADs incidences,*

especially in populations harboring HLA-B*08:01, HLA-A*024:02, HLA-A*11:01 and HLA-B*27:05. The Southeast Asia, East Asia, and Oceania are at higher risk of AD development."[21] (The human leukocyte antigen (HLA) system is a complex of genes on our chromosome 6 which encode cell-surface proteins responsible for the regulation of the immune system)
- *"This immune survey reveals evidence of a compartmentalized immune response in the CNS of individuals with COVID-19 and* ***suggests a role of autoimmunity in neurologic sequelae of COVID-19.***"[22]

Aspects of autoimmunity have also been noted in those suffering from severe COVID-19. One study showed that **those who suffered worse had higher circulating levels of autoantibodies than those with a mild infection**, highlighting the important point that not all antibodies are made equally.[23] This was further reinforced in another study that noted that the **majority of SARS-CoV-2-specific antibodies in COVID-19 patients with obesity were autoimmune and not neutralising.**[24]

Certain autoantibodies have also been related to clotting and bleeding disorders.[25,26] And autopsies of Chinese citizens who died from COVID-19 showed evidence of lung scarring, again suggesting an autoimmune basis for COVID-19.[27]

So do these shots cause autoimmune diseases?

We know that COVID-19 patients who are very sick have less Treg cells and their CD8+ T cells don't work as well.[28,29] We know that traditional vaccines are linked to autoimmune diseases. We know that the basis of *these* mRNA jabs relies on autoimmune attacks. We know that the virus and its spike protein are structurally very similar to many human proteins. We know that high levels of autoantibodies correlate with disease severity.

So going by what we know so far, it would be unwise to answer that question with a simple "no."

It would be further unwise (and plain wrong) to answer "no," because we have real-life evidence that these shots *do* trigger autoimmune diseases, sometimes fatally.

Vaccine-induced thrombotic thrombocytopenia (VITT) is a blood disorder that is characterised by widespread blood clots, predominantly in atypical sites like the brain and lungs, in combination with low platelet counts after receiving the COVID-19 shot.

Studies and VAERS reports have highlighted many cases of VITT, and the majority of people affected were previously healthy and had no personal or family history of thromboembolic events.[30] VITT has a mean time to onset of symptoms after inoculation of 8 days and predominantly affects females, most commonly ages 27 to 62 years old. Blood tests on people with VITT show that their D-dimer levels are high, their fibrinogen levels are low, and they have PF4 antibodies.

It is theorised that VITT occurs via a platelet-targeted autoimmune reaction that occurs as the contents of the mRNA jabs travel to the spleen.[31] The spleen is the largest secondary lymphoid organ in humans and it contains as much as 1/3 of the body's platelet supplies.

To give you an idea of how serious VITT can be, I present to you one study that described in detail the clinical and laboratory profiles of 22 patients in whom VITT developed.[32]

*"Among these 22 patients, 14 cases were women, with an age range of 21–77 years, and 21 had elevated D-dimer levels, positive PF4 antibodies and abnormal fibrinogen levels. In addition, 1****3 of these 22 patients had cerebral venous sinus thrombosis; four cases had pulmonary embolism, one case had deep vein thrombosis and bilateral adrenal haemorrhage, two cases had ischaemic stroke affecting the middle cerebra*****l artery region, and two cases had portal vein thrombosis**."[32]

Brain clots, lung clots, clots in the veins of the legs, adrenal bleeding, and more Autoimmunity is no joke. Other types of autoimmune diseases have also been described post-jab.

Immune thrombocytopenic purpura (ITP) is an autoimmune condition characterised by a lowered platelet count, which leads to inappropriate bleeding from various biological sites. Again, many cases of ITP after COVID-19 jabs have been described in the literature.[30]

One case in the literature describes a 28-year old male who presented to the Emergency Department around three weeks after his first dose of the AstraZeneca shot due to **oral bleeding and the appearance of pinpoint bruising from broken capillaries** (medically termed "petechiae" over his body, arms, and legs for three days.[33]

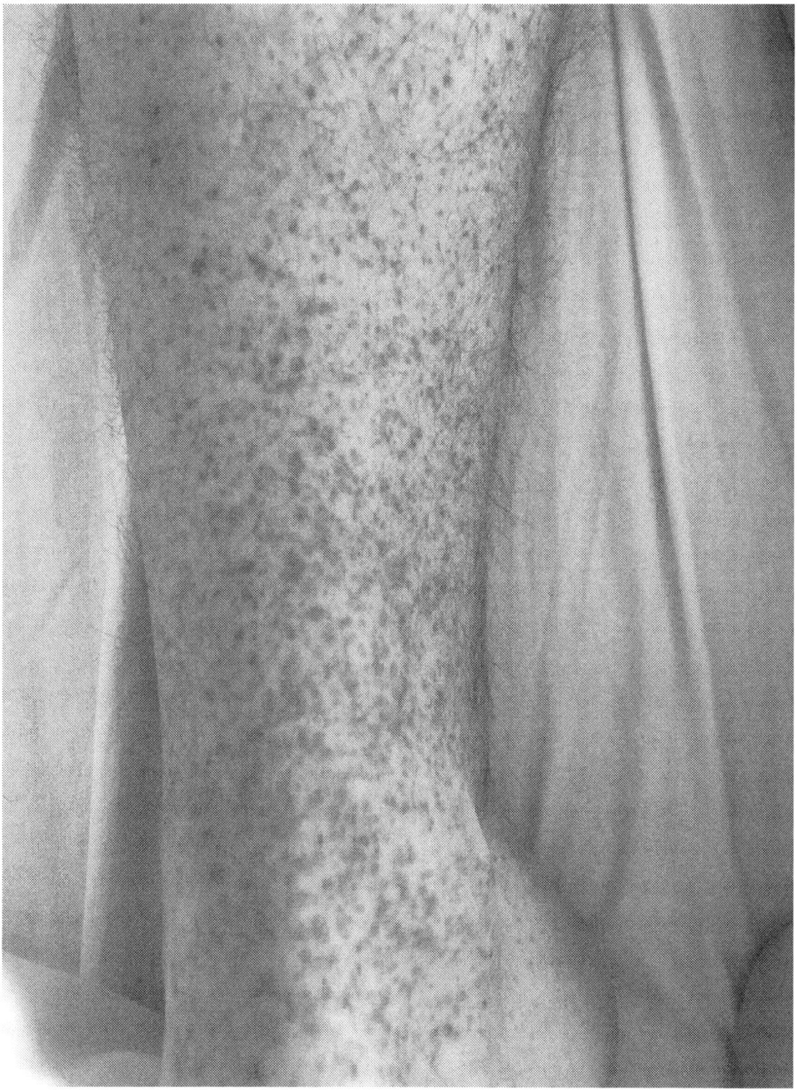

Pinpoint bruising from broken capillaries, medically termed "petechiae," from: https://www.ncbi.nlm.nih.gov/pmc/articles/PMC8239819/figure/bjh17508-fig-0001/

It is thought that ITP happens when pathogenic antibodies bind to platelets and megakaryocytes, which are cells that help make platelets.[34] This lowers the number of platelets through various immune pathways.

Autoimmune liver disease has also been reported post-jab repeatedly in the scientific literature. People present with deranged liver function, elevated blood tests, and even jaundice. The mean time from inoculation to the onset of symptoms is 13 days.[30]

Guillain–Barré syndrome (GBS) is a rare autoimmune neurological disorder that affects the nerves, causing limb weakness and changes in sensation. And again, this has been written about many times after people have had these mRNA shots.[30]

In addition to the complications described above, other autoimmune manifestations have been reported in some cases, such as[30]

- **IgA nephropathy** - a kidney disease that occurs when IgA deposits build up in the kidneys, causing inflammation that damages kidney tissues.
- **Inflammatory arthritis** - joint inflammation caused by an overactive immune system.
- **Systemic lupus erythematosus** - a widespread autoimmune condition causing systemic inflammation.
- **Graves' disease** - an autoimmune condition where your immune system mistakenly attacks your thyroid, which causes it to become overactive.

Autoimmune phenomena	Vaccine type
Vaccine-induced immune thrombotic thrombocytopenia	Adenovirus vector vaccine and mRNA vaccine
Immune thrombocytopenic purpura	mRNA vaccine
Autoimmune liver diseases	mRNA vaccine and Adenovirus vector vaccine
Guillain–Barré syndrome	mRNA vaccine and Adenovirus vector vaccine
IgA nephropathy	mRNA vaccine
Autoimmune polyarthritis	mRNA vaccine
Rheumatoid arthritis	mRNA vaccine and Adenovirus vector vaccine
Graves' disease	mRNA vaccine
Type 1 diabetes mellitus	mRNA vaccine
Systemic lupus erythematosus	Adenovirus vector vaccine

Genetic shot-related autoimmune diseases, from:
https://onlinelibrary.wiley.com/doi/10.1111/imm.13443

It looks like those prone to autoimmune diseases may be at greater risk of developing said diseases post-jab. And remember, too, that autoimmunity requires chronic antigen stimulation. This may mean that those who have had more shots and/or COVID-19 infections are more likely to suffer from autoimmune diseases in the future.

Women may also be more likely to suffer autoimmune side effects for a number of reasons. Firstly, women are more susceptible to autoimmunity in general, and this is looking like the case post-jab too. This is thought to be due to skewed "X-chromosome inactivation" and the involvement of female sex hormones.[35,36]

Females have two X chromosomes; X-inactivation is where one of the copies of the X chromosome is inactivated. This is normal, as X-inactivation prevents them from having twice as many X-chromosome gene products as males.

Skewed X-chromosome inactivation occurs when the X-inactivation of one X chromosome is favoured over the other. Some will have extreme skewing, however, and this is deemed medically important due to the increased potential for the expression of disease genes present on the X chromosome that are normally not expressed due to random X-inactivation. Growing evidence suggests that this plays a part in certain autoimmune conditions, including autoimmune thyroid disease (ATD) and scleroderma.[37,38]

WHAT IS LONG COVID?

Shortly after the 1918 flu pandemic, a global, decade-long epidemic of encephalitis lethargica—a neurological condition involving movement disorders, sleep issues, and lethargy—coincided with the flu and lasted for the 10 years following. Encephalitis lethargica is now thought to be a post-viral sequelae.[1]

Long COVID, technically termed "post-acute COVID-19 syndrome" (PACS), renders sufferers with symptoms such as fatigue, shortness of breath, chest pain, brain fog, changes in smell and/or taste, fevers, and a milieu of other symptoms beyond four or twelve weeks after initial infection (time length depending on which institution you ask).[2,3]

Long COVID sufferers can have a wide range of symptoms, and thus different individuals with long COVID can present differently. The wide range of presentations is thought to occur due to the fact that the SARS-CoV-2 virus enters cells via the ACE2 receptor, which is present in numerous cell types throughout the human body, including the oral and nasal mucosa, lungs, heart, gastrointestinal tract, liver, kidneys, spleen, brain, and arterial and venous endothelial cells.[4] Not only that, but SARS-CoV-2 has been shown to damage blood vessels, the architecture that allows life to exist.[5]

Though scientific evidence continues to verify its existence, some still remain sceptical with regard to whether or not long COVID is an actual condition, but sufferers would beg to differ. Irritable bowel syndrome, postural tachycardia syndrome (POTS), myalgic encephalomyelitis/chronic fatigue syndrome (ME/CFS), and fibromyalgia are some other conditions where this was once the case too, but emerging evidence over time has cemented their reality.

Studies continue to mount every day, showing biological characteristics unique to long COVID sufferers. And for many, it looks like long COVID will become a greater concern than the infection itself going forward.

We still don't know the root cause of long COVID and why only a certain number of people suffer from it, sometimes reportedly for months. Potential mechanisms contributing to the pathophysiology of PACS are theorised to be a combination of virus-specific pathophysiologic changes, inflammatory damage in response to the acute infection, and the expected result of post-critical illness.[6]

What we do know is that long-term COVID appears to be fueled by immune dysfunctions in some people.[7] More precisely, it has been found that the introduction of the S1 protein (a subunit of the spike protein) in certain individuals creates long COVID-like symptoms, which are caused by CD16+ monocytic vascular inflammation.[8] Monocytes are a type of white blood cell that turns into other types of white blood cells in tissues.

What increases the levels of spike protein within us? COVID-19 and genetic agents. And thus it makes sense why scientists have now found out that breakthrough infections after having a jab increase the risk of death and chances of acquiring long COVID.[9]

Another study that followed up on a large group of people who suffered with COVID-19 over a period of up to 12 months showed that in some there was persistence of moderate T cell activation for up to 1 year after SARS-CoV-2 infection rather than recovery back to baseline. They speculated that the cause of this increased immune activation could be associated with residual tissue damage or persisting SARS-CoV-2 antigen, resulting in ongoing T and B cell immune responses. And they note, ***"Ongoing immune activation detected up to 12 months after mild and severe COVID-19 could potentially be related to long-term post-viral symptoms termed post-acute COVID-19 syndrome or long-COVID."***[10]

Others have noted autoimmunity as a key characteristic of long COVID. In one study, latent autoimmunity (i.e., one IgG autoantibody) and PolyA (i.e., two or more IgG autoantibodies) were found in 83% and 62% of patients with long COVID, respectively. They found that IgG anti-SARS-CoV-2 antibodies were related to age and BMI, and they thought that many autoantibodies may have been present before the disease started.[11] An autoantibody is an antibody produced by the immune system that is directed against one or more of the individual's own proteins.

Extracellular vesicles (EVs), which are small packages of cargo released by different types of cells, may help SARS-CoV-2 get to distant tissues and organs and may also play a role in clot formation.[12] EVs may also play a "Trojan horse" role in the return of viral RNA in COVID-19 patients who have been thought "cured".[13] Combine this with the fact that endothelial dysfunction is an independent risk factor for long COVID syndrome,[14] and you can see why long COVID has been described as essentially a "thrombotic sequela."[12]

It seems like multisystem persistent immune dysregulation caused by autoimmunity and/or viral persistence, which in turn leads to vascular endothelial inflammation and microclot formation, may be the underlying pathophysiology of long COVID. But there's more.

And one reason for viral persistence may be the fact that bits of the virus continue to live in the gut of those with long COVID. As one study of those with inflammatory bowel disease noted, ***"only patients who displayed viral RNA expression in the gut reported symptoms compatible with postacute COVID-19 sequelae****. Patients without evidence for viral antigen persistence in our cohort did not display postacute COVID-19 symptoms."* The study also says that anti-nucleocapsid IgG antibodies were less likely to be found in patients with persistent viral antigen in the gut.[15]

Not very reassuring if you remember that data from the UK Health Security Agency (UKHSA) showed that N antibody levels appear to be lower in individuals who acquire infection following 2 doses of the shot.[16] In addition, patients with long COVID had lower levels of nucleocapsid-specific IFN-producing CD8+ T cells, according to another study.[17]

A recent study further cemented the link between a poor gut microbiome and acquiring PACS after COVID-19 infection, and stated, *"Gut dysbiosis in these patients (long COVID) did not fully recover.* ***Both bacteria diversity and richness of patients with COVID-19 were still significantly lower than that of controls.****"*[18]

The diagram below, from a paper titled, "The immunology and immunopathology of COVID-19" demonstrates the current working hypotheses of long COVID beautifully.[19]

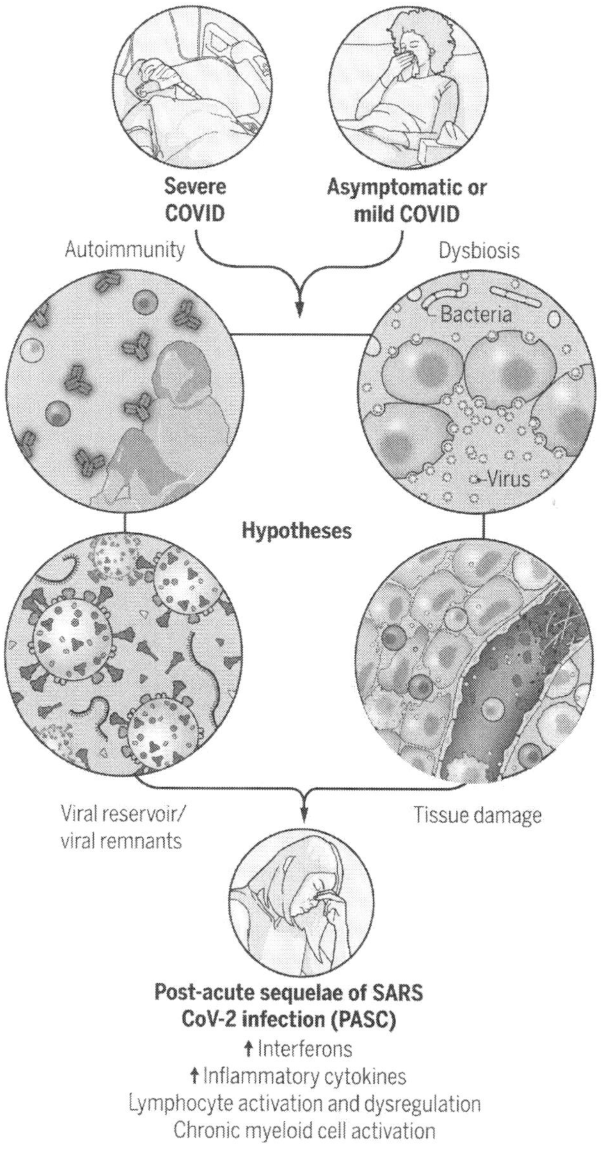

Immunopathology of COVID-19, from: https://www.science.org/doi/10.1126/science.abm8108

In addition to the current working hypotheses, a study of 215 individuals using machine learning methods distinguished key novel biological features unique to long COVID sufferers.[19] Some of these were (taken from a Twitter thread by one of the study's authors, Prof. Iwasaki):[20]

- An increase in **non-conventional monocytes,** activated B cells double-negative B cells, and decrease in conventional dendritic cells.
- Reduced central memory T cells and increased **exhausted CD4 and CD8 T cells**. "The exhausted T cells suggest chronic antigens stimulating these T cells."
- Increases in **CD4 T cells that secrete IL-2, IL-4 and IL-6**, as well as some that secrete both IL-4 and IL-6. These T cells correlated with the levels of **EBV reactive antibodies**.
- **Higher levels of IgG against Spike** in those with Long COVID who were jabbed. And in those with Long COVID without the jabs, these individuals had higher IgG against nucleocapsid. Possibly suggestive of persistent antigen.
- Long COVID group had **lower plasma cortisol levels** than control groups, with no elevation in adrenocorticotropic hormone (ACTH), a hormone made by the brain which in turn controls the level of cortisol (the "stress hormone")
- **No difference in the level of autoantibodies** compared to controls, but a subset of those with Long COVID had e**levated autoantibodies to sodium ion transporters**. Those with tinnitus and nausea had elevated levels of these autoantibodies.
- **Elevation in IgG against herpes virus antigens**. In particular, antibody reactivity to glycoproteins and early antigens of Epstein-Barr virus and Varicella zoster virus. And data suggesting recent reactivation of EBV and VZV in Long COVID.
- **Low serum cortisol being the strongest predictor for both defining Long COVID status and predicting disease severity**.

Cortisol is a hormone made by the adrenal glands. It is released in small amounts regularly, in larger amounts twice during the day, and at other times in response to stress or low blood glucose concentrations. It functions primarily to increase blood sugar levels and act as an anti-inflammatory hormone. When used as a medication, it is known as hydrocortisone, a drug used to dampen inflammation used commonly in autoimmune diseases.

Cortisol is colloquially known as the "stress hormone," but its relationship with our immune system is less appreciated. Cortisol has been shown to shift T-helper status from Th1 to Th2 dominance, favouring a "humoral" B-cell-mediated antibody immune response.[21] Cortisol has also been shown to inhibit natural killer cell activity; however, its relationship with NK is a little bit more complicated than this.[22]

Cortisol and other anti-inflammatory pathways are important for our bodies to work right because they help keep our immune systems in balance and act as buffers so that inflammation doesn't get too out of hand. Small spikes secreted at the right time are important; the problem arises when either the body makes too much, which can lead to the immune system becoming "resistant," or not enough, as we can see in the case of long COVID.[23]

Low levels of cortisol are also seen in those with a condition termed "adrenal insufficiency." Interestingly, both VZV and EBV are noted in the literature as causing adrenal insufficiency.[24,25] Moreover, Chronic fatigue syndrome (CFS), a clinical condition characterised by persistent debilitating fatigue, neurological problems, and a combination of flu-like symptoms ranging from at least 6 months up to several years, a condition similar to long COVID, has been noted to be staggeringly similar to Addison's disease, also known as primary adrenal insufficiency.[26]

One study suggested that a persistent EBV infection could cause chronic fatigue syndrome by dysregulating immune system response.[27] Noting that if some people are exposed to Epstein–Barr virus antigens for too long, internal immunological correlations may form, which can cause the immune system to stay active even after the virus is gone.

It is well known that mortality rates in patients with primary adrenal insufficiency are significantly higher, with respiratory infections being the leading cause of death.[28] In fact, one study in patients with Addison's disease found a two-fold increased risk ratio for death and a five-fold higher mortality rate from infections than in the general population, with pneumonia being the major cause of infection-related death.[29] Patients with adrenal insufficiency have also been reported to have a four- to five-fold increased risk of hospital admission for infections of all kinds.[30]

Immune dysfunction in those with adrenal insufficiency has been postulated to occur due to natural killer (NK) cell dysfunction. NK cells are part of the innate immune system, where they provide first-line defence against acute infection and cancer, as well as a critical role in immune balance.

In particular, NK cells rapidly eliminate virally infected cells via antibody-dependent cytotoxicity, a process where NK cells recognise antibodies that have been bound to target cells and, in effect, kill them.

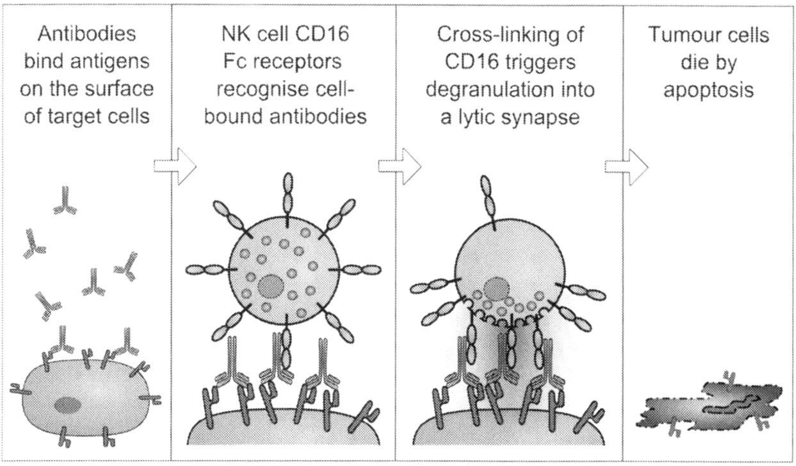

Antibodies bind antigens on the surface of target cells
NK cell CD16 Fc receptors recognise cell-bound antibodies
Cross-linking of CD16 triggers degranulation into a lytic synapse
Tumour cells die by apoptosis

Antibody-dependent cellular cytotoxicity, from: https://en.wikipedia.org/wiki/Antibody-dependent_cellular_cytotoxicity#/media/File:Antibody-dependent_Cellular_Cytotoxicity.svg

SARS-CoV-2 infection has been shown to impede NK cell function.[31] Severe COVID-19 can also make people feel tired and reduce the number of NK cells in their bodies.[32] And interestingly, those with adrenal insufficiency also show dysfunction in NK cells.[28]

And so, adding it all together, it seems to me like long COVID is a condition characterised by a multisystem persistent immune dysregulation (with possible NK cell dysfunction) driven by adrenal insufficiency that was possibly originally brought on by VZV and/or EBV, which results in autoimmunity, which in turn leads to vascular endothelial inflammation and microclot formation.

In effect, due to low levels of cortisol, those with Long COVID may have immune "overshooting," creating an environment perfect for long-term inflammation, subsequent damage, and immune fatigue. This again highlights the importance of immunological balance.

With all that being said, a huge new study of over a million people from the UK measuring the incidence of long COVID symptoms showed that the risk of long COVID was associated with several risk factors, including being a younger female, belonging to a black, mixed-ethnicity, or other ethnic minority group, having socioeconomic deprivation, smoking, having a high BMI, and the presence of a wide range of comorbidities.[33]

What's more interesting, and slightly controversial, is that the study found that in those with long COVID, 5.4% had a history of COVID-19 infection, and 4.4% had *no* history of COVID-19 infection.

Before the Long COVID sceptics come out in full force (and yes, they exist), the data from this study comes from GP primary care records, and so many may have had COVID-19 either knowingly or unknowingly and not seen a GP for this to be recorded as a case.

Interestingly, another prospective study with over 3,000 participants discovered that pre-infection psychological distress was associated with the risk of developing long COVID.[34]

When I worked in healthcare, I did encounter a couple of patients with Long COVID, but I saw more with jab-related injuries for sure. Jab-related injuries outnumbered Long COVID injuries by a factor of ten in my limited experience. Furthermore, I noticed that those with long COVID had also taken the shot. As a result, I've always wondered if long COVID was a type of jab-related injury rather than a separate condition in some people.

We need more data, and high-quality, trusted data at that, especially when an early and influential paper on long COVID that appeared in The Lancet has been recently flagged with an expression of concern while the journal investigates "data errors" brought to light by a reader.[35]

It's hard to know what's going on, especially when the scientific data is dubious.

WHAT DOES IMMUNE DYSFUNCTION MEAN FOR HUMANITY?

Anything that goes against the natural laws of complex systems will definitely and inevitably result in multiple negative consequences. Examples of this in everyday life include monoculture farming, the printing of fiat money, wearing masks, looking at our phones at night, not regularly exercising, and ingesting processed foods. The list is nearly endless and continues to grow. But I believe that injecting a large number of people in the population with a previously minimally tested new form of genetic technology has got to be up there as one of the most disruptive things we have ever done to ourselves and humanity as a whole.

Disruptive, not only because we are witnessing never-before-seen levels of side effects and deaths since the introduction of these jabs, but also because we literally have no idea what these jabs will do to recipients in the long term.

These mRNA agents work in a completely new way by teaching the body to make a highly toxic surface protein and causing a form of autoimmunity to fight it. These mRNA agents have quite a few other "firsts" too.[1] **They were the first "vaccines" to use polyethylene glycol; the first time Moderna had brought any products to the market; the first to have public health officials tell those receiving the jab to *expect* adverse reactions; the first to be implemented publicly with nothing more than preliminary data; the first to make no clear claims about reducing infections, transmissibility, or deaths; the first coronavirus "vaccine" ever attempted in humans; and the first injection of genetically modified polynucleotides in the general population.**[1]

These "firsts" pose a problem with regards to cultivating future cures for side-effects, as the causative agent is unlike anything human biological science has come across before. Moreover, these mRNA jabs were purposely tampered with genetic modifications like 1-methylpseudouridine substitutions, GC enrichments, microRNAs, and GP120 and Staphylococcus enterotoxin B gene inserts, and we are told that these were added to both increase "vaccine efficiency" as well as downregulate our own immune system.

Despite this, evidence continues to mount that these mRNA jabs retain none of the previously touted infection-prevention claims and all of the previously unknown immune downregulating properties.

There are countless studies showing that these jabs are nowhere near as effective as acquiring a natural infection;[2] that they can *enhance* the transmission of highly virulent pathogens;[3] that those jabbed recover slower from COVID-19 and remain contagious for longer than people who are not jabbed at all;[4] and that they may cause negative effectiveness by six months.[2]

"Negative effectiveness" is the complete opposite of "effective," in that those who are injected become *more* likely to get infected than those who haven't been inoculated.

Real-life data is mounting and reflecting study findings. **Official figures from the Netherlands and Canada show that the effectiveness of the COVID shots against serious diseases declines to zero and turns negative within 12 months.**[5,6] And New Zealand, one of the most jabbed nations in the world, also has one of the highest COVID-19 case rates on Earth (at the time of writing this). [7]

I understand that population figures can only ever be used to conclude correlations, not causation. But if you understand that the risk of suffering from COVID-19 increases after receiving the jab, then it all begins to make sense.

The rebuttal I've heard to this claim is that the more people you jab, the higher the total number of cases, but the total number of those hospitalised would be a fraction of what it would be otherwise – claiming that these jabs "reduce disease severity." As explained previously, we don't know if they do this either. The *only* scientifically blinded information we have about this is the pivotal clinical trial by Pfizer, which showed that the mRNA jabs did nothing to reduce the overall risk of death.[8] *Nothing.*

In the trial, 15 patients who received the jab and 14 who received a placebo died. *Yes, you read that right—more people died in the vaccine group.* This is the only controlled information we will ever get, as the trial blind is broken now.

Africa has gone fairly unscathed throughout the pandemic. Many will say this may be because data collection in African nations is less stringent than in Western nations. But first, explain Kenya.

If you go back to March 2021, it was estimated that almost half of Kenya's adult population had evidence of a past SARS-CoV-2 infection. Between March and June, 2% of the population was jabbed against COVID-19, and the country experienced a third epidemic wave.[9]

Given the evidence, it is easy to conclude that these vaccines cause both short- and long-term immunocompromisation. The contents of the jab were designed to evade our immune system and cause autoimmunity, and the risks of immune-wiping, T-cell fatigue, and potential OAS and ADE grow with every shot.

This is obviously bad news for recipients, but it's particularly bad news for the blindly unaware who continue to become or stay unwell and reach out for another shot marketed as being the only cure. With this, a perpetual cycle is set up, benefiting pharmaceutical companies and the COVID-19 narrative while harming recipients immensely.

You don't have to take this from me; a paper in *The Lancet* showed that i**mmune function among vaccinated individuals 8 months after the administration of two doses of COVID-19 vaccine was lower than that among unvaccinated individuals.**[10] And according to the European Medicines Agency's recommendations, frequent COVID-19 booster shots could adversely affect the immune response and may not be feasible.[11]

This is disastrous news. Once a person's immune system has been hurt, both outside and inside threats are more likely to hurt them. COVID-19 and its variants aren't your only problem; suffering from other infectious diseases and the reactivation of previously dormant infections become commonplace too. Future pandemics caused by other pathogens are more likely to occur in sicker populations.

Also, keep in mind that our immune system is connected to many other parts of our bodies. Clotting factors, autoimmune diseases, atherosclerosis (the hardening of arteries that can eventually lead to heart attacks), fertility, brain function, metabolic diseases, cancer, and even weight gain are all partly immune-driven,[12] and thus I worry that we may see a rise in related conditions in the future.

To give you some context, people with HIV, a virus that damages the cells in your immune system, are significantly more likely to be diagnosed with a range of cancers compared to those who are uninfected.[13] And a recent paper showed Epstein-Barr virus (EBV) as the leading cause of multiple sclerosis.[14] *What will the future entail for many millions of people?*

As more people receive boosters, more will inevitably catch COVID-19. In turn, looking for "protection" or via coerced mandates, some may get another shot and subsequently become more unwell. Cases of infections, side effects, related disease states, and deaths will all increase.

mRNA agents make conventional lab-grown vaccines seem natural in comparison. With every shot given, we face a rising risk of a colossal human health crisis that will dwarf the pandemic many times over.

HOW MANY PEOPLE HAVE BEEN INJURED?

The main bulk of this book has been dedicated to the immune system, partly in efforts to teach and show you the wonders of our natural-born immunological defences. I believe that only through collective understanding can we change current narratives for the better. And only once we have understood what is going on can we begin to think about the future intelligently and not get bamboozled when the next pandemic arrives. Only once we understand ourselves can we appreciate the biological strengths we hold, and only then can we begin to think without fear and think about freedom.

Just look at the complexity of the intercellular wiring of our immune system.[1]

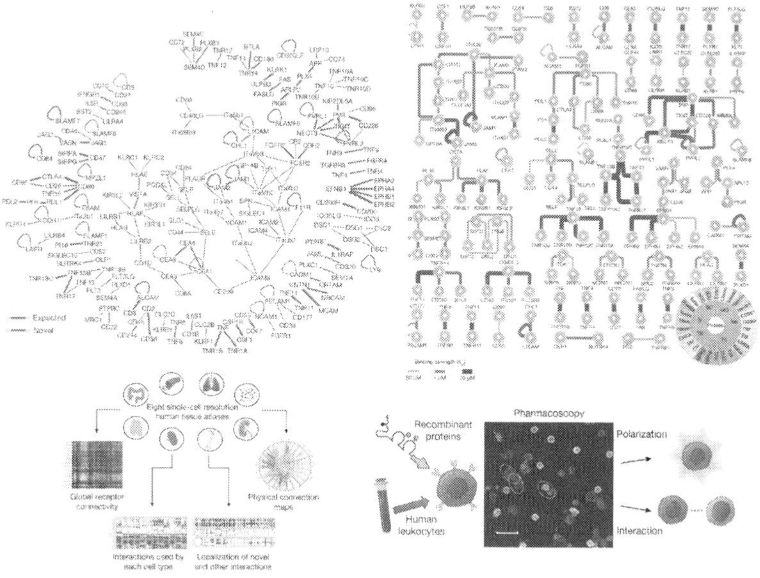

A physical wiring diagram for the human immune system, from: https://www.nature.com/articles/s41586-022-05028-x

The other reason for devoting most of this book to the immune system is that we are dealing with a virus and a proposed treatment that both primarily affect our immunological defences. The pathology caused by the disease and the side-effects of the shots overlap greatly and are both driven by and cause harm to our immune system.

Because the immune system is intimately involved in all aspects of our biological functioning, it is not surprising that its interference causes widespread and seemingly unrelated harm. But it seems like regulatory bodies either cannot or will not see these consequences.

The British National Formulary (BNF) is a pharmaceutical reference book that offers a variety of suggestions and information on pharmacology and prescribing. It's what I used to scroll through to find out medication information so I could safely prescribe the right drugs to my patients.

Well, if you go on there and look under "COVID-19 vaccine," you will note that the "common or very common" and "uncommon" side effects are mild and sparse in number.[2] More serious and life-threatening conditions like Guillain-Barré syndrome and myocarditis are placed in the "rare" or "very rare" category, and a handful of others have been assigned the "Frequency not known" label. Note also how "death" is not listed as a side effect. I have added a screenshot of the page below.

For COVID-19 vaccine

Common or very common

Axillary lymph node tenderness; chills; influenza like illness; pain in extremity

Uncommon

Asthenia; dizziness; drowsiness; insomnia; sweat changes

Rare or very rare

Angioedema; facial paralysis; Guillain-Barre syndrome (following AstraZeneca vaccine); myocarditis (following Moderna and Pfizer/BioNTech vaccines); pericarditis (following Moderna and Pfizer/BioNTech vaccines); sensation abnormal

Frequency not known

Arterial thrombosis (following AstraZeneca vaccine); capillary leak syndrome (following AstraZeneca vaccine); cerebral venous sinus thrombosis (following AstraZeneca vaccine); extensive swelling of vaccinated limb; thrombocytopenia (following AstraZeneca vaccine); thromboembolism (following AstraZeneca vaccine); transverse myelitis (following AstraZeneca vaccine); venous thrombosis (following AstraZeneca vaccine); visceral venous thrombosis (following AstraZeneca vaccine)

BNF side-effects for COVID-19 vaccine, from: https://bnf.nice.org.uk/drugs/covid-19-vaccine/#side-effects

I am unsure how the frequencies of each side-effect were determined and grouped into the subsequent categories in the BNF. As we have already appreciated, the VAERS and the UK Yellow Cards system paint a very different picture.

VAERS is "a national early warning system to detect possible safety problems in U.S.-licensed vaccines," and according to the CDC, it is "especially useful for detecting unusual or unexpected patterns of adverse event reporting that might indicate a possible safety problem with a vaccine."

The Yellow Card scheme is run by the MHRA and is the UK system for collecting and monitoring medication-related safety concerns. Like VAERS, the scheme relies on the voluntary reporting of suspected side effects by health professionals and the public.

It is reported that fewer than 1% of all vaccine-related adverse events are reported to VAERS.[3] While it is estimated that only 10% of serious reactions and between 2 and 4% of non-serious reactions are reported to the Yellow Card scheme.[4]

I should point out that because both systems are open to the public, anti-vaccination activists *could* fill VAERS and the Yellow Card scheme with fake reports to make it look like there is a higher risk of adverse events.

Saying this though, during the time period 2011-2014, healthcare professionals submitted 38% of U.S. reports, patients and parents submitted 14%, vaccine manufacturers submitted 30%, and others (e.g., friends or acquaintances of the patient, 3rd party reporters who became aware of adverse events from the media, lawyers, etc.) submitted 12%, indicating that the majority of reports were historically submitted by "professionals."[5]

The data in the last two years from both systems is shocking. **In the 31-year history of VAERS up until February 3, 2022, there were a total of 10,321 deaths reported as a "symptom" in association with any vaccine, and 8,241 (80%) of those deaths were linked to COVID-19 shots.**[6] And **in the year 2021, COVID-19 shots represented 93% of the total cases reported for any vaccine that same year;**[6] that's 737,689 events reported in VAERS for COVID-19 vaccines that year.

The total number of adverse event reports for COVID-19 injections is far greater than if you were to add up all reported side-effects from all other vaccines in all prior years. And as one study reviewing VAERS data notes, ***"there are 27 times as many reports for COVID-19 vaccines as would be expected if its adverse reactions were comparable to those from the flu vaccine."***[6]

Recent VAERS data analysis shows that the total number of deaths associated with the COVID-19 shots is more than triple the number of deaths associated with all other vaccines combined since the year 1990.[7]

More than triple.

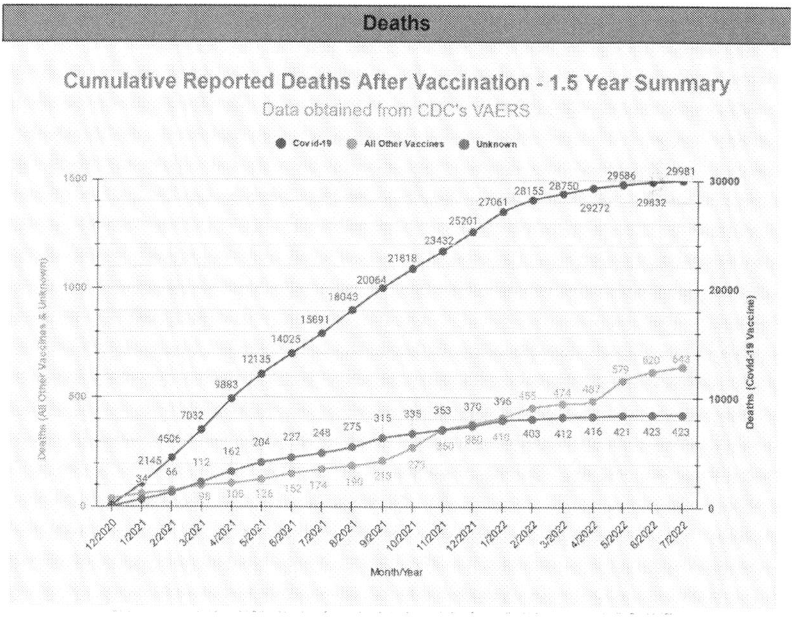

Cumulative reported deaths after vaccination, COVID-19 vaccines versus all other vaccines, from: https://vaersanalysis.info/2022/08/05/vaers-summary-for-covid-19-vaccines-through-7-29-2022/

And it's not like the US got a bad batch. As of July 2022, in the UK, there have been 460,533 Yellow Cards reported for the Pfizer/BioNTech, AstraZeneca, and Moderna vaccines combined.[8] Taking into account that only 2–10% of reactions are normally reported, this places the number of actual possible side effects at around 4.6 million to over 23 million cases in the UK.

There are so many different kinds of side effects reported to VAERS that they make the BNF side-effect profile look small.

To paint a clearer picture of what reality has been like and continues to be like for many millions of people, I've combined all VAERS information collected in 2021 using the study titled "Innate immune suppression by SARS-CoV-2 mRNA vaccinations: The role of G-quadruplexes, exosomes, and MicroRNAs" to populate the number of side-effects in descending order of occurrence linked to mRNA agents in comparison to all other vaccines VAERS that year.[6]

SYMPTOMS	COVID-19 SHOTS	ALL OTHER VACCINES	% COVID-19 SHOTS
Nausea	69,121	2,154	97
Dyspnea	39,551	836	97.9
Vomiting	27,885	1,070	96.3
Syncope	14,701	567	96.3
Tinnitus	13,275	247	98.2
Mobility decreased	8,975	768	92.1
Migraine headache	8,872	187	97.9
Vertigo	7,638	181	97.7
Bell's Palsy/facial palsy	5,881	248	96
Dysphagia	4,711	124	97.4
Thrombosis	3,899	52	98.7
Anosmia	3,657	20	99.5
Anosmia	3,657	20	99.5
Pulmonary embolism	3,100	37	98.8
Deafness	2,895	138	95.5
Myocarditis	2,322	39	98
Deep vein	2,275	22	99

thrombosis			
Myocardial infarction	2,224	48	97.9
Dysphonia	1,692	59	96.6
Memory impairment	1,681	39	97.7
Arrest	1,319	52	96.2
Cardiac failure	1,156	34	97.1
Arrhythmia	1,069	18	98.3
Cognitive disorder	779	36	92.1
Bradycardia	673	26	96.3
Pulmonary thrombosis	631	15	97.7
Neoplasm	428	24	94.7
Cancer	396	7	98.3
Breast cancer	246	8	96.8
Liver function test increased	238	7	97.1
Cerebral thrombosis	211	4	98.1
Carcinoma	176	11	94.1
Metastatic/metastasis	175	4	97.8
Leukaemia	155	6	96.3
Lymphoma	144	9	94.1

Liver function test abnormal	90	4	95.7
Portal vein thrombosis	89	1	98.9
[Acute] hepatic failure	86	2	97.7
Liver disorder	83	4	95
Parkinsonian symptoms	83	6	93.3
Superficial vein thrombosis	81	0	100
Peripheral artery thrombosis	74	0	100
Hepatic cirrhosis	67	2	97.1
[Drug-induced] liver injury	65	0	100
Lung cancer	64	2	97
Mesenteric vein thrombosis	55	1	98.2
Brain neoplasm	53	2	96.4
Prostate cancer	50	2	96.2
Venous thrombosis	41	0	100
Colon cancer	40	1	97.6
Alzheimer's dementia	37	2	94.9

Hepatic function abnormal	34	0	100
Hepatic cyst	33	1	97
Bladder cancer	30	0	100
Ovarian cancer	27	0	100
Pancreatic cancer	24	0	100
Hepatic cancer [metastatic]	12	0	100
Haemangioma of liver	10	0	100
Liver abscess	7	0	100
Liver transplant	6	0	100
Brain neoplasm	53	2	96.4
Prostate cancer	50	2	96.2
Venous thrombosis	41	0	100
Colon cancer	40	1	97.6
Alzheimer's dementia	37	2	94.9
Hepatic function abnormal	34	0	100
Hepatic cyst	33	1	97
Bladder cancer	30	0	100
Ovarian cancer	27	0	100
Pancreatic cancer	24	0	100

Hepatic cancer [metastatic]	12	0	100
Haemangioma of liver	10	0	100
Liver abscess	7	0	100
Liver transplant	6	0	100

When I was a GP trainee, I noticed an increase in the number of patients with jab-related side effects at work. Presentations included a frozen shoulder (of the jabbed arm), systemic inflammation, blood clots, excessive facial sweating, total body fatigue, heart damage, early menopause, and missed menstrual periods.

These patients were once "fit and healthy," and though some suspected that the shots may have had something to do with their new ailment, the majority were either in denial or completely oblivious to any link between the two. Others have even asked me how they'd go about booking a booster. Cognitive dissonance was alive and kicking.

Since I quit my job, some of my family members and friends of friends have been diagnosed with cancer, and some of them have died soon after getting their shots. Others close to me have said that they now feel more tired than before, are more susceptible to illness, and suffer from brain fog.

The table above really helps put everything into perspective, and I was actually given a suspension that eventually led to a permanent ban on Twitter for posting it on their platform.

I hope you can appreciate the sheer range and number of reported side effects post-COVID-19 shots. For example, there were 30 reported cases of bladder cancer, 1681 reports of memory impairment, and over 27,000 cases of vomiting post-jab. I can't think of anything else, pharmaceutical or not, that has caused this much harm. This is not normal.

It is also important to question whether seemingly atypical side effects post-jabs like cardiac arrests are being underreported due to the lack of a link between the two being made. Other side effects, like cancer, may take months or weeks to manifest, and by then too much time may have passed for anyone to connect the dots unless they were clued up beforehand. *And even then, will it have been reported in VAERS or the Yellow Card reporting system? Who knows?*

It is difficult to know who to believe. The BNF only has a small page of side effects, and yet people have reported them differently.

Worse yet, in documents sent to the FDA, Pfizer included a table that took up five and a half A4 pages and listed all of the people in their trial who had at least one serious side effect from the first dose to one month after the second dose.[9] The range of side effects is astonishing, and most of the time, they happen to people who got the shot and not to those who got the placebo.

Pfizer's trial reported no serious adverse events occurring more than one month after dose two. But as one study notes, *"this reporting threshold may have led to an undercounting of serious AESIs in the Pfizer trial."*

It's been hard to get clear-cut evidence of possible jab-related deaths. Secondary sources of information, like the CDC and other government-funded organisations, are full of pro-vaccine bias, skewed information, and false information.

In the UK, the definition of a "COVID death" is anyone who has died with a laboratory-confirmed positive COVID-19 test within (equal to or less than) 28 days of the first positive specimen date.[10] Many have died with the virus, not from it. The UK doesn't have the data of those who have been harmed or have suffered illness from a COVID-19 vaccination, as this is not recorded on the death certificate.[11]

With this information, I can only suspect that many thousands are inappropriately having the wrong cause of death written on death certificates. This is not only unscientific and deeply undignified, but it also allows others to suffer in the future. We must have begun post-mortems a lot sooner.

At every level of the playing field, from pharmaceutical companies to the health-care professionals administering the jabs, the data has been corrupted and fails to tell the jab recipient what really is going on. There has been and still is a clear manipulation of scientific facts to fit a story, which is called "propaganda."

Many have been maimed and killed, and I worry that this is only the tip of the iceberg. Even so, major news outlets and pharmaceutical companies have been complicitly silent about it all.

CAN WE TRUST THE PHARMACEUTICAL INDUSTRY?

Throughout my first few years as a doctor, I remember prescribing a medication called "ranitidine" (Zantac), an anti-reflux medication used to treat those with peptic ulcer disease or gastroesophageal reflux disease.

In early 2020, the FDA requested all ranitidine products be pulled from the market immediately, as ongoing investigations uncovered traces of N-Nitrosodimethylamine (NDMA), a *probable* human carcinogen, in ranitidine products from a number of manufacturers.[1]

In medical school, we were taught about Thalidomide, a medication first marketed in the 1950s in West Germany as having beneficial effects on anxiety, insomnia, and morning sickness. Though the drug's toxicity was examined in several animals, it was never tested on pregnant women.[2] At that time, scientists did not believe that any drug taken by a pregnant woman could cross into the placenta and harm the developing foetus.

In the UK, thalidomide was sold as a cure for morning sickness under the brand name Distaval. Their advertisement claimed that "Distaval can be given with complete safety to pregnant women and nursing mothers without adverse effect on mother or child... Outstandingly safe Distaval has been prescribed for nearly three years in this country." By the mid-1950s, thalidomide was marketed worldwide.[3]

In the late 1950s and early 1960s, more than 10,000 children in 46 countries were born with deformities, such as phocomelia, a condition that involves the malformation of limbs, as a consequence of thalidomide use. Thalidomide also damaged the eyes, ears, and brain of children. The disaster prompted many countries to introduce tougher rules for the testing and licensing of drugs.[4]

Thalidomide, which is now only used to treat multiple myeloma (a type of blood marrow cancer), can only be given to women once pregnancy is excluded with a medically supervised pregnancy test performed on, or within 3 days prior to, initiation and repeated every 4 weeks thereafter. Women of childbearing potential must use effective contraception during treatment, and men are advised to use condoms too.[5]

A news article from The Guardian reads, *"On Thursday in Brisbane magistrates court, coroner John Hutton found that a commonly prescribed drug named Champix – manufactured by Pfizer and sold internationally under the name Chantix – contributed to the death of a 22-year-old Brisbane man, Timothy John, who died by suicide soon after he began taking a medication that he had hoped would cut his smoking habit from eight cigarettes a day down to zero."*[6]

Chantix is a medication used for smoking cessation that was brought to the market by Pfizer. About 3,000 Chantix lawsuits were filed against Pfizer by people who said they had suicidal thoughts and mental illnesses after taking the drug. Pfizer set aside about $288 million, and some cases were settled.[7]

In 2021, Pfizer recalled all in-date batches of Champix as a precautionary measure due to the presence of levels of N-nitroso-varenicline (a potential carcinogen) above the acceptable level of intake.[8]

Pfizer agreed to pay $2.3 billion to settle charges of fraud, civil and criminal liability, and promotion of off-label use of four drugs in 2009.[9] It was the largest health care fraud settlement and criminal fine in history at the time. Though groundbreakingly large, The New York Times noted that $2.3 billion amounted to less than three weeks of Pfizer sales.[10]

Purdue Pharma, the maker of the opioid painkiller OxyContin, agreed to plead guilty to criminal charges and face penalties of approximately $8.3 billion in 2021 for its role in the opioid epidemic.[11]

As you can see, the pharmaceutical industry does not have a flawless record, so when the same culprits continue to reassure that their minimally tested new form of therapy is safe and effective, I would argue that it would be unnatural *not* to be even a little wary.

Combine this with the fact that medical errors are the third leading cause of death in the US after heart disease and cancer, and you've really got a recipe for disaster.[12,13]

There's a reason why genetic injectables weren't a thing before the pandemic; it's not because no one was working on them; in fact, many were; it's because mRNA technology ran into a lot of safety issues.

The online article titled *"Lavishly funded Moderna hits safety problems in bold bid to revolutionize medicine"* written in 2017, portrays these problems better, straight from Big Pharma's mouth.[14] I have included pertinent sections from the article below and highlighted in bold those that I found particularly interesting.

"...Exactly one year ago, Moderna CEO Stéphane Bancel talked up his company's "unbelievable" future before a standing-room-only crowd at the annual J.P. Morgan Healthcare Conference here. He promised that Moderna's treatment for a rare and debilitating disease known as Crigler-Najjar syndrome, developed alongside biotech giant Alexion Pharmaceuticals, would enter human trials in 2016."

"...But the Crigler-Najjar treatment has been indefinitely delayed, an Alexion spokeswoman told STAT. ***It never proved safe enough to test in humans,***

according to several former Moderna employees and collaborators who worked closely on the project. Unable to press forward with that technology, Moderna has had to focus instead on developing a handful of vaccines, turning to a less lucrative field that might not justify the company's nearly $5 billion valuation."

"...His presentation instead focused on four vaccines that the company is moving through the first phase of clinical trials: two target strains of influenza, a third is for Zika virus, and the ***fourth remains a secret****."*

"...Founded in 2012, Moderna reached unicorn status — a $1 billion valuation — in just two years, faster than Uber, Dropbox, and Lyft, according to CB Insights. The company's premise: Using custom-built strands of messenger RNA, known as mRNA, it aims to turn the body's cells into ad hoc drug factories, compelling them to produce the proteins needed to treat a wide variety of diseases."

"But ***mRNA is a tricky technology. Several major pharmaceutical companies have tried and abandoned the idea, struggling to get mRNA into cells without triggering nasty side effects."***

"...The ***indefinite delay on the Crigler-Najjar project signals persistent and troubling safety concerns for any mRNA treatment that needs to be delivered in multiple doses, covering almost everything that isn't a vaccine****, former employees and collaborators said."*

"...In order to protect mRNA molecules from the body's natural defenses, drug developers must wrap them in a protective casing. For Moderna, that meant putting its Crigler-Najjar therapy in ***nanoparticles made of lipids****. And for its chemists, those nanoparticles created a daunting challenge:* ***Dose too little, and you don't get enough enzyme to affect the disease; dose too much, and the drug is too toxic for patients****."*

"...From the start, Moderna's scientists knew that using mRNA to spur protein production would be a tough task..."

"...Yet Moderna could not make its therapy work, former employees and collaborators said. ***The safe dose was too weak, and repeat injections of a dose strong enough to be effective had troubling effects on the liver in animal studies.****"*

Working as a doctor for many years, I totally appreciate the wonders of modern medicine and how pharmaceuticals can not only transform lives for the better but save them too.

But I am also not blind to the negatives of polypharmacy, the growing burden of chronic disease, and the increasingly overbearing role that the medical-industrial complex is having on our lives.

Pre-pandemic, pharmaceutical technology worked within the realm of biological laws, and even then we faced problems like antibiotic resistance and disastrous medical side effects.

I am concerned that mRNA technology is a step too far, completely disconnected from what we consider normal and thus safe. It is so different from our regular biological physiology that at best it will prove ineffective, and at worst it will be life-threatening.

I think that our constant need for the next cool thing and our tendency to put all of our weight on one answer, especially in times of crisis, will turn out to be catastrophically bad in the long run.

CTV NEWS LIVE

CORONAVIRUS | News

Moderna CEO says COVID vaccines will evolve like 'an iPhone'

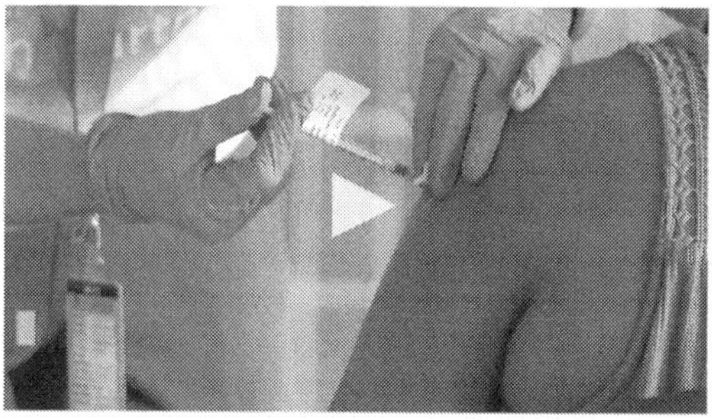

News article on how the Moderna CEO envisages a future where jabs evolve like 'an iPhone', from: https://www.ctvnews.ca/health/coronavirus/moderna-ceo-says-covid-vaccines-will-evolve-like-an-iphone-1.6023144

Putting genetic material that hasn't been tested into a new particle that was made just for it and giving it to people in a new way will cause new diseases and disease states to happen more often and in age groups that haven't been affected by them before. We have entered the age of "unknown cause," "sudden death," and "once rare."

In times of crisis, it is tempting to reach for the thing marketed as the "cure-all," but I'd advise next time maybe stepping back and taking a little longer to evaluate your situation, other forms of available treatment, preventive measures, and the history of those seemingly acting a little too friendly.

Just because something is new doesn't automatically make it good, especially when introducing it to a biological system that has been evolving and working fine without it for around 3.7 billion years and counting.

WHAT IS POLYETHYLENE GLYCOL?

Human beings are evolutionarily hardwired to *want,* as well as being particularly drawn to novelty. These traits proved beneficial for us in the harsh African savannas, but in today's world, these underlying traits have been exploited by Big corporations to drive consumerism.

In 2019, the world was introduced to a never-before-seen deadly virus, and for many, only a new seemingly high-tech solution would qualify as the perfect elixir to this novel threat.

It's easy to forget that millions of people around the world lined up to get not just one but several shots of a drug that had only been minimally tested. Most people didn't pedantically analyse the risks and benefits of getting jabbed. Rationalisation does not exist when fear is involved. And irrationality is normalised when everyone else is collectively irrational.

It felt like the minds of the majority were taken over by the mantra, "*new virus, new rules, new threat, and only one solution.*" A solution that has catastrophically failed, as evidenced by no other than the CEO of Pfizer himself, Albert Bourla.

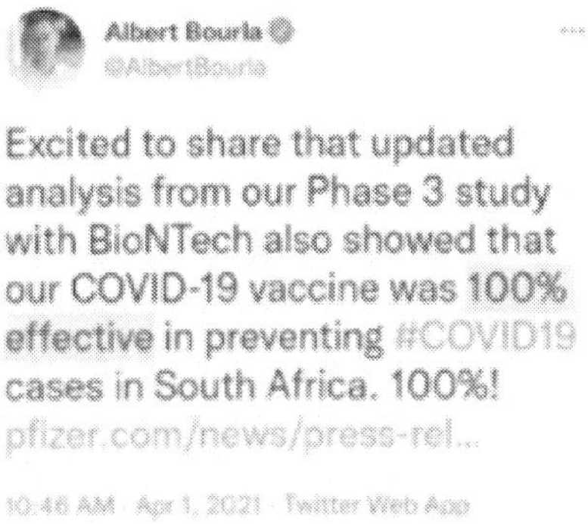

Albert Bourla
@AlbertBourla
Excited to share that updated analysis from our Phase 3 study with BioNTech also showed that our COVID-19 vaccine was 100% effective in preventing #COVID19 cases in South Africa. 100%!
pfizer.com/news/press-rel...
10:46 AM · Apr 1, 2021 · Twitter Web App

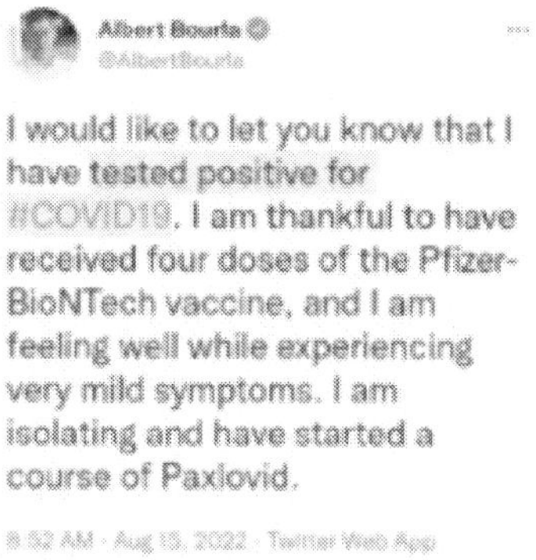

Albert Bourla
@AlbertBourla
I would like to let you know that I have tested positive for #COVID19. I am thankful to have received four doses of the Pfizer-BioNTech vaccine, and I am feeling well while experiencing very mild symptoms. I am isolating and have started a course of Paxlovid.

Tweets from Albert Bourla, CEO of Pfizer, from: https://twitter.com/albertbourla/status/1377618480527257606?lang=en https://twitter.com/albertbourla/status/1559145992594784256

More than two years later, I guarantee that the average "vaccinated" person still does not know what was actually injected into them. In fact, if you were to go up to a hundred "vaccinated" people and ask them what "mRNA," "polyethylene glycol," and "spike protein" are, how many do you think would be able to competently answer that question?

This lack of knowledge was the primary driver for this book, and hopefully by now, you, the reader, feel a little more confident in explaining two out of the three scientific terms. The one I haven't gone through properly as of yet is *polyethylene glycol (PEG).*

PEG is a compound derived from petroleum and used in various industries, from industrial manufacturing to medicine. In medicine, PEG is frequently used in medicines to treat constipation.[1]

Up until three years ago, PEG was never used in vaccines. Moderna and Pfizer–BioNTech changed this with the introduction of their mRNA products that use bubbles, called lipid nanoparticles (LNPs) coated with stabilising molecules of PEG.

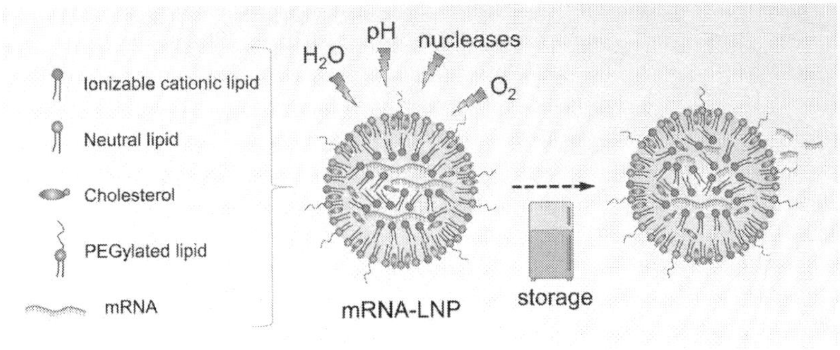

LNP structure, from: https://ars.els-cdn.com/content/image/1-s2.0-S0378517321003914-ga1_lrg.jpg

For a long time, PEG was classified as a non-immunogenic polymer,[2] however, recent evidence suggests that nanoparticles with PEG molecules *can* interact with circulating antibodies and serum components.[3] One study found that 65–76% of the general population had anti-PEG antibodies, for example.[4]

In 2020, concerns over PEG triggering allergic reactions were raised.[5] Researchers noted that one-third of those who experienced anaphylaxis after being jabbed had a previous history of allergic or anaphylactic reactions, suggesting that anti-PEG antibodies formed after exposure to PEGylated compounds may play a role.[6]

Women are more likely to experience allergic reactions after mRNA inoculation and have also been shown to have higher anti-PEG antibodies.[6]

Luckily for us, though the risk of anaphylaxis exists, it is seemingly rare. During December 14, 2020, through January 18, 2021, a total of 9 943 247 doses of the Pfizer-BioNTech vaccine and 7 581 429 doses of the Moderna vaccine were reported administered in the US. During this time, 66 reports of anaphylaxis were sent to VAERS, which the CDC looked at.[6]

However, we are not yet out of the woods; PEG may cause biological harms other than anaphylaxis. One study presented the case of a 45-year-old female patient who developed kidney injury and required emergency dialysis one week after receiving the second mRNA jab. The patient also required steroid treatment. Her kidney inflammation and subsequent kidney damage were attributed to PEG.[7]

A study on mice in which PEG was injected into the abdominal cavity noted, "*Based on the common assumption that polyethylene glycol (PEG) is non-toxic, our local regulatory authorities recently recommended the use of PEG instead. However, mice injected..with PEG 200..did not tolerate PEG 200 well, and **half of the animals had to be euthanized**.*"[8]

Worryingly, too, what happens to the "vaccine" syringe and vial before inoculation may also play a cardinal part in what happens to the mRNA recipient. In one study, shaking syringes of mRNA caused lipid nanoparticles to stick together and mRNA to break down.[9]

Remember that PEG has never been injected into so many people in history. And on this point, I agree with a review that notes, ***"The PEG adjuvant in mRNA vaccines, an established chemical fusogen, was never a component of approved vaccines previously therefore, its exact interaction with viral fusogens is currently unknown. Thus, more studies are needed to evaluate the spectrum of rare interactions at the molecular level, and whether PEG is the ideal vaccine component."***[10]

WHY DO ONLY SOME PEOPLE HAVE SIDE-EFFECTS?

If you ignore the fact that death is a very likely side effect of these shots and that we are witnessing a global, officially "unknown," increase in excess mortality figures, [1] ·

if you discount the fact that contracting COVID-19 is a side effect of these mRNA jabs,

if you discount the point that many may ignore new illnesses post-jab due to a time delay and/or a seemingly unrelated aetiology,

if you discount VAERS ever existing, and ignore the fact that in 2021 the total number of adverse event reports for COVID-19 injections was far greater than if you were to add up all reported side-effects from all other vaccines in all prior years,

if you discount the evidence of manipulation of pharmaceutical studies to fit certain narratives and underplay "vaccine" harms,

if you discount the fact that there is widespread myopia and willful blindness amongst healthcare workers to ignore or dissociate post-jab side effects from the causative agent out of fear of potential repercussions,

if you discount the point that we are only a few years into this and do not know what the downstream effects of these mRNA agents are,

if you discount these facts, then it may seem that only a handful of people seemingly suffer with side effects post-jab.

Are they just unlucky or is there something going on?

Marc Girardot, a tech executive, senior advisor and member of PANDA (Pandemics Data & Analytics),[2] explains this question with his “Bolus theory”.

WHAT IS THE BOLUS THEORY?

The Bolus theory is a type of domino theory, a theory made up of multiple other theories that requires their coordination to work. There are seven dominoes to the **Bolus theory**.[3]

1. **Inadvertent IV injection**

Vaccines are injected into the deltoid muscle and are meant to drain primarily to the lymph nodes around the armpit (axillary lymph nodes) and stay there - where the body recognises the vaccine contents and forms immunological memory.

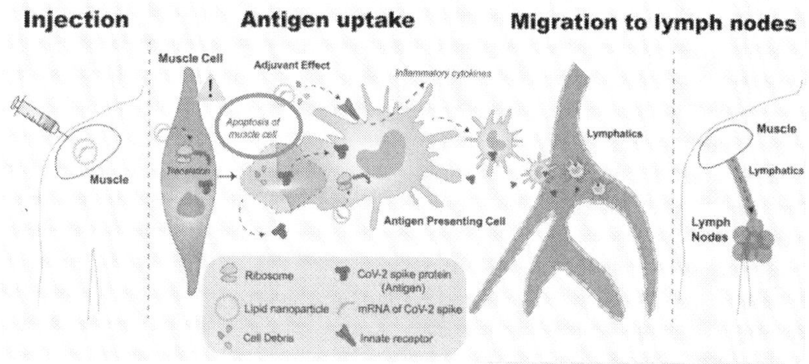

Vaccines are injected into the deltoid muscle and are meant to drain primarily to the lymph nodes around the armpit, from: https://covidmythbuster.substack.com/p/vaccine-russian-roulette-why-some#footnote-1

And so, theoretically, the LNPs in which the mRNA is encapsulated *should* have a very restricted biodistribution,[4] only targeting the draining axillary lymph nodes.[5] However, studies performed by Pfizer for the Japanese regulatory agency as well as assessment reports by the European Medicines Agency (EMA) show that the LNPs display an off-target distribution in rodents, accumulating in organs such as the spleen, liver, pituitary gland, thyroid, ovaries, and other tissues.[6,7]

Girardot believes this occurs because mRNA agents are accidentally administered to the veins rather than the muscle.[8] This is because jab givers aren't usually trained to pull the syringe back to check for blood, a process called "aspiration," to make sure they aren't in the vasculature. But when they are trained to aspirate, as they are in Denmark, there are 60% fewer adverse effects.[9]

Other studies have shown that intravenous (into the vein) injection of genetic agents can induce inflammation of the heart in mice, as well as thrombocytopenia (a condition of low levels of platelets, cells that help with clotting).[10,11]

Why all international health regulatory bodies continue to not promote the aspiration technique is beyond me.

. . .

2. **The Bolus effect**

Instead of giving "vaccine" contents slowly, most practitioners push the "vaccine" plunger quickly, administering the contents in a very short period of time—a term called a "bolus dose."

This highly concentrated hit probably makes endothelial damage worse and starts a chain reaction of cell death and damage.[13]

3. **Trapped in the vascular system**

The way mRNA agents are supposed to work is through a process called "transfection," which involves deliberately introducing naked or purified nucleic acids (genetic material) into cells.

Whether given into the muscle or veins, Girardot believes that the vast majority of lipid nanoparticles end up in the bloodstream, and thus those who are jabbed are exposing the lining of their blood vessels to vaccine particles and to subsequent transfection.

4. **Immune destruction of transfected cells**

Traditional vaccines do not induce our cells to produce viral proteins, but mRNA agents do so via transfection. Transfected cells produce spike proteins and are killed by our immune system.

If most of the mRNA in our bodies moves through our blood vessels, our immune system will damage these cells and organs.[13]

5. **Concentrated damage**

Depending on the percentage of the dose administered into the vessels, the concentration of nanoparticles coming into contact with the endothelial wall will vary.[14] Higher concentrations may cause vessel wall damage and leakage.

6. **Arterial damage**

Damage to vessel endothelial walls leads to further destruction of other vessel wall layers, like smooth muscle cells. This in turn can lead to bleeding, clots, strokes, and heart disease.

Girardot quotes one study where mice were given the mRNA jab, and this later triggered calcification of the sac around the heart in just 2 days—a sign of damage and attempted healing by the body.[15]

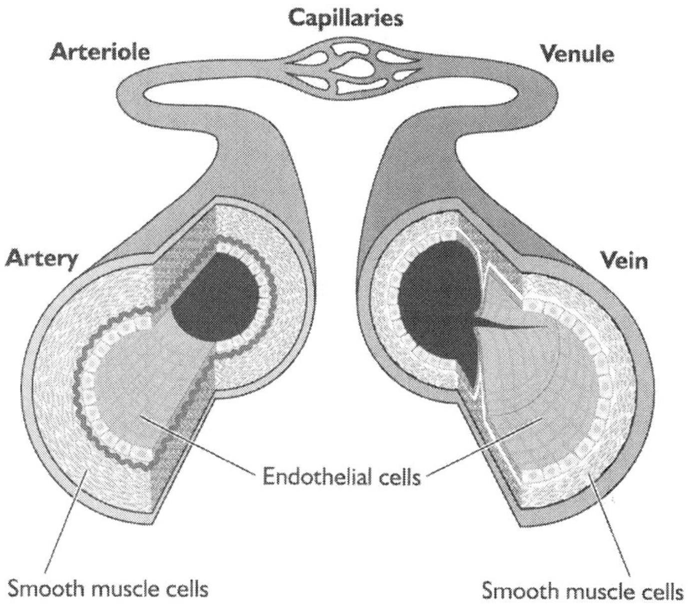

The vascular endothelial system, from: https://bioscience.lonza.com/lonza_bs/GB/en/what-are-endothelial-cells-and-their-function

7. **Blood-Tissue Barrier damage**

The blood-brain barrier (BBB), as the name suggests, is a barrier of specialised cells that exists between the circulating blood and the central nervous system.[16] This highly selective, semipermeable border of endothelial cells prevents certain components in the blood from non-selectively crossing into the fluid that bathes our brain and spinal cord.

Cognitive conditions like Alzheimer's disease are related to a breakdown of the BBB.[17] And Girardot believes that these mRNA jabs likely transfect BBB endothelial cells, causing them to be leaky and thus causing a breakdown of the BBB.[16]

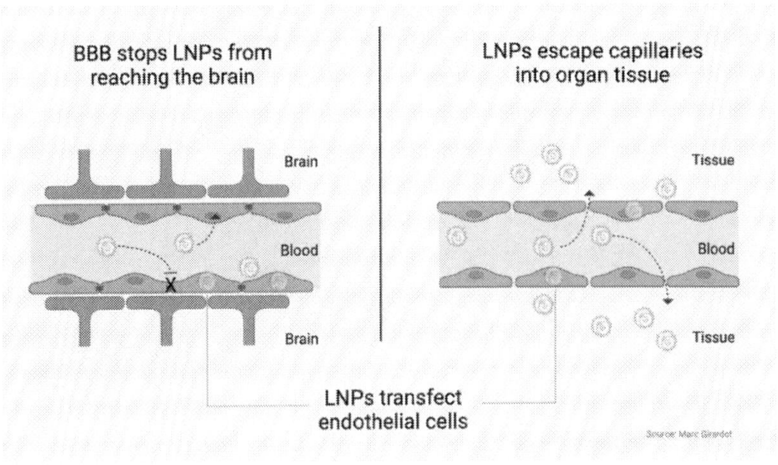

Endothelial cells becoming transfected, from:
https://covidmythbuster.substack.com/p/poking-holes-in-the-brain-blood-barrier

Leaky vessels post-jab have been demonstrated by a Japanese study of the heart.[18] Studies on the effect of mRNA jabs on the BBB are lacking, but we know that the spike protein can cross the BBB in mice.[19]

Girardot also says that leaking blood vessels in the blood-tissue barriers of the testes or ovaries will always cause sterility and problems with reproduction.[20]

Using Girardot's Bolus Theory, I have come up with an all-encompassing theory called the **"Three Causes Three Effects"** hypothesis to explain how I believe genetic agents harm us.

WHAT IS THE "THREE CAUSES THREE EFFECTS" HYPOTHESIS?

Girardot's Bolus theory highlights the pivotal importance of the vaccine administration technique and suggests that a lot of damage could have been avoided if injections were given using the "aspiration technique" and given slowly. *This is independent of the growing evidence that the mRNA agents themselves are harmful, useless, and unnecessary.*

The Bolus theory also highlights the importance of our vascular system, a system that is often taken for granted and disregarded for sexier end organ problems. But one mustn't forget that these end organs and their accompanying problems would not exist without the blood and other nutrients that flow to and from them.

History suggests that empires fall when barriers to cities and trading routes are destroyed. And blood has been spilled throughout history to protect these vital geographical areas.

The destruction of our vascular system causes all sorts of problems, from vessel inflammation to heart attacks. Injecting agents that target the very infrastructure of life is not very wise.

How something is given is as important as *what* it contains, especially if it is toxic. Using the Bolus theory, I have come up with my own COVID-19 shot side effect theory called the 'Three Causes Three Effects' hypothesis.

I believe that there are three components of these mRNA agents that pose particular harm to us (in no particular order):

1. **Spike protein (made via transfection of mRNA)**
2. **Nanoparticles**
3. **Mode of delivery**

And I believe all related side effects can be explained by three biological dysfunctions (in no particular order):

1. **Endothelial damage**
2. **Immune dysfunction**
3. **Cell death and ageing**

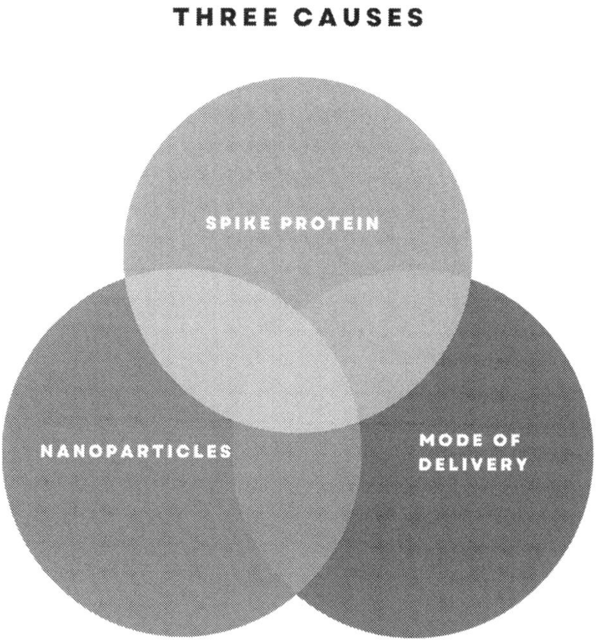
THREE CAUSES
SPIKE PROTEIN
NANOPARTICLES
MODE OF DELIVERY

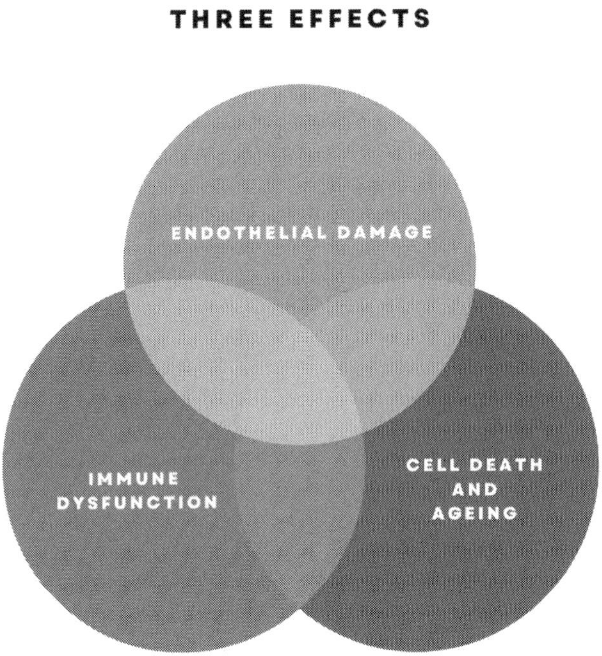
THREE EFFECTS
ENDOTHELIAL DAMAGE
IMMUNE DYSFUNCTION
CELL DEATH AND AGEING

THREE CAUSES

1. **Spike Protein**

Anyone who still denies the dangers of spike proteins doesn't know what they are talking about. Though structurally non-identical, the spike proteins found both on the virus and made by mRNA jabs are similar, and a major cause of pathology in those infected and/or inoculated.

So far, we know that the spike protein shares similar protein regions with our own cells, resulting in autoimmunity against endothelial cells.[1] It has also been speculated that the spike protein mutates in our body to infect our cells more efficiently.[2]

The spike protein has been shown to damage cells;[3] disrupt mitochondrial (our cellular batteries) function;[4] cause lung inflammation;[5] cross the blood-brain barrier in mice and cause nerve damage;[6] be prion-like in structure (prions are "proteinaceous infectious particles" that causes diseases such as mad cow disease and Creutzfeldt Jakob disease);[7] significantly inhibit DNA damage repair;[8] cause cardiac damage;[9] cause vascular cell dysfunction;[10] cause clot formation and increased blood thickness;[11,12] cause amyloid microclots;[13] induce cell senescence (a process where cells stop dividing);[14] interact with tumour suppressor proteins - p53 and BRCA;[15] and increases the expression of ACE2 receptors - which in turn has been shown to promote DNA damage and ageing.[16,17,18] The list goes on.

This toxin has been noted to be everywhere in autopsy studies of those who died from COVID-19, from the lungs to the testis.[19]

Now what if your body was trained to make spike proteins repeatedly?

2. **Nanoparticles**

It has been recently found out that exposure to lipid nanoparticles (LNP) of these mRNA agents can lead to inflammation and immune exhaustion.[20]

In another study, mice exposed to mRNA-LNPs or LNP alone showed long-term inhibition of adaptive immune responses.[21] These mice had diminished resistance to the fungus *Candida albicans*, which correlated with a general decrease in blood neutrophil percentages. Mice that had been exposed to mRNA-LNP before got sick with the flu virus less often, and this was a trait they could pass on to their offspring.

According to the study's authors, "*pre-exposure to the mRNA-LNP platform has long-term effects on both innate and adaptive immune responses, with some of these traits even being inherited by the offspring.*"[21]

Polyethylene glycol (PEG) is part of the LNP structure. I have gone over the concerns raised by PEG, predominantly anaphylaxis, in the section titled "What is polyethylene glycol?"

3. **Mode of delivery**

I believe Marc Girardot's Bolus theory explains why *how* mRNA jabs are given plays a central role in their pathophysiology.

If mRNA is injected into vessels, then it will not only travel further around the body but also cause vascular damage via transfection. In some cases, this can be fatal.

More specifically, Bolus theory may explain why some people suffer severe vascular-related side effects soon after inoculation and others don't.

THREE EFFECTS

1. **Endothelial damage**

Subversion of our mucosal membrane and, in turn, our mucosal immune system, consisting of SIgA antibodies and resident TRM cells, was the first mistake.

Instead of allowing controlled virus exposure against a backdrop of supplementary medications or the development of a mucosal live attenuated vaccine, we were forced to wear masks (in ways that vilified the existence of our mucous membrane) and were told to be injected with mRNA technology.

Many people who were injected either didn't need it (they already had mucosal immunity) or were unprepared physiologically. Those inoculated were promised protection via a newly designed technology that circulated the body using our blood vessels and totally ignored the location where natural infection actually took place.

Some commonly proposed mechanisms for genetic-shot-induced vascular inflammation and injury include immune dysfunction and blood clotting (coagulation) via molecular mimicry;[22] endothelial damage via transfection (and subsequent T cell response);[23] and direct spike protein damage to endothelial layers.[24]

We've even got a study saying it out in the open: ***"Our study shows that the mRNA vaccine causes a prominent increase in inflammatory markers, especially after the 2nd dose, and a transient deterioration of endothelial function at 24h that returns to baseline at 48h. These results confirm the short-term cardiovascular safety of the vaccine."***[25]

Returning to the baseline is great and all, but a system-wide deterioration of our vascular system even for a minute is a cause for concern, let alone for longer than one day.

Microvessel damage in the brain is related to dementia;[26] damage to large vessels is related to aneurysms;[27] and damage to the vessels of the heart is related to pump failure.[28] Endothelial damage is also linked to fibrosis (tissue scarring) and cancer.[29] *Are the risks of these conditions increased after every shot?*

As vessels, both large and small, make up arguably the most important system in our body, trauma may likely lead to the emergence of chronic diseases and even be the underlying reason for recent fatalities.

2. **Immune dysfunction**

A recent Icelandic paper of over 11,000 PCR-positive people showed COVID-19 reinfection rates *rise* with the number of vaccine doses.[30]

If you have been connecting the dots so far, then you wouldn't be surprised by that result. But if you're not sure what that sentence means, think back to 2018 and ask yourself, *"If I were to be injected with something and it made me more likely to get sick with the pathogen it was supposed to protect me from, would I take it?"*

I bet (and hope) that nearly all of you would say "no."

And if I asked you, *"Why do you think this happens?"*

I'd hope that you have now learned that these shots mess with our immune systems.

I've come to think that underlying individual differences, the number of shots taken, and prior infection status play a significant role in the severity of immune dysfunction post-jab. This leads to a spectrum of immune-related side effects.

And if you combine this with the fact that our immune system plays a vital part in nearly all biological processes, then you may appreciate the depth of this problem.

To simplify matters, I think there are two (not mutually exclusive) forms of immune dysfunction one may suffer with post-jab: "SARS-CoV-2-specific" and "SARS-CoV-2-non-specific."

SARS-CoV-2-specific dysfunction refers to things that make it more likely to get SARS-CoV-2 but not other pathogens. These include the "hook effect," ADE, original antigenic sin OAS, chronic antigen stimulation, molecular mimicry, antigenic drift, and non-stimulation of mucosal immunity.

SARS-CoV-2-non-specific immune dysfunction is a broader issue that increases the likelihood of contracting SARS-CoV-2, *as well as* other pathogens and causing immune-related pathology like cancers.

The processes related to genetic jabs that cause SARS-CoV-2-non-specific immune dysfunction include innate immune suppression via type I IFN signalling impairment; T cell exhaustion; mRNA caps; GC enrichments;GP120 HIV-1 gene inserts; and the addition of N1-Methylpseudouridine.

N1-Methylpseudouridine is the methylated derivative of pseudouridine, an isomer of the nucleoside uridine. N1-Methylpseudouridine, a form of genetic engineering, has been used in these genetic shots to reduce our body's natural immune response to the mRNA by reducing the innate immune response as well as increasing (spike) protein output.[31]

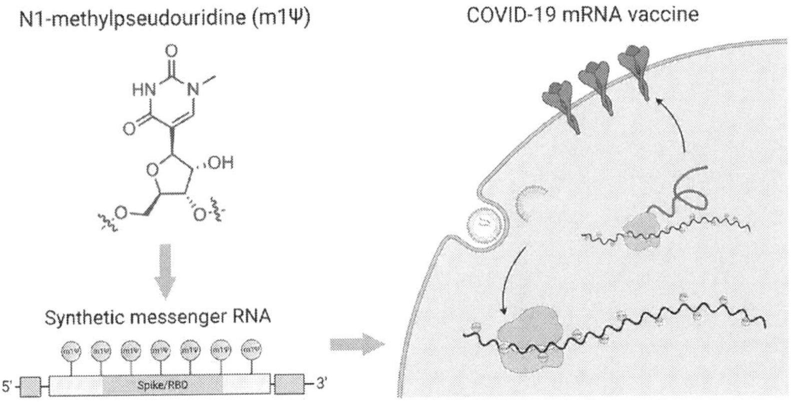

N1-Methylpseudouridine reduces mRNA immunogenicity, whilst also increasing protein production from synthetic mRNAs, from: https://pubs.acs.org/doi/10.1021/acscentsci.1c00197

Many of the mechanisms mentioned above are yet to be proven, but taken together, whichever way you look at it, it seems like immune dysfunction is not something to take lightly or to be unexpected.

If jabbed, the best one can hope for is a SARS-CoV-2 infection post-jab due to a lack of mucosal stimulation; the worst is a combination of the mechanisms highlighted above leading to increases in all types of infections, autoimmune conditions, and cancers.

3. **Cell death and ageing**

I have heard comments from people who have noted that many of their friends and families seemed to have aged rapidly over the last three years. Their observations may have scientific validity due to a number of reasons.

Cellular senescence is the process by which cells cease to divide and is a key biological process underlying ageing and disease formation.

It is thought we age due to cells progressively losing their ability to divide, which is essential to replace damaged cells that naturally accumulate over time.[32]

Just like everything else, senescence isn't all bad. *Biology is all about balance, remember?* Cellular senescence is a process that is important for normal development early in life and for tissue repair and stopping cancer growth later in life.[33]

This balance in the function of senescent cells is dependent on their elimination by the immune system once their beneficial functions have been performed.[33] Problems arise when cellular senescence is unwanted, however.

One problem with senescent cells is that they can express pro-inflammatory, tissue-destructive molecules; when this happens, they develop into a version called "senescence-associated secretory phenotype" (SASP). SASP can have deleterious effects on the tissue microenvironment as well as promoting tumour progression.[34]

Other than being unable to divide, senescent cells are also resistant to a process of programmed cell death called "apoptosis" and thus continue to "live."[35] You will agree that the fact that they can't die is not helpful when they are in a state that makes them more likely to get cancer and makes them more prone to inflammation.

Unwarranted cellular senescence occurs in response to many different triggers, including DNA damage and other cellular stressors, including coming into contact with cancer cells, spike protein,[36] and immune dysregulation.[37]

In one study, it was found that SARS-CoV-2 caused senescence in human cells that weren't already senescent and made the SASP worse in human cells that were already senescent.[36] Another study noted that the spike protein amplifies SASP in senescent cultured human cells.[38]

Cells, which have been either infected with SARS-CoV-2 or come into contact with mRNA, produce spike proteins on their surfaces. In some people, fusion of the infected cells with neighbouring cells occurs, which causes rupture of the nuclear membranes and the formation of a clump of cells called "syncytia."

Syncytia formation has been linked with more severe COVID-19 outcomes.[39] It seems like those who produce syncytia may have a lack or dysfunction of the IFN-Induced Transmembrane Proteins, a class of proteins that work with type I IFN and block many viruses by inhibiting virus–cell fusion. [40,41]

I bring this point up as syncytia can activate immunological pathways (cGAS and STING), which in turn can activate SASP as well as play a significant role in tissue fibrosis.[42,43]

Aside from causing some of the effects of ageing, ageing itself is linked to a weaker immune system and more infections. Thus, the relationship between senescence and immunity is likely to be bidirectional.[44]

If we're talking about ageing, we can't forget about prions and amyloid proteins, which are both linked to neurodegeneration, spike proteins, and ageing.

Prions, short for "proteinaceous infectious particles," are misfolded proteins that have the ability to transmit their misfolded shape onto normal variants of the same protein, causing fatal brain diseases that affect both animals and humans. They include the familiar mad cow disease (bovine spongiform encephalopathy) and scrapie in sheep, as well as chronic wasting disease (CWD) in deer. The primary human prion disease is known as Creutzfeldt-Jakob disease (CJD), a fatal neurological condition.

Amyloids are another type of protein that forms as a result of normal proteins losing their structure and thus their physiological functions. Amyloids are linked to a great number of diseases, including amyloidosis, Alzheimer's disease, and Parkinson's disease.[45] Amyloids are prion-like. Prions are an infectious form of amyloid proteins.[46]

The SARS-CoV-2 spike protein is prion-like, and thus it has been proposed that it could cause prion-like diseases.[47]

One study proposed that the spike protein's S1 component is prone to acting as a functional amyloid and forming toxic aggregates. They write that S1 has the ability ***"to form amyloid and toxic aggregates that can act as seeds to aggregate many of the misfolded brain proteins and can ultimately lead to neurodegeneration."***[48]

The authors of another study found a **prion-like domain in the RBD of the SARS-CoV-2 spike protein, which was missing from the original SARS-CoV virus.**[49] Asparagine (Q) and glutamine (N)-rich regions are a characteristic feature of many prion proteins and were found in SARS-CoV-2 but not in the original SARS-CoV virus.

Another study showed amyloid-like fibrils with evident branching were formed during the first 24 hours when spike protein was left co-intubated with another enzyme, protease neutrophil elastase *in vitro*.[50]

Worryingly too, the European Medicines Agency (EMA) Public Assessment Report—a document submitted to gain approval to market the vaccine in Europe—highlights one concerning finding, which is the presence of ***"fragmented species" of RNA in the injection solution***.[51] There is concern that these fragments would generate incomplete spike proteins, resulting in altered and unpredictable three-dimensional structures and a physiological impact that is at best neutral and at worst biologically detrimental.

Pfizer claims however that the RNA fragments *"likely... will not result in expressed proteins"* due to their assumed rapid degradation within the cell.[52] No data was presented to rule out protein expression, though, leaving the reviewers to comment, ***"These [fragmented RNA] forms are poorly characterised, and the limited data provided for protein expression do not fully address the uncertainties relating to the risk of translating proteins/peptides other than the intended spike protein."***[53]

The eye-opening review titled "SARS-CoV-2 Spike Protein in the Pathogenesis of Prion-like Diseases" further highlights the likelihood of prion-like protein and neurodegeneration formation by the spike protein and other components of the mRNA jab. In fact, they state, *"We explain why these prion-like characteristics are more relevant to vaccine-related mRNA-induced spike proteins than natural infection with SARS-CoV-2."* [54]

The authors of this paper go on to conclude, ***"In light of these considerations, the risk/benefit ratio for the mRNA vaccines needs to be reevaluated. With every vaccine comes a flood of spike protein released into the circulation, further advancing the potential for amyloidogenic effects and increasing the risk of future neurodegenerative disease."***[54]

To drive the point home further, I present to you a case study of a previously healthy woman in her 60s after her second jab.[55]

"A previously healthy woman in her 60s ***developed social isolation and behavioural abnormality in the form of moving around un-purposefully, irrelevant verbal responses and refusal to take food, one day after receiving the second dose of ChAdOx1 nCoV-19 vaccination***...*Over the next two days,* ***the patient developed difficulty in walking and echolalia*** ...*However, overall neurologic deterioration continued over the next two weeks, and* ***she developed respiratory distress and shock to which she finally succumbed after one month of admission***... *Although radiological and EEG findings in our patient are suggestive of a* ***prion disease like pathology****, we could not perform measurement of 14-3-3 protein in*

cerebrospinal fluid or post-mortem studies of the brain to confirm the diagnosis in this patient."[55]

She was diagnosed with rapidly progressive dementia before dying.

Cell death, senescence, and related tissue scarring have the potential to result in sudden fatality, cancer, and irreversible damage if located in high-risk areas of the body. If the vascular system is affected, then this can predispose the individual to atherosclerosis, strokes, and heart attacks.[56] If the reproductive organs are affected, this may lead to infertility.[57] And if the heart is affected, then this may result in scarring and/or enlargement of the heart muscle and result in sudden cardiac death.

Because spike proteins are similar to prions, there is a very real chance that many thousands of people in the future will get prion-like diseases and then die from them. And the process of ageing will bring about diseases more commonly associated with the elderly and early death.

HOW DOES THE SPIKE PREY ON WEAKNESS?

"Germ theory" is the currently widely accepted theory that specific microscopic organisms are the cause of specific diseases.[1]

The main idea behind this theory is that microorganisms, which are also called "germs" or "pathogens," infect the body and cause infectious diseases.

Tuberculosis (TB) is thought to be caused by a type of bacterium called *Mycobacterium tuberculosis*; polio is thought to be caused by one of three types of the poliovirus; malaria is thought to be caused by single-celled microorganisms of the *Plasmodium* group; COVID-19 is thought to be caused by SARS-CoV-2; and so on.

"Terrain theory," described as a "fringe set of beliefs" by one online article,[2] is the opposing theory that views pathogens as a consequence of disease, itself caused by other factors.

Simplifying it greatly, germ theory states that to avoid infectious diseases, one must avoid causative pathogens and find ways to eliminate them. Whereas terrain theory argues that if our biological systems are healthy and well-balanced, then germs are a natural part of life and will be dealt with by the body without causing disease.

Asymptomatic carriers of disease, the increased susceptibility to infection in certain types of people, similar disease presentations attributed to various pathogens, and infectious disease states worsening in those with additional exposure to other environmental toxins all support the terrain theory.

In one Danish study, it was found that people with higher levels of perfluorinated alkylate substances in their blood were more likely to have a worse case of COVID-19.[3]This is a good example of terrain theory. Perfluorinated alkylate substances are environmental toxins that are used as stain, water, and grease repellents in carpets, clothing, and cooking tools like nonstick coatings.

On the other hand, the efficacy of antibiotics, the pathognomonic features of some infectious diseases, and the success of traditional vaccines (some of which may be put down to improvements in population-wide living conditions too)[4] are some examples supporting germ theory.

Just like other areas of science, I believe the compartmentalisation of the complex interplay between us, pathogens, and the environment into two distinct theories is too reductionist. These two theories appear to me to be on opposite ends of the spectrum, when in fact the real answers are somewhere in the middle.

In reality, I don't think humanity can claim to know even 1% of the human immune system, so I'm hedging my bets, playing it safe, and sticking to the middle using the available evidence. *I mean, how can I be so confident with absolute claims when it's hard to know whether or not viruses actually cause disease?*

Remember Kary Mullis, the Nobel Prize-winning inventor of PCR? Well, he earned a reputation for being labelled an "AIDS denier" for asking his colleagues if they could provide him with one scientific reference showing that HIV probably caused AIDS. They couldn't.

This is what he writes in his autobiography titled "Dancing Naked In The Mind Field":

"I did computer searches. Neither Montagnier, Gallo, nor anyone else had published papers describing experiments which led to the conclusion that HIV probably caused AIDS. I read the papers in Science for which they had become well known as the AIDS doctors, but all they had said there was that they had found evidence of a past infection by something which was probably HIV in some AIDS patients. They found antibodies."[5]

Antibody detection isn't always cut and dry, however, even with regards to HIV and the symptoms of AIDS. Take the case of a 71-year-old homosexual man who came to the hospital with a fever and lots of tick bites that had been going on for four days. HIV tests came back (falsely) positive for him, yet he was actually diagnosed with *Babesiosis,* a parasitic infection caused by deer ticks, not HIV. The case study abstract concludes with, ***"the positive HIV serology turned negative after successful treatment of babesiosis."***[6] Antibodies aren't always reliable for inferring causation.

One way to establish a causal relationship between a microbe and a disease is by using Koch's postulates, four rules that scientists Robert Koch and Friedrich Loeffler came up with in 1884.[7] These are:

1. The organism must be shown to be invariably present in characteristic form and arrangement in the diseased tissue.
2. The organism, which from its relationship to the diseased tissue appears to be responsible for the disease, must be isolated and grown in pure culture.
3. The pure culture must be shown to induce the disease experimentally.
4. The organism should be re-isolated from the experimentally infected subject (this postulate was added after Loeffler).

But because there are some exceptions to these rules and because the rules were originally made for living things, particularly bacteria, scientists have come to realise that they are hard to apply to pathogens that are not alive, like viruses and infectious proteins.[8]

Did you know that it has been noted that SARS-CoV-2 does not fulfil Koch's postulates?[9] The link between the virus and the disease isn't as absolute as germ theory advocates say it is. In other words, SARS-CoV-2 may not *cause* COVID-19. *Shock, horror.*

It can be appreciated why germ theory is popular today. If specific microorganisms cause specific diseases, this means specific treatments need to be developed. And in turn, preventative measures are sidelined or viewed as quack medicine.

But playing devil's advocate, if the extreme take on germ theory *was* correct with regards to COVID-19, then we would all be dead and you wouldn't be reading this book right now.

Though Koch's postulates are not met, it appears (until better quality counter-evidence is presented) that there is no other explanation than that we require the "germ" SARS-CoV-2 to achieve COVID-19. *But why do some people get sick or have side effects while others don't?*

This is a key question to ask, especially as the spectrum of COVID-19 and jab-related symptoms ranges from death to being completely seemingly unaffected. **If the virus is the same, then the differences in disease states must be due to individual variabilities.**

We have already learned that immunological imbalances can not only increase one's systemic susceptibility to SARS-CoV-2 but can also predispose the individual to sustained inflammatory responses.

Those who were already unwell are more likely to become unwell with COVID-19. Risk factors associated with those with COVID-19 *not* returning to "usual health" include having high blood pressure (hypertension), obesity, a psychiatric condition, or an immunosuppressive condition.[10]

Risk factors for severe COVID-19, hospital admission, and death as a result of COVID-19 include older age, male sex, non-white ethnicity, being disabled, and pre-existing comorbidities including obesity, cardiovascular disease, respiratory disease, hypertension, and diabetes.10,11

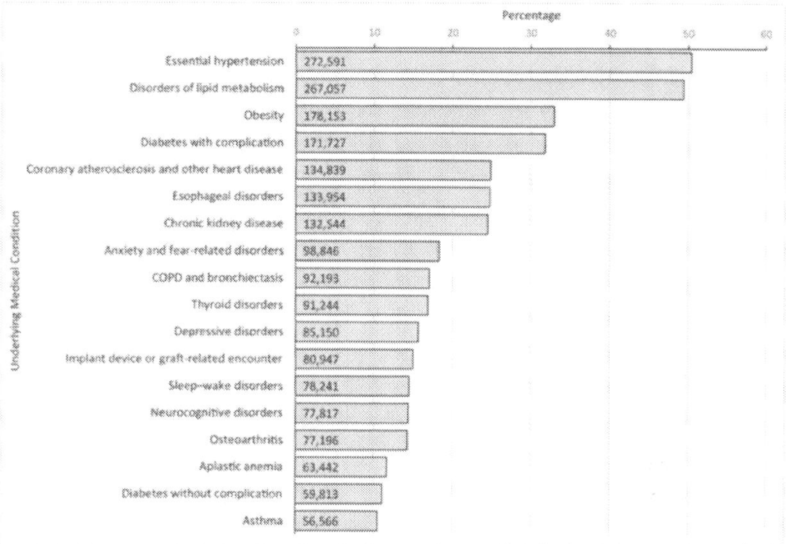

The prevalence of the most frequent underlying medical conditions in a sample of US adults hospitalised with COVID-19, March 2020–March 2021. https://www.cdc.gov/pcd/issues/2021/21_0123.htm

In addition to the way the injection is given, I think that the spike protein (and other viral and genetic components) uncovers and speeds up individual biological risk factors and weaknesses (you could say "faulty terrain"), which causes the wide range of disease states after the jab and COVID-19.

Let's say you were already at risk of developing dementia, for example, and had a leaky BBB. Well, if you got COVID-19 and/or had the jabs, the BBB damage would probably get worse, and the brain and blood vessels around it would get inflamed.[12] This could lead to a full diagnosis of the neurodegenerative disease.

This could also be true for cancers, in which precancerous cells become cancerous when they come into contact with the spike protein, other parts of the jab, or/and via immunodysregulation.

And if you already had low-level pancreatic abnormalities, then your chances of developing diabetes may have increased with post-spike exposure too,[13] and so on and so forth.

When and how these side effects show up depends on a number of things, such as the severity of any underlying pre-existing disease, the number of times a person has been sick with COVID-19 and/or had the jabs, how long each bout of illness lasted, whether or not a person has biological reserves to repair damage, other lifestyle factors, and where in the body the damage happened.

The fact of the matter is that we will never be able to infer *direct causation* between spike proteins and new illnesses. Also, the longer it takes for a disease to show up after being infected or immunised, the more likely it is that other things played a role in it.

Even so, I must remind you that there are no direct randomised controlled trials "proving" that smoking causes cancer, even though the link has been established using all other types of data and is now widely accepted.

Whether you are team "germ" or team "terrain," I hope you can appreciate that the full acceptance of germ theory predisposes the individual to look externally for help, whereas the terrain theory forces the individual to look within, accept potential flaws, and mitigate these before they become unwell. One is inherently reactive and externally seeking, while the other is proactively self-reliant.

The last three years should have shown you that the vast majority of people are only reactive to problems as they arrive, rushing to buy toilet paper and not preventing illness. In a way, this way of thinking is not their fault; most people either don't have the time, urgency, or knowledge to know what to do.

It also doesn't help that during the peak of the pandemic, institutions were promoting donuts,[14] cannabis,[15] burgers,[16] and prostitutes,[17] completely ignoring the importance of our health terrain. If you try searching for terrain theory on Wikipedia, you will find it under "Germ theory denialism." This reflects the state of society we currently live in.

Popularity and a near-religious belief in germ theory led most people to embrace a so-called "therapeutic" that had not been thoroughly tested while ignoring other methods of staying healthy.

It seems like human nature has not changed. This is what Pierre Jacques Antoine Béchamp, the French scientist and father of terrain theory had to say over two hundred years ago:[18]

> **"THE GENERAL PUBLIC, HOWEVER INTELLIGENT, ARE STRUCK ONLY BY THAT WHICH IT TAKES LITTLE TROUBLE TO UNDERSTAND. THEY HAVE BEEN TOLD THAT THE INTERIOR OF THE BODY IS SOMETHING MORE OR LESS LIKE THE CONTENTS OF A VESSEL FILLED WITH WINE, AND THAT THIS INTERIOR IS NOT INJURED – THAT WE DO NOT BECOME ILL, EXCEPT WHEN GERMS, ORIGINALLY CREATED MORBID, PENETRATE INTO IT FROM WITHOUT, AND THEN BECOME MICROBES.**
>
> **"THE PUBLIC DO NOT KNOW WHETHER THIS IS TRUE; THEY DO NOT EVEN KNOW WHAT A MICROBE IS, BUT THEY TAKE IT ON THE WORD OF THE MASTER; THEY BELIEVE IT BECAUSE IT IS SIMPLE AND EASY TO UNDERSTAND; THEY BELIEVE AND THEY REPEAT THAT THE MICROBE MAKES US ILL WITHOUT INQUIRING FURTHER, BECAUSE THEY HAVE NOT THE LEISURE – NOR, PERHAPS, THE CAPACITY – TO PROBE TO THE DEPTHS THAT WHICH THEY ARE ASKED TO BELIEVE."**
>
> PIERRE JACQUES ANTOINE BÉCHAMP

I hope that recent years have forced the scientific community to reconsider concepts that we have long taken for granted. And maybe one day we will get to a stage where we will appreciate or even disprove the role of spike proteins in disease occurrence. But until that happens, it's all pointing towards the fact that the spike preys on our weaknesses.

As I was taught in medical school, *"If it walks like a dog, wags its tail like a dog, and barks like a dog, it's a dog until proven otherwise."*

STEPHEN'S STORY

My name is Stephen and I'm 49 years old. Prior to the vaccine I was working as a service delivery supervisor for an offshore oil company in Aberdeen, Scotland.

I have 5 children (2 are stepchildren) and 2 grand-children who I try to spend as much time with as I can. I worked as much as I could to help support my family and enjoyed my free time on the weekends. I love to go to watch Aberdeen at Pittodrie stadium.

I got the vaccine solely because I wanted to protect my elderly mother who suffered a stroke around 20 years ago and has had ill health ever since. I thought It was the right thing to do as we were told COVID was a massive threat to people who were already compromised.

I got my first AstraZeneca vaccine on the 7th of April 2021, in my left arm.

It was just a usual day like any other and I was on my way to work when I began feeling a lot of pain at the top of my back and chest and was experiencing tingling all down my arms with pins and needles in my fingers.

I was driving one of the young lads I work with into work that day when I had to explain to him he would have to walk the rest of the way. I knew I needed to go to the hospital right away.

Me being me, I cracked open a can of energy drink and sparked a cigarette to calm my nerves and drove myself to the hospital.

I'd never experienced something like this happen to me before. The journey was a blur, I was running on adrenaline.

Arriving at the hospital, I somehow managed to reverse into a parking space. I was beginning to experience noticeable muscle weakness in my left arm, I actually had to use both hands to get the gear stick into reverse.

I walked myself into the Accident and Emergency, gave the receptionist my details and sat in the waiting area.

After a few minutes, a voice called me "Mr Bowie, you can go down to the ward now". As I tried to stand up, nothing would move. I just couldn't get my legs to work.

"I'm sorry'. I replied. "I canna stand up, I think I'm going to need some help"

They transferred me to a bed via wheelchair as I was now paralysed from the neck down for almost two weeks, including two nights in ICU as my heart rate had dipped dangerously low.

Medical staff were bamboozled and mentioned a stroke but because a stroke usually only affects one side, they continued to deliberate.

I was in blind panic; the doctor could only reply with "I don't know,I don't know "

After many tests, they told me I had suffered an extremely rare type of spinal stroke.

I did not leave that hospital for 1 month. Only to be transferred to Woodend's neurologist rehabilitation department.

There, I had to learn how to walk unaided again, feed myself, pick things up, everything again. Neurology tests confirm my left arm is blocked and although I can now make a fist I cannot grasp or use as normal. My left hand is gone.

I had to be fed for 2 weeks, all this gave me depression and anxiety to add to my problems.

Whilst in the first hospital, A doctor told me someone else had come in two weeks after me with the same symptoms. They had suffered the very same spinal stroke.

It was such a rare injury that to see two of them in the same hospital within two weeks of each other was unheard of in the medical world.

We both had received the AstraZeneca vaccine within 4 weeks of our strokes.

The same doctor came to see me, accompanied by a student or junior. They closed the curtains round my bed and confirmed with me verbally that the stroke was indeed a reaction to the vaccine.

He told me he had filled out a form for the yellow card scheme, the UK system for recording adverse effects through medicine and vaccines.

My head was spinning during this interaction and I did not think to ask for the statement in writing.

Whilst in the rehabilitation hospital, they arranged to get a 2nd vaccine.

Initially I refused. I point blank refused to take AstraZeneca anyway. When challenged, they asked why and I replied that the 1st COVID vaccine was what put me in hospital in the first place. To which, they didn't say much.

I was discharged with a 5 week Course of Physio and occupational therapy, coming to my house 4 days a week between them both.

Now I get an occasional appointment at Woodend but nothing routine. I go to RGU University to be the subject of student training when trainee physios start. Its finished right now,as there is usually around a 3 week break in between, I value this treatment because it's one of the few things which gets me out the house now.

I am ashamed to admit but a few days after I left the hospital on the 30th of July 2021 I took my 2nd COVID vaccine. Pfizer this time. The nurse even questioned my decision due to my notes showing vaccine injury from the first time around.

Things were so bad at this point, I was very depressed, I didn't see how it could possibly get worse and didn't care if it finished me off this time.

Some people won't understand why but I got it because they were still saying we couldn't see our loved ones without being fully vaccinated (at the time that meant 2) and I hadn't seen mum in months.

If the nurse could see this, I question why I wasn't discharged with any notes myself.

I asked for all my backdated notes from the doctor,

for 2 years before this happened to hold evidence that the vaccine did this, not my previous state of health which was always pretty good.

I have 2 blood clots, in my neck and my left lung. My notes will clearly show I had chest x-rays a few months before that were clear. All evidence points to the COVID vaccine.

I am taking clopidogrel for the clots, no MRI was ordered and no observations to monitor their size or severity.

The hospital told me "That's not something we do here" I would have to arrange and pay for my own scans or go private which I can't afford.

I thought that it was strange that they themselves wouldn't want to know what the cause was for this or how they were developing. They cause me pain, stress and a lot of worry.

My injury has affected every aspect of life, I can't even go for a pint before the footie anymore.

I'm using crutches and a wheelchair which my family must push as I can't wheel myself around.

My father bought me a mobility scooter which I use to go see my mum who stays 20 mins away and it gives me some type of control.

I feel anxious leaving the house, I don't want to bump into people I know as I'm not as confident as I used to be. The difference in me is like day and night.

I lost my job in April 2022 after holding my position for 8 years, almost a year after I took the vaccine.

I have friends and family who give me support,my amazing partner Julie is there for me day and night,I couldn't do this without her support.

I'm on twitter but it's a mine field of negativity and scammers.

One day I noticed a post about benefits grants and left a comment asking where the support was for vaccine injured persons?

Kirsty Blackman, a Scottish MP privately messaged me, and I am currently waiting for her to get back to me in hope of helping, not just me but all those suffering vaccine injury. I am grateful for her help.

It's not often you get help from people in a position of authority.

I also use Backup trust, a London based charity where they pair you with a mentor whose injury is as close to your own as possible, however not many people have such a rare condition as I do

It only ran for 10 weeks but I try to keep in touch with the people I have met there.

I haven't even thought about the future because this feels like this is it, a disabled future with such uncertainty.

I am so far away from what I was hoping my future to be like.

If I could say anything to others out there it is fight. Fight for help.

If you're not sure, reach out and ask, I hope there will be something positive that comes from this.

HOW MANY MORE EXCESS DEATHS?

If you've been paying attention recently, you may have noticed an increasing number of news reports outlining the sudden tragic deaths of previously healthy individuals. One notable example is Shane Warne, the legendary Australian cricket player who sadly passed away on March 4, 2022, from a suspected heart attack.[1]

Another is mountain biker Rab Wardell, who died in his sleep at the age of 37, just two days after winning the Scottish championship. He even appeared on BBC Scotland's The Nine programme, on Monday the 22nd August, the day before his death. *"Olympian Katie Archibald said she tried desperately to save her partner Rab Wardell as he suffered a fatal cardiac arrest in bed beside her."*, one BBC article notes.[2]

Some news reports state that these individuals had been fully jabbed, whilst others do not delve into this detail. And mainstream media aren't the only ones shying away from giving us the full picture.

It's been hard to get clear-cut evidence of possible jab-related deaths. Secondary sources of information, like the ones provided by the CDC and other government-funded agencies, are littered with pro-vaccine biases, skewed information, and straight-up lies.

And as we know, the UK doesn't have the data of those who have been harmed or suffered illness from a COVID-19 shot, as this is not recorded on the death certificate.[3] I would also like to add that even if jabs were suspected to have been the primary cause of death in a particular case, it is more likely than not that the healthcare bureaucratic powers that be will not allow such a controversial and blastformous entry to be written in legal documents.

Politics aside, we know that younger people are more likely to experience side effects post-jab compared to their older counterparts.[4] And people in general who have had a previous COVID-19 infection are almost twice as likely to experience side effects post-jab too.[5]

What no one wants to talk about is why there is a rise in excess mortality in all or nearly all of the genetic-agent-jabbed countries.

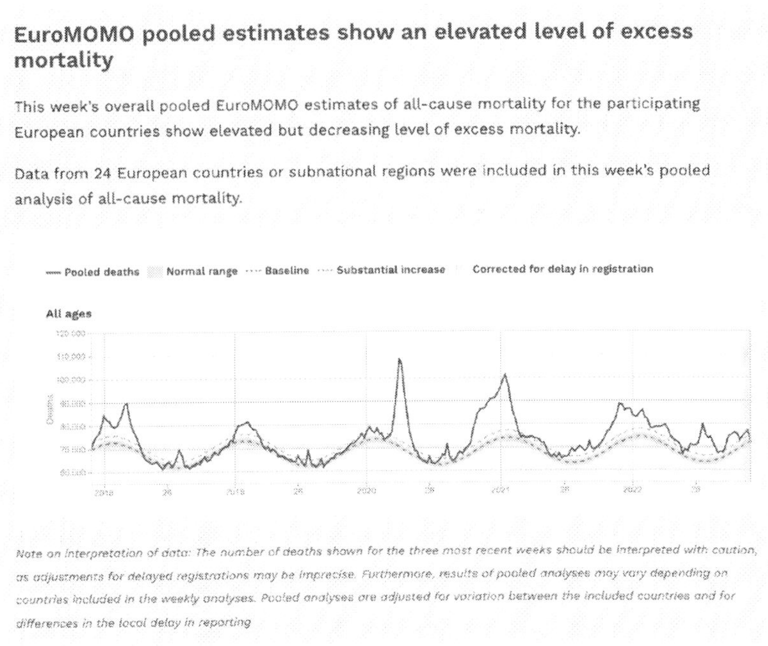

EuroMOMO pooled estimates show an elevated level of excess mortality

This week's overall pooled EuroMOMO estimates of all-cause mortality for the participating European countries show elevated but decreasing level of excess mortality.

Data from 24 European countries or subnational regions were included in this week's pooled analysis of all-cause mortality.

Note on interpretation of data: The number of deaths shown for the three most recent weeks should be interpreted with caution, as adjustments for delayed registrations may be imprecise. Furthermore, results of pooled analyses may vary depending on countries included in the weekly analyses. Pooled analyses are adjusted for variation between the included countries and for differences in the local delay in reporting

Note the excess deaths (dark line) above the others from European data, from: https://www.euromomo.eu/

What is causing the 148,479 non-COVID deaths registered in England and Wales from December 28, 2019 to August 19, 2022? A 17.8% increase in the number of deaths registered in the UK above the five-year average for that week.[6]

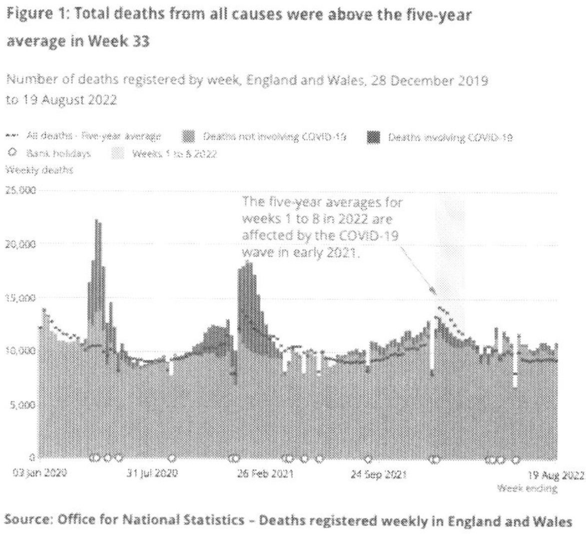

Excess deaths in the UK, from: https://www.ons.gov.uk/

Why are Native Americans, who led the way in the US vaccination effort, disproportionately dying?[7]

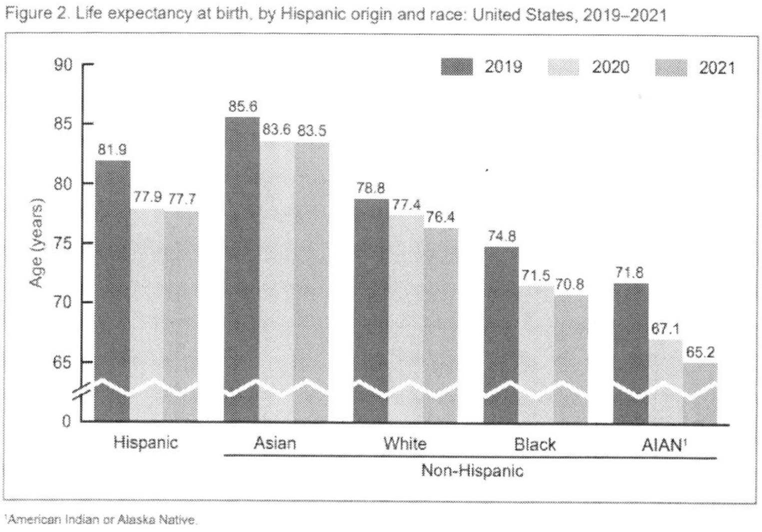

Dramatic drop in life expectancy of American Indian or Alaska native people year after year throughout the pandemic, from: https://www.cdc.gov/nchs/data/vsrr/vsrr023.pdf

Why is there a correlation between the spring fourth dose booster rollout among over-75s in England and a wave of now over 15,300 non-Covid excess deaths?

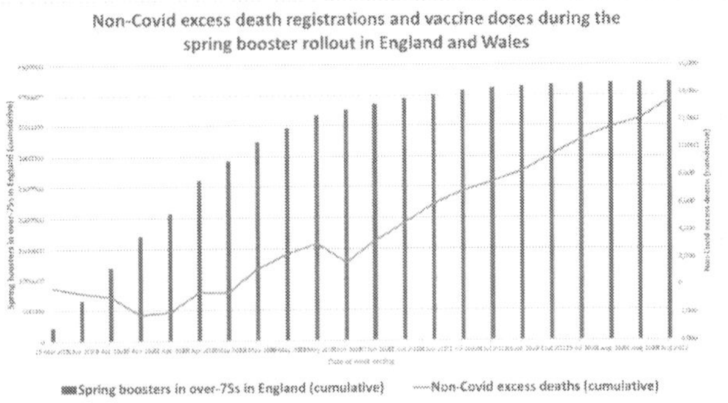

Non-COVID excess death and vaccine doses during spring booster rollout in England and Wales, from: https://dailysceptic.org/2022/09/01/excess-non-covid-deaths-top-15300-in-17-weeks-as-mysterious-wave-of-heart-deaths-continues/

Why has 80% jabbed Australia suffered with 15,000 excess deaths since October 2021?

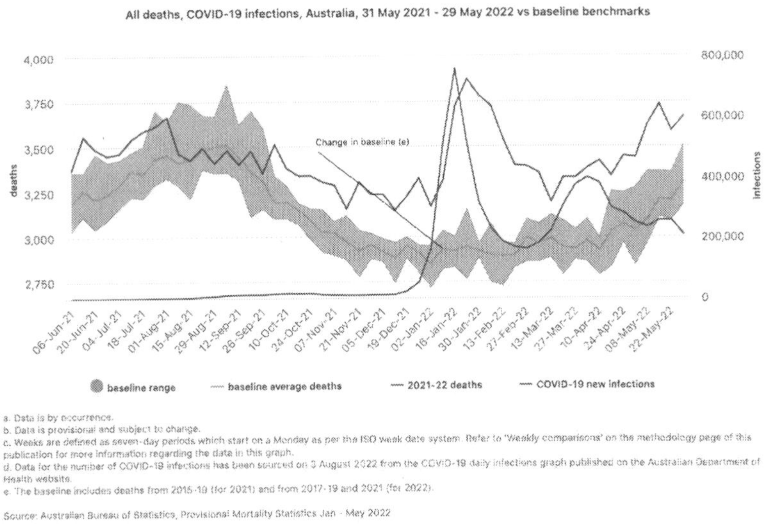

A dramatic increase in baseline average deaths in Australia, from: https://www.abs.gov.au/statistics/health/causes-death/provisional-mortality-statistics/latest-release

Why are people dying, and why are the mainstream media shying away from reporting this? They were only eagerly reporting minute-by-minute COVID-19 related deaths a year and a half ago. *What happened?*

I understand that there are a plethora of causes, such as lockdowns, increased psychological stress, financial stress, and poorer metabolic health, over the pandemic period that could have contributed to some of the increase in death that we are witnessing now. But what about the rise in mortality among the young and the 769 men and women who collapsed with heart issues during competition over the course of 2021 and early 2022?[8]

At the moment, to avoid biases, it may be best to include anecdotal evidence as well as raw figures when analysing data. And both of these tell a sorry story.

WHY ARE THERE MORE PEOPLE DYING SUDDENLY?

Mortality data from the Office for National Statistics (ONS) for England and Wales from the 1st of May 2021 until the 17th of September 2021 showed a significant excess, particularly in the 15–19 year age group. This is between 16% or 47% above expected levels, depending on the baseline chosen.[1] The data also shows that a disproportionate number of these excess deaths were among males.[2]

Could it be attributed to suicides? Well, I don't think so. I don't disagree with the fact that lockdowns and quarantines had an effect on the mental health of the country as a whole. During my placement in Children & Adolescence Mental Health Services in the summer of 2021, I was deeply saddened by the sheer number of attempted suicides I was seeing on the ward. Some children as young as 13 years old were on the ward for serious attempts on their lives—an age where I was mostly preoccupied with video games.

I don't think this rise in excess deaths is solely due to suicides due to the timing of the rise in deaths among young people. Studies have shown that suicides among young people happened after a month of the implementation of lockdown.[3] We instead saw a rise in deaths among young men and teenagers since the beginning of May-June 2021 (using UK data), as indicated by the graph below. People aged 18 and over in England were being invited to book their first COVID-19 jab in June of 2021.[4] 16 and 17-year-olds were invited two months later, in August.[5]

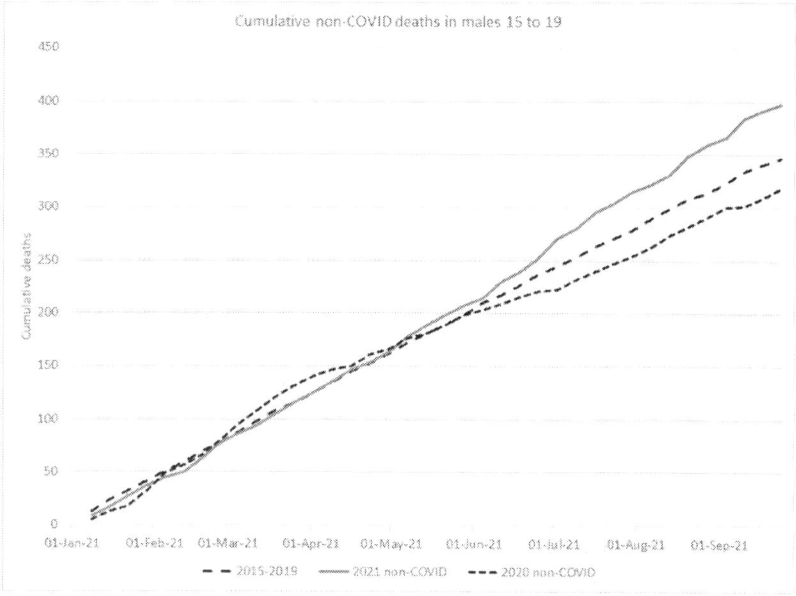

Cumulative non-COVID deaths in males 15 to 19 in 2021 England, from: https://www.hartgroup.org/recent-deaths-in-young-people-in-england-and-wales/

Even if we ignore the raw data, we can't ignore the rise in sudden deaths among young athletes, most of whom are men. In 2021, a German news agency made a list of 75 European athletes who died "suddenly" after being fully jabbed in the second half of the year.[6] By November 2021, there had been 54 collapses reported in sports games in the four and a half months since Christian Eriksen collapsed shortly before halftime in Denmark's opening Euro 2020 game against Finland.7 Thirty of the 54 collapses resulted in deaths, almost all of which occurred in players aged 15 to 19.

Avi Barot, 29, pro cricketer, cardiac arrest, dies. Abou Ali, 22, pro footballer collapses on pitch.Fabrice NSakala, 31, Besiktas defender collapses on pitch.Jens De Smet, 27, footballer collapses on field, dies of heart attack.Jente van Genechten, 25, footballer - heart attack.Frederic Lartillot, pro footballer dies of heart attack after game. Benjamin Taft, 31, pro footballer dies of heart attack. Rune Coghe, 18, pro footballer - cardiac arrest on pitch. Helen Edwards, referee, heart issues World Cup qualifier. Dimitri Lienard, 33, midfielder collapses during game. Sergio Aguero, 33, pro footballer - cardiac exam after match. Emil Palsson, 28, midfielder, cardiac arrest during game. Antoine Mchin, 31, triathlete, pulmonary embolism following Moderna. Luis Ojeda, 20, football player unexpectedly passes away. Greg Luyssen, 22, Belgian pro cyclist ends career - heart issues.Pedro Obiang, 29, ex-West Ham star - myocarditis post vaccine.Cienna Knowles, 19, equestrian star, blood clots.

Only a handful of athletes who succumbed to a number of conditions, collapsed and even died in 2021.

It is not uncommon for people to die from sudden cardiac death. Between the years of 2012 and 2017, one study of more than 2 million inhabitants showed that the annual incidence of sudden cardiac death ranged from 36.8 to 39.7 per 100,000.[7]

But why have so many footballers gone on to suffer in an industry that is known to screen for cardiac abnormalities? And sports aside, I just worry that we are recently seeing more of these occur than we should, especially with excess mortality figures on the rise.

What could possibly be going on?

WHAT IS MYOCARDITIS?

Myocarditis is an inflammation of the heart muscle, a serious condition linked to fatal misfiring of the heartbeat, heart failure, and even sudden death. Pericarditis is an inflammation of the pericardium, the saclike tissue that surrounds the heart. We know that these jabs are linked to both conditions. Some countries noted this risk early on and halted the use of these jabs in young people,[1] not the UK or US though.

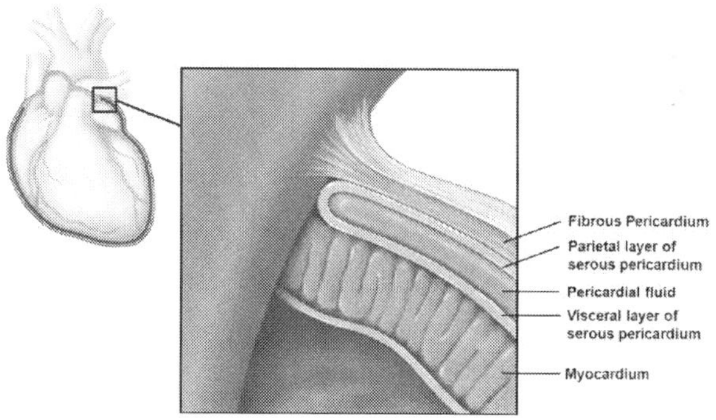

The layers of the heart, from: https://www.clevelandclinicmeded.com/

The worrying thing about myocarditis is that it can lay dormant, affecting people asymptomatically until it is too late.[2] It is a condition with a mortality rate of 7-15% and accounts for up to 17% of sudden cardiac death in children younger than 16 years.[3]

It seems like individuals who are jabbed are more likely to develop myocarditis than those who haven't. One Isreali study showed that individuals vaccinated with Pfizer's mRNA shot had a 3.24-fold increased risk of myocarditis within 21 days of either the first or second dose compared to unvaccinated individuals.[4] A US study showed that those aged 12-39 years old had a 9.8-fold increased risk of myocarditis/pericarditis at days 1–21 of vaccination compared to those at days 22–42 of vaccination.[5]

And recently, a Thai preprint of 301 students aged 13–18 years old found one case of myopericarditis, four cases of subclinical myocarditis, and two cases of pericarditis among the 301 participants.[6] That's heart inflammation in one in 43 young people. In the same study, 54 participants (18%) had a rapid heart rate or abnormal heart rhythm. Of these, 39 reported symptoms such as palpitations or chest pain. Fifteen reported no symptoms at all.[6]

Due to the relatively short period of time in circulation as well as the lack of post-mortems, the underlying pathophysiological mechanisms of COVID-19 jab-induced myocarditis are still unknown. Current theories of why some people suffer from myocarditis post-vaccination include:

REINFECTION

We mustn't forget that myocarditis is normally commonly caused by viral infections, including SARS-CoV-2.[7] We also know that individuals who've been vaccinated are still able to suffer from COVID-19. As we have now learned, jabbing against the SARS-CoV may actually enhance the disease with reexposure. This is what was found in early animal studies for SARS-CoV-1 and the Middle East respiratory syndrome coronavirus.[8] Vaccinated animals had enhanced disease with reexposure to wild-type virus after vaccination, likely due to non-neutralising antibodies resulting in ADE of immunity.[8]

This also brings up the importance of checking immunity status before getting injected, something that we did not do. Many of us would have unknowingly been naturally immune from the virus before getting jabbed, but many likely became unwell post-jabs. In theory, that's exposure to the spike or pathogen four times if unwell with COVID-19 after two shots.

Compounding damage cannot be ruled out.

INCREASED AUTO-ANTIBODIES AND MOLECULAR MIMICRY.

A case report of a patient with myocarditis post-jab noted that the patient had higher levels of antibodies against some self-antigens.[9] And it should be noted that in the past, people with myocarditis have been more likely to have heart-reactive autoantibodies in their blood. Autoantibodies are found more frequently in first-degree relatives of patients with cardiomyopathy than in the healthy population.[10]

Another proposed mechanism for myocarditis is molecular mimicry between the spike protein of SARS-CoV-2 and self-antigens.[11] The antibodies that the jabbed produce against SARS-CoV-2 spike glycoproteins have been shown to cross-react with structurally similar human peptide protein sequences, including α-myosin. α-myosin is a type of cardiac muscle involved in active force generation. Mutations in α-myosin have been shown to be linked with congenital heart defects, dilated cardiomyopathy and hypertrophic cardiomyopathy (pathological enlargements of the heart.)[12,13]

MODE OF INJECTION

Going back to the Bolus Theory, a study examining the hearts, blood, and other organ profiles of mice injected with Pfizer's mRNA shot via the intramuscular (muscle) route compared to the intravenous (vein) route showed that mice that were given the shot intravenously suffered from ***"multifocal myopericarditis with elevated serum troponin, cardiomyocyte degeneration, and changes of both necrosis and apoptosis, adjacent inflammatory infiltrate of mononuclear cells, interstitial edema, and visceral pericardial calcification within two days post injection."***[14]

Basically, excessive cardiac damage.

Concerningly, the study also revealed ***"histopathological changes of myopericarditis deteriorated and became rather diffuse after the second dose boosting with either IV or IM administration 14 days after the first dose of priming."*** Repeated vaccinations may cause further cardiac damage.[14]

INCREASED CARDIAC INFLAMMATION

A recent study showed that the vaccines may directly damage heart muscles by dramatically increasing inflammation on the endothelium and T cell infiltration of cardiac muscle. The study concluded that this ***"may account for the observations of increased thrombosis, cardiomyopathy, and other vascular events following vaccination.'"***[15]

ADRENALINE SURGE

Autopsies of two teenage boys who were found dead in bed three and four days after receiving the second dose of the Pfizer-BioNTech COVID-19 shot showed the presence of catecholamine-induced myocardial injury.[16] This is not typical myocarditis in this age group.

Catecholamines are hormones important in stress responses and nerve system function. Examples of them include epinephrine (adrenaline), norepinephrine (noradrenaline), and dopamine. The release of the hormones epinephrine and norepinephrine from the adrenal medulla of the adrenal glands is part of the fight-or-flight response.

The autopsy study goes on to note that what was seen were "***areas of contraction bands and hypereosinophilic myocytes distinct from the inflammation. This injury pattern is instead similar to what is seen in the myocardium of patients***

who are clinically diagnosed with Takotsubo, toxic, or "stress" cardiomyopathy, which is a temporary myocardial injury that can develop in patients with extreme physical, chemical, or sometimes emotional stressors."[17]

In plain English, jabs may harm certain people's hearts when associated with a surge of adrenaline. The combination of the two may stress the heart, causing cardiac damage.

Another study reviewing the epidemiological and biological findings of mRNA-induced sudden cardiac death also agreed that catecholamine-triggered myocarditis played a pivotal role in the condition.[18] They discovered that SARS-CoV-2 mRNA and spike protein are found in higher concentrations in the area of the adrenal glands that produce adrenaline; that SARS-CoV-2 mRNA leads to an enhanced conversion of dopamine into noradrenaline; and that younger, fitter men had higher physiological catecholamine levels than older, heavier men.

In combination, they note, "***All this evidence was fully concordant, which supported the proposed hypothesis that catecholamines are a key player in the SARS-CoV-2 mRNA vaccine-induced myocarditis and the consequent apparent increase in sudden deaths."***[18]

And:

"It is unlikely that the enhanced catecholamine release, response, receptor sensitivity, and overall activity acted alone to provoke the vaccine-induced, catecholamine-triggered myocardial complications. ***The catecholamines possibly acted synergistically with other dysfunctions, including abnormal immunological and inflammatory responses, as they alone may cause myocarditis only during extreme catecholamine exposure."***[18]

Free radicals are unstable atoms that have the potential to harm cells, resulting in disease and ageing. Free radicals have been linked to ageing as well as a variety of diseases, including shot-induced cardiac death.

Surges in catecholamines, like adrenaline, can affect heart tissue directly and are also a potential source of oxygen-derived free radicals. There is also a feedback loop between catecholamines and cytokines.

LIPID NANOPARTICLE

One review speculated on the role of LNP in causing deleterious effects on myocardial cells, whether as a result of an immune response to it or its aggregate with the mRNA strand within the jab preparations.[19]

PEG has been shown to be implicated in other hypersensitivity reactions, which could in theory cause cardiac damage. But the autopsy report discussed above noted that *"A hypersensitivity reaction is in the differential diagnosis, however, infrequency/lack of eosinophils would be unusual."*,[17] making the cause of myocarditis in that case less likely.

More studies are needed.

SEX DIFFERENCES

There are many possible reasons why young men unfavourably develop jab-induced myocarditis compared to women.

Firstly it is thought that oestrogen (the predominantly female sex hormone) may have inhibitory effects on pro-inflammatory T cells, resulting in a decrease in the body's inflammatory immune responses.[20] Pericarditis incidence is also higher in women during the postmenopausal period, where oestrogen levels are lower.[20]

Women also carry more body fat. One mouse study suggested that white adipose tissue (a type of body fat) may serve as a reservoir for SARS-CoV-2, sparing the lungs from the viral burden and infection severity.[21] They note, *"It is well documented that females have higher body fat content compared to males and the fat distribution pattern differs between the sexes, which constitute one reason why males are more susceptible to pulmonary CoV2 infection."*[21] More data is needed to confirm whether this is true with regard to cardiac damage.

It is looking like younger fitter men (e.g. pro-football players) are more likely to suffer from post-jab myocarditis due to a combination of reasons. Young healthy men naturally tend to have lower body fat percentages, higher circulating testosterone levels, greater heart muscle mass and increased vascularity (increasing the risk of intravenous inoculation). Combining the other reasons mentioned above, young men may also metabolise the mRNA shots "better", creating more spike proteins than the average person. This may be why the Moderna vaccine is linked with a 2.5-times increased risk of myocarditis than Pfizer's.[22] Moderna's mRNA jab dose (100 micrograms) is higher than Pfizer's (30 micrograms).[23]

THRESHOLD THEORY

Sudden cardiac deaths were happening long before the pandemic, no one is arguing with that. Various risk factors and triggers have been noted in the literature of increasing one's likelihood of this fatal condition. These include everything from congenital cardiac abnormalities[24] to exposure to heavy metal toxins like arsenic,[25] and recreational drugs like cannabis.[26]

Our environment is becoming increasingly polluted and with that our risk of diseases like sudden cardiac death rises. It seems to be that some are not able to handle further exposure to the contents of the mRNA jabs and/or SARS-CoV-2, as if they had reached their biological limit.

Surprisingly heavy metals like caesium, chromium, iron, aluminium, and gadolinium have been *apparently* found in the jabs.[27] Whether or not these heavy metals contribute to sudden cardiac death is another question. For now, more independent molecular analyses of mRNA jabs need to be carried out.

Though it looks like all organs are affected by the mRNA jabs, the heart may be particularly vulnerable due to structural and size limitations, as well as unfortunately not having the ability to regenerate (although the consensus is slowly changing)[28,29]. Once cardiac cells are damaged, they are damaged forever.

There are also genetic differences that make some people more likely to get heart damage than others. The SCN5A gene encodes the alpha subunit of the main cardiac sodium channel, and one small study noted that SCN5A variants may be associated with sudden unexplained death *"within 7 days of COVID-19 vaccination, regardless of vaccine type, number of vaccine dose, and presence of underlying diseases or post-vaccine fever."*[31]

For us to live, the heart has to keep pumping all the time, and it has to do so in perfect time and rhythm. Excessive damage or damage to the wrong areas can be fatal, especially when environmental toxins and underlying genetic differences render it more prone to damage to start off with.

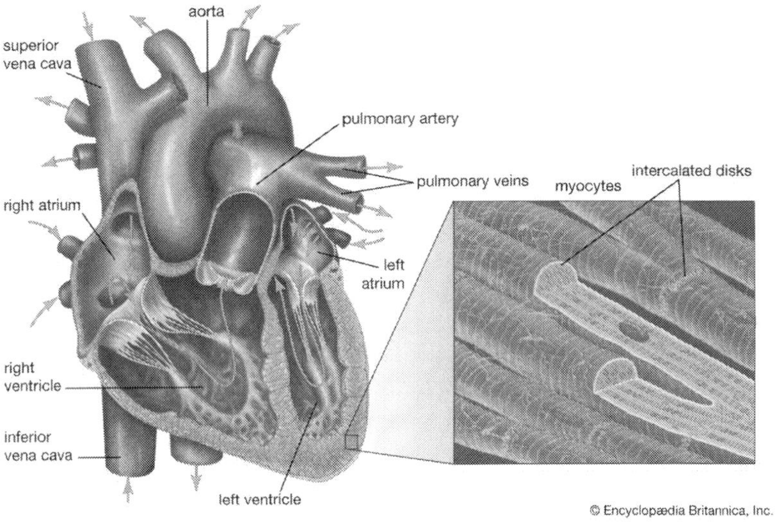

Cardiac muscle, from: https://www.britannica.com/science/cardiac-muscle

WHAT IS THE RISK OF A DAMAGED HEART?

Due to a lack of data, specifically post-mortems, the link between the shots and the increase in excess deaths in people remains a correlation rather than a cause. The correlation is strong, however, and it's fair to assume that these jabs have a significant role with regards to cardiac death, even if this hasn't been said out loud officially. You don't have to be an "expert" to see that there is a link.

Plus, don't shrug and dismiss myocarditis as a transitory condition. One study noted **persistent cardiac MRI findings in a cohort of teenagers with post-COVID-19 mRNA shot myopericarditis.**[1] Another study found that in a cohort of 18 patients with myocarditis, nearly 70% had persistent cardiac MRI changes at a median follow-up time of **7 months**.[2]

50% of the 357 patients in another study by the CDC reported in the Lancet, continued to report at least one symptom potentially associated with myocarditis after COVID-19 inoculation. And among a subset of 151 patients who had follow-up cardiac MRI results, **54% had an abnormal finding**.[3]

A review of sixty-two studies noted that 21.5% of people with mRNA-jab-induced myocarditis had significant pump failure and a **mortality rate of 2%**.[4]

The State Surgeon General of Florida, Dr. Joseph A. Ladapo has since recommended new guidance regarding mRNA shots. Recommending against males aged 18 to 39 from receiving mRNA COVID-19 shots, after an independent analysis found that there was an ***"84% increase in the relative incidence of cardiac-related death among males 18-39 years old within 28 days following mRNA vaccination."***[5]

In this scenario, it seems like the extremely fit and healthy are *more* prone to death, a population-wide phenomenon I never thought of ever happening. This is all because the heart is an extremely precious organ, and once damaged, it can prove fatal.

Note: Late gadolinium enhancement (LGE) is an imaging technique where gadolinium-based contrast agents are administered intravenously and delayed imaging is performed at least 10 minutes later to achieve optimum contrast between normal and damaged heart tissue. The presence of LGE is an indicator of cardiac injury and fibrosis and has been strongly associated with a worse prognosis in patients with classical acute myocarditis.

CAN THE SHOTS CAUSE BRAIN DAMAGE?

We must keep in mind that myocarditis is only one of 1,291 officially reported side effects of these shots.[1] It is said that Pfizer understood these implications firsthand, as their documents reveal that they needed to employ six hundred more people to process the overwhelming amount of jab-related injuries.[2]

Injuries from mRNA shots are diverse and appear to differ from person to person, depending on the agent used, the dosage, and the timing. One must also understand that the SARS-CoV-2 virus is biologically detrimental too, and that these shots increase the risk of becoming ill with COVID-19, only adding fuel to the fire and accumulating damage in the process.

So far, we've talked about the major side-effect profiles of immune-mediated dysregulation (which can lead to diseases like autoimmunity, immunodeficiency, and cancer), myocarditis, and other types of damage to blood vessels and clotting that happens as a result. The results of clotting and heart damage seem to present more rapidly than cancers, but there is another common side effect that is underappreciated: neurological decline.

The brain is one of the most energy-consuming organs in the body and is protected from the external world by the BBB.[3] We have, however, learned that the spike protein is able to cross the BBB and thus cause brain damage.[4] But it doesn't stop there.

Other than the various unnatural gene inserts (GP120 HIV-1 and SEB) that the spike protein possesses, we have also learned that the spike protein contains prion-like domains too. In fact, SARS-CoV-2 is the *only* coronavirus with a prion-like domain found in the receptor-binding domain of the S1 region of the spike protein.[5]

Other than helping the virus adhere and enter our cells, these prion-like domains have been postulated to play a role in the formation of an abnormal protein called amyloid,[5,6] which in turn may drive inflammation and the formation of pathogenic lesions in the brain and central nervous system.

Prion-like domains are known to clump together and clump with other prion-like proteins and contribute to diseases that include, but are not limited to, Alzheimer's dementia and human prion diseases.[6]

Creutzfeldt-Jakob disease is a fatal neurodegenerative prion disorder in humans. It has been noted to occur in those with COVID-19,[7] as well as in some after receiving the jab.[8]

In one case study, a 64-year-old woman was described as having rapidly declining memory loss, behavioural changes, headaches, and walking disturbances one week after receiving the second dose of the Pfizer-BioNTech mRNA COVID-19 shot. She was diagnosed as having sporadic Creutzfeldt-Jakob disease.[8]

Brain fog, cognitive decline, and memory impairment are common symptoms post-COVID-19, all linked to neuroinflammation and brain damage. Though various factors from the "Three Cause Three Effects" hypothesis have a part to play here, the spike protein, with its unusual inserts and high ability to form pathological proteins within the brain, is particularly neurologically worrisome.

How many people will be diagnosed with dementia many years before they would have been otherwise, naturally? How many people are living lives that are more cognitively impaired than they were before? What does this mean for those who rely on high mental acuity for work? How many people have died due to diseases of the nervous system?

Well, the last question has been partially answered by the ONS. They have shown that from March 2020 to June 2022, there was an excess of more than 15,000 deaths related to "diseases of the nervous system," the highest cause of excess death compared to all other categories.[9]

5. Excess deaths by cause grouping

Figure 3: Diseases of the nervous system had the highest number of excess deaths

Number of excess deaths registered by ICD-10 chapter, England and Wales, March 2020 to June 2022

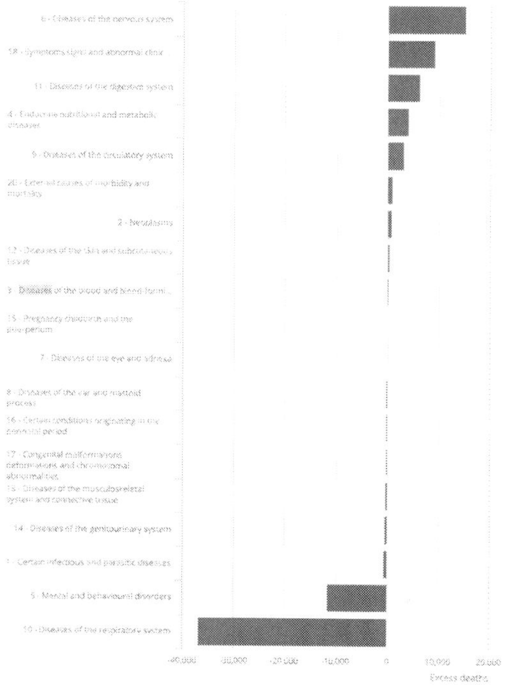

Excess deaths by cause grouping, England and Wales, March 2020 to June 2022, from: https://www.ons.gov.uk/

WHY IS JABBING CHILDREN ALL RISK AND NO BENEFIT?

On September 30, 2021, I risked my career and reputation by sending an open letter to the GMC, pleading with them to reconsider the decision to introduce the COVID-19 jab to children aged 12 to 15 in England.

My clinical experience in paediatrics and general practice during the second wave, as well as months of research, told me clearly that most children did not suffer from COVID-19 like adults did and were extremely unlikely to die from it.

So when it was confirmed that children around the country were about to be jabbed, I was more than confused; I was mortified.

In a hurry, I wrote the letter, hoping that someone had made a mistake, and sent it to the GMC, hoping that they would protect the children.

To accelerate the process, I posted the letter online along with a petition that was gaining traction fast. Others obviously felt what I felt. However, in no less than a few hours, the petition got taken down by the website, and a few days later, the GMC replied with a generic response, pretty much saying that it could not do anything about it.

I felt defeated.

To those who want to understand why the inoculation of children is all risk and no benefit, I will provide you with what I wrote to the GMC below:

"Dear members of the General Medical Council,

I write this open letter to you as a matter of urgency from a concerned doctor and public citizen. My name is Dr. Eashwarran Kohilathas, I am a GPST3 trainee and someone who has worked on the front line in various patient-facing specialties throughout the pandemic.

In the last two years I have tried my best to keep up-to-date with emerging scientific evidence regarding COVID-19, and the various ways we have been told to manage the virus. The primary reason for my ongoing pursuit of scientific understanding is so I can provide my patients with information so they are well-informed and kept safe during these uncertain times. Furthermore, as you highlight in your 'duties of a doctor registered with the General Medical Council'[1], doctors should 'make the care of your patient your first concern' and 'provide a good standard of practice and care...by keeping professional knowledge and skills up to date'. I am merely doing what is expected of me.

Under the title 'Safety and quality', you also state that doctors should 'Take prompt action if you think that patient safety, dignity or comfort is being compromised.' I strongly believe, with scientific evidence, that the safety of the children in our nation is being compromised. Please take this open letter as my 'prompt action' in highlighting this to you. I plead that you read the next section carefully and understand the grave unscientific and unethical harm we may be subjecting many millions of our children to.

The decision to offer the first dose of the COVID-19 (Pfizer BioNTech) vaccine to children aged 12-15 years old was made by our Health Secretary, Sajid Javid, earlier in September. He based his decisions on the recommendation of the chief medical officers (CMOs) of the four UK nations. The CMOs recommendation was supposedly based on "public health grounds". They have stated that it is "likely vaccination will help reduce transmission of COVID-19 in schools" and that "COVID-19 is a disease which can be very effectively transmitted by mass spreading events, especially with Delta variant.". They also stated that "They [vaccines] will also reduce the chance an individual child gets Covid-19. This means vaccination is likely to reduce (but not eliminate) education disruption.".

Under scientific scrutiny, the comments made by the CMOs and the subsequent decision made by Sajid Javid do not hold up. The overwhelming evidence we currently have suggests that offering vaccines to 12-15-year-olds provides extremely marginal or no benefit whilst potentially subjecting many millions to life-threatening risks. I am not a contrarian in my beliefs, the Joint Committee on Vaccination and Immunisation (JCVI) also did not recommend mass vaccinating this age group.[2]

Here is why I, along with many others believe vaccinating 12-15-year-olds is unscientific, unethical and extremely dangerous:

- *Although it was initially claimed that they would reduce infections (which appears not to be happening), the current position appears to be that the COVID-19 vaccines have been rolled out to reduce the severity of symptoms; initial trials suggested that vaccinated people suffered less symptomatic COVID-19 than the unvaccinated [3]. Vaccines are therefore only theoretically useful for individuals who are at risk of potentially fatal or debilitating COVID-19; children do not fall under this category.* ***Children are in fact extremely unlikely to have symptomatic COVID-19, and extremely unlikely to die from it****. [4],[5]. Statistically speaking, children are more likely to be hit by lightning than die of Coronavirus. [6]*

This fact is further demonstrated by the low absolute risk reduction (1.59%) of the Pfizer vaccine in children. [7]

- ***Vaccines do not stop spread** - A recent Oxford study showed that adults who had been fully vaccinated against SARS-CoV-2 can carry the similar viral loads of the delta variant as those who are unvaccinated. [8] Vaccines are there to protect the vaccinated individual; not even the manufacturers are claiming they reduce spread. Theoretically, by blunting symptoms without reducing the likelihood of infection and infectiousness, it is possible they are contributing to increased spread. As stated previously, children do not need protection from a condition that poses very little risk to them, especially given that complete sterilising immunity may ultimately require infection anyway.*
- ***Many children would have acquired natural immunity already especially with the reintroduction of schools**. One must remember that one does not need to be symptomatically affected by the virus to acquire natural immunity. [9] Natural immunity is likely to last longer than vaccine-induced immunity, allow protection against a broader range of variants and contribute to herd immunity. [10][11][12]*
- ***Children are not drivers of transmission**. Being a low-risk group, children catch and transmit the virus less than adults, schools have not been shown to be drivers of transmission and teachers are at no higher risk from COVID-19 than the rest of the population. [13],[14],[15],[16],[17].*
- ***These vaccines are completely new forms of therapy with no medium or long-term data**. Pfizer also excluded COVID-19 recovered 12-15-year-old from its study submitted to the FDA. In essence, adverse events in COVID-recovered adolescents were not studied.[18] There is the worry that vaccinating previously infected children will lead to more adverse events. As mRNA vaccines are a new technology, longer-term side-effects remain speculative. Vaccine manufacturers also have zero liability over adverse events.*
- ***Serious and fatal adverse reactions have been reported.** The Yellow Card data reports that "As of 15 September 2021, for the UK, 114,752 Yellow Cards have been reported for the Pfizer/BioNTech vaccine, 231,920 have been reported for the COVID-19 Vaccine AstraZeneca, 15,916 for the COVID-19 Vaccine Moderna and 1088 have been reported where the brand of the vaccine was not specified." [19] The US voluntary reporting system (VAERS) has higher rates of vaccination-associated death than all other vaccines combined over the past 20 years.[20] The risk of cardiac adverse events in boys receiving their second dose of the vaccine has been shown to be 2 to 6 times higher than the 120-day risk of hospitalisation in boys 12-17 without underlying medical conditions [21]. Another study [22] found a 3-fold increased risk of post-vaccination myocarditis in those who had previously been infected with SARS-CoV-*

2. Myocarditis carries a mortality rate of 7%-15%, and accounts for up to 17% of sudden cardiac death in children younger than 16 years.[23]

As you can see above, there is overwhelming evidence against the mass vaccination of children. Vaccinating children could cause serious harm to many whilst providing very little benefit. The CMOs have reportedly said that offering vaccines to this age group may also alleviate mental health issues. [24] I am yet to see how vaccinating children can improve their mental health, when in fact it is the policy-driven reaction to the virus - lockdowns, testing and masking - that has caused disruption to their education and livelihood. Vaccines will not fix these.

Excess deaths in the UK are now climbing, bed spaces are being filled, many millions are awaiting medical therapies - if we continue with the mass vaccination of children, we will only add to these horrific numbers. The GMC was formed more than 150 years ago, with the primary aim to protect patients. As an extremely worried doctor, I beg for you to look at the science and protect the children of our nation.

Respectfully,

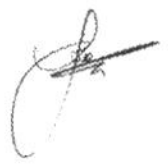

Dr. Eashwarran Kohilathas"

Since then, I have always wondered why the government not only allowed, but promoted the inoculation of children. It seemed evil. But it didn't stop there; in 2022, the COVID-19 jabs were made available to 5- to 11-year-olds, and then to infants aged six months to four years old a few months later.

"Emergency Use Authorization" (EUA) made it possible for the FDA to quickly give the jabs to millions of Americans. It is said that these jabs were offered to children to justify the EUA and thus protect the major pharmaceutical companies from liability further down the line.

In America, the CDC had unanimously approved the childhood vaccine schedule. And thus, Pfizer and Moderna are thought to immediately enjoy permanent liability protection, as their current liability protection ends when EUA expires.

The go-ahead for the inculcation of children from the very start has been the most disturbing aspect of this whole ordeal for me; it changed my perspective of global "elites" wanting only profit to something much more sinister. Children are being used as human sacrifice.

The CDC's addition of the jabs to the childhood immunisation schedule makes the jabs mandatory for kids to attend school. *An emergency use authorization product will be added to the childhood schedule. Make that make sense.*

For people in the UK, the NHS seems to have added the jabs to the schedule for children in June 2022,[25] but a recent update to their website page seems to have taken them off the list. We await further clarification, but it does look promising.

We must protect our children.

CAN THESE SHOTS MAKE ME INFERTILE?

All living things and things that are seemingly living all have one trait in common. They all live to reproduce. Everything from a tiny virus to a forest mushroom to the elephants at your local zoo, your parents, and yes, even you, all inherently live to reproduce.

Do not misunderstand where I am coming from. Our *desire* to reproduce as humans exists deeper than on a psychological level. You may not *want* to have a child; that choice is up to you, but understand that that choice exists only on a thought-processing level. Biologically, every cell and living fibre we possess has been optimised to help us spread our DNA when we're ready. Our ancestors, who were best at reproducing and looking after children, lived on. We are merely vessels for our DNA. Without reproduction, there would be no life, and so every organism eats, sleeps, moves, and lives to eventually one day fulfil this purpose and do it well.

Human fertility is clearly a very complex trait that is influenced by both physiological and behavioural factors. But it could be said that infertility is even more complicated because its causes are mostly unknown from a physiological and an evolutionary point of view.

It is reported that infertility affects nearly 7% of all couples and is rising.[1,2] And yet, no one can confidently say why. What we do know is that lifestyle factors play a big part in becoming infertile, and mitigating reversible ones sometimes leads to success.

Psychological stress, smoking, caffeine, and alcohol consumption, the Western diet, lack of exercise, and associated obesity, as well as environmental pollutants and cancer therapy, all contribute to the increased risk of infertility in both men and women.[2]

Also, gynaecological problems that cause menstrual problems, like polycystic ovary syndrome (PCOS), uterine fibroids, and endometriosis, can make it hard for women to get pregnant. Orchitis (testicular inflammation); testicular trauma, torsion, and cancer; varicocele; genital inflammation; hormonal changes; and being systemically ill, on the other hand, can significantly reduce male fertility.

Even though there are common health problems and ways of living that can lead to infertility, it is thought that nearly 50% of infertility cases are caused by genetic defects.[1] Even though hundreds of studies with animal knockout models show that infertility is caused by problems with genes, it has been hard to use this information in people. The vast majority of people who are infertile are left with no answers as to why they are.

Questions everyone wants answered now include *"whether or not these gene therapies are linked to fertility-related issues?"* And, *"Is it fair to now add mRNA technology to the list of fertility disruptors?"*

The short answer to both questions is, *"We don't know."*

This is what we do know. Let's start with the bad news, in no particular order:

- **Bill Gates, a huge proponent of population growth control**, has committed more than $2 billion to address the pandemic via the Bill & Melinda Gates Foundation.[3]
- The UK government recently updated information regarding the use of these shots in pregnant women, noting, ***"it is considered that sufficient reassurance of safe use of the vaccine in pregnant women cannot be provided at the present time****: however, use in women of childbearing potential could be supported provided healthcare professionals are advised to rule out known or suspected pregnancy prior to vaccination. Women who are breastfeeding should also not be vaccinated."*[4] This goes against their previous recommendation of, *"COVID-19 vaccination is strongly recommended for pregnant and breastfeeding women."*[5]
- The UK government website has further contradictory information regarding fertility, noting, *"There is no evidence that COVID-19 vaccines have any effect on fertility or your chances of becoming pregnant."* As well as, ***"A combined fertility and developmental study (including teratogenicity and postnatal investigations) in rats is ongoing****."*[4]
- A study of nearly 40,000 participants noted that **42% of people with regular menstrual cycles bled more heavily than usual after having the shot**. And that among people who typically do not menstruate, 71% of people on long-acting reversible contraceptives, 39% of people on gender-affirming hormones, and 66% of postmenopausal people reported breakthrough bleeding.[6] (This reflects what I was seeing in clinic).
- **Early menopause, also known as premature ovarian insufficiency has been documented to occur after COVID-19 infection.**[7] (Again, this reflects what I was seeing in clinic).

- Studies performed by Pfizer for the Japanese regulatory agency, as well as assessment reports by the European Medicines Agency (EMA) show that the **LNPs display an off-target distribution on rodents, accumulating in organs such as the ovaries and testes**.[8,9]
- A 2018 scientific review noted that **lipid nanoparticles had the ability to cross the placental barrier as well as accumulate in both male and female reproductive organs**. Here they are thought to **cause reproductive toxicity via oxidative stress, cell death, and DNA damage**.[10]
- Exposure to e**thylene glycol ethers has been linked to reproductive toxicity.**[11]
- **COVID-19 infection has shown to temporarily impair male fertility**.[12,13]
- **COVID-19 jabs have been shown to impair semen concentration and total motile count among semen donors**.[14]
- Pfizer notes that their product shows **no evidence of reproductive toxicity based on a study of 44 female rats and *untreated* male rats**.[15] This study was funded by Pfizer.[16]
- 2022 first quarter data from various regions around the world have shown a **drop in birth rates**. Examples include Hungary,[17] Germany,[18] North Dakota,[19] Singapore[20] and Taiwan.[21] Taiwan, where it is reported that as of September 2022 93% of the Taiwanese population has received at least one shot,[22] have reported a 23.25% decrease in birth rates from May 2021 to May 2022.[21]
- **There is some evidence that COVID-19 infection increases the risk of miscarriage.**[23] And preterm birth and stillbirth are more common than normal in pregnant COVID-19 patients, and their babies are more likely to be admitted to the neonatal unit.[24]
- Based on its own study,[25] the CDC calls vaccination in pregnancy "safe and effective."[26] But an independent analysis of this data notes, ***"Our re-analysis indicates a cumulative incidence of spontaneous abortion 7 to 8 times higher than the original authors' results"***.[27]

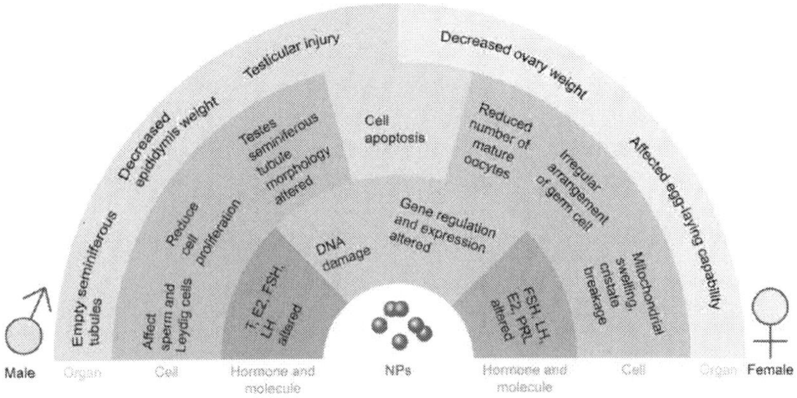

Adverse effects of nanoparticles on reproductive cells, organs, and molecules, from: https://www.ncbi.nlm.nih.gov/pmc/articles/PMC6294055/

Adverse effects of nanoparticles on reproductive cells, organs, and molecules are outlined in the diagram above.

Reassuring data includes:

- Pregnant people were not included in the first round of trials, and participants were asked to avoid becoming pregnant, **but nonetheless a number of people became pregnant by accident**. In the Pfizer trial there was a higher proportion of miscarriages in the control group.[28]
- **By June 14, 2021, 27,370 Americans had reported post-vaccination pregnancies to the CDC**, and by July 31, 2021, 10,178 Americans who had received at least one dose of the COVID shots had informed one of the country's nine major healthcare organisations of their pregnancy.[29]
- One study showed a statistical **significant *increase* in all sperm parameters after doses of COVID-19 mNRA shot**.[30]
- And a handful of other studies found **no concerning changes to sperm count or quality associated with the shot**.[31,32,33]
- A study of **48 placentas collected shortly after the shot was unable to detect any Spike protein or mRNA in samples**.[34]
- A meta-analysis of various studies reviewing the pregnancy outcomes post-jab across various countries found that COVID-19 jabs actually **reduced the rate of stillbirth by 15%.**[35]
- The Swiss COVI-PREG registry followed 1012 people vaccinated during pregnancy and found **no increased risk of miscarriage, preterm birth, stillbirth, or babies needing intensive care or dying**.[36]
- A case-control study looking at 18,950 pregnancies in Norway found that people who experienced a **miscarriage were no more likely to have received a COVID-19 shot in the previous three or five weeks, that those who did not miscarry**.[37]
- The COVID-19 shots are associated with changes to menstrual periods but recorded changes have been small and cycles return to normal in most. Studies have shown that the shots are associated with a small (0 - 2.3d) delay to the next menstrual period, but that cycle timings **returned to normal within one or two months**.[38,39,40]
- Another study noted that *In vitro* fertilisation (IVF) parameters like number of eggs and mature eggs retrieved, fertilisation rate and the ratio of top-quality embryos (TQEs) per fertilised egg, **did not significantly differ between the pre- and post-shot groups**.[41]

At the moment, it seems like everyone agrees that COVID-19 infection likely harms our reproductive system, but whether or not mRNA does it is still yet to be finalised. Severe COVID-19 disease is noted to lead to a reduction in sperm concentrations and motility and an increase in morphological abnormalities.[42] But the overall side effects of COVID-19 on the female reproductive system have remained unclear.[43] Menstrual changes commonly do occur after mRNA jabs, but we are told reassuringly that data suggests that these changes are *"short-lived and small compared with natural variation in normal cycles."*[44]

I find this an interesting take, as for one, mRNA jabs are linked to an increased likelihood of becoming ill with COVID-19, and secondly, both mRNA agents and COVID-19 similar in nature. In fact mRNA agents contain additional supposed fertility toxins such as lipid nanoparticles and PEG; and these are given intramuscularly, and so theory the jabs should be *more* harmful.

Regardless, most of the reproductive studies we do have so far look promising. And it must be noted that miscarriage rates and raw data fertility figures are prone to seasonal differences and other behavioural determinants of childbirth, like the impact of lockdowns over the last two years.

Who knows, perhaps fewer people had sexual relations because they were concerned about further burdening the healthcare system or raising a child during difficult times. Maybe others who were more conservative couldn't begin a family as weddings were postponed? And could a drop in fertility rates be attributed to increased psychological stress?

I do indeed hope that any fertility changes, in both men and women, are short-lived, whether that's after a COVID-19 infection or mRNA jab. But longer, better-quality data is needed to properly and confidently come up with a definitive "yes" or "no.. This is especially the case when government information is prone to doing a 180 in a matter of months.

Again, like the heart, fertility issues post-jab may be present in those who already had or have the beginnings of underlying issues to start with. This phenomenon is noted similarly in women who use hormone replacement therapy (HRT).[45]

HRT is avoided by some women due to its link with certain cancers. But there is some evidence to suggest that HRT does not *cause* breast tissue to become cancerous, but that the use of combined HRT for more than 5 years may promote the growth of cancer cells that are already present in some women.[45]

In terms of fertility, we don't know if the cellular process of ageing caused by infection and/or jabs has shortened fertile time windows for both men and women. We also have no data on whether or not these shots affect development or increase the likelihood of certain conditions in children born to parents who have taken them.

The data on male fertility compared to female fertility post-jab seems more negative and is sparser in number. This lack of information needs to be mitigated, especially as the male reproductive system is particularly sensitive to a broad variety of reproductive and developmental toxicants, including many environmental pollutants. And in this sense, human semen can be viewed as an early and sensitive environmental and health marker.[46] Environmental pollution impairs female fertility in all mammalian species, too.[47]

The absolute number of couples affected by infertility worldwide increased from 42.0 million in 1990 to 48.5 million in 2010.[48] This is likely to keep going up because of the growing number of environmental toxins that get into our bodies and the rising number of people with obesity.

We will only know the true impact of these jabs in years to come, as fertility data takes time to agglomerate. Though initial studies seem reassuring, I hypothesise that repeated inoculations and subsequent bioaccumulation of mandated products will prove to be a net negative to population reproductive rates and pregnancy outcomes in the future.

But the data we will collect may take longer to come in than we expect, and it may also be changed in ways that give a false picture of reality. For example, at the end of 2021, official figures from Scotland revealed that 21 infants died during September within 28 days of birth, causing the neonatal mortality rate to go past an upper warning threshold known as the "control limit" for the first time in at least four years.[49] This was also encountered in March 2022.

These two incidences were *investigated* by health authorities, and we were reassured that there was no plausible link between unusually high levels of mortality among newborns and maternal jab status.[50] Shockingly, health officials never looked into the jab status of the notwomen whose babies died.

As the Herald notes, *"Public Health Scotland (PHS) said its consultants had given "careful consideration" to the "potential benefits and harms" of carrying out such as analysis as part of its probe into the tragic deaths of 39 infants, but concluded against doing so because "**it was not possible to identify a scenario that would have resulted in a change to public health policy or practice" given that vaccination policy was already "appropriately informed by good-quality population-level evidence and safety data."***[50]

In plain English, the health officials didn't look into a possible link between material jab status and newborn deaths because they didn't want to change the health policies that were already in place.

Though our focus is currently on more severe end points like fertility rates and neonatal deaths, one must not forget about the possible long-term health consequences of children born to those who were injected.

Consider paracetamol (acetaminophen), a medication used to treat fever and pain that is commonly used during pregnancy and is listed by the BNF as "not known to be harmful" in pregnancy.[51] Well, recent studies are now linking paracetamol use in pregnant mothers to an increased risk of autism spectrum disorders (ASD) and attention-deficit hyperactivity disorder (ADHD) in the children born to them.[52,53]

Now what about mRNA shots?

What will the world be like in 50 years?

HEALING THE INJURED.

HOW CAN WE TREAT THOSE INJURED?

Post-jab injuries are extremely diverse and can present without warning due to various physiological mechanisms. To make matters worse, they are being ignored by the mainstream media, politicians, and the scientific community. I believe this is being done to avoid the legal suing frenzy that would ensue if the connection was made official, bankrupting major corporations and destroying all remaining trust in health-care services and politicians.

This willful blindness and planned silencing of mRNA-related injuries causes people to suffer alone, often without knowing what's wrong or getting the right medical help. *How can medical staff treat those injured by these genetic agents if they are unsure of the cause of the injury? What treatments can be provided if the scientific community hasn't studied the various ways that these agents cause disease?*

And so, causes of death are written as "unknown" or what the patient died with (not from), for example, "bladder cancer." But what caused the rare cancer in a young patient is not investigated. And even if it is, as the link is not widely accepted, most pathologists do not make that connection or are too afraid to document it, fearing downstream hospital bureaucratic consequences.

What this all means is that more and more people will begin to die, be inflicted with rare conditions, or become unusually unwell with diseases that did not regularly occur to people like them before the pandemic. The longer the obvious is avoided, the less likely it is that these people will fully recover. And to appease the masses, increasingly deranged reasons will be put forward to explain these hellish trends, like changes in the climate, for example.

To make matters worse, the pharmaceutical industry, to whom we usually turn for medication, is the sole cause of the current crisis. They cannot be trusted.

Instead, the future of humanity, I believe, is in the hands of those who have proven to be trustworthy over the last three years, and for now, we must use natural products for treatment.

Natural remedies and supplements have been belittled in the last 50 years or so, but I believe this negative sentiment towards them exists because they are not handed out by those with a stethoscope around their neck. There is no reason to belittle them, especially when up to 50% of the approved drugs during the last 30 years were either directly or indirectly made from them.

Synthetic therapeutics have been popularised during the current age of mass consumerism and crony capitalism due to their reduced production cost, time effectiveness, easy quality control, and quick therapeutic effects. They are so popular, in fact, that more than 131 million Americans take at least one prescription medication.[1]

The vast majority of people taking them will defend their benefits, but one cannot ignore the fact that prescription drugs are the third leading cause of death after heart disease and cancer.[2] The other two conditions are also becoming more common, which raises more questions about how well mainstream drugs work.

Nature has had millions of years to make and perfect an endless number of molecular entities. This is in contrast to synthetically made medicines, some of which were only tested on a few mice for a year or so, as we now know.

Humans have been using time-tested herbal drug preparations for thousands of years, and so it can be argued that modern pharmaceuticals, and especially synthetic drugs, are evolutionarily unnatural for us. This is no better reflected than the disaster of mRNA technology, being both ineffective and dangerous to our health.

Natural products, like anything else, come with risks and can prove ineffective in some cases. They are certainly not cure-alls. However, with the corrupt powers of those involved in the medical-industrial complex on the rise and the failure to address mRNA-related injuries, the only form of therapy that can be trusted is tried and tested natural products.

In the following sections, I will be going through a handful of potential supplements, herbal medicine, and various lifestyle modifications that may help improve natural immunity, reduce risk of future disease states, and aid certain individuals who have been injured post-jab. Please be aware that these are all pretty much in their experimental infancy and lack a great deal of evidence.

For this reason, I must state that:

I cannot guarantee success if you wish to try these supplements, and I take no responsibility for adverse outcomes if you do. I have added them for educational purposes only. Please exercise caution, inform medical personnel if you wish to try these substances, and seek immediate medical help if you experience side effects.

WHAT DO WE NEED TO DO BEFORE USING SUPPLEMENTS?

Natural products and supplements, for most, will not be the elixir that fixes all mRNA-related injuries. *I'm just being realistic here*. This is especially the case if other regular, long-term lifestyle changes aren't implemented by the individual in accordance with popping pills.

The vehicle of aid is only as effective as the quality of roads it must traverse, and in that sense, using natural remedies on a background of poor baseline health is not only near futile but also a waste of money. For some, due to whatever reason, supplementing may be the only realistic first step, but it is important to note that to squeeze as much benefit from natural supplements as possible, lifestyle changes must be implemented as soon as humanly possible too.

The human body is extraordinarily able to heal itself, but it must be provided with the right stimuli to do so. We do not blame the death of an overly shaded house plant due to inherent underlying flaws that it may possess; no, we blame ourselves for not sitting the plant by the window.

Like a houseplant, we must first and foremost provide for our basic needs before reaching for Miracle-Gro®. This is even more pertinent to get right if you'd like to increase your chances of remaining well during the next pandemic. For some, lifestyle changes alone may be sufficient to alleviate various side effects.

HOW TO IMPROVE IMMUNITY NATURALLY?

Worried about SARS-CoV-2 after seeing what it was doing to my patients in the hospital, I made it my duty to thoroughly learn everything I could about the virus, the immune system, and ways to enhance our natural defences, so I could protect my loved ones and my own health.

I understood early on that washing groceries, double-masking, and wearing a visor were not only delusional behaviours but utterly useless against an inevitability. The only way to protect oneself against a constant threat was to improve one's terrain.

Well, it sure has paid off, as it's been nearly three years and counting, and my parents and I have yet to have suffered from COVID-19 or even a common cold in that time.

To add some context to that, I worked day-in and day-out in an emergency department during the first peak, sometimes maskless, and then in various other healthcare settings for a year and a half after that. And though many of my colleagues were off sick with COVID-19, sometimes more than once, I did not take one day of sick leave during that time.

My parents, who are both deemed "high risk," have been well and have not even had the beginnings of the sniffles for nearly three years now. That was my intended goal, and I am grateful for the results.

Are we enigmas or anomalies? Maybe. *But as our friends and extended family members fell ill with COVID-19, why didn't we?*

With emerging evidence[1] showing not only that the effectiveness of the Pfizer shots becomes negative within five months but that the shots destroy any protection a person has from natural immunity and that immune disruption places individuals at greater risk of conditions like cancer and autoimmunity, it wouldn't be a bad idea to improve your natural defences now.

And whether you're jabbed or not, it may also be best to start improving your natural immunity as soon as possible to detach your reliance on the pharmaceutical industry just before the next pandemic arrives. As I hope you have learned, your freedoms are directly tied to your health. To remain free, you must remain healthy.

Just like muscles, I believe our immunity can be trained. And just like muscles, it can also be overtrained without adequate rest. But unlike muscles, which need weighted stimuli to grow, a well-functioning immune system needs a lot of different things to keep going. Eleven of the most important ways to maintain a healthy immune system include:

1. **Adequate exposure to sunlight**
2. **A good amount of sleep**
3. **Moderate-intensity exercise**
4. **Reduced carbohydrate consumption**
5. **Fasting**
6. **Fixing micronutrient deficiencies**
7. **Reduce stress**
8. **Frequent exposure to pathogens**
9. **Healthy gut microbiome**
10. **Removal of toxins**
11. **Medicinal mushrooms**

The eleven factors listed above form the foundations of not only a healthy immune system but also a healthy body in general. They are the main part of the metaphorical iceberg that is under the water, and any other herbal supplements or therapies won't work optimally until this foundation is built and kept up.

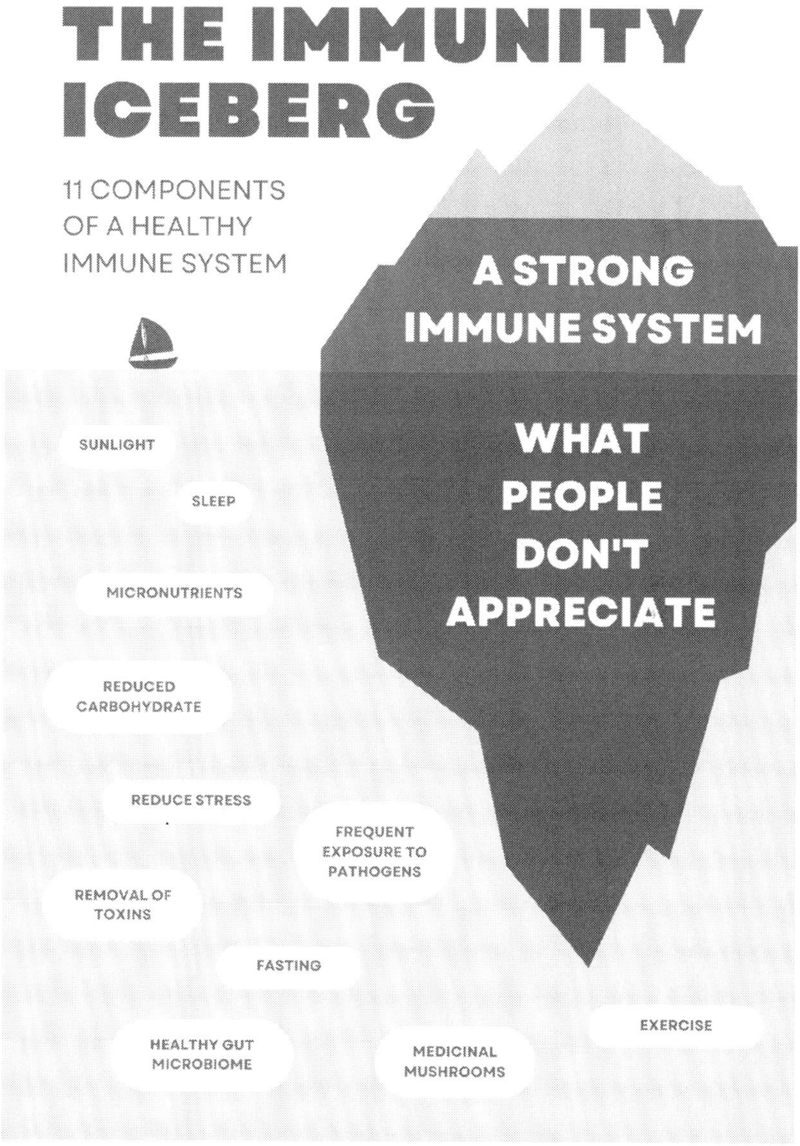

ADEQUATE EXPOSURE TO SUNLIGHT

Sunlight and its effect on immunity and general health have been a hotly debated topic for a while now (pun intended). Most public health messages of the past century have focused on disparaging sun exposure. We're continually told to not spend too much time out in the sun, and if we are, to apply a good slathering of sunscreen for protection.

But is all this sun-fear warranted or useful? Out of all the organisms that inhabit this planet, why is it only us humans that have to worry about our 4 billion-year-old star?

Dermatologists will tell you that increased intermittent exposure to sunlight and increased occurrence of burning increases the risk of developing malignant melanoma,[2] the most aggressive type of skin cancer. They'd also tell you that increased exposure to sunlight raises the risk of developing other types of skin cancer.[3] And they'd be right.

Sunlight is made up of ultraviolet (UV), visible, and infrared radiations. And though essential for life, light, and warmth on this planet, these components of sunlight *have been* shown to damage skin and DNA, creating free radicals in the process.[4] Exposure to sunlight has also been shown to cause immunosuppression.[5] It is thought that these mechanisms contribute to the formation of skin cancer.

What they don't tell you is that while the disease burden from overexposure to sunlight was estimated to be 50 000 deaths and 1.6 million disability-adjusted life years (DALYs) in the year 2000, representing 0.1% of the total global disease burden, the disease burden from very low exposure to UV radiation was estimated to be 9.4%, nearly one hundred times more.[6]

One DALY represents the loss of the equivalent of one year of full health. DALYs for a disease or health condition are the total of years of life lost to premature mortality and years spent with a disability as a result of the disease or health condition's widespread occurrence in a population.

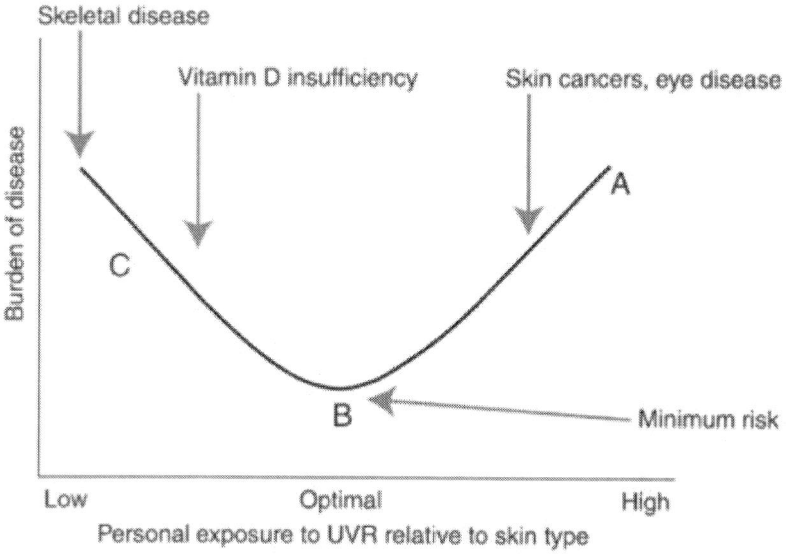

Optimal UVR exposure lay in the middle, from: https://academic.oup.com/ije/article/37/3/654/743622

Most of us do not get enough sunshine, and this increases our risk of certain cancers, including breast, colon, prostate, and non-Hodgkin lymphoma;[7,8,9,10] and increases our risk of diseases and autoimmune disorders such as multiple sclerosis and type 1 diabetes.[11,12] In fact, it has been said that sun avoidance is a risk factor for death of similar magnitude to smoking.[13]

Dermatologists will also forget to mention that *continuous* exposure to sunlight is *negatively* associated with malignant melanoma.[14] And in fact, one study noted people tend to survive *longer* with melanomas the more sunshine they have been exposed to.[15] The sun is not all bad, and various other factors like genetics must be considered too.

Immunosuppression after sunlight exposure is true, but it's a little more complicated than that. Even though it has only been seen in animal studies and in men, it is thought that this mechanism controls autoimmunity and is what makes sunlight good for people with a wide range of autoimmune conditions.[17]

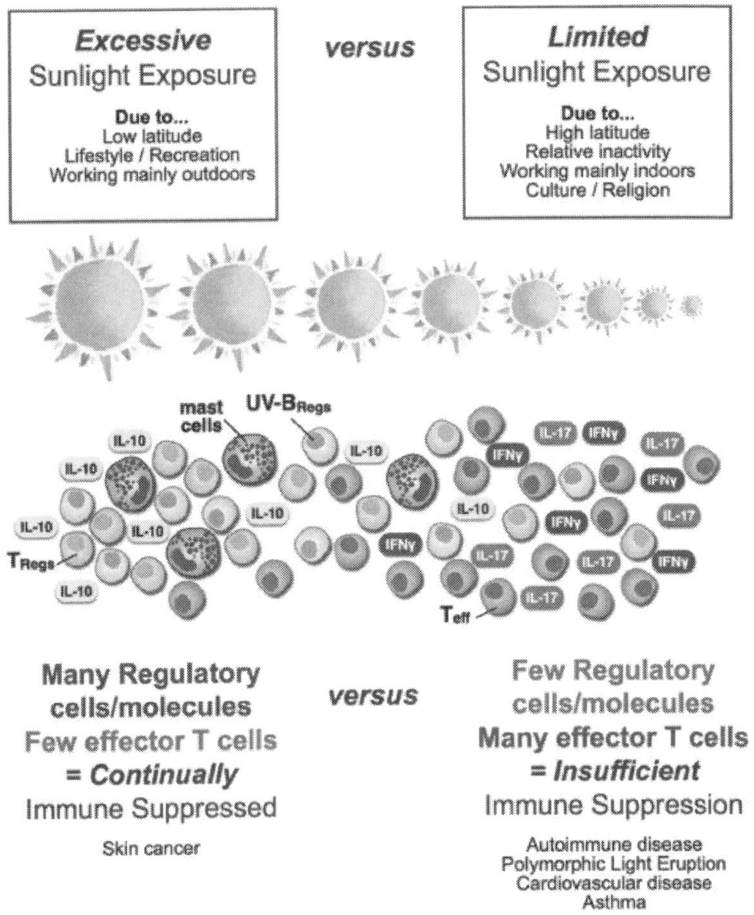

Both excessive and limited sunlight exposure can lead to immune suppression with varying outcomes, from: https://pubmed.ncbi.nlm.nih.gov/24770340/

And it's not like exposing yourself to the sun will increase your risk of skin infections. This is because other innate immune system proteins (antimicrobial peptides) are made to combat pathogens while sunlight shines on your skin.[18] Tanning is also accompanied by the generation of local antifungal defences on the skin.[19] Light itself helps T cells move.[20] And one of the best-known benefits of sunlight is that it makes us make more vitamin D.

Vitamin D was a furiously debated hormone at the start of the pandemic, and health institutions only begrudgingly began recommending it to patients many months later. Those not on board with vitamin D supplementation said that the small number of studies undertaken didn't show much benefit in reducing disease risk for COVID-19.

This is partly true, as vitamin D supplementation initially was not concretely proven to be effective. But this may have been the case because the quality of studies on this topic was initially low,[21] plus taking high doses of vitamin D supplementation for a few weeks is not the same as achieving good levels of this hormone naturally via the sun. Furthermore, vitamin D levels are thought to drop when we are unwell,[22] skewing the data.

Regardless, vitamin D *has* been noted to play a vital role in maintaining the healthy running of our immune system.[23] Vitamin D is known to impact the innate immune system by enhancing the barrier function of epithelial cells in the eyes and intestinal tract,[24,25] by enhancing the anti-pathogenic activities of key innate immune cells,[26] and by helping to express antimicrobial peptides in epithelial cells of the respiratory tract and gut barrier.[27,28,29]

With regards to the adaptive immune system, vitamin D helps to facilitate the differentiation of naïve T cells into effector T cells,[30] including "killer" or "helper", as well as regulating inflammation by altering the cytokine balance in favour of anti-inflammatory cytokines,[31,32] and promoting regulatory T cells that suppress inflammation.[33] In this sense, vitamin D acts like a helpful immunomodulator.

There are studies supporting its role in COVID-19 too.[34] In one study involving patients who were tested for COVID-19 infection, vitamin D3 supplementation acted as a defensive agent when taken right before COVID-19.[35] It was also related to decreased severity and an improved survival rate. And a meta-analysis of 27 studies revealed that 64% of severe COVID-19 patients were suffering from low levels of vitamin D.[36]

The most up-to-date evidence also supports the important role of vitamin D with regards to COVID-19 protection. In a paper released in November 2022, researchers note that the use of **Vitamin D2 and D3 were associated with reductions in COVID-19 infection of 28% and 20%, respectively.**[37] Mortality within 30-days of COVID-19 infection was similarly 33% lower with Vitamin D3 and 25% lower with vitamin D2. Plus, veterans who received larger Vitamin D dosages benefited more from supplementing than those who received lower dosages. And with supplementation, Black veterans experienced bigger related COVID-19 risk reductions than White veterans. The authors of this study note, ***"When we extrapolate our results for vitamin D3 supplementation to the entire US population in 2020, there would have been approximately 4 million fewer COVID-19 cases and 116,000 deaths avoided."***[37]

As well as vitamin D status, there are many other studies concluding that increased sun exposure is linked to better COVID-19 outcomes. So you could say that the pandemic restrictions negatively impacted vitamin D uptake by limiting exposure to sunlight.[38]

How much sunlight and/or vitamin D one should have is dependent on the person, what they do, and where they live. That being said, most of us are both sunlight and vitamin D deficient. The most problematic, and arguably the most important, is a lack of sunlight. This is because we know that food sources of vitamin D and supplements are second only to UV light.

Vitamin D produced in the skin may last at least twice as long in the blood compared with ingested vitamin D.[39] One study showed that when an adult in a bathing suit was exposed to UV radiation(giving them a slight pinkness to the skin 24 hours after exposure), the amount of vitamin D produced is equivalent to ingesting between 10,000 and 25,000 IU.[40]

At latitudes above 37°N and below 37°S, sunlight is insufficient to induce cutaneous vitamin D3 synthesis during the winter months.[41] That sucks for most of us, but even more for those with darker skin, as increased skin pigmentation has been shown to reduce cutaneous vitamin D3 production by as much as 99.9%.[41]

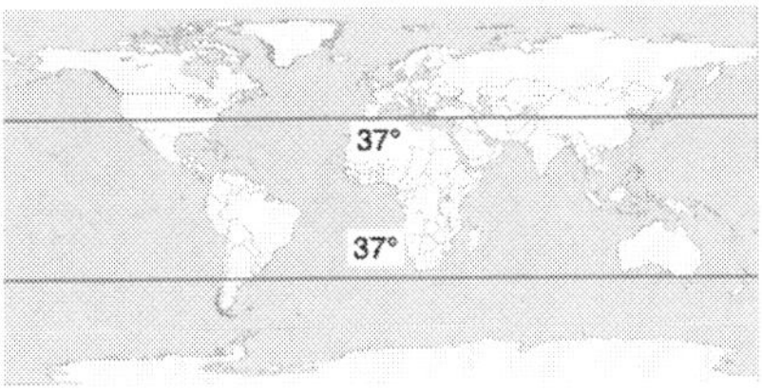

Latitudes above 37°N and below 37°S

Vitamin D measurements may be used as a proxy marker of sunlight exposure and is easier to measure than time spent out in the sun. But more vitamin D isn't better. With regards to sufficient levels, a prospective cohort study of 365,530 participants showed a reverse J-shaped association between serum vitamin D levels and all-cause mortality.[42]

Vitamin D levels of less than 45 nmol/L and anything above60 nmoll/L were associated with an increased risk of cardiovascular disease, cancer and all-cause mortality. **Therefore, this study suggested a serum Vitamin D 'sweet-spot' of 45 to 60 nmol/L.**[42]

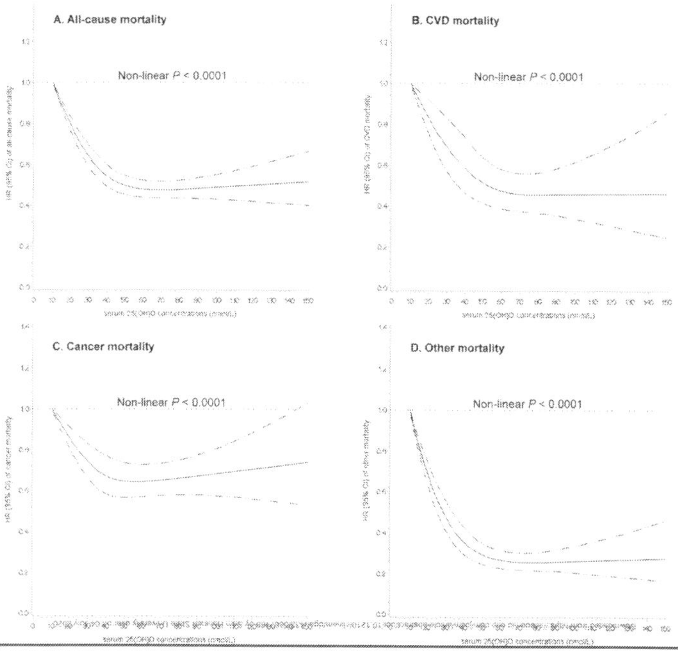

Vitamin D status and mortality, from: https://pubmed.ncbi.nlm.nih.gov/32620963/

Other similar studies have revealed a U-shape association between serum vitamin D levels and mortality rates, with similar sweet spots, but some have noted figures at the higher end at 120nmol/L.[43] An extensive review stated that ***"practically all persons are sufficient at levels of 50 nmol/L (20 ng/mL) and above. Serum concentrations of 25OHD above 75 nmol/L (30 ng/mL) are not associated with increased benefit."***[44]

But it's not all about vitamin D. We must also remember that sunlight exposure is involved in regulating many other hormones, including nitric oxide (NO), serotonin, cortisol, and melatonin.[45] Bright exposure during the day and total darkness at night optimises melatonin levels and improves our quality of sleep.[46] Melatonin has also been shown to act as a potent anti-inflammatory hormone.[47]

NO is involved with endothelial cell relaxation, but confusingly, at other times, it also plays a key role in the inflammatory pathway. It is made by many cell types involved in immunity and inflammation, acts as a major defence molecule, and regulates the functional activity, growth, and death of many other immune cells.

If you have no risk factors for acquiring skin cancer, then exposing yourself to an adequate amount of sunshine throughout the year *without* the use of sunscreen (there is some evidence suggesting sunscreens may enhance your risk of cancer, by the way),[48] and taking precautions to not get burned may help boost your immune system, reduce autoimmunity, and improve your overall health.

For those worried about burning, it has been said that the risk of burning may be reduced if your overall health is improved and if your diet is full of protective antioxidants and omega-3 fatty acids.[49,50] More studies are needed in this regard, so always be careful out in the sun.

Since the Second World War, developments such as cars, Netflix, computers, video games, indoor sports, etc. have meant we are spending more and more time indoors. German and Danish studies revealed that indoor workers on average expose their hands and faces to less than 3% of the total available amount of sunlight.[51,52]

Let's break the cycle. Go outdoors, get sun-kissed, and improve your health and immunity.

A GOOD AMOUNT OF SLEEP

Though it may not feel like it, sleep is not a passive condition but a vital biological state where both the brain and body are highly active and go through various stages (characterised by different brain wave patterns and body movements) to help the overall functioning of all physiological systems.

Sleep consists of two main stages: rapid eye movement (REM) and non-rapid eye movement (NREM) sleep. REM sleep makes up about 20% of total sleep time and is when most of the dreaming episodes seem to occur. It is called REM due to the typical rapid eye movements that occur only during this sleep stage. The biological function of REM sleep still largely remains a mystery, but proposed theories suggest that REM sleep plays a role in memory improvement and in processing emotional information.[53]

The other ~80% of total sleep time is made up by NREM sleep. NREM is known for its beneficial effect on long-term memory formation and immune memory (we'll get to that in a bit). And NREM is also where slow wave sleep (SWS), the most restorative sleep stage, associated with sleep quality and maintenance of sleep occurs.[54] An average night with 8 hours of sleep contains around five of these NREM-REM sleep cycles, which each last ~90 min.

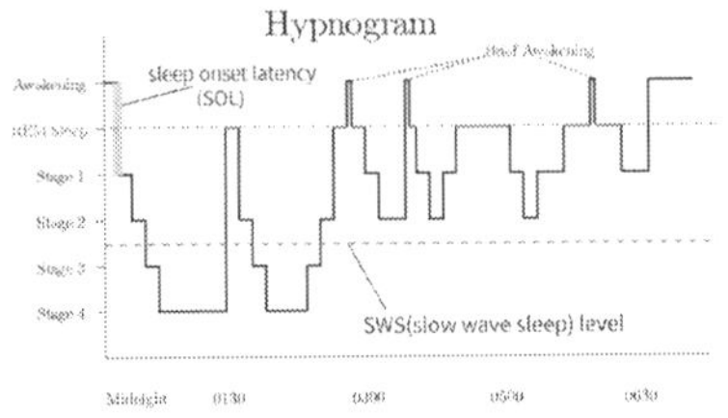

Sleep stages and brain waves, from:
https://en.wikipedia.org/wiki/Rapid_eye_movement_sleep#

It goes without saying that being sick makes us sleepy, which is why getting a good night's sleep is sometimes referred to as "the best cure" for infectious diseases.

And it may come as no surprise that an inadequate amount of sleep may increase our risk of becoming ill in the first place.

Though the link between sleep, infection risk, and recovery is commonly known, the science behind why exactly this is the case is still in its infancy. What we *do* know is that both sleep and immunity are bidirectionally linked: immune system activation alters sleep, and sleep in turn affects our body's defence system.

Hypnotoxins are chemicals that make you sleepy when you're awake and get rid of you when you're asleep. In the 1980s the first hypnotoxin was discovered.[55] This hynotoxin was the bacterial cell wall component muramyl peptide and was noted in animal models to contribute to the regulation of SWS,[56] the deepest form of sleep. Muramyl peptide was shown to induce sleepiness by activating the immune system and releasing sleep-regulatory substances like the cytokines TNF and IL-1β.

Since then, though other cytokines have shown to have sleep-regulating properties,[57] these cytokines have received much less attention than IL-1 and TNF, especially in animal models.[58,59] In humans, circulating levels of IL-1, TNF, and IL-6 have often been found to naturally peak during sleep or in the early morning hours.[60,61] One study noted a reduction in SWS amount and intensity in the beginning of the night following administration of granulocyte colony-stimulating factor (a growth factor that stimulates neutrophil increase), which in parallel led to an increase of the molecular promoters of IL-1 and TNF.[62] But human studies are still severely lacking in this area, and not all human studies have been as clear-cut as the ones noted above.[63]

Prostaglandins are molecules made from omega-6 fatty acids and mediate some of the cardinal symptoms of inflammation, such as fever and pain. Ibuprofen and aspirin, both nonsteroidal anti-inflammatory drugs (NSAIDs), work by preventing the formation of prostaglandins by inhibiting cyclooxygenase (COX) enzymes.[64]

Interestingly, again in the 1980s, work by another group of scientists identified prostaglandin D2 (PGD2), the most abundant prostanoid in the brains of rodents, as a potent, sleep-promoting substance in rats and mice.[65,66] Infusion of PGD2 into the brain space in rats substantially increased NREM sleep,[67] and the inhibition of PGD2 reduced spontaneous and TNF-induced increases in NREM sleep in animal models.[68]

Human studies are also lacking in this area, but NSAID administration to humans has been shown to cause sleep disruption. It has been noted that the acute administration of aspirin at the recommended daily dose range in healthy participants decreased sleep efficiency,[69] increased the number of awakenings, and decreased SWS.[70] Acute administration of ibuprofen, in addition to its sleep-disturbing effect, also led to a delay in SWS.[69]

Over the years, evidence has also accumulated indicating that pathogens, including bacteria, viruses, fungi, and parasites, increase the amount and intensity of NREM sleep while decreasing the amount of REM sleep.[71] These pathogens likely affect our sleep via our physiological responses to them via the direct and/or indirect manipulation of immune mediators, IL-1, TNF, and PGD2.[59,66,72]

Enhanced NREM sleep is thought to occur to benefit host defences and/or recovery. For example, in one study,[73] rabbits inoculated with *Escherichia coli* bacteria had less morbidity and mortality when NREM sleep was *enhanced* in response to the infectious challenge. A potential explanation for this immune-supportive effect is that sleep may facilitate energy allocation to the immune system.[74]

Other than sleeping more or deeper when unwell, not sleeping enough or sleeping too much are both linked to an increased risk of death and risk of infection.[75,76]

Self-reported short habitual sleep (≤5 h per night), in one study,[77] was associated with an increased risk for the development of pneumonia within the next 2 years. Researchers from another study showed that those who reported a short sleep duration in the weeks before they received nasal drops containing a rhinovirus had an increased risk of developing a cold.[77] And another study of adolescents showed that short sleep duration was associated with a higher number of reported illness events, which included symptoms of cold, flu, and gastroenteritis.[78]

Interestingly though, how well-rested you feel after a short duration also plays a part in infection risk, as participants reporting a habitual sleep duration of ≤5 h per night, but indicating that they feel their sleep duration is adequate, did not have an increased pneumonia risk in one study.[76]

The graph below outlines the relationship between sleep and risk of death beautifully. It is from a meta-analysis of prospective cohort studies that indicates 7 hours of sleep a day being associated with the lowest risk of all-cause mortality among adults.[59]

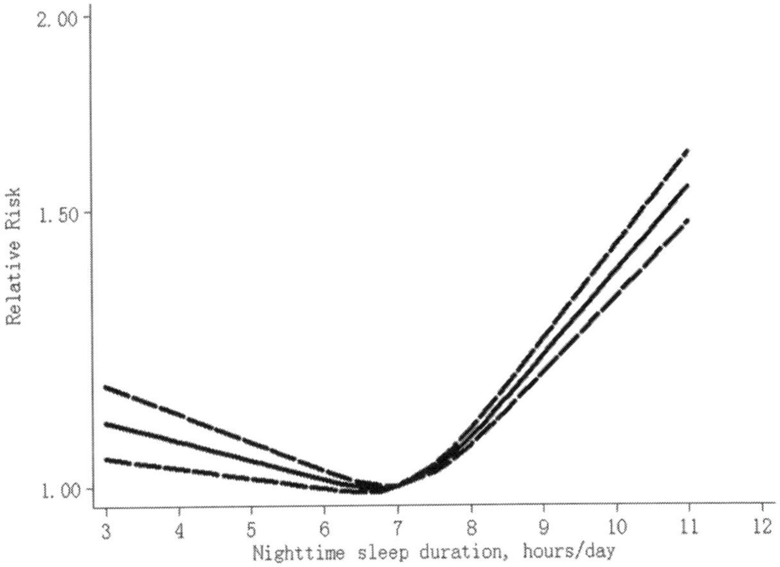

Sleep duration and risk of death, from: https://www.nature.com/articles/srep21480/figures/1

Longer sleep may be indirectly linked to death and infection risk due to other variables such as underlying diseases mediating this association;[59] in other words, someone who is already unwell may be more likely to sleep longer, skewing the data. Regardless, in this day and age, shorter sleep duration times are more likely than longer ones. And likely for this reason, there are more studies on sleep-loss-related immunocompromise than on excessive sleep.

There are various reasons why we think sleep loss is related to poor immunological outcomes. For one, evidence suggests that nearly all circulating forms of white blood cells are reduced by adequate sleep compared to sleep reduction in humans.[59] **It is thought that sleep helps with the redistribution of cells from the circulation to different tissues and organs, and an impairment in this process causes circulating levels to be higher than normal.**

Sleep loss is also associated with increased or unchanged levels of TNF levels in the various tissues, including the spleen, liver, brain, adipose tissue, and peritoneum.[59]

Remember the Th1/Th2 balance? **Well sleep, and especially the early sleep period, is thought responsible for establishing a predominant Th1 cytokine response. One study noted sleep restriction in humans caused an unfavourable shift in the Th1/Th2 cytokine balance towards Th2 activity that was strongest during the daytime.**[80]

Furthermore, just as sleep can improve one's psychological memory, sleep may also help us form immunological memory to new pathogens by directing white cells to appropriate training sites in the body such as lymph nodes.

One study also noted that the amount of SWS as well as accompanying changes in certain hormones (increases in growth hormone and prolactin and reductions in cortisol levels) in the night following vaccination correlated with the percentage of antigen-specific CD4 T cells measured up to 1 year later.[81]

The migration of white cells to lymph nodes and accompanying changes in hormones during SWS post-vaccination or contact with a pathogen are thought to increase the likelihood of interactions between antigen-presenting cells (APCs) and T cells, which results in a stronger immunological memory. And thus working backwards, an inappropriate amount or poorer quality of sleep likely reduces immunological memory. *Fascinating if you ask me.*

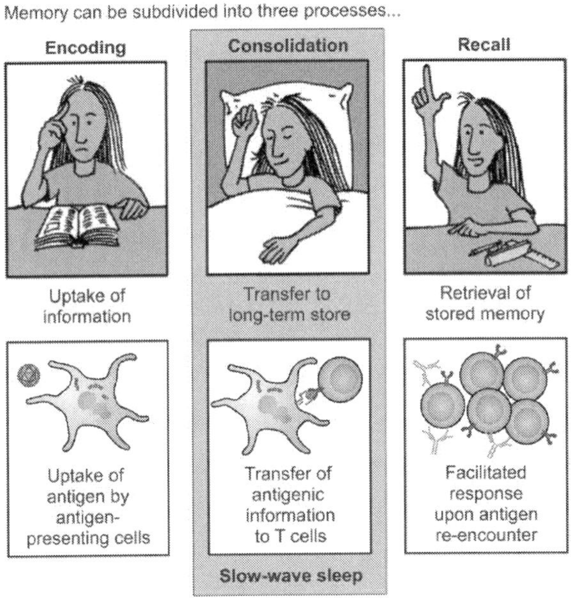

Sleep and immune memory consolidation, from: https://www.ncbi.nlm.nih.gov/pmc/articles/PMC6689741/

To wrap it up, habitual short sleep duration and long-term sleep disturbances are related to a variety of diseases, including cardiovascular diseases, metabolic diseases, chronic pain conditions, some forms of cancer, neuropsychiatric diseases, and an increased risk of infectious diseases.[82]

A lack of sleep is linked to an increased risk of COVID-19 too. In one study of nearly three thousand high-risk healthcare workers from six countries, every 1-hour increase in sleep duration at night was associated with 12% lower odds of COVID-19 while conversely, having severe sleep problems was associated with 88% greater odds of COVID-19.[83]

The study goes on to state, ***"Lack of sleep at night, severe sleep problems and high level of burnout from work may be risk factors for COVID-19 among healthcare workers, highlighting the importance of healthcare professionals' well-being during the pandemic."***[83]

If you'd like to work optimally throughout the day and reduce your risk of death and infection, then improving your sleep should be paramount. A lack of sleep is associated with higher underlying inflammation, poorer immunological memory, and even increases in allergic reactions.[84] And if you can't get a full 7-8 hrs sleep overnight, then try napping, it has been shown to be helpful.[85]

MODERATE-INTENSITY EXERCISE

During lockdown, gyms were closed, and many outdoor workout stations in local parks were barred from use and wrapped up with police tape, resembling mini crime scenes. UK government rules in early 2021 noted that exercise *"should be limited to once per day, and you should not travel outside your local area."* So though not totally banned, exercise was severely limited by the state. Alas, if logic and science were truly upheld, exercise should have been greatly encouraged.

Many of us know that exercise is good for our heart and lungs, but the vast majority of people probably don't know how good it is for our immune systems. A single bout of exercise has a profound effect on the total number and composition of circulating white cells.[86] It is not uncommon for the total lymphocyte count to increase two- to threefold after a short period of exercise and even up to fivefold during prolonged endurance exercises.[87] This highlights that the acute immune response to exercise depends on the intensity and duration of effort.

Even though higher levels of lymphocytes are usually a sign of infection or inflammation, the increase in circulating lymphocytes caused by exercise is only temporary. Within 6–24 hours after stopping exercise, normal levels return to what they were before exercise.[88] This, however, only happens after a period of undershooting (especially in endurance-based exercises), where blood white cell counts may reach clinically low levels by falling 30–50% below pre-exercise values and may remain diminished up to 6 hours later.[88]

The rise of lymphocyte levels during exercise is thought to be due to the relocation of these lymphocytes, which are normally adhered to the vascular endothelial surface, from reservoirs such as the liver, lung, and spleen to the circulation.[89] This is thought to happen because exercise increases cardiac output, blood flow, and vasodilation (dilation) of the blood vessels. It also increases sympathetic nervous system activity, which causes catecholamines to be released.

Exercise seems to preferentially mobilise cytotoxic (cell-killing) cells such as NK cells, CD8+ T cells, and γδ T cells;[90] produce substantial amounts of Th1-type and pro-inflammatory cytokines via the Toll-like receptor signalling pathways;[91] and raise neutrophil counts and increase neutrophil phagocytosis too.[92,93] In fact, the lymphocyte mobilisation response observed during exercise appears to broadly mirror the differential expression of beta-2 adrenergic receptors on lymphocytes, with natural killer cells expressing it the most, followed by CD8+ T cells, then B cells, and finally CD4+ T cells, including regulatory T cells.

Over time, these transient, exercise-induced changes in white cells are thought to enhance immunosurveillance (a process by which immune cells look for and recognise foreign pathogens, such as bacteria and viruses, or precancerous and cancerous cells in the body) and lower inflammation.[94]

In this way, both short bursts of exercise and moderate-intensity exercise done over a longer period of time can be called "immuno-enhancing." Vaccine studies using influenza, tetanus toxoid, diphtheria, pneumococcal, and meningococcal vaccines on healthy young adults and elderly people living in the community have shown that exercise mostly improves immune responses to vaccination.[88] Also, it's interesting that most of these studies found that exercise improved the immune response to the vaccine strains that made the control group's immune response weakest. This means that exercise probably boosts the immune system's response to vaccine antigens that don't cause a strong immune response.

Those who regularly exercise have been shown to have fewer self-reported chest infections, and one study of 11 elite endurance athletes over a period of 3–16 years showed that the total number of training hours per year was inversely correlated with the number of sickness days reported.[95,96] Regular exercise also appears to help clear out aged (senescent) immune cells.[97]

But it's not all good. Though the rise in exercise-induced circulating white cells is thought to be immunologically beneficial, the sudden drop in white cell levels after exercise is thought to place the individual in an immunocompromised state for a period of time, an "open window" for opportunistic infections, one might say.

This is the premise of the highly debated "open-window" hypothesis, which notes that if successive bouts of exercise are performed during the window (i.e., without adequate recovery),[98] then the exercise-induced enhancement in immunity is blunted and the postexercise immune depression is more severe and prolonged, rendering the athlete more susceptible to infection.

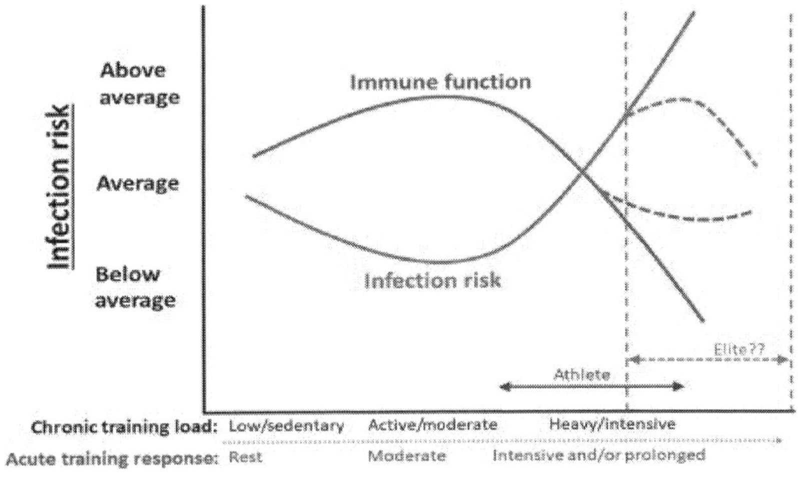

Exercise intensity and infection risk, from: https://www.ncbi.nlm.nih.gov/pmc/articles/PMC7149380/figure/f0010/

Indeed, there is evidence to suggest that athletes engaging in marathon and ultramarathon race events and/or very heavy training are at increased risk of upper respiratory tract infections (URTI). For example, in the week after the Los Angeles Marathon, nearly 13% of endurance athletes got sick, while only 2.2% of control athletes did.[99] Furthermore, in a study of Olympic athletes, all participants reported at least one illness symptom in the previous month.[100] There are many more examples like these.

The J-curve model, taken from work carried out at the start of the century, summarises the differences between the increased sickness risk associated with prolonged and intense exercise and the preventive effect of moderate activity on illness incidence.[101]

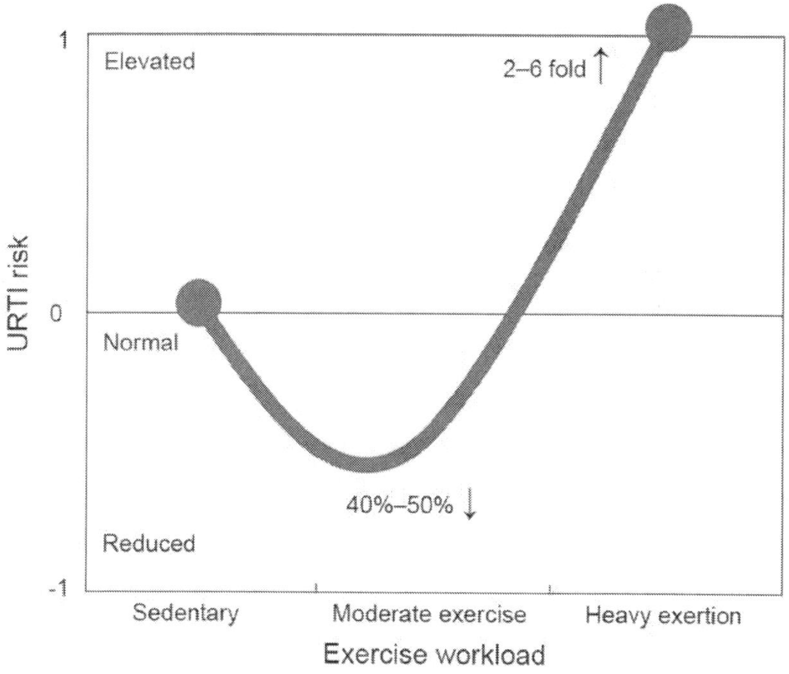

Risk of URTI and exercise workload, from:
https://www.ncbi.nlm.nih.gov/pmc/articles/PMC6523821/

Though a heavy exercise workload seemingly increases one's risk of infection, other factors such as travel, pathogen exposure, sleep disruption, mental stress, environmental air pollutants, and dietary patterns may likely influence this relationship. The International Olympic Committee has also warned that high training loads are not always linked to an increased risk of disease and that the right side of the model may not apply to elite athletes at the highest level.[102]

A more modern perspective notes that this acute and brief reduction in white blood cells 1-2 hours after exercise is advantageous to immune surveillance and regulation rather than stifling immunological competency.[103] In fact, it is widely believed that exercise redeploys immune cells to peripheral tissues (such as mucosal surfaces) to carry out immunological surveillance, a highly specialised and systematic response. The acute stress/exercise immune-enhancement concept states that these immune cells are thought to recognise and eliminate other cells contaminated with pathogens, as well as damaged or cancerous cells. And so **the drop in white cells post-exercise is in fact beneficial for the host**.

In support of this, one study noted that T cells redistributed in huge numbers to peripheral tissues, including the gut, lungs, and bone marrow.[104] Plus, this redistribution of white cells post-exercise may in fact be why regular exercise is linked to reduced rates and better outcomes of cancer. In another study,[105] the presence of natural killer cells (but possibly also T cells) in tumour sites, redeployed by adrenaline during exercise stress, was noted to **"*provides a spark*" for tumour elimination, in what could be considered a form of "*exercise immunotherapy,*"** as evidenced by the significant increase in the number of natural killer cells in tumours from active versus inactive rodents.

The jury is still out with regards to both the "open-window" hypothesis and J-curve distribution. Even though there is a lot of evidence that doing heavy workouts over and over again makes you more likely to get sick, most of that evidence comes from self-reported questionnaires. And though low levels of lymphocytes are noted after heavy exercise, this may in fact be a physiological feature and not the reason for a possible increase in the associated infection risk.

This beautifully highlights the importance of terrain health. It seems speculative to isolate exercise as a sole factor and exclude other non-exercise factors that contribute, including long-haul air travel, sleep disruption, altered diet, and psychological stress. This is especially true when studies look at a large group of nasopharyngeal swabs from athletes with URTI symptoms and find no isolable pathogens.[106]

We can say with some certainty that short-term changes in cell number and function after exercise are a sign of immune surveillance, that lifelong exercise and physical fitness might help get rid of senescent immune cells, and that being physically inactive is linked to a higher risk of COVID-19 outcomes that are more severe.[107]

With data suggesting that more than one in four adults globally (28% or 1.4 billion people) are physically inactive,[108] it is more likely than not that you reading this would benefit from regular exercise to help your overall health and immunity.

For those already engaged in regular physical exercise, the key, it seems, is to avoid overtraining and excessive inflammation. To reduce your risk of infection, make sure other areas of your health and environment are optimum, and take regular rest days. Eat well, sleep well, and supplements like magnesium and quercetin *may* help too.[109,110]

One way to measure overtraining or the risk of it is by measuring one's heart rate variability (HRV).[111] HRV is the variance in timing between the beats of your heart and can be measured using various heart rate monitors and even an Apple Watch. A drop in HRV is indicative of overtraining and an increased risk of infection.[112]

It seems to me that as one gets physically fitter, immunological strength also improves overall. The key is getting fit safely.

REDUCED CARBOHYDRATE CONSUMPTION

Diabetes mellitus, colloquially known simply as "diabetes," is an important public health issue, affecting an estimated 451 million people worldwide.[113] There are two main forms of this condition, both characterised by the disruption of the hormone insulin that controls circulating blood sugar levels. And thus, both types of diabetes are characterised by unnaturally high blood sugar levels over a prolonged period of time.

Diabetes is associated with kidney disease, blindness, loss of nerve function, heart disease, dementia, and a whole host of other negative health implications, including an increased risk of infection.[114] **And due to underlying physiological mechanisms, those with type 2 diabetes are suggested to be more susceptible to severe SARS-CoV-2 infections than those who aren't.**[115]

But it's not just diabetes. A multicentre retrospective study from China showed that **high fasting glucose levels at admission were an *independent* predictor of increased mortality in patients with COVID-19 who did not have diabetes mellitus.**[116] In other words, if you don't have diabetes but have an increased blood sugar level, you may still be at greater risk of contracting symptomatic COVID-19.

Interestingly, virus aside, blood glucose taken on the admission of those who suffered heart attacks has also been shown to be an *independent* predictor of long-term mortality in patients with *and* without known diabetes.[117]

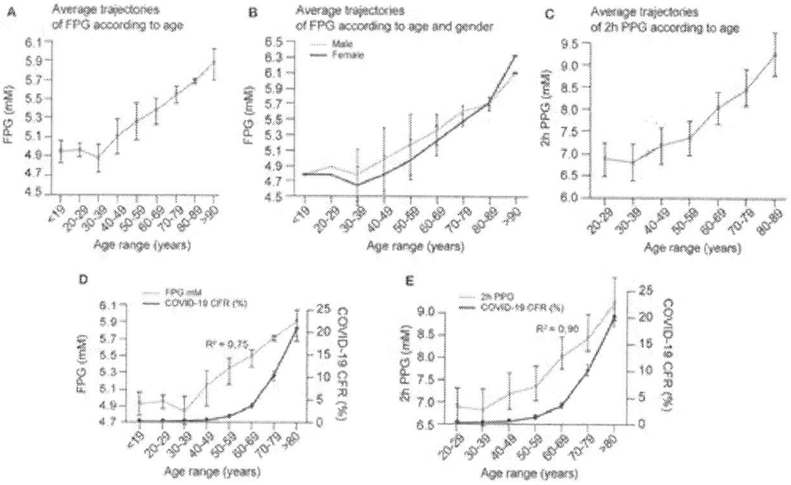

Blood sugar levels and risk of COVID-19, from:
https://www.frontiersin.org/articles/10.3389/fpubh.2021.695139/full

A fantastically in-depth study using machine learning went through nearly a quarter-million articles on SARS-CoV-2 and repeatedly noted that **elevated blood glucose was a key facilitator in the progression of COVID-19.**[118] The study found evidence linking elevated glucose to each major step of the life-cycle of the virus, progression of the disease, and presentation of symptoms.

They state, ***"elevations of glucose provide ideal conditions for the virus to evade and weaken the first level of the immune defence system in the lungs, gain access to deep alveolar cells, bind to the ACE2 receptor and enter the pulmonary cells, accelerate the replication of the virus within cells increasing cell death and inducing a pulmonary inflammatory response, which overwhelms an already weakened innate immune system to trigger an avalanche of systemic infections, inflammation and cell damage, a cytokine storm and thrombotic events."***[118]

The paper is science-heavy,[118] but I would recommend you have a read. These are some other points they highlighted:

- Elevated blood glucose is the **most likely single risk factor** to explain why, in otherwise healthy patients, disease severity is associated with age and known comorbidities.
- **Elevated blood glucose can facilitate virtually every step of the SARS-CoV-2 infection.**
- Elevated blood glucose increases glucose in the pulmonary airway surface liquid (ASL), which breaks down the primary innate antiviral defences of the lungs and facilitates viral infection and replication.
- Elevated blood glucose **causes dysregulations in the immune response** that facilitates the cytokine storm and acute respiratory distress syndrome (ARDS).
- Elevated glucose levels act synergistically with SARS-CoV-2-dependent inactivation of angiotensin-converting enzyme 2 (ACE2) to **escalate the disease to multi-organ failure and thrombotic events**.

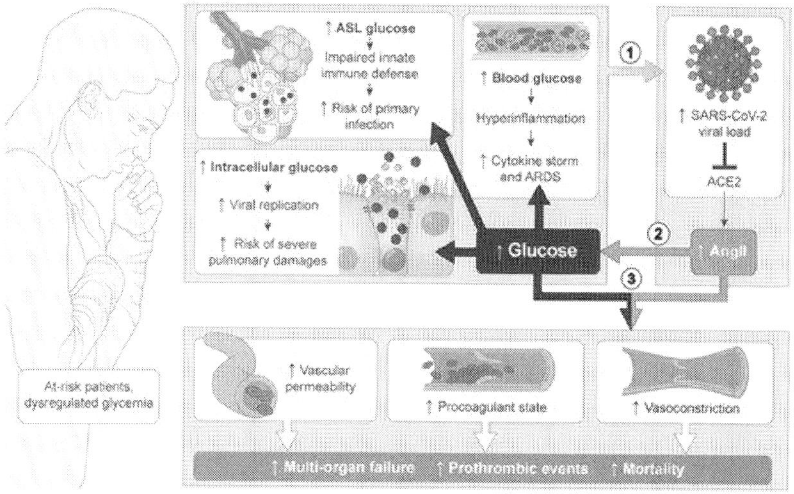

How glucose helps with the risk of infection, from:
https://www.frontiersin.org/articles/10.3389/fpubh.2021.695139/full

The problem of diabetes continues to rise worldwide in parallel with an increased incidence of obesity. This makes sense considering that there is a seven-fold greater risk of diabetes in obese people compared to those of healthy weight and a threefold increase in risk for overweight people.[119]

But as the China study noted above points out, one cannot be falsely reassured that just because one is not diagnosed with diabetes that one is protected from SARS-CoV-2 (and other infections). This is especially true when large numbers of the population are inflicted with insulin resistance.

Insulin is a hormone secreted by the pancreas regularly and in response to food. Its main function is to regulate the metabolism of carbohydrates, fats, and proteins by enhancing the absorption of blood glucose from the circulation into fat cells, muscles, and the liver to be used as a source of energy. However, excess blood sugar levels and increased underlying inflammation over a long enough period of time cause the body to not respond to insulin and/or not produce insulin like it once did. This is insulin resistance.

When it is associated with uncontrolled blood sugars, it is called type 2 diabetes, but we are all on a spectrum of insulin resistance. Some people have better blood sugar control than others. Plus, insulin resistance doesn't always present as diabetes.

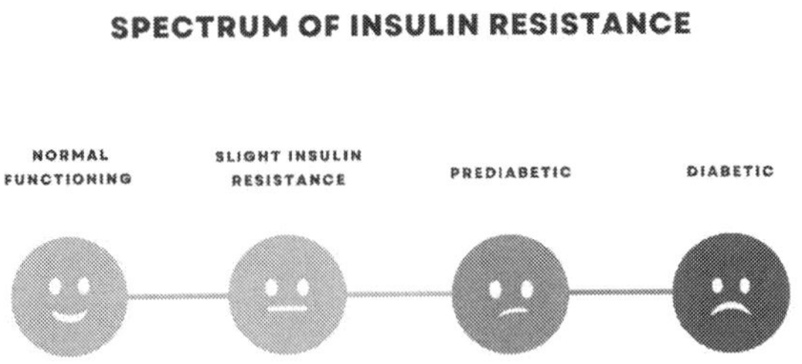

Obesity, high blood pressure, low cholesterol levels, nonalcoholic fatty liver, neurocognitive disorders,[120] polycystic ovarian syndrome, and virtually all other common chronic conditions are now widely accepted to be linked to insulin resistance in some way.[121] Our immunity is negatively impacted by insulin resistance too.

T cells, like all other components of our body, need energy to work effectively. Upon the recognition of an antigen, naive T cells become activated, turn into effector T cells, and rapidly expand to the numbers required to mount immunity against microbial and other antigen-driven stimuli.[122] Different types of T cells require unique energy demands for this to happen, with Th1 and Th17 cells both having high energy needs.[123]

Insulin, a metabolic hormone, plays a vital role in regulating energy demands around the body, and this holds true for the immune system. It has been known since the late 1970s that T cells and other immune cells express insulin receptors.[124] But its precise role in immune function has only recently begun to be established.

A 2018 study titled "Insulin Receptor-Mediated Stimulation Boosts T Cell Immunity during Inflammation and Infection" showed that insulin and its downstream signalling through its insulin receptor shape adaptive immune function through modulating T cell metabolism.[125]

In essence, they found that insulin signalling acted as a stimulatory pathway or "boost" on T cells, driving proliferation, cytokine production, and glycolytic and aerobic metabolism, which ultimately result in strengthening the host's defence against infection. The researchers go on to say that insulin receptors are essentially worn out and/or don't work as well in people with insulin resistance and may be one important reason for immunocompromisation caused by insulin resistance.

An unenergized T cell response, a sluggish innate immune response,[126] cytokine impairment,[127] defects in pathogen recognition, and inhibition of antibodies are some of the ways that insulin resistance and higher than normal circulating levels of sugar impair the immune system.

Both of my parents have type 2 diabetes. To keep them from getting sick, I learned early on how important it was to control their blood sugar levels. To help them, I advised and encouraged them to start the ketogenic diet. I began eating ketogenically too.

Ketogenic diets (KDs) are high-fat, low-carbohydrate (typically below 50 g of carbohydrate per day) diets that have been primarily used to treat epilepsy in children since the 1920s.[128] Though now a somewhat popular weight-loss diet, the KD is emerging as an effective way to counteract obesity and its associated comorbidities like T2D,[129] deranged cholesterol results,[130] insulin resistance, inflammation,[131] fatty liver disease,[132] and even polycystic ovary syndrome.[133]

The benefits of the KD extend beyond just weight loss. KDs have also been shown to improve cognitive function and stabilise mood.[134,135] These benefits and the KD's ability to help with a vast range of chronic diseases are primarily down to two things: reducing and stabilising circulating blood sugar levels (and hence improving insulin resistance) and the generation of ketone bodies. It has been hypothesised that these characteristics of the KD may aid in tackling COVID-19 too.[136]

The unique thing about the KD is its ability to increase blood levels of ketone bodies, acetoacetate, and beta-hydroxybutyrate (ßOHB). Ketone bodies are molecules produced from fatty acids by the liver through a process called ketogenesis. The body uses ketone bodies as fuel when sugar stores in the liver have been depleted. Other than being a fuel, ketone bodies have been shown to exert genetic-level changes that reduce oxidative stress and can display immunomodulatory and anti-inflammatory properties.[137,138]

There are many proposed ways in which ketone bodies may help reduce the likelihood of infection as well as decrease the resultant inflammatory reaction. These include:

- **Inhibiting NLRP3/inflammasome activation**[139] - NLRP3/inflammasome is an important immunity sensor, activating virus-induced inflammation through the induction of inflammatory cytokines.
- **Increasing T-cell expansion**[140] - mice on the KD for seven days had better T cell response and displayed a better blood O2 saturation compared to control chow-fed mice.
- **Indirectly inhibiting NF-κB**[141] - nuclear factor kappa-light-chain-enhancer of activated B cells (NF-κB) is a protein complex responsible for copying parts of gene sequences, producing cytokines and regulating the immune response to infection. Ketone bodies have shown to indirectly inhibit NF-κB.
- **Inactivating SARS-CoV-2 spike protein**[142] (theoretical) - acetoacetate may act similarly to other biocidal agents (formaldehyde and glutaraldehyde) that appear to interact with specific parts of the spike protein of some coronaviruses resulting in spike inactivation. This is highlighted by the illustration below.

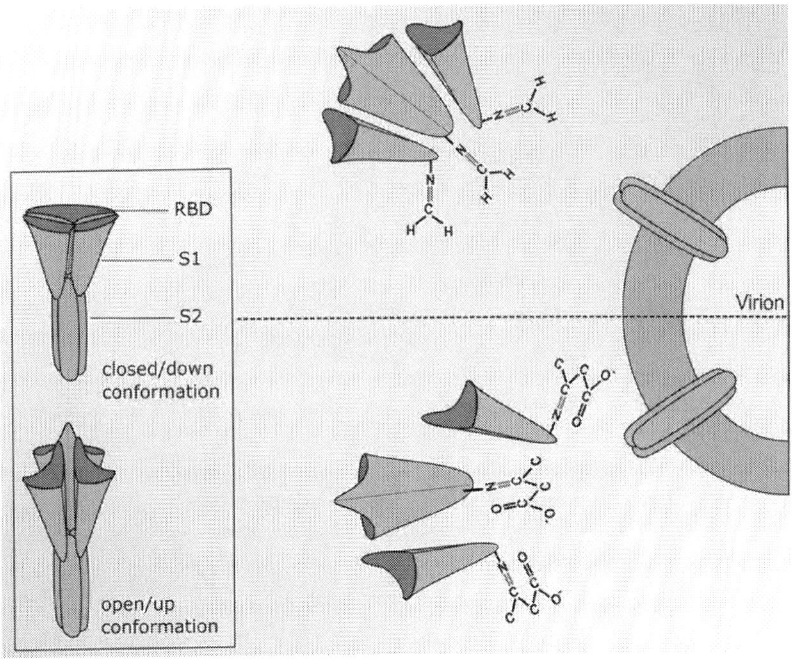

Theorteical binding of spike protein by ketones, from: https://www.ncbi.nlm.nih.gov/pmc/articles/PMC8250295/figure/bies202000312-fig-0004/

- **Upregulating expression of antioxidant genes and directly scavenging free radicals**[143] - ROS are highly reactive chemicals formed from oxygen. In low quantities they are needed for proper cellular functioning, but high quantities can cause irreversible damage to DNA. Antioxidants counteract ROS. Studies have shown ketones being able to heal somewhat damaged organs and prevent oxidative stress. β-hydroxybutyrate functions as a direct antioxidant and can inhibit mitochondrial reactive oxygen species (ROS) production.
- **Closing mitochondrial permeability transition pore**[144] - the mitochondria are parts of the cell that produce energy. Mitochondria have pores and these are used by some viruses (including the influenza virus) to promote cell death and disrupt the energy-making process. Ketone bodies can help close these pores.
- **Preserving and improving organ function, tissue resistance and tolerance**[145] - which may favour survival with few or no long-term complications. This has been replicated in one study of patients with COVID-19 who were ventilated. Results showed a statistically significant difference in survival and need for the intensive care unit by those on the KD compared to those on a standard diet.[146]

I'm sure that the KD played a direct role in keeping my parents from getting COVID-19, in addition to lowering their risk of infection indirectly by making them take less diabetes medicine and lose weight. My mother and I continue to eat a ketogenic diet, while my father has since opted to go a little less extreme and has reduced his carbohydrate consumption, particularly his refined sugar intake.

Worldwide, the prevalence of insulin resistance ranges from 15.5 to 46.5% among adults.[147] And evidence suggests not only that those who are diabetic and/or overweight are at greater risk of infectious diseases but that the risk of diabetes also rises after even mild SARS-CoV-2 infections.[148] Lockdowns surely did not help, but I presume that COVID-19 also further pushed those at risk of diabetes into full diabetes via inflammatory processes likely predominantly mediated by spike proteins.[149]

While working during the pandemic, I felt a little more confident knowing that my blood sugars were stable and my body was producing healthy amounts of ketones. I am thankful for not squandering it all by eating junk that was handed out on the wards. It is also very comforting to read about new studies that prove what I already thought.

"...ketone bodies profoundly impact human T-cell responses. CD4+ , CD8+ , and regulatory T-cell capacity were markedly enhanced, and T memory cell formation was augmented.", a 2021 study reports.[150]

A goes on to conclude, ***"Our data suggest a very-low-carbohydrate diet as a clinical tool to improve human T-cell immunity. Rethinking the value of nutrition and dietary interventions in modern medicine is required."***[150]

FASTING

In a world where food consumption is endlessly promoted, fasting may seem not only a little strange but also counter-cultural. Though abstinence from eating and sometimes drinking is common practice in various religions, its history in modern medicine has been a turbulent one. Fasting has a history of being labelled as a fad diet, a path to "digestive ruin," and those who promote it as faddists and quacks.[151] But emerging scientific evidence is beginning to paint a very different picture.

Before we carry on, I must note that fasting is not for everyone, and like everything else in this book, what is contained here is for educational purposes only. I must also note that fasting is not the same as starvation.

Fasting is defined as *"abstinence from food or drink or both for health, ritualistic, religious, or ethical purposes. The abstention may be complete or partial, lengthy, of short duration, or intermittent."* [152]

Whilst starvation is defined as, *"widespread or generalized atrophy (wasting away) of body tissues either because food is unavailable or because it cannot be taken in or properly absorbed."* [153]

In other words, fasting is a short period of time of food or water abstinence that *you* have control over, in our case, used for biological optimisation. The "short period of time" varies depending on what you read and who you talk to.

Intermittent fasting (IF) is an increasingly popular dietary practice that consists of regular alternating periods of unrestricted dietary consumption and abstinence from food intake. One group of researchers has defined IF as the umbrella term to mean *"eating patterns in which individuals go extended time periods (e.g., 16–48 h) with little or no energy intake, with intervening periods of normal food intake, on a recurring basis."*[154]

Time-restricted eating (TRE) is a type of IF with continuous short periods of fasting and food consumption typically within an 8- to 10-hour window period. Other versions of IF include reducing food consumption over 2-3 days per week or on alternate days.[155] As you can see, the definition of fasting is loose.

The majority of research looking into IF has focused on weight loss, and the results here look very promising.[156] IF has also been shown to improve markers of metabolic health and insulin sensitivity.[157]

But the reported benefits don't stop there. Many people who practise IF claim that going without food for extended periods of time has positive effects on their psychological and spiritual well-being. And according to recent research, fasting may also have physiological advantages.[155] For example, studies on mice have shown that fasting extends life expectancy,[158] lowers the production of reactive oxygen species,[159] improves inflammatory marker profiles (TNF-α and ceramides)[160] and metabolic profiles (lower body weight and fat mass),[161] as well as being associated with DNA repair and immune system optimisation.[162]

The ketogenic diet (KD) is commonly also referred to as a "fast-mimicking" diet as both KD and fasting use fats, which turn into ketone bodies, for energy. Though fasting and KD are similar, fasting comes with additional benefits, including:

Activating autophagy

Autophagy is a process whereby the body degrades unnecessary or dysfunctional cellular components for energy.[163] A cellular clearing mechanism, if you will. Though KD can also activate autophagy,[164] fasting is thought to do so with greater intensity. Autophagy is a potential therapeutic target for a diverse range of diseases, including metabolic conditions, neurodegenerative diseases, cancers, infectious diseases,[165] and prion disease,[166] and has even been shown to reverse an advanced form of cardiomyopathy.[167]

Activating sirtuins

Sirtuins are a family of proteins that regulate cellular health, promote DNA repair, and promote longevity. More specifically, sirtuins regulate telomere length.[168] Telomeres are sections of DNA found at the ends of our chromosomes. They protect the ends of our chromosomes by forming a cap (similar to the plastic tips of shoelaces). Each time a cell divides, its telomeres shorten. Oxidative stress also contributes to telomere shortening. When telomeres become too short and reach a "critical length," a process called apoptosis takes place; this is programmed cell death. Telomere length shortens with age, and shorter telomeres have been associated with an increased incidence of diseases and poor overall survival.[169] And thus, by activating sirtuins, fasting can aid in DNA repair and protection and somewhat ameliorate the effects of ageing.

Reduced systemic inflammation

The Oxidative Stress Hypothesis postulates that free-floating radicals are reduced during fasting.[170] This is thought to happen due to lower mitochondrial energy production, which ultimately lowers the body's oxidative stress. This means less overall inflammation.

Iron-removing

Iron is required for life and is what makes our blood red. Anaemia and related immunological dysfunction can be caused by a lack of iron (as discussed further in this book). But too much iron is not good either.

A variety of diseases, including fungal infections,[171] can flourish in the presence of too much iron,[172] especially when it is free-floating in the blood. Iron overload is also linked to oxidative damage, and this has been noted to occur when red blood cells are destroyed by the spike protein.[173]

Ferritin, an iron storage and buffering protein, is an indirect marker of the total amount of iron stored in the body. It has been noted that those with severe COVID-19 disease have extremely high ferritin levels.[174]

Fasting has been shown to both reduce levels of iron and ferritin concentrations as well as decrease the expression of genes associated with iron storage and export and increase the expression of genes involved in iron acquisition.[175]

Levels of serum ferritin are directly linked with elevated fasting blood glucose, serum insulin, and diagnosed diabetes, suggesting that serum ferritin may be a marker for insulin resistance.[176] And thus, fasting likely reduces inflammation via reducing iron too.

Interestingly, turmeric, the yellow spice, can also reduce iron levels.[177] It is thought that turmeric can inhibit iron absorption by 20–90% in humans and that curcumin, the active ingredient in turmeric, binds ferric iron to form a ferric-curcumin complex that is dose-dependent and may have other therapeutic benefits. [178,179]

I bring turmeric up because, like fasting, it also increases sirtuins and is known to have anti-inflammatory properties. As a result, both may help with severe COVID-19 and related iron overload diseases through iron depletion. One review even went to the extent of calling COVID-19 part of the *"hyperferritinemic syndromes"*.[180]

Changes in P-gp expression

Permeability-glycoprotein (P-gp) is a cell transporter that plays a major role in pumping many bodily substances and foreign material out of cells. P-gp function is critical for drug detoxification in both healthy and diseased tissues.[181]

P-gp has been mostly studied in cancer research, as the proper and optimised function of P-gp could reduce intracellular drug accumulation and, as a consequence, chemotherapeutic toxicity.[182] But it's not just chemotherapy that P-gp can move out of cells.

P-gp has also been shown to transport amyloid-β, a protein that is associated with Alzheimer's disease.[183] Low levels of P-gp in brain capillaries are inversely related to amyloid- deposition in the brain.[184] Plus, endothelial BBB expression of P-gp reduces as humans age, and this decrease in P-gp expression is accompanied by reduced functioning of the BBB.[185]

Those with Crohn's disease, the inflammatory bowel disease, are also noted to have a reduced expression of P-gp in their colon.[186]

12 to 24-hour fasting has been shown to increase the liver levels of P-gp in male mice,[187] and thus it was alluded to in another paper that proper feeding patterns might up-regulate toxin transporters in healthy tissues, thus reducing the side effects of chemotherapy (and theoretically, other toxin build-up).[188]

Boosting immunity

Fasting is a great biological resetter and anti-aging tool, and though these help with overall physiological functioning, the only reason fasting was added to the list was because of its direct effect on our immune system.

Cycles of fasting have shown to reduce autoimmunity,[189] activate lymphocyte-dependent killing of cancer cells,[190] promote stem cell activation,[191] regenerate immune cells and reverse immunosuppression,[192] ameliorate pathology in various mouse autoimmunity models,[193] trigger T cells to move to the bone marrow,[194] promote survival and enhanced protective function, and enhance memory T cell development,[195] maintenance, and function via reduced mammalian target of rapamycin (mTOR) activity - (mTOR is a protein that supports cell growth, it's suppression leads to longevity). This is by no means an exhaustive list, but it is impressive, as you will agree.

One study showed that a 72-hour fast not only protected against chemotherapy-related immune system damage but also induced immune system regeneration, shifting stem cells from a dormant state to a state of self-renewal.[192] Because the body needs time to fully switch to a fat- and ketone-based metabolism, it was thought that a long fast would cause more significant changes to the body than a fast of 24 hours or less.

Whatever the ketogenic diet can do, prolonged fasting can do too, and ketones, as we now know, have a vast array of anti-inflammatory properties.

A new 2022 study also found that the ketone - β-hydroxybutyrate (BHB) promoted both the survival of and the production of interferon-γ by CD4+ T cells. Mice in this study that were fed a ketogenic diet and delivered BHB as a ketone ester drink restored CD4+ T cell metabolism and function, ultimately reducing their mortality rate when infected with SARS-CoV-2.[196]

Programmed cell death protein 1 (PD-1) is a protein found on the surface of T and B cells that helps prevent autoimmune diseases by down-regulating the immune system and promoting self-tolerance by suppressing T cell inflammatory activity. PD-1 is also associated with T-cell exhaustion or dysfunction in many clinical settings.[197] BHB in the 2022 study noted above was shown to reduce PD-1 expression on T cells *in vitro* and *in vivo*.[196]

Real-life evidence seems to highlight the benefits of IF too. One prospective study showed that, ***"Routine periodic fasting was associated with a lower risk of hospitalisation or mortality in patients with COVID-19."*** [198]

And a review looking at the anti-inflammatory properties of Ramadan fasting speculated, ***"dawn to sunset fasting has the potential to optimize the immune system function against SARS-CoV-2 during the COVID-19 pandemic*** fast***as it suppresses chronic inflammation and oxidative stress, improves metabolic profile, and remodels the gut microbiome."***[199]

Timing and what is eaten before and after a fast seem to be as important as the fast itself. Water-only fasting cycles, for example, have been shown to only promote *limited* changes in the gut microbiota and result in increased gut leakiness in mice.[200] And another mouse study showed better protection against infections and tumours when only a 50% calorie restriction was applied instead of water-only fasting. More studies are needed.[201] But we aren't mice.

As you can agree, fasting has far-reaching benefits for our health and immunity. But it must be highlighted again that not everyone will find prolonged fasting easy (especially if you have underlying thyroid issues, for example),[202] nor may it be safe for you to undergo fasting (if you're prone to suffer from low blood sugar levels, for example).

And so I must reiterate: please, for your own safety, seek professional medical advice before thinking of going without food for a prolonged period of time.

FIX MICRONUTRIENT DEFICIENCIES/INADEQUACIES

If I walked down my local high street and asked random passers-by which populations of people they thought were most malnourished around the world, they'd likely describe an emaciated villager from a developing country. Though it's likely that this villager would be deficient in certain nutrients and vitamins, it may come as a surprise that a lot of people in the West and even themselves would be micronutrient deficient too.

While undernutrition continues to be a well-known threat to health and well-being in developing countries, obesity in these countries and other nations around the world is also driving malnutrition. You heard that right. Many people who are either obese or overweight are very likely malnourished.

Though obesity is associated with a state of "overfeeding" and thus presumed overnourishment, it is in fact associated with micronutrient deficiencies and inadequacies. To be precise, a very low dietary intake of a vitamin or nutritionally essential mineral can result in deficiency disease, also known as micronutrient deficiency, which is more common in developing countries. Whereas, micronutrient inadequacies are defined as nutrient intake less than the Estimated Average Requirement (EAR),[203] these are more common in the developed countries.

The WHO estimates that more than 2 billion people worldwide suffer from micronutrient deficiencies.[204] Those undernourished in developing countries are primarily iodine-, iron-, vitamin A-, and zinc-deficient due to poor micronutrient availability in food sources.[205] Whilst studies have shown that many people with obesity are low in iron, calcium, magnesium, zinc, copper, folate, and vitamins A, C, D, E, and B12. But the list of macromineral deficiencies in both groups is likely much longer. [206,207]

Being overweight or obese appears to impact the bioavailability, utilisation, absorption, excretion, storage and distribution, and metabolism of micronutrients. Plus, those with excess weight have increased physiologic requirements and generally eat lower amounts of micronutrients.[208]

Food is more than a means of providing energy; though it is vital for that purpose, it is also a vessel for various minerals, vitamins, and peptides that our bodies need for proper functioning. The public health implications of micronutrient disorders are huge.

What makes this matter worse is that, due to the nonspecific presentation of many inadequacies,[203] the vast majority are unaware that they are micronutrient inadequate or deficient until it's too late. It is a silent epidemic that affects people of all ages and genders. It causes a wide range of nonspecific physical problems that slow or stop physical and psychomotor development and make people less resistant to infections and metabolic diseases.[209] In addition to worsening infectious and chronic diseases, malnourishment also directly contributes to specific disease conditions and has a major negative influence on morbidity, mortality, and quality of life.

Getting back to the main topic, numerous studies have shown that micronutrient deficiencies and insufficiencies can affect immune responses and immunological function, which can raise the risk of infections and other immune-related diseases and disorders.[207] It may also be one major factor in why obesity is one of the biggest risk factors for suffering from severe COVID-19.[210]

We have already covered the various vital roles that vitamin D plays with regards to our immune system in the "Adequate exposure to sunlight" section, but did you know that almost 1 billion people around the world have low vitamin D levels, regardless of ethnicity or age?[211]

To highlight the growing problem of other micronutrient deficiencies and to educate you on why this negatively impacts our immune system, I have gone over some of the most common deficiencies that impact our ability to fight off infections.

Vitamin A

Vitamin A is a fat-soluble vitamin that plays an essential role in maintaining vision (low light and colour vision), embryonic development, immune function, and reproductive health. Technically speaking, it is a group of organic compounds that includes retinol, retinal (also known as retinaldehyde), retinoic acid, and several provitamin A carotenoids (most notably beta-carotene [β-carotene]).

Vitamin A deficiency (VAD) is one of the four major nutritional deficiencies worldwide.[212] It predominantly affects developing nations, causing growth and developmental deficits in children, loss of vision, and increases the risk of infection.[213] According to a report from the WHO, 190 million preschool children and 19 million pregnant women were exposed to VAD globally.[214]

Though deficiency is rare in developed nations, vitamin A inadequacy is not so uncommon here. It has been estimated that 45% of the U.S. population has an inadequacy for vitamin A,[215] a major problem considering vitamin A has been associated with resistance to infection from its early days of discovery in the early 20th century, when it was referred to as "the anti-infective vitamin." [216]

More studies since then have confirmed that vitamin A plays various roles in maintaining our innate and adaptive immunity. These include:

- Helping to maintain skin and epithelial mucosal cells of the respiratory and GI tract.[217]
- Directing innate immune cells to intestinal mucosa.[218]
- Playing a vital role in the regulation of various innate immune cells.[219]
- Regulating the function of NK cells and macrophage phagocytosis.[220]
- Helping to develop and differentiate Th1 and Th2 cells and the normal function of B cells.[220]
- Reduce the toxic effects of ROS.[221]

Vitamin A deficiency can cause:

- Altered integrity of mucosal epithelium.[222]
- Impaired T and B cell movement in the intestine.[222]
- Impaired gut microbiome composition.[223]
- Impaired innate immunity.[224]
- Suboptimal neutrophil and eosinophil function.[222]
- Reduced number and killing activity of NK cells.[222]
- Impaired ability of macrophages to phagocytose pathogens.[222]
- Diminished antioxidant activity of macrophages.[222]
- Induces inflammation and potentiates existing inflammatory conditions (increases production of TNF-α)[218]
- Decreased number and distribution of T cells.[225]
- Altered Th1/Th2 balance, decreasing Th2 response.[222]
- Impaired antibody-mediated immunity.[218]

What about COVID-19? Well, one multicentre study noted, ***"Taken together, we conclude that vitamin A plasma levels in COVID-19 patients are reduced during acute inflammation and that severely reduced plasma levels of vitamin A are significantly associated with ARDS (Acute respiratory distress syndrome) and mortality."***[226]

With regard to natural sources of vitamin A, your body can make vitamin A from carotenoids found in certain plants and vegetables. These carotenoids include beta-carotene and alpha-carotene, which are collectively known as provitamin A. Both beta-carotene and alpha-carotene give plants their red or orange colour, which is why carrots are usually associated with vitamin A and better night vision.

Though vegetables like sweet potatoes, winter squash, and carrots contain a good amount of carotene, nearly half of people carry a genetic mutation that significantly reduces their ability to convert provitamin A into vitamin A.[227]

Vitamin A1, also known as retinol, is only found in animal-sourced foods, and you'll find the most retinol in beef and lamb liver. And thus, when it comes to vitamin A, eating liver significantly outcompetes carrots. One slice of beef liver contains 6,421 mcg of vitamin A.

The RDA for vitamin A is 700–900 mcg/day.[228]

Vitamin B6

Vitamin B6 is a water-soluble vitamin that is actually a group of six chemically similar compounds (called "vitamers") that can be interconverted in biological systems.[229] Its active form, pyridoxal 5′-phosphate (PMP), serves as a coenzyme in more than 140 enzyme reactions in protein, glucose, and fat metabolism. Pyridoxal 5' phosphate (PLP) is the other active form of vitamin B6.[230]

Other than being vitally important in the metabolism of macronutrients, B6 also plays a role in cognitive development via the production of neurochemicals and in maintaining normal levels of homocysteine, a molecule that, when present in high levels in the blood, is associated with an increased risk of cardiovascular disease and other pathologies.[231]

Vitamin B6 is also involved in the production of haemoglobin, a protein found in red blood cells that transfers oxygen from the lungs to the tissues, as well as giving blood its red colour.[229]

Vitamin B6 deficiency is diagnosed when the plasma PLP level is lower than 20 nmol/L.[232] Suboptimal vitamin B6 status may be considered when plasma PLP concentrations are between 20 and 30 nmol/L.

When blood levels of PLP were used by the CDC in the analysis of data from the 2003–2006 National Health and Nutrition Examination Survey (NHANES), over 10% of US population over 1 year old was found to be vitamin B6 deficient (plasma PLP < 20 nmol/L).[233] Other studies have noted B6 deficiencies from 51% to 75% in elderly people in institutions and hospitals.[234,235]

As vitamin B6 is present in all foods, a low overall food intake is one risk factor for poor overall status. Plant sources have less bioavailable B6 than animal sources, and some foods can lose some of their B6 value when they are processed or stored.[236] Furthermore, some groups, like the elderly and women (compared to men), have a higher risk of vitamin B6 deficiency due to both low intake and higher requirements.

Those who have type 2 diabetes, colorectal cancer, rheumatoid arthritis, renal disease, and renal transplant also are at greater risk of vitamin B6 deficiency.[236]

Vitamin B6 is a concern as it is also needed for proper immune functioning. Within the immune system, vitamin B6:

- Promotes lymphocyte and IL-2 production.[229]
- Helps with the migration of lymphocytes into the intestine.[237]
- Maintains or enhances NK cell cytotoxic activity. [220]
- Helps to form the building blocks of cytokines and antibodies.[225]
- Helps to regulate inflammation (higher levels of the active form result in lower rates of inflammation).[220]
- Is involved in lymphocyte proliferation, differentiation, maturation, and activity.[225]
- Maintains Th1 immune response.[238]

B6 deficiency can cause:

- Decreased IL-2 production.[218]
- Reduced lymphoid tissue weight and low circulating white blood cells.[239]
- Suppression of a Th1 response and promotion of a Th2 response.[238]
- Decreased lymphocyte growth and proliferation.[238]
- Decreased NK cell activity; and decrease in proinflammatory cytokines IL1β IL-2, IL-2 receptor.[238]
- Lowered antibody response.[239]

It is worth noting that supplementation of B6 has shown to restore cell-mediated immunity as well as improve lymphocyte maturation and growth and increase the number of T cells in those who were previously deficient.[218,240]

Vitamin B6 deficiency is associated with lower immune function and higher susceptibility to viral infection,[241] but though one review highlighted the potential role of vitamin B6 in ameliorating the severity of COVID-19 and its complications,[242] the author of this book is not aware of any direct studies between B6 and COVID-19 outcomes that have been performed at the time of writing this.

The RDA for vitamin B6 in both men and women aged 19 to 50 years is 1.3 mg/day. The RDA for pregnant women is 1.9 mg and 2.0 mg for those lactating.[229]

Vitamin B6 is found in a variety of foods, with one cup of chickpeas having the highest content of 1.1 mg of B6. Then three ounces of beef liver containing 0.9 mg and three ounces of yellowfin tuna containing 0.9 mg.[229]

High intakes of vitamin B6 from food sources have not been reported to cause adverse effects. However, long-term administration of 1–6 g of oral pyridoxine per day for 12–40 months has been shown to cause severe and progressive sensory nerve tingling characterised by a loss of control of body movements. The severity of symptoms seems to be dose-dependent and subsides when supplements are stopped.[229]

You may also find it interesting to hear that vitamin B6 deficiency may also increase one's risk of heart disease,[243] certain cancers and worsen age-related cognitive function.[244,245] While B6 supplementation has been shown to possibly reduce the symptoms of premenstrual syndrome,[246] help with nausea and vomiting in pregnancy, as well as treat irritable bowel syndrome.[247,248]

Vitamin B12

Vitamin B12, also known as cobalamin, is the most chemically complex of all vitamins, and the only vitamin that *must* be derived from animal-produce or from supplements.[249,250]

Vitamin B12 is needed to form DNA and preserve DNA integrity, to preserve the conductive wrapping (myelin sheath) around nerve cells, to help red blood cells mature, and needed (along with folate and B6) to metabolise homocysteine.[249]

The elderly and those who do not eat animal products are at greater risk of vitamin B12 deficiency. In the US and the UK, approximately 6% of adults younger than 60 have vitamin B12 deficiency, but the rate is closer to 20% in those older than 60.[251]

Vitamin B12 deficiency can cause symptoms including tingling of the fingers and toes, soreness of mouth and tongue, weakness, fatigue, loss of appetite, weight loss, and constipation. And as B12 is vital for proper red cell turnover, a B12 deficiency can also cause anaemia.

Other than its wide array of biological properties, adequate levels of vitamin B12 are also essential for optimum immune function. Vitamin B12:

- Regulates NFκB via the regulation of NO, which plays a key role in regulating the immune response to infection.[252]
- Increases CD8+ T cells and NK cells.[253]
- Maintains the balance of CD4+/CD8+ ratio.[253]
- Modulates the gut microbiome.[254]

Vitamin B12 deficiency can cause:

- Suppressed NK cell activity.[253]
- CD4+/CD8+ imbalance leading to abnormally high CD4+:CD8+ ratios.[255]
- Reduced T cell proliferation.[239]
- Decreased number of white blood cells.[218]
- Impaired antibody response.[256]

One review ranked vitamin B12 among the top four substances for potential use in treatment for COVID-19, on the basis of findings from a study carried out with the help of molecular modelling and virtual screening tools, using data on US FDA approved drugs.[257]

Studies on COVID-19 outcomes and vitamin B12 deficiency are lacking, however. But I did manage to find one case study of a man who complained of a wide array of neurological symptoms post-jab. This 43 year old man complained of sudden onset dizziness, limb weakness, brain fog, facial numbness, and tingling of the lips post-second jab, and was noted to have a B12 deficiency. Treatment with intramuscular vitamin B12 and later oral B12 tablets helped with symptom resolution.[258]

One review noted that those with *too much* vitamin B12 were linked to poorer COVID-19 outcomes.[259] But these results may have been due to the fact that certain conditions like liver disease and certain blood cancers can *raise* B12 levels in the blood.[260] Regardless, this prompts me to add, though B12 is usually removed in the urine, you should always be careful supplementing it (and any vitamin).

The biggest dietary source of vitamin B12 is liver,containing 70 mcg per serving. Other sources include meat (3–10 mcg), dairy foods (0.3–2.4 mcg), eggs (1–2.5 mcg) and poultry (trace amounts to mcg) in 100 g wet weight. Bonito fish and clam extracts contain considerable amounts of free vitamin B12, 41 mcg and 132 mcg/100 g wet weight, respectively.[261]

The RDA of vitamin B12 is 2.4 mcg/day.[262]

Vitamin C

Vitamin C, also known as ascorbic acid or ascorbate, is a water-soluble vitamin found famously in citrus fruits, but also in other fruits and vegetables.

It is involved in the repair of tissues, the formation of connective tissue (called collagen), the production of certain neurotransmitters, and immune system function.[263] It also functions as an antioxidant.[264]

Smokers, fruit and vegetable avoiders, and those with long term conditions like end-stage kidney disease on haemodialysis are at higher risk of vitamin C deficiency.[254,265] One study noted vitamin C deficiency occurring among 5%–17% of Americans.[266] Another noted that 46% may have inadequate amounts.[215]

In the 1970s, it was suggested that vitamin C could successfully treat and/or prevent the common cold.[267] But though subsequent controlled studies have been inconsistent, fueling confusion and controversy, it is now thought that the use of vitamin C supplements might shorten the duration of the common cold and reduce symptom severity in the general population.[264]

What the scientific community at large agrees on is that vitamin C contributes to both the innate and adaptive immune systems through a variety of mechanisms that include:

- Supporting the epithelial barrier though synthesis of collagen and protection from ROS.[268]

- Stimulating the production and function of leukocytes and helps with the killing and clear up of pathogens (thus reducing associated tissue damage).[268]
- Modulating cytokine production and decreases histamine levels.[268]
- Helping to regenerate the antioxidants glutathione and vitamin E.[215]
- Maintains or enhances NK cell activities.[220]
- Playing a role in T cell differentiation and proliferation.[268]
- Increasing circulating immune system defences including antibodies and complement proteins.[268]

Vitamin C deficiency can cause:

- Increased oxidative damage.[269]
- Impaired wound healing.[268]

Almost 150 animal studies have shown that vitamin C may alleviate or prevent bacterial or viral infections.[269] And though a Cochrane review that included 24 trials found that vitamin C (at least 200 mg) did *not* significantly reduce the risk of the common cold in the general population, it *did* find a 52 percent reduction in the risk of the cold in five trials with 598 marathon runners, skiers, and soldiers engaged in subarctic exercises, indicating a higher need for those exposed to physical stress.[270]

Aside from those who are under extreme physical stress, vitamin C may be beneficial to the elderly because it may help prevent age-related immune function impairments by inhibiting thymic involution (thymic shrinkage).[271]

Results from studies reviewing vitamin C and COVID-19 have not been clear-cut. This is primarily due to a scarcity of high-quality studies; more high-quality randomised controlled trials are required.[272]

Foods high in vitamin C include raw red peppers (half a cup contains 95 mcg of vitamin C), orange juice (93 mg per ¾ cup), oranges (70 mg per orange), kiwifruit (one containing 64 mg) and broccoli (51 mcg per half a cup).[273]

The RDA for vitamin C is 75–90 mg/day. While the optimal daily intake is at least 200 mg/day, this higher amount is thought to be required to help achieve vitamin C levels of 60 mol/L for optimal cell and tissue function, and it is the lowest dose found to reduce the duration of the common cold.[274,270]

Just to add, it has been noted that both glucose (sugar) and vitamin C both compete for the same glucose transporter,[275] and so high blood glucose levels inhibit vitamin C uptake. This likely means that those who are insulin resistant need more vitamin C,[276] but it would be counterintuitive to get it from sugary sources like certain fruits. This conundrum can be alleviated by improving insulin resistance and/or consuming vitamin C from non-sugar sources. This also likely means that those on a lower carbohydrate diet need less vitamin C to function optimally compared to those who eat normal or high amounts of carbs.

• • •

Vitamin E

Vitamin E exists in eight fat-soluble chemical forms that include four tocopherols and four tocotrienols (alpha-, beta-, gamma-, and delta-tocopherol and alpha-, beta-, gamma-, and delta-tocotrienol). While they all have varying levels of biological activity, alpha- (or α-) tocopherol is the only form that is recognised to meet human requirements.[277]

Vitamin E is a potent antioxidant that protects cells from free radical attack.[278] It has been found that alpha-tocopherol mainly inhibits the production of new free radicals, while gamma-tocopherol traps and neutralises the existing free radicals.[278] Vitamin E also improves cell stability as well as inhibiting platelet aggregation.[278]

Vitamin E deficiency is rare, but one study found that 84% of people got less than the EAR of vitamin E,[279] which suggests widespread inadequacy. Even though vitamin E deficiency is rare, taking more than the recommended amount has been shown to improve immune system function and lower the risk of infection, especially in older people.

Vitamin E's importance in immune function is evident by the fact that it is found in concentrations thirty times higher in white blood cells than in red blood cells.[280] Vitamin E has various immunomodulatory properties including:

- Protecting cell membranes from damage caused by free radicals and supporting the integrity of epithelial barriers.[281]
- Maintaining or enhancing NK cell activity.[220]
- Inhibiting certain prostaglandin production by macrophages and thus indirectly protecting T-cell function.[282]
- Enhancing lymphocyte proliferation and T-cell-mediated functions.[238]
- Optimising and enhancing Th1 response.[238]
- Suppresses Th2 response.[238]
- Helping to form effective immune synapses between and Th cells.[283]
- Increasing the proportion of antigen-experienced memory T cells.[284]

Vitamin E deficiency can cause:

- Impaired humoral and cell-mediated aspects of adaptive immunity, including B and T cell function.[225]
- Reduces T cell maturation.[285]

Because of thymic involution, our T-cell-mediated immunity goes down as we age. But intriguingly, one of vitamin E's most studied effects on immunity is the prevention of this immunosenescence that comes with ageing.[286]

This mechanism has also been shown to be beneficial in HIV/AIDS patients with low T cell counts. In one study, at a dose of 400 IU, vitamin E was shown to restore delayed skin hypersensitivity reactions and interleukin-2 production, and at high doses, it was shown to stimulate T helper cell (CD4 T-cell) proliferation. [287]

And a study on mice with AIDS showed that a fifteen-fold increase in dietary vitamin E normalised immune parameters that are altered in HIV/AIDS.[289]

Other than this, it seems like vitamin E intake also helps prevent (and kill) certain cancers, cataracts, and Alzheimer's disease.[278]

When it comes to treating or preventing COVID-19, there isn't enough information about vitamin E use to make a recommendation.[289] Even so, because of how it affects the immune system, many researchers say that vitamin E should be studied to see if it lowers the risk of COVID-19 or makes the disease less severe.

In a small Mexico trial, 22 hospitalised adults with COVID-19 pneumonia were given 800 mg of vitamin E (as alpha-tocopheryl acetate) every 12 hours for 5 days, along with the drug pentoxifylline. They found that the inflammatory markers interleukin-6 and procalcitonin were much lower in patients who took both vitamin E and pentoxifylline than in those who took pentoxifylline alone.[290]

Supplementing with vitamin E is suboptimal compared to getting it naturally for many reasons. First of all, most vitamin E supplements only have alpha-tocopherol. However, there are "mixed" products that have other tocopherols and even tocotrienols. Second, it has been shown that the natural structure of alpha-tocopherol is twice as effective as the all-racemic (synthetic) structure of other alpha-tocopherols when it comes to certain biological activities.[291] And thirdly, high doses of alpha-tocopherol supplements can cause bleeding and interrupt blood coagulation in animals, and *in vitro* data suggest that high doses stop platelets from sticking together.[277] Research has not found any adverse effects from consuming vitamin E in food.[292]

It is important to note that vitamin E is heavily dependent on vitamin C, vitamin B3, selenium, and glutathione (a natural antioxidant). It is said that a diet high in vitamin E cannot have an optimal effect unless it is also rich in foods that provide these other nutrients.[278]

The need for vitamin E may be higher in people with metabolic syndrome too, and since more than a third of the US population has metabolic syndrome, the need for adequate vitamin E status across the population cannot be stressed enough.[293,294]

Vitamin E is a common nutrient found in most foods. Gamma-tocopherol, which is found in soybean, canola, corn, and other vegetable oils and food products, makes up the majority of vitamin E in American diets, while nuts, seeds, and vegetable oils are among the best sources of alpha-tocopherol.[295] The highest source of alpha-tocopherol is wheat germ oil (one tablespoon contains 20.3 mg).[277] Wheat germ oil also contains octacosanol, a molecule that may aid in weight loss as well as having anti-parkinsonian and anti-inflammatory effects.[296,297,298]

The RDA for vitamin E is 15 mg/day (22.4 IU), and the optimal daily intake for immune health in older adults is 134 mg/day (200 IU).[228,299]

I must note that sources high in vitamin E are also high in omega-6 fatty acids, which in turn can cause a pro-inflammatory state if enough omega-3 fatty acids aren't also consumed in the diet. So overconsumption of seed oils may become counterintuitive. We'll expand on this later on.

• • •

Copper

Copper is an essential mineral that is vital to the health of all living things. It is an essential element for a variety of vital enzymes (known as "cuproenzymes") involved in energy production, iron metabolism, neuropeptide activation, connective tissue synthesis, and neurotransmitter synthesis.

Copper is also important for the development of new blood vessels, the balance of hormones that affect our mood, brain growth, the colour of our skin, the control of gene expression, and the health of our immune systems.[301]

95% of the total copper carried in healthy human plasma is in the form of ceruloplasmin, an enzyme involved in iron metabolism.[302] And our antioxidant defences depend mainly on the copper-containing superoxide dismutases.[303]

Though deficiency is uncommon, copper levels in the Western diet have been declining since the 1930s. It is estimated that half of the adult population consumes less than the amount recommended in the European Communities and the United Kingdom. And least 25% of adults consume less than the estimated average requirement published for the United States and Canada.[304]

Other causes for copper deficiency and/or inadequacies include elevated levels of dietary zinc,[305] and simple sugars (fructose and sucrose) which both inhibit the dietary absorption of copper.[306,307] High-dose vitamin C and iron supplementation can both also reduce copper status.[308,309]

Others at greater risk of copper deficiency include those with genetic defects for Menkes disease (a genetic copper deficiency syndrome),[310] individuals with malabsorption syndrome (impaired dietary absorption),[311] diabetics,[312] people with chronic diseases that lead to low food intake (such as alcoholics), people with eating disorders, low-birth-weight infants, infants fed cow's milk instead of breast milk or fortified formula, pregnant and lactating mothers, and patients receiving total parenteral nutrition.

Copper and its relationship with immunity have been noted for a long time. Copper-containing devices have been used as antimicrobial devices since the ancient Egyptian and Roman civilizations.[313] And early studies from the 1970s linked that mild copper deficiency in humans and animals was often characterised by low levels of neutrophils.[314]

We now know that copper does more than just help us deal with oxidative stress. It also has a number of immunomodulatory effects, such as:

- Accumulating in macrophages to combat certain infectious agents.[313]
- Enhancing NK cell activity.[220]
- Maintaining intracellular antioxidant balance, suggesting an important role in inflammatory response.[218]
- Being involved in the differentiation and proliferation of T cells.[218]
- Inducing autophagy and in turn maintaining the cell's antiviral defence.[315]

Whilst copper deficiency can result in:

- Abnormally low neutrophil levels and reduced phagocytic ability.[316]
- Reduced IL-2 and decreased T-cell proliferation, even in slight deficiencies.[285]
- Ineffective immune response to infections.[218]
- Increased viral virulence.[218]

In a study about COVID-19, people in critical condition had lower copper levels in their blood, but this was not linked to how they ended up.[316] But other than this, the data around copper and COVID-19 treatment or prevention is sparse.

As a side note, one scientific review did postulate using sodium copper chlorophyllin (SCC), a specific mixture of chlorophyll (the light-absorbing molecule that gives leaves their green colour), to help with COVID-19-related low levels of white blood cells.[317] Copper is thought to be the major contributing factor here. SCC has also been demonstrated to have skin healing properties.[318,319]

It is important to note that *too much* copper can also negatively impact the immune response and our health.[218] Copper toxicity is commonly caused by consuming acidic foods cooked in uncoated copper cookware or by exposure to excess copper in drinking water or other environmental sources.[320]

But though copper toxicity is a real risk, in 1996, the International Program on Chemical Safety, a WHO-associated agency, stated "*there is greater risk of health effects from deficiency of copper intake than from excess copper intake.*" [321]

A healthy human body is capable of regulating copper levels by excreting excess copper if given the right tools, which is likely why long-term toxicity of copper is not frequently observed in the population.[322]

The food source containing the most copper is liver (again). Beef liver contains 12400 mcg in a 3 ounce or 85 gram serving. Next is oysters (4850 mcg per 3 ounces), followed by chocolate (938 mcg per ounce). To avoid both copper and vitamin A toxicity, it is frequently advised not to eat liver more than once a week.[323]

The RDA for copper is 900 mcg/day.[300]

Iron

Iron is extremely abundant in our body; it is predominantly found in red blood cells as it is an essential component of haemoglobin.[324] It has been predicted that there are about one billion atoms of iron in a single human red blood cell.

Iron is also necessary for physical growth, neurological development, cellular functioning, the production of various hormones, and the proper functioning of our immune system.[324]

Anaemia is a condition where there are not enough healthy red blood cells to carry adequate oxygen to our body's tissues. The WHO estimates that approximately half of the 1.62 billion cases of anaemia worldwide are due to iron deficiency.[326] And in 2002, the WHO characterised iron deficiency anaemia as one of the 10 leading risk factors for disease around the world.[324]

In the developing world, iron deficiency often results from intestinal pathologies and blood loss associated with gastrointestinal parasites. Whereas in countries like the US, iron deficiency is associated with poor diet, malabsorptive disorders, and blood loss.[324]

In developed countries, iron deficiency is not uncommon, especially among young children and women of reproductive age. In fact, a 1997 study noted that approximately 700,000 toddlers and 7.8 million women had iron deficiency; of these, approximately 240,000 toddlers and 3.3 million women had iron deficiency anaemia in the US.[327]

Others at risk of iron deficiency include women who suffer from heavy menstrual periods,[328] frequent blood donors,[329] people with cancer (likely due to long-term blood loss),[330] those with gastrointestinal disorders,[331] and people with heart failure.[332]

Iron's interaction with the immune system is complex and poorly understood. Iron deficiency has been reported to be associated with increased susceptibility to infection,[333] but the results of many of these studies have been conflicting and hard to interpret due to other coexisting nutritional problems. What we do know, is that iron is:

- Essential for differentiation and growth of epithelial tissue and components of enzymes critical for functioning of immune cells.[238]
- Involved in the regulation of cytokine production and action.[238]
- Involved in the killing process of bacteria by neutrophils through the formation of highly toxic hydroxyl radicals.[238]
- Involved in macrophage polarisation.[234]
- Involved in the proper functioning of neutrophils.[234]
- Involved in the development, proliferation, activation and function of NK cells.[234]
- Involved in producing IFNγ.[268]
- Important in differentiation and proliferation of T cells.[225]
- Important in regulating the ratio between T helper cells and cytotoxic T cells.[238]
- Needed as fuel for activated T cells.[335]

Iron deficiency can cause:

- Cytokine secretion impairment.[225]
- Reduction in NK cell activity.[334]
- Impaired microbial killing by macrophages.[225]
- Impaired cellular immunity (e.g., decreased T helper cells, increased cytotoxic T cells).[225]
- Decreased white cell bactericidal activity.[225]
- Impairment of memory immune responses.[335]
- Inhibition of T and B cells.[335]

It must be noted that though iron deficiency may increase one's likelihood of infection, too much iron (as a result of over supplementation and/or underlying genetic disorders like haemochromatosis) can result in the excess of ROS,[336] leading to injury of DNA and other biological molecules.[337]

Too much iron, especially free floating in the blood, also acts as a growth medium for a whole host of pathogens,[334] including fungi.[325] To counteract this, we have developed an evolutionary mechanism for reducing the uptake of iron from the intestine and increasing the expression of iron storage proteins during an infection. This mechanism is known as "nutritional immunity."[338]

Excess iron also shifts the balance between Th1 and Th2 cells towards the latter, resulting in increased production of IL-4 as well as having a profound impact on macrophage functions.[334]

This detrimental effect of too much iron or iron in the wrong place is no better reflected by studies carried out in Sub-Saharan Africa, where iron supplementation to infants and young children *increased* morbidity and mortality from infections,[325] possibly due to iron-induced growth of *Plasmodium*, the causative agent of malaria, or expansion of pathogenic *E. coli*.

On the other end of the spectrum, some individuals with long-term diseases become anaemic, a term called "anaemia of chronic disease (ACD)". ACD is a common feature of long-lasting immune activation due to chronic infections, autoimmune and autoinflammatory disorders, chronic kidney disease, and cancers. It is thought these individuals have low levels of iron due to the suppression of red blood cell formation,[325] the destruction of circulating red blood cells by autoantibodies or autoreactive T cells, and macrophages trapping recycled iron.[339]

Many of the pathophysiologic features of ACD are thought to indicate that this type of anaemia is an intended mechanism of defence against infections that aims to withdraw iron, oxygen, or both from pathogens.[325]

All in all, I hope you can appreciate the diverse role that iron plays in our immune system and its propensity to play a "double-edged sword" role in cells.

In the case of COVID-19, anaemia has been identified as an independent risk factor associated with the disease's severe illness.[340] But one must remember that an acute infection itself can manifest anaemia too.[341] In contrast, another study found that high iron levels may contribute to the progression of SARS-CoV-2 viral infection.[342]

Both too much and too little iron (and iron in the wrong places) can increase one's risk of infection. With anaemia becoming more common and one study claiming that lockdowns exacerbated iron deficiency anaemia in the population, most of you reading this will most likely need a way to increase iron levels rather than decrease them.[343]

Natural foods high in iron include oysters (3 ounces contain 8 mg of iron), white beans (1 cup contain 8 mg), and beef liver (3 ounces contain 5 mg).[324]

The RDA for iron in people aged 19 to 50 is 8 mg/day for men and 18 mg/day for women (27 mg/day for pregnant women and 9 mg for lactating women).[324]

Remember that iron *balance* confers the best immunological defence. So instead of scrupulously trying to reach daily RDAs, it may be best to eat foods naturally high in iron while also donating blood once in a while in efforts to dump the "excess" of it. Interestingly, giving away iron may be one reason why those who donate blood tend to live longer than those who don't.[344,345]

Iodine

Iodine is an essential component of the thyroid hormones thyroxine (T4) and triiodothyronine (T3). Thyroid hormones, made by the thyroid gland, regulate a vast array of biological processes, including protein synthesis and enzymatic activity, and are critical determinants of metabolic activity. Thyroid hormones are also vital for proper skeletal and central nervous system development in foetuses and infants.[346]

Inadequate intake of iodine can lead to thyroid dysfunction and a related lump or swelling at the front of the neck caused by a swollen thyroid called a goitre. To prevent this, iodized salt was introduced to the US in the 1920s, and since the 1940s, the US overall has been considered iodine sufficient. But since the 1970s, U.S. dietary iodine intakes have decreased by 50%, and recently, mild iodine deficiency has reemerged in some population groups.[347]

Around 2 billion people are at risk of iodine deficiency, according to the WHO.[348] Pregnant and breastfeeding women, children, and those eating a vegan, vegetarian, or gluten-free diet are particularly susceptible.[349]

Other than being vital for thyroid function, a significant amount of iodine in the body is non-hormonal and is concentrated in areas other than the thyroid, where its biological function is only a little understood.[350]

It is thought that iodine has various antioxidant functions by attaching to the double bonds of some polyunsaturated fatty acids in cell membranes, making them less reactive to ROS.[351] Iodine also binds to the omega-6 fatty acid arachidonic acid and turns it into 6-iodolactone, a molecule thought to be a key mediator of the antitumoral properties of iodine.[352] Depending on where and which form of it is taken up, iodine can act as an anti-inflammatory or proinflammatory agent.[353]

The effects of iodine deficiency on the immune system, as well as the effects of iodine outside of its involvement with thyroid hormones, remain relatively unexplored. What we do know is that iodine is:

- Considered an ancestral antioxidant and an inhibitor of lipoperoxidation.[353]
- Able to inhibit the formation of prostaglandins (with equivalent intensity to that observed with Celecoxib, a NSAID). [354]
- Able to decrease neutrophil movement.[355]
- Able to inhibit complement, mast cell degradation, NO and TNF-α production by macrophages.[356]
- Involved in the production of thyroid hormones that can enhance various types of white cells.[356]
- Able to increase white cell survival.[356]

- Able to induce stronger cytokine and chemokine responses by altering transcription immune signatures.[356]
- Able to improve Th1 response in leukocytes from normal subjects by increasing the release of IL2 and IFN-γ cytokines.[356]
- Able to increase IgG antibodies.[357]

Though research on iodine supplementation and COVID-19 is limited, iodine-based products for mouthwash, gargles, and nasal sprays have been shown to reduce nasopharyngeal viral load in COVID-19 patients.[358]

One study noted that the use of Essential Iodine Drops (EID) on SARS-CoV-2 *in vitro* reduced the viral titre by 99%. The authors of the study conclude, "***...demonstrating that Iodine-V in EID is effective at inactivating the virus in vitro and therefore suggesting its potential application intranasally to reduce SARS-CoV-2 transmission from known or suspected COVID-19 patients.***"[359]

The average consumption of iodine in the Japanese population ranges from 1200 to 5280 mcg per day, compared to 166 and 209 mcg per day in the United Kingdom and the United States, respectively.[360] And some have speculated that this may be one reason why the Japanese fared better during the pandemic than their Western counterparts.[361]

Like everything else, the proper amount of iodine consumption is important. Other than immunocompromise, a diet deficient in iodine can lead to mental retardation, underactive thyroid disease, congenital anomalies, a swelling of the neck called "goitre," or low IQ, whereas iodine excess can result in iodine-induced overactive and underactive thyroid disease and thyroid cancer.[349,346] But it must be noted that, despite the high nutritional intake of iodine, Asia does not differ from the rest of the world in the prevalence of thyroid disorders.[362]

According to the International Council for Control of Iodine Deficiency Disorders (ICCIDD), the recommended dietary allowance of iodine is 150–299 mcg/day for normal thyroid functioning, and the maximum limit of iodine intake with the lowest observed adverse effect level is 1700–1800 mcg/day.[353] Dose-response studies in humans have demonstrated that iodine at concentrations of 1 to 6 mg/day exhibited significant beneficial actions in pathologies like fibrocystic breast disease, prostatic hyperplasia and polycystic ovaries, without additional side effects.[353,363]

The official RDA for iodine is 150 mcg/day for adults, 120 mcg/day for children (between 9 and 13 years of age), 220 mg/day for pregnant women, and 290 mcg/day for lactating women.[354]

The best natural sources of iodine include seaweed (such as kelp, nori, kombu, and wakame), fish, oysters, and eggs. Three ounces of cod contain 158 mcg of iodine, while 5 g of seaweed contains 116 mcg of iodine, and 3 ounces of oysters contain 93 mcg of iodine.

Magnesium

Cofactors are non-protein compounds that help enzymes do their jobs. Magnesium is a cofactor in more than 300 enzyme systems, and it is thought that more than 3000 human proteins bind to it.[365]

This vital mineral is involved in fundamental processes like energy production, DNA synthesis, glucose utilisation, formation of fat, proteins and nucleic acids; muscle contractions and relaxation, the release of neurotransmitters, maintaining normal neurological functions, regulation of vascular tone, heart rhythm, platelet-activated thrombosis, bone formation and immunity.[366]

It is estimated that between 56 and 68% of Americans do not obtain enough magnesium in their diet on a daily basis.[367] Other research suggests that around 10-30% of a given population has subclinical magnesium deficiency based on serum Mg levels <0.80mm/L.[368]

One of the largest studies on this subject, a cross-sectional study of over 16 000 subjects in Germany, discovered a 14.5% prevalence of hypomagnesaemia (magnesium levels below 0.76 mmol/L).[369]

Magnesium deficiency has been found in 84% of postmenopausal women with osteoporosis. Magnesium deficiency is also commonly found in diabetics and the elderly.[370] The prevalence of magnesium deficiency ranges from 9% to 65% in hospitalised patients.[371,372,373]

Chronic magnesium deficiencies over time have been linked to atherosclerosis, heart attacks, high blood pressure, malignant tumours, kidney stones, and alterations in blood cholesterol levels.[374,375]

There are numerous reasons why many of us are magnesium deficient. First of all, the food we eat now has less magnesium than the food our ancestors ate. This is due to monocropping, the use of certain pesticides, soil mineral depletion, certain cooking methods, and heavily processed food manufacturing methods.[365]

Smoking, gastrointestinal absorption disorders, calcium supplementation, and too much or too little vitamin D can all lower our magnesium levels.[365]

And finally, insulin resistance, drinking too much alcohol, diabetes, and some kidney diseases can all cause more magnesium to leave the body and less magnesium to be stored.[376]

It is also important to know that stress, whether physical (i.e., exercise, cold, heat, burns, trauma) or emotional (i.e., pain, depression, excitement), increases the need for magnesium.[377] It can be argued that our stressful lives deplete magnesium stores, and this, along with a reduced input, may potentiate the risks of unabated stress. Magnesium deficiency may mean we are not optimally handling stress which in turn can deplete magnesium stores even more

It probably wouldn't come as a surprise that a mineral involved in over 300 enzyme systems and over 3000 human proteins would be involved in our immune system. Plus, all of the enzymes that metabolise vitamin D seem to require magnesium, and we know how important vitamin D is with regards to our immunity.[378] This is what else magnesium can do:

- Acts as a cofactor of enzymes of nucleic acid metabolism and stabilises structure of nucleic acids; involved in DNA replication and repair.[379]

- Help protect DNA against oxidative damage.[379]
- High concentrations can reduce superoxide anion production - a ROS.[380]
- Has a role in antigen binding to macrophages.[381]
- Regulates leukocyte activation.[382]
- Involved in the regulation of cell death.[379]
- Acts as a cofactor in the formation of antibodies.[383]
- Involved in the antibody-dependent dissolution of cells.[383]
- Needed for the proper docking and thus antipathogenic effects of CD8+ T cells.[384]

While magnesium deficiency can result in:

- Decreased numbers of monocytes.[385]
- Decreased NK-cell activity.[385]
- Increased oxidative stress after strenuous exercise.[385]
- Increased levels of cytokines such as IL-6.[386]
- Increased inflammation.[386]
- Decreased T-cell ratios.[387]

Even though magnesium is an important mineral, only a small amount of scientific research has looked into how too much or too little magnesium may affect the immune system.

Recent discoveries have noted that those with mutations in magnesium transport systems found in certain genetic conditions (human hypomagnesemia with secondary hypercalcemia, and X-linked immunodeficiency with magnesium defect) are likely to suffer from severe and chronic EBV infection and cancer formation, suggesting an important role for magnesium as a second messenger in immunity.[388]

With regards to COVID-19, one review noted that adequate magnesium levels were associated with lower mortality rates and less severe symptoms.[389] And this was reflected by a cross-sectional study that noted, ***"We found that higher intake of dietary magnesium was inversely associated with COVID-19 severity and symptoms."***[390]

The RDA for magnesium for men aged 31–50 years is 420 mg and 310 mg for women.[391]

Intoxication is rare but not impossible, and side effects in the digestive system are often the first sign that magnesium levels may be too high.[365] These side effects can be different depending on the type of magnesium salt that is taken. (It is important to note that those with renal disease are at higher risk for adverse effects)

The Institute of Medicine (IOM) has set the upper tolerable limit of magnesium supplementation with no side effects at 350 mg/day (no risk of gastrointestinal side effects in almost all individuals).[365] With this limit, there is a substantial margin of safety; intoxication with magnesium is rare.

Foods containing the highest content of magnesium are seeds and nuts.[391] One ounce of roasted pumpkin seeds contains 156 mg of magnesium. One ounce of chia seeds contains 111 mg of magnesium, and one ounce of almonds contains 80 mg.

Due to monocropping, the cooking and processing of food, and the fact that most of us live stressful lives, it can be argued that the amount of magnesium ingested is low, whereas the amount needed is high.[392] Furthermore, some of us may need more magnesium than others and at specific times. Magnesium is depleted during heavy exercise, for example, and may be one reason for the possible immunological changes observed after strenuous exercise.[383]

Due to the high need and low natural supply, some people may find it helpful to take magnesium supplements.

Magnesium glycinate has good bioavailability with fewer gastrointestinal side-effects as the compound is absorbed in different areas of the intestine. Along with magnesium taurinate, there is some evidence (case histories) that magnesium glycinate may help with rapid recovery from major depression in less than 7 days.[393]

The presence of glycine in magnesium glycinate may aid sleep. Ingestion of glycine before bed has been shown to improve sleep quality.[394,395]

The modern age has brought about a way of life that is accompanied by poor sleep habits, a poor diet, an abundance of stress, decreased physical exercise, and alcohol misuse. All of these elements have a negative impact on the human genome by increasing inflammation and oxidative stress. It's never been more important than now to look after your DNA and immunity, and magnesium helps both.

Omega 3s

It is more important to consume some fats than others. And a group of fats called "essential fatty acids" *must* be consumed because the body requires them for proper functioning and cannot make them naturally.

Only two fatty acids are known to be essential for humans: alpha-linolenic acid (ALA), an omega-3 fatty acid, and linoleic acid (LA), an omega-6 fatty acid. The distinction between omega-6 and omega-3 fatty acids is based on the location of the first double bond, counting from the methyl end (CH3 side) of the fatty acid molecule.

Because they *must* be consumed, their influence on our health and food choices is greater than that of other fats. The proper consumption and ratio of consumption of both are vital.

LA is plentiful in nature and is found in the seeds of most plants except for coconut, cocoa, and palm. ALA, on the other hand, is found in the chloroplasts of green leafy vegetables and in the seeds of flax, rapeseed, chia, perilla, and walnuts.

Before you run off to your local whole foods store to buy bags of chia seeds and buckets of rapeseed oil, I have to warn you that it gets a little more complicated than that. First, it seems that ALA's main job is to make other omega-3 fatty acids with longer chains. These include eicosapentaenoic acid (EPA) and docosahexaenoic acid (DHA). In humans, however, this conversion process is inefficient.[396] On average, only 0.22–21% of ALA is converted into EPA and 0.5–5% into DHA.[397]

LA, on the other hand, is metabolised to arachidonic acid (AA). These secondary fatty acids are also found in our food. AA is found predominantly in the phospholipids of grain-fed animals, dairy products, and eggs. EPA and DHA are found in the oils of fish, particularly fatty fish.

Studies have shown that EPA and DHA are important for proper foetal development, including brain function, eye health, immune function, and many other biological functions. And in mammals, including humans, the cerebral cortex, retina, testis, and sperm are particularly rich in DHA.[398]

On the other hand, AA plays a vital role in cell-to-cell communication, plays a role in inflammation, and helps make a molecule called anandamide. Anandamide is a molecule that is transmitted across different regions of the brain and is part of a network called the endocannabinoid system.

You'd hope that our amazing body would have a way of just sorting out what we eat into the various forms of fat, but unfortunately, this does not happen. Instead, there is competition between omega-6 and omega-3 fatty acids for enzymes that help them turn into their longer forms. The enzymes we process prefer ALA to LA, but this is where we face a problem. Western diets contain so much LA that it interferes with the conversion of ALA to EPA and DHA.

The theory goes that one cause of excessive inflammation and cardiovascular disease in modern man is due to an imbalance of omega-3 to omega-6 fats—essentially, that an excessive intake of omega-6s and an inadequate intake of omega-3s predisposes us to exaggerated inflammatory responses. The ratio of omega-6:omega-3 in a normal modern diet has been estimated to be between 4:1 (in Japan) and a whopping 50:1 (in urban India). The UK and US are estimated to have ratios of 15:1 and 16.74:1, respectively.[399]

Our late Palaeolithic ancestors, who lived on Earth 3.3 million years ago with minimal heart disease, had diets with estimated ratios of 1:0.79 (that's more omega-3 than omega-6).[399] Recent population studies have shown that nations with low levels of omega-3 and high levels of omega-6 are at greater risk of heart disease.[400]

This *ratio* of omega 3:omega 6 is important because, as we have noted, omega 3s and omega 6s have different roles in the body yet compete for the same enzymatic spot. LA converts to AA, which is later used to make inflammatory molecules, which can cause or exacerbate inflammation,[399] increase blood viscosity, increase the likelihood of clot formation, and cause vessel constriction. ALA and EPA are involved in anti-inflammatory mechanisms.

If we consume too many omega-6s and not enough omega-3s in our diet, then it is accepted that this excessive amount will prevent ALA from being converted to EPA and DHA, thus reducing their anti-inflammatory properties and possibly promoting an inflammatory environment.[401]

Using this theory, one scientific review suspected that omega fatty acid ratios, as well as genetic differences in their formation, were why certain races were affected more than others during the pandemic and why obesity was such a big risk factor for both severity and death from COVID-19. The author of this review concludes with, ***"A proper diet (with a balanced omega-6/omega-3 fatty acid intake) and exercise,***

along with drugs, and eventually vaccines, should be able to conquer the pandemic of COVID-19."[402]

Other than reducing omega-6 consumption, the other way to improve omega ratios is to increase omega-3s. This is especially true because omega-3s have been shown to have other direct effects on the immune system, such as:

- Being able to reduce inflammation.[403]
- Reducing macrophage cytokine production and secretion.[404]
- Polarising macrophages towards M2 phenotype.[404]
- Increasing macrophage and neutrophil phagocytosis.[404]
- Reducing T cell activation.[404]
- Increasing Treg differentiation.[404]
- Increasing IgM production.[404]

With regards to COVID-19, one self-proclaimed "scoping review" noted that ***"severe COVID-19 patients have low levels of omega 3 in their blood. Omega 3 was considered to reduce the risk of positive for SARS-CoV-infection and the duration of symptoms, overcome the renal and respiratory dysfunction, and increase survival rate in COVID-19 patients. Omega 3 fatty acid supplementations were thought to have a potential effect in preventing and treating COVID-19."***[405]

Though it is understandable to want to go out and buy a year's supply of omega-3 tablets, you might want to know that they may in fact cause more harm than good. This is because omega-3s are extremely fragile.

They get damaged easily through oxidation, and this results in harmful bioproducts called lipid peroxides being formed. Not only that, but lipid peroxides are also unstable and further degrade to form secondary oxidation products, including aldehydes such as 4-hydroxyhexenal (HHE) and malondialdehyde (MDA), which are toxic chemicals.

One study on this matter explains that *"...even oil stored in the dark at 4°C may oxidize unacceptably within a month of storage . Added antioxidants reduce but do not prevent oxidation...Significant peroxidation is highly likely to occur in over-the-counter supplements which are commonly kept at room temperature both in retail shops and in the home."*[406]

And these harmful byproducts are no joke. Long-term lipid peroxidase consumption may be a mechanism in the formation of cancer, atherosclerosis and in the pathogenesis of Alzheimer's disease. The study mentioned above further explains that *"chronic feeding of oxidized PUFAs to rats led to growth retardation, intestinal irritation, liver and kidney enlargement, haemolytic anaemia, decreased vitamin E, increased lipid peroxides and inflammatory changes in the liver, cardiomyopathy, and potentially malignant colon cell proliferation".*[406]

If you still want to supplement with omega-3s, high-quality krill oil products may be best because they are more resistant to oxidation due to the presence of an antioxidant called astaxanthin.[407] Also, it may be best to try to purchase products that have either the GOED standard for purity or a third-party seal. And try to also buy krill oil supplements from the Marine Stewardship Council, the Environmental Defense Fund, or a similar certified organisation.

It is also best to keep your supplements in a dark container away from light and in a cool place, and to use them as soon as possible. Also remember to check the label for high levels of DHA and EPA too (some omega-3 pills have higher levels of the less useful ALA).

The other, and arguably less stressful, method is to get your omega-3s from natural sources, with fish being the primary source. Salmon is the best with regards to omega-3 content, with three ounces of it estimated to contain 1.24 g of DHA and 0.59 g of EPA.[408]

The RDA for omega-3s for those aged 19–50 years is 1.6 g/day in men and 1.1 g/day in women. Women who are pregnant are recommended 1.4 g/day, and those who are lactating are recommended 1.3 g/day.[408]

One potential way to normalise omega-3:6 ratios is to include the possible use of cannabidiol (CBD), an active ingredient in cannabis that is derived from the hemp plant and does not cause a high or have addictive properties. But nothing works better than reducing omega-6 intake by a lot while increasing omega-3 intake at the same time.[409]

Selenium

Selenium is an essential micronutrient that plays a vital role in various physiological processes such as contributing to growth,[410] supporting healthy muscle activity,[411] supporting reproductive organs,[412] supporting the immune system,[413] helping with thyroid function,[414] and even delaying the spread of certain viruses like influenza, Ebola, and HIV.[415]

There are several enzymes in which the active centre contains selenium; one of them is glutathione peroxidase, a critical enzyme involved in protecting the body from oxidative damage.[416] Glutathione peroxidase changes ROS into more manageable molecules, reducing its harmful effects.[417] And selenium, through its role in helping glutathione peroxidase helps neutralise certain toxins, has shown to inhibit the growth of cancer cells as well as fight infections. [418,419]

Selenium deficiency and inadequacy are rare in countries like the US.[420] But the elderly, the overweight, and those eating a vegan diet are more likely to have lower selenium blood concentrations.[420,421,422] Worldwide, it has been estimated that up to 1 billion people are affected by insufficient selenium intake.[423]

Selenium deficiency can lead to various forms of illness. One of these is Keshan disease, a cardiomyopathy that occurs in those who are selenium deficient and are affected by a second stress, usually a viral infection.[424] Selenium deficiency is also associated with cardiomyopathy in general,[420,425] male infertility,[426] various cancers,[427] cognitive decline,[428] thyroid disease,[429] and iodine deficiency.[430]

Selenium is vital for the proper function of our immune system; its roles include:

- Being part of selenoproteins, which are important for antioxidant host defence systems, affecting leukocyte and NK cell function.[285]
- Supporting the structural integrity and intactness of the respiratory epithelial barrier, which lowers viral entry to respiratory cells.[431]
- Helping to form defensive proteins and antioxidant enzymes present on the mucosal surface.[431]
- Required to help phagocytic white blood cells surround and engulf pathogens.[432]
- Increasing IFNγ production.[433]
- Having roles in in differentiation and proliferation of T cells, and helping to improve Th cell counts.[434,435]
- Helping to maintain antibody levels.[285]

While selenium deficiency has been linked to:

- Suppression of immune function.[239]
- Diminished NK-cell cytotoxicity.[281]
- Impaired humoral and cell-mediated immunity.[225]
- Decreased immunoglobulin titers.[281]
- Impaired cell-mediated immunity.[281]
- Increased viral virulence.[281]
- Decreased response to vaccination.[281]

With regards to COVID-19, one systematic review on the subject noted that, ***"In most cases, selenium deficiency was associated with worse outcomes, and selenium levels in COVID-19 patients were lower than in healthy individuals."*** and went on to note, ***"Thus, it could be concluded that cautious selenium supplementation in COVID-19 patients may be helpful to prevent disease progression."*** [436]

In one South Korean study, selenium deficiency was associated with higher mortality in COVID-19 patients.[437] Another study in China showed that better selenium status was associated with better cure rates in COVID-19 sufferers.[438]

Interestingly, too, diseases such as HIV, influenza, and Ebola are more likely to evolve and spread in areas where soils are deficient in selenium.[439] This may be because selenium deficiency has been shown to promote viral mutations, replication, and the emergence of a more pathogenic form of RNA viruses.[440] This is yet to be confirmed to be the case with SARS-CoV-2, but sheds some light on who may be at risk of being true "super spreaders."

The RDA for selenium in those aged 19–50 years is 55 mcg in both men and women, 60 mcg in those who are pregnant, and 70 mcg in lactating women.[420]

The food highest in selenium are brazil nuts, with an estimated 544 mcg of selenium per 6–8 nuts. Next are yellowfin tuna and halibut, three ounces of each containing 92 mcg and 47 mcg of selenium, respectively.[420]

Though deficiency and inadequacy are rare in the West, those who are obese are usually more deficient in a vast array of micronutrients and vitamins compared to those who are not; this likely applies to selenium too.[422,441] We all know that obesity is an extremely strong risk factor for COVID-19 morbidity and mortality, and selenium deficiency may play a part as to why.

Selenium appears to be effective in preventing COVID-19, and adequate amounts may also help reduce the risk of certain heart conditions and infertility. There is also data showing the combination of selenium and niacin (vitamin B3) to be effective in blunting the effects of infection in the lung.[442,443]

Zinc

Zinc is an essential mineral involved in many aspects of biological metabolism. It is required for the speeding up of hundreds of enzymes, and it plays a role in enhancing immune function, protein and DNA synthesis, wound healing, and cell signalling and division.[444]

The WHO says that zinc deficiency affects 31% of the world's people, with rates ranging from 4% to 73% in different parts of the world.[445] Others estimated that 17.3% of the global population is at risk of inadequate zinc intake.[446] And another study of a US population showed zinc inadequacy in 15% of participants.[447]

Because zinc has many functions throughout the body, a zinc deficiency affects many different tissues and organs. One of these symptoms associated with zinc deficiency includes a lack of smell and taste.[448] This feature, along with the fact that zinc has been hypothesised to reduce the severity and duration of colds by directly inhibiting rhinovirus binding and replication in the nasal mucosa,[449] is likely why it became a popular go-to supplement for many during the pandemic.

Recent evidence with regards to the lack of smell and taste during a COVID-19 infection suggests that sensory changes during the infection aren't *directly* related to zinc deficiency but may occur due to a possible indirect link through reduced odorant receptor levels in response to innate immune signalling.[450]

The role of zinc on our health has been mainly studied in the context of our immune system and there is some promising evidence suggesting that the supplementation of it can reduce the duration of colds;[451] reduce the prevalence of pneumonia in children;[452] decrease the rates of opportunistic infections in HIV sufferers;[453] shorten the duration of infectious diarrhoea in children;[454] slowing the progression of age-related macular degeneration;[455] and possibly helping with the progression of type two diabetes.[444]

Zinc is vital for the proper function of our immune system; its roles include:

- Helping to maintain integrity of skin and mucosal membrane.[456]
- Maintaining or enhancing NK cell cytotoxic activity.[433]
- Having a central role in cellular growth and differentiation of immune cells that have a rapid differentiation and turnover.[209]
- Improving the phagocytic activity of macrophages and monocytes.[433]
- Being involved in complement activity; role in IFNγ production.[268]

- Helping to modulate cytokine release.[457]
- Having antioxidant effects that protect against ROS and reactive nitrogen species.[457]
- Induces the production of cytotoxic T cells.[458]
- Supporting Th1 response.[433]
- Being required for T cell development, differentiation, and activation.[457]
- Inducing development of Treg cells and is thus important in maintaining immune tolerance.[433]
- Being involved in antibody production, particularly IgG.[459]
- Important in maintaining immune tolerance (i.e., the ability to recognise "self" from "non-self").[286]

Zinc deficiency is linked to:

- Impaired survival, proliferation and maturation of monocytes, NK cells, T and B cells.[460]
- Impaired NK cell activity.[218]
- Impaired phagocytosis by macrophages and neutrophils.[218]
- Unfavourable cytokine response, contributing to greater oxidative stress and inflammation.[461]
- Increased thymic shrinkage.[462]
- Alterations in the expression of genes related to proliferation, survival, and response of T-cells even with moderate deficiency.[463]
- Th1/Th2 imbalance.[460]
- Impaired antibody response to T cell-dependent antigens.[218]

With regards to COVID-19, one meta-analysis noted that zinc supplementation was associated with a lower mortality rate in COVID-19 patients. They concluded with, ***"Zinc supplementation could be considered as a simple way and cost benefit approach for reduction of mortality in COVID-19 patients."***[464] But the evidence is still mixed.[465]

The RDA for zinc in those aged 19 years and above is 11 mg in men and 8mg in women, 11mg in those who are pregnant and 12mg in women who are lactating.[466]

The richest food sources of zinc include meat, fish, and seafood. The highest source of zinc are oysters, three ounces of which contain 32 mg of zinc. Next is beef which contains 3.8 mg of zinc per three ounces.[466]

A summary of micronutrients

The list of micronutrients noted above is in no way exhaustive, but I believe they are both the most immunologically essential and some of the least consumed throughout the world.

The unfortunate reality is that, while the quantity and variety of food available to us are greater than they have ever been, the quality has declined significantly due to monoculture, battery farming methods, and ultra-processing. To make matters worse, the rates of obesity and metabolic syndrome are continuing to rise worldwide. And the cherry on top is that a growing vegan/plant-based philosophy is taking over the world.

I believe that it is always best to get essential nutritional components naturally, and only with a few exceptions, the foods highest in these micronutrients are organ meats, fish, and oysters. This is best illustrated by the table below, which is from a study comparing the nutritional content of various foods.[467]

	Overall density	Iron	Zinc	Vitamin A	Calcium	Folate	Vitamin B_{12}
Liver	Very high	Very high	Very high	Very high	Low	Very high	Very high
Spleen	Very high	Very high	Very high	Low	Low	Low	Very high
Small dried fish	Very high	Very high	Very high	Very high	Very high	Low	Very high
Dark leafy greens	Very high	High	Low	Very high	Very high	Very high	Low
Bivalves	Very high	Very high	Very high	High	Very high	Moderate	Very high
Kidney	Very high	Very high	Very high	High	Low	High	Very high
Heart	Very high	Very high	Very high	Low	Low	Moderate	Very high
Crustaceans	Very high	High	Very high	Low	Moderate	Low	Very high
Goat	Very high	Very high	Very high	Low	Low	Low	Very high
Beef	Very high	Very high	Very high	Low	Low	Low	Very high
Eggs	Very high	High	High	Very high	Low	High	Very high
Cow milk	Very high	Low	High	Very high	Very high	Low	Very high
Canned fish w/ bones	Very high	High	High	Low	Very high	Low	Very high
Lamb/mutton	Very high	Very high	Very high	Low	Low	Low	Very high
Cheese	High	Low	Very high	High	Very high	Low	Very high
Goat milk	High	Low	Moderate	High	Very high	Low	Low
Pork	High	High	Very high	Low	Low	Low	Very high
Yoghurt	Moderate	Low	Low	Low	Very high	Low	Very high
Fresh fish	Moderate	Moderate	Moderate	Low	Low	Low	Very high
Pulses	Moderate	Very high	Moderate	Low	Low	Very high	Low
Teff	Moderate	Very high	Moderate	Low	Low	High	Low
Canned fish w/o bones	Moderate	Moderate	Moderate	Low	Low	Low	Very high
Vit A-rich fruit/veg	Low	Low	Low	Very high	Low	High	Low
Other vegetables	Low	Low	Low	Low	Low	Low	Low
Quinoa	Low	High	Moderate	Low	Low	Very high	Low
Fonio	Low	Very high	Moderate	Low	Low	Moderate	Low
Seeds	Low	High	High	Low	High	High	Low
Millet	Low	Very high	Moderate	Low	Low	Moderate	Low
Unrefined grain prod	Low	Moderate	Moderate	Low	Low	Moderate	Low
Chicken	Low	Low	High	Low	Low	Low	Moderate
Other fruits	Low	Low	Low	Low	Low	Low	Low
Sorghum	Low	Very high	Low	Low	Low	Low	Low
Roots/tubers/plantains	Low	Low	Low	Low	Low	Low	Low
Whole grains	Low	Moderate	Low	Low	Low	Low	Low
Nuts	Low	Low	Low	Low	Low	Low	Low
Refined grain products	Low	Low	Low	Low	Low	Low	Low
Refined grains	Low	Low	Moderate	Low	Low	Low	Low

Food micronutrient densities, from:
https://www.frontiersin.org/articles/10.3389/fnut.2022.806566/full

All in all, this means that many of us, some more at risk than others, are malnourished even though we're "well fed." And the push to go "plant-based" is likely just adding fuel to the fire, especially when many plants, if not cooked properly, can reduce the bioavailability of certain micronutrients too.

We are literally what we consume, and thus it is no wonder why many of us suffer from chronic illnesses and immunological dysfunction. Vitamins, minerals, and essential macronutrients are not only essential for the smooth running of our immune system but for our biology as a whole.

Food is medicine.

HEALTHY GUT MICROBIOME

A typical man contains on average about 30 trillion human cells and 39 trillion bacteria.[468] And the majority of the bacteria found in the body live in the human gut.

It has been estimated that between 15,000 and 36,000 individual species of bugs live in the intestines.[469] And the microflora genome is estimated to contain more than 100 times as many genes as the human genome.[470]

By the way, it's not just bacteria either; the gut microbiome (GM) is the totality of all the bacteria, viruses, protozoa, fungi, and their collective genetic material present in the gastrointestinal tract.

Being vastly abundant, and in fact out-numbering our own cells, it may come as no surprise that the GM has been linked to a whole host of biological processes such as vitamin production,[471] regulating the immune system, protection from "bad" bacteria and even having a part to play with our mood and personality.[472] One's GM is a good reflection of one's overall health, and the GM also affects our health. It's a bidirectional relationship.

A recent study of 100 patients with laboratory-confirmed SARS-CoV-2 infection showed that gut microbiome composition was significantly altered in patients with COVID-19 compared with non-COVID-19 individuals, irrespective of whether patients had received medication. The study notes that ***"several gut commensals with known immunomodulatory potential such as Faecalibacterium prausnitzii, Eubacterium rectale and bifidobacteria were underrepresented in patients and remained low in samples collected up to 30 days after disease resolution."***[473]

The study further explains that those with unfavourable GM also had concordant elevated concentrations of inflammatory cytokines and blood markers and in fact that, ***"GM dysbiosis after disease resolution could contribute to persistent symptoms."***[473]

In other words, those with poorer GM had worsened COVID-19 outcomes, and an altered GM after the initial infection could lead to chronic symptoms, aka long COVID.

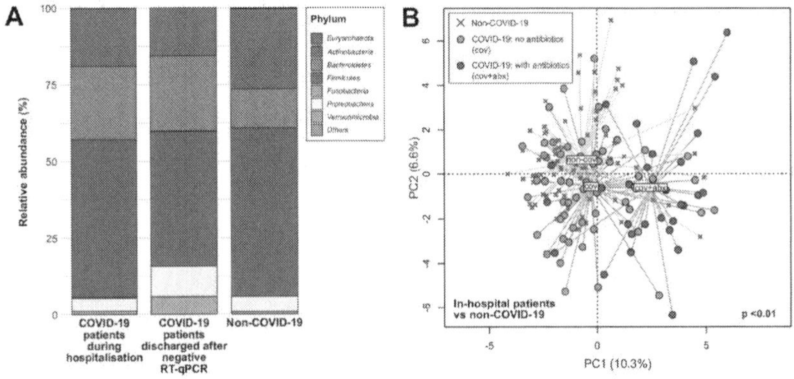

Differences in gut microbiome in COVID-19 patients (in and out of hospital) and non-COVID-19 patients, from: https://gut.bmj.com/content/70/4/698

But how does the gut affect the immune system, you may ask? Well, disease-causing bugs can make us sick by producing toxins that directly affect normal bodily functions. But as we have hopefully understood by now, the severity of a disease is also determined by our immune response to it. This is why some of us remained asymptomatic throughout the pandemic, while others faced multiorgan failure and even death.

The GM has been noted to play a role in modulating the host immune response and potentially influencing disease severity and outcomes. The lack of certain strains and the enrichment of other bacteria in the GM are linked to worsened COVID-19 disease, indicating that this imbalance may have a role in exacerbating overly aggressive inflammation.

Ratios are everything. Depleted gut commensals such as *B. adolescentis*, *F. prausnitzii*, *E. rectale*, *R. (Blautia) obeum,* and *D. formicigenerans* have been separately linked to reduced host inflammatory response in other inflammatory-related diseases too.[474] *F. prausnitzii* has been shown to help activate T-cells in the colon.[475] *E. rectale* in the is are linked to reduced inflammation in Alzheimer's disease,[476] and *B. adolescentis* is able to suppress activation of NF-κB (similar to what ketone bodies do).[477]

On the other hand, the enrichment of *Ruminococcus gnavus*, *Ruminococcus torques*, *Bacteroides dorei* and *Bacteroides vulgatus* in COVID-19 is consistent with microbial-mediated immune dysregulation. Which is not so surprising, considering that *R. gnavus*, *R. torques*, *B. dorei* and *B. vulgatus* population levels have all been reported to positively correlate with inflammatory bowel disease.[478,479,480,]

Another study comparing those non-infected with others who had severely symptomatic COVID-19 showed again that, compared with controls, **severely symptomatic SARS-CoV-2-infected patients had significantly less bacterial diversity, and positive patients overall had lower relative abundances of *Bifidobacterium*, *Faecalibacterium* and *Roseburium*, while having increased *Bacteroides*.**[481]

A lot of the protection from severe disease was thought possibly due to the higher presence of *Bifidobacterium*. Unfortunately though, due to the nature of the study design, it was not possible to determine whether the differences in *Bifidobacterium* and other bacterial strain levels observed between patients and exposed controls preceded or followed infection.

What we do know, though, is that the abundance of *Bifidobacterium* decreases with increasing age and BMI,[482] and that these bacterial strains are linked to various biological processes such as:

- Enhanced cellular energy production.[481]
- Immune modulation.[483]
- Mucosal barrier integrity.[481]
- Restriction of bacterial adherence to and invasion of the intestinal epithelium.[481]
- Modulation of central nervous system activity.[484]
- Decreasing pro-inflammatory cytokines.[483]
- Promoting Th1 while inhibiting the Th2 immune response.[485]
- Increasing Treg responses and reducing cell damage by inhibiting TNF-α and macrophages.[486]

Gut microbiome modulation is a relatively new and growing area of science. But regardless, with this information, some of you are likely wondering how one could improve gut health. Well firstly, both fasting and ingesting fibre have shown to increase *Lactobacillus* and *Bifidobacterium*.[487,488] The other way may be through the use of probiotics, in particular kefir.[489]

Kefir is a fermented probiotic drink made from milk that is renowned for its health properties. Unlike other types of fermented milk, kefir is unique in that it is made with kefir grains. Kefir grains are groups of bacteria and yeast that live together in a matrix of protein and fat. The grains ferment the milk by breaking down lactose into lactic acid and other beneficial vitamins and minerals.

This ancient drink was patented first in Eastern Europe, the Balkans, and the Caucasus. Traditionally, milk kefir was made by combining fresh milk and kefir grains inside goatskin bags. During the daytime, goatskin bags were hung in doorways, and prodded or pushed by those walking through. As people consumed the drink, more fresh milk was added to the goatskin bag, forming a continuous fermentation cycle.

The people of the Caucasus mountains have been making kefir for hundreds or even thousands of years, and kefir grains are known by the name "Grains of the Prophet." Legend has it that the prophet Mohammed gifted kefir grains to the Orthodox Christians in this region. Mohammed is said to have taught the people how to make kefir, and the people revered kefir as a health-promoting food.

Ounce for ounce, kefir might be the most nutrient-dense drink around. Kefir possesses several health benefits associated with its microbial community and their metabolic yields. The main polysaccharide (complex sugar molecules) in kefir grains is the heteropolysaccharide kefiran (also known as kefiran). Kefiran has been shown to have important antitumor, antifungal, and antibacterial properties, as well as immunomodulatory or epithelium-protecting, anti-inflammatory, healing, and antioxidant properties.[490,491]

Kefir grains can contain up to 61 strains of bacteria and yeast, making them a very rich and diverse probiotic source.[471] The most common bacteria in kefir grains and milk are *Lactococcus, Streptococcus, Lactococcus lactis subspecies lactis, Lactobacillus delbrueckii subspecies bulgaricus, L. helveticus, L. casei subspecies pseudoplantarum, L. skefiri, L. kefir, L. Brevis,* and *Streptococcus thermophiles*.

In addition to the large and variable bacterial population in kefir grains, there is an abundant yeast population that exists in a symbiotic relationship with the bacteria. Three common types of yeasts found in kefir grain or milk include *Saccharomyces*, *Kluyveromyces*, and *Candida.*

Aside from containing a vast number of beneficial microorganisms, these organisms also ferment milk, producing various nutritionally beneficial biomolecules and metabolites. Some of them include vitamins B1, B2, B5, C, calcium, magnesium, potassium, sodium, and amino acids such as serine, threonine, alanine, lysine, valine, isoleucine, methionine, phenylalanine, and tryptophan. These components have important roles in improving immunomodulation, digestion, metabolism, energy balance, healing, aiding the central nervous system, and maintaining normal bodily functions.[491]

Kefir supplementation may be able to restore GM balance while also providing other nutrients to help fight infection and reduce overall inflammation.

In animals, probiotics/kefir have been shown to suppress viral activity and virus entry into host cells;[491] protect the host against influenza (*Bifidobacterium breve* strain);[492] reduce the population of nasal pathogens;[493] reduce the risk of acquiring common-cold infections (*L. plantarum* and *L. paracasei* strains);[494] have inhibitory activity against herpes poliovirus-1 (*L. lactis* subspecies *lactis*);[495] enhance the healing response to treatments of infection by the hepatitis-C virus (HCV) (*Lactobacillus acidophilus* and *Bifidobacteria*);[496] reduced levels of reactive oxygen species; decrease expression of proinflammatory cytokines; benefit the outcomes of chronic HCV infection; possibly enhance the immunogenicity of influenza vaccines; reduce viral levels in lungs (*L. lactis* subspecies *Cremoris*);[497] have significant activity against the respiratory syncytial virus (RSV) (*Lactobacillus gasseri*);[498] have anti-swine influenza virus activity (*Saccharomyces cerevisiae*)[499] and the list goes on and on.

All in all, those with worse COVID-19 outcomes are more likely to have an unfavourable GM. Drinking kefir may aid this and in turn help prevent COVID-19, other infectious diseases, and even treat long COVID, but more studies are needed. And more specifically, more *human* studies are needed, as most of the current evidence comes from animal models.

Before you go out and start purchasing kefir from your nearest supermarket, it may be best to make your own at home using milk (raw or raw goat is said to be better). Supermarket kefir is significantly underwhelming in comparison to the real thing, as well as containing additional sweeteners and preservatives (like maltodextrin)[500] that are ironically harmful to the gut. Also, keep in mind that the GM is also a measure of your overall health, so drinking kefir without making changes to other parts of your life is pretty pointless.

The interplay between our gut, metabolism, and immunity is a fascinating one. This area of research is only growing and may even help us understand the root causes of common ailments like obesity. A recent study on mice showed microbiota imbalance induced by dietary sugar disrupted immune-mediated protection from metabolic syndrome. Sugar eliminated protective Th17-inducing microbes and promoted the outgrowth of *Faecalibaculum rodentium* which displaced Th17-inducing microbiota. Eliminating sugar from high-fat diets protected mice from obesity and metabolic syndrome in a manner dependent on commensal-specific Th17 cells.[501]

Is this another reason to reduce our consumption of refined sugar?

As our GM works bidirectionally with us and is thus a reflection of our internal and external environment, it may not be too unhinged to say that it also works as an amplifier of our biological status. A healthy GM will help us feel better and promote healthier behaviours to promote its growth, while an unfavourable GM may do the opposite. And thus, kefir should be consumed as part of an overall healthy lifestyle. And it is recommended to start off with a little and slowly.

REDUCE STRESS

Life for all living things' is, and has always been stressful. Stress is necessary; you wouldn't be here without it.

The world, for the majority of time for all organisms, has been a dangerous place with unpredictable natural disasters and predators to look out for, and the ability to respond to these environmental stressors meant either survival or death. The ones who lived were better at sensing and responding to these threats, and these helpful traits were passed on to their offspring.

Organisms have evolved various mechanisms to handle stress and fend off threats. We humans, like other mammals, have two main stress-signalling pathways: the autonomic nervous system (ANS) and the hypothalamic-pituitary-adrenal (HPA) axis. The ANS is a component of our central nervous system (CNS) and is in charge of our immediate response to threats, our "fight or flight" response. The HPA axis, on the other hand, causes the release of stress hormones like adrenocorticotropic hormone (ACTH), cortisol, growth hormone, prolactin, epinephrine, and norepinephrine.[502]

The CNS, endocrine (hormone) system, and immune system are complex "sensing" systems that interact with each other and the world to optimise our survival and function. The problem we face now is that the world is not how it once was; it is not the place we were evolved to live in, and this causes biological imbalances and immune dysregulation.

As Sapolsky writes in his famous book, "Why Zebras Don't Get Ulcers," *"Stress-related disease emerges, predominantly, out of the fact that we so often activate a physiological system that has evolved for responding to acute physical emergencies, but we turn it on for months on end, worrying about mortgages, relationships, and promotions."*[503]

It's all about timing, though. Short-term stressors have been noted to *increase* immune responses. One study showed that when mice were subject to short-term stress, T cells were selectively redistributed into the skin, where they contributed to the enhancement of the immune response.[504] And elements of the innate immune system, such as natural killer cells and neutrophils, have also been shown to become activated during short bursts of stress.[503]

Evolutionarily speaking, this upregulation of the immune system (and especially the innate immune system) in response to short-term stressors makes sense. Back in the day, fighting or fleeing a threat would have carried an additional risk of injury and subsequent entry of infectious agents into the bloodstream or skin, and thus stress-induced changes in the immune system that could accelerate wound repair and help prevent infections would have been beneficial for our long term survival.

The problem we have now is that we rarely come across many of the things that used to make our ancestors want to fight or run away. Instead, most of our stresses are psychological and long-term. Many of us worry about various aspects of our lives for a long time and have to deal with less than ideal living and working conditions. To make matters worse, we are constantly bombarded with environmental pollutants and given stress-promoting foods to eat.

Though short-term stress upregulates certain parts of our immune system, long-term stress has been shown to negatively impact our immune system via a number of mechanisms. Studies in the late 1990s and early 2000s reported that chronic forms of stress were accompanied by reduced NK cell cytotoxicity, suppressed lymphocyte proliferation, and blunted antibody responses to immunisation.[505,506,507] And this diminished immune response in chronically stressed individuals is assumed to be responsible for the heightened incidence of infectious and neoplastic diseases in these people.[508]

Chronic stress has also shown to alter cytokine secretion patterns from Th1 to Th2. This shift can occur via the effects of stress hormones such as cortisol. Cortisol is ordinarily anti-inflammatory, but chronic elevations can lead to the immune system becoming "resistant," causing an accumulation of stress hormones, and increased production of inflammatory cytokines.[509] This has shown to cause an overall Th2 response that may explain the increased vulnerability to infectious, autoimmune disease and neoplastic disease in those chronically stressed.[510]

The link between cortisol and our immune system is more complex, as stress itself can be broadly classified into two main groups:[503] bereavement and trauma. Maternal separation in animals and bereavement in humans are commonly associated with increased cortisol production,[511] which is in turn associated with decreased natural killer cell cytotoxicity; whereas trauma is associated with non-significantly increased cytotoxicity and increased proliferation of natural killer cells but decreased numbers of T cells. Trauma and post-traumatic stress disorder are commonly associated with decreased cortisol production.[512]

Other than cortisol, the release of catecholamines like adrenaline can have immunomodulatory effects too. Animal studies have shown that stress-induced suppression of cytolytic CD8+ T cell responses during influenza virus infection is caused by adrenaline stimulation.[513]

Another way stress negatively impacts our immune system is through its effects on our GM. According to one study, when rhesus monkeys were separated from their mothers and thus appropriately stressed, their levels of "beneficial" *Lactobacillus* decreased while gut pathogens *Shigella flexneri* and *Campylobacter jejuni* increased.[513] During stressful times, college students also have less lactobacilli, but it's important to remember that big changes in diet can happen during stressful times, which can also affect the GM.[513]

Other than a difference in food intake, the GM is thought to be affected by stress in numerous other ways. The activation of our "flight or fight" response suppresses stomach acid production, and this has been hypothesised to alter GM populations.[515] Another possible explanation is that stress-related changes in the microflora are caused by changes in sIgA and/or defensins.[515] Defensins are small molecules made by white blood cells that help fight pathogenic bacteria, fungi, and many viruses.

As well as changing how our intestines move, stress hormones can directly change the number of commensal bacteria and how "leaky" the wall of our intestines is, which can affect how bacteria move through our bodies.[515] All of this can cause GM imbalances, which in turn have been shown to cause immune dysregulation and even autoimmune disorders.[516]

Overall, chronic stress is not good for us. It has been shown to impair wound healing, cause reactivation of latent viruses, reduce CD4 counts in HIV-infected persons, contribute to the early emergence and progression of atherosclerosis, help develop insulin resistance, enhance both tumour progression and metastasis, and age us and our immune system.[517-522]

And to make matters worse, people's efforts to manage the demands of stressful experiences sometimes lead them to engage in unhelpful behaviours—such as alcohol use or changes in sleeping patterns—that also usually negatively impact our immune system processes.[523] A vicious cycle is formed.

Concerning COVID-19, an interesting study on mice found that short-term stress sent neutrophils to sites of injury, but stress that caused stress hormones to be released protected against autoimmunity but made the body less resistant to SARS-CoV-2 and influenza infection.[524] **This may be why another study of nearly half a million subjects showed that late-life anxiety increased the risk of developing COVID-19.**[525]

If you've been very stressed, you might have been advised to breathe slowly and deeply. Though it may sometimes feel like annoying advice, it does have some scientific merit because this type of breathing activates the vagus nerve.

The vagus is the longest nerve of the autonomic nervous system. It supplies parasympathetic fibres to all the organs (except the adrenal glands), from the neck down to part of our small intestine, which in turn helps us "rest and digest." It also helps regulate our heartbeat and plays an important part in other bodily processes like sweating and speech.

One way to stimulate it is through deep breathing. In one study,[526] COVID-19 patients were asked to perform a 20-minute breathing exercise three times a day with six breaths per minute and an inhalation to exhalation ratio of 4:6 seconds. Though the participant size was small, results showed that the intervention reduced the pro-inflammatory cytokine IL-6 in these patients. **The breathing also alleviated the participants' "feeling of being helpless and without control, introducing the feeling of self-efficacy."**[526]

There are many other ways to break the stressful cycle other than through deep, purposeful breathing. Non-traditional therapies, including yoga, tai chi, acupuncture, spiritual practises, and meditation, have been linked to improvements in natural killer cells and leukocytes, as well as changes in cortisol, adrenaline, and norepinephrine levels, as well as IL-6 and TNF levels.[527]

Exercise, eating correctly, and adequate sleep must also not be forgotten for not only their direct effect on immunity but also for indirectly improving immunity via helping with stress.[528,529] Loneliness and past unresolved psychological issues can worsen our immunological function too. So find someone to speak to.[530,531] Go visit your mother if you can. Turn off the news. Breathe deeply and de-stress.

This once again highlights the detrimental immunological impacts of lockdown, mainstream media fear-mongering, and our treatment of the elderly during the pandemic. All that stress made some of us literally worry sick.

REMOVAL OF TOXINS

Other than being less chronically psychologically stressful, the world that our ancestors were used to was also a lot less polluted and thus a lot less physiologically stressful.

Globalisation and corporatisation since the Industrial Revolution have meant that a greater proportion of the global population can enjoy the fruits of convenience, but this has come at a massive cost. The world is becoming increasingly desecrated, and so is our health.

Convenience and crony capitalism in combination have been an ecological and biological nightmare. Poisons that have been birthed via cut corners, lacklustre safety precautions, and the need to meet high wasteful demands lurk in the foods we eat, the water we drink, and even in our clothes.

Just like mRNA technology, the main problem with these chemicals is that they are foreign to our biological systems. Some of them also have a tendency to bioaccumulate in our body, whilst others affect various receptors causing detrimental downstream effects at even low concentrations.

Because these environmental toxins are physiologically foreign in nature, we usually do not know what the long-term effects will be on us or the environment until it is too late. And by the time the damage is done, the accumulation of various other variables has tainted the water, obscuring cause and effect. This means that many environmental toxins aren't prohibited early on if obvious concerns don't arise and stay within circulation until a massive fuss is made about them. Even so, because corporate structures have become reliant on their circulation, and many of these chemicals have a long half-life, banning does not always result in immediate clearance.

The list of environmental toxins grows every day, as does the list of their related health issues. We are beginning to learn that everything from autism, obesity, inflammatory bowel disease, and asthma to mental disorders and the risk of premature birth can be linked to various environmental toxins one way or another.[532-537]

Our immune system, along with our nervous and endocrine systems, is thought to be primarily influenced by these toxins. Immunological interference by these toxins can result in immune dysfunction, autoimmunity, asthma, allergies, and malignancies.[538]

The list of environmental toxins and related immunological problems is gargantuan and ever-growing. In the interest of time, I have gone over some of the most common environmental toxins that impact our immune system below.

Ultra-processed foods

Next time you visit your local supermarket, take a stroll around and note the different types of food on offer. If your supermarket is anything like mine, then fresh whole food products will be found on the outside, while most of what you will encounter will be ultra-processed "foods."

One scientific analysis of over two hundred thousand American food products found 71% of products such as bread, salad dressings, snack foods, sweets, sugary drinks, and more were ultra-processed. And of the 25 companies with the most sales, 86% of their products were considered to be ultra-processed.[539]

And so it is not surprising that a cross-sectional study of just under ten thousand American participants published in the BMJ found that ultra-processed foods comprised 57.9% of energy intake and contributed 89.7% of the energy intake from added sugars.[540]

I'm going to the extent of calling ultra-processed foods environmental toxins and biological poisons. Hence why they are on this list. Foods should be the transporters of vitamins, minerals, and energy, but processing changes a food from its naturally beneficial state and instead puts the profits of major food corporations before our health.

Processing involves the use of additives such as sugar, salt, fat, emulsifiers, artificial colours or preservatives, and deodorizers (in the case of cooking oil) to make the end product last longer and be more addictive and palatable.

All of this causes global environmental havoc, contributing to colossal agrobiodiversity loss, as well as coming at the expense of the cultivation, manufacture, and consumption of traditional foods, cuisines, and diets, comprising mostly fresh and minimally processed foods.[541]

Other than harming our planet, ultra-processed foods also wreak havoc on our health. They have been linked to a greater risk of cancer, heart disease, and even death.[542,543,544] **Recent research has also found that eating more ultra-processed foods is linked to a higher chance of getting COVID-19.**[545]

Processed foods are also associated with an increased risk of obesity and insulin resistance, both of which have been linked to immunocompromisation.[546,547] Ultra-processed foods may also harm our immune system directly in a number of different ways, including by:

- Increasing overall oxidative stress and inflammation, and thus could implicate a lower tolerance of the immune system and an increased risk of infections.[548]
- Hyper-activating the complement system as well as promoting intestinal leakiness.[549]
- Increasing gut leakiness which in turn causes bacteria to end up in places they should not be, this in turn causes inflammation and higher than normal levels of endotoxins in the blood.[550]
- Disrupting the gut microbiome leading to dysbiosis, increased mucosal inflammation and an increased risk of autoimmunity. [550, 552,553]
- Directly and indirectly causing micronutrient deficiencies leading to immune dysfunction and increased susceptibility to infection.[550,554]

For these reasons and more, just like not calling mRNA and genetic agents "vaccines," I do not personally call ultra-processed foods "foods." To keep your immune system strong, it might be best to stick to the real foods that are mostly found on the edges of grocery stores. Remember, you are literally what you eat.

Microplastics

Microplastics are defined as "synthetic solid particles or polymeric matrices, with regular or irregular shape and size ranging from 1 μm to 5 mm, of either primary or secondary manufacturing origin, which are insoluble in water."[555]

The distribution and abundance of microplastics in the world are becoming increasingly extensive. So extensive in fact that many scientists are using them as key indicators of the recent and contemporary period defining a new historical epoch: The Plasticene. *Sad, right?*

The recent pandemic has certainly not helped either. One study showed that more than eight million tonnes of pandemic-associated plastic waste had been generated globally, with more than 25,000 tonnes entering the global ocean. 87% of this waste came from hospitals, including plastic gloves, gowns, and masks, with only about 8% of the waste generated by individuals.[556]

Nanoplastics and other harmful pollutants have been found in disposable face masks that are released when submerged in water. The other pollutants within the silicon-based and plastic fibres of common disposable face masks included lead, antimony, and copper.[557]

And a study from the University of Portsmouth found mask litter increased by

9,000% in the first seven months of the pandemic and could have led to further spread of the virus.[558]

Microplastics are everywhere, and they have recently been found in people's lungs.[559] This suggests that they can be inhaled. This is worrying, as exposure to them has been hypothesised to be linked with neurotoxicity, reproductive toxicity, oxidative stress, carcinogenicity, and immune disruption.[560]

Recent research has alluded to various mechanisms by which microplastics cause immunotoxicity, including:

- Increasing oxidative stress of cells, the release of immune modulators, and the inappropriate activation of immune cells - which in turn may result in the production of antibodies against self-antigens.[561]
- Causing temporary immunosuppression due to increased production of anti-inflammatory cytokines, suppression of T-helper cells, and decreased production of T-effector cells.[560]
- Causing DNA damage in human peripheral lymphocytes.[562]
- Causing alterations in the expression of immune system genes and the down-regulation of genes correlated with epithelium integrity and fat metabolism in zebrafish.[563]
- Causing hormonal dysfunction and downstream immune dysfunction.[564]
- Altering the intestinal microbiota profile of certain crab species.[565]

Though a great and growing health and environmental concern, human trials with regards to how microplastics affect our biological systems and immunity are severely lacking. At the time of writing this, there has been no direct study comparing the risk of COVID-19 and levels of microplastics in one's body. But a very recent study notes that oral feeding of nanoplastics reduces brain function in mice by triggering gut interleukin-1 beta (IL-1β)-producing macrophages, thus further highlighting the gut-brain-immunological axis.[566]

Another review notes that the increased human exposure to microplastics during the pandemic may have contributed to increased population-wide DNA damage.[562] This is likely made worse by the consumption of unhealthy food and sleep deprivation.

BPA

Bisphenol A (BPA) is an industrial chemical that is used to make epoxy resins and polycarbonate plastics. It is found in common household products like plastic food containers and water bottles. It's also found in credit cards and DVDs. It has been used since the 1960s to produce strong plastics for food packaging and home kitchen use.[567]

BPA is a worry because it seems like this industrial chemical is leaching into our biological systems and causing pathology. Its exposure is so widespread that it is becoming difficult to run away from.

Diet is the most common source of BPA intake. Baby food seems rife with it too; one study noted BPA detection in infant food is as high as 76%, and in the same study, 85% of Korean children had detectable levels of BPA in their urine.[568]

BPA exposure has been linked to a number of health issues, which may be due in part to the fact that it mimics the structure and function of the oestrogen hormone. As a result, BPA and a few other chemicals are referred to as "environmental oestrogens."

BPA, as an environmental oestrogen, is also classified as an "endocrine disruptor" or "hormone disruptor." And, despite being initially thought to be a weak environmental oestrogen, recent research suggests that BPA may be as effective as natural estradiol in stimulating some cellular responses.[569]

Furthermore, it is extremely important to note that a lot of endocrine disruptors, BPA included, work in an inverted U-shaped dose-response manner, meaning that extremely high and low doses have minimal effects, while mid-range doses are enough to activate receptors. You may find this relationship between endocrine disruptors and receptors described as having a "non-monotonic dose response."[570]

Endocrine disruptors are also thought to cause the most biological damage during specific time windows and specifically to endocrine organs. These time windows include pre-conception, foetal development, pregnancy, breastfeeding, and puberty. One of the most studied groups of endocrine organs that are affected by BPA are the reproductive organs, but growing evidence is showing that nearly all parts of the body are affected by this chemical.

Several studies conducted in animals and humans have reported that exposure to BPA during the gestational period affects brain development and behaviour.[571] It has been elucidated that exposure to BPA can induce anxiety, an increased risk of autistic behaviours, impaired memory and learning, as well as changes in social behaviours.[572]

Being an oestrogen-mimicking endocrine disruptor, BPA looks like it affects males and females differently. In one long-term study,[573] the amount of BPA found in the urine of mothers was linked to more anxiety and depression in boys at age 7 but not in girls. Boys who were exposed to higher levels of BPA *in utero* were also found to have a higher likelihood of shorter anogenital distances, indicating BPA had antiandrogenic (anti-male hormone) effects *in utero*.[574]

The list of pathological effects, including immunotoxic effects of BPA, is long, so I've picked excerpts from various studies to highlight this point more clearly.

- *"Exposure to BPA is linked to the hyperandroginism present in polycystic ovary syndrome."*[575]
- *"Exposure to BPA impairs cardiac performance in a dose-dependent manner, and has a strong negative impact on electrical conduction, intracellular calcium movement, and ventricular contractility."*[576]
- *"BPA exposure ...favouring the development of insulin resistance in adult male rats"*[577]

- *"Developmental Exposure to Bisphenol A Modulates Innate but Not Adaptive Immune Responses to Influenza A Virus Infection."*[578]
- *"Exposure to BPA appears to be linked to the higher incidence of various cancer types, namely breast, uterus, ovarian, prostate, and testicular."*[571]
- *"...suggesting food intolerance and impaired immune response to parasitic infection in rats exposed perinatally to BPA doses".*[579]

Other potential ways BPA may contribute to immune dysfunction include its impact on simulating higher-than-normal levels of prolactin, oestrogenic immune signalling, cytochrome P450 enzyme disruption, immune signal transduction pathway alteration, cytokine polarisation, activation of Th-17 receptors, molecular mimicry, macrophage activation, lipopolysaccharide activation, and antibody pathophysiology.[580] All of this is thought to have an impact on the pathogenesis of autoimmunity.[580]

In recent years, a lot of attention has been paid to how BPA affects the endocrine system. However, it now seems that BPA also affects the immune system by activating many immune pathways that are involved in both the development of autoimmune diseases and the triggering of autoimmune reactions.[580]

So it appears that if you want to reduce hormone and/or immune disruption, you should limit your BPA consumption.

PFAS

Per- and polyfluoroalkyl substances (PFAS), also called "forever chemicals," are made to never break down in the environment. Because of this, they build up in the soil, water, animals, and human blood. In fact, extensive human exposure to PFAS is so widespread that it has resulted in quantifiable PFAS in the blood of nearly the *entire* population in developed countries, with associated global health impacts.[581]

PFAS are used in industrial and home appliances specifically for their grease-repelling properties. They are found in non-stick cookware, fire retardants, stain and water repellents, some furniture, waterproof clothes, pizza boxes and take-out containers, food packaging, carpets and textiles, rubbers and plastics, electronics, and some dental floss.[582]

PFAS negatively impacts nearly all parts of our biology, causing kidney and liver dysfunction, thyroid disease, fertility issues, and even increasing the risk of cancer.[583,584,585]

If you remember, I have already highlighted one Danish study that showed that **those with greater blood concentrations of PFAS substances were associated with an increased risk of a more severe course of COVID-19.**[586] The authors of this study highlight that the findings make an association of PFAS exposure with disease severity ***"biologically plausible."*** This was a concerning finding considering Denmark has low background PFAS exposure levels compared to other parts of the world.[586]

PFAS-related immunotoxicity is even more biologically possible considering other studies have also noticed its effect on our immune system. Some of them include:

- One study assessing the impact of PFAS on vaccine response noted that *"2-fold greater concentration of major PFCs [perfluorinated compounds] in child serum was associated with a difference of −49% in the overall antibody concentration."*[587]
- A recent review on a similar topic noted that there was *"Strong evidence of PFAS exposure on diminished childhood antibody vaccination response"*.[588]
- *"A pregnancy cohort study prospectively detected an increased risk of airway and throat infections and diarrhoea in children through age 10 yr, correlated with umbilical cord-blood PFAS measurements."* [589]
- A worker study of over three thousand participants found a higher prevalence and incidence of ulcerative colitis and rheumatoid arthritis with increasing perfluorooctanoic acid (PFOA) serum concentrations. The study also noted suggestive positive trends for prostate cancer, non hepatitis liver disease and male thyroid disease with increased PFOA concentrations.[589]

It is thought that the immunotoxic effects of PFAS are primarily due to its disruption of antigen-specific antibody responses.[591] This might be more of a concern for the elderly, who generally have higher PFAS levels than the young.[592] It has also been put forward by another study that, ***"While it is important not to infer causality from the higher levels of PFAS observed in elderly populations that also have higher serious adverse events from COVID-19 infections, it is also reasonable to assume that these events are not wholly unrelated."***[593]

I'll leave you with an excerpt from an extensive review on this matter, which states, ***"Taken together, we find that results of epidemiological studies, supported by findings from toxicological studies, provide strong evidence that humans exposed to PFOA and PFOS are at risk for immunosuppression."***[591]

Fluoride

Water fluoridation was once heralded as one of the best public health achievements of the twentieth century. But this sentiment is rapidly changing as major concerns over excessive fluoride intake and related toxicity have been raised worldwide, leading several countries to ban fluoridation.

It cannot be denied that there is a known association between low fluoride intake and the risk of dental caries.[594] Fluoride ion is thought to be anticarcinogenic, antimicrobial and reduces oral pH - all thought to contribute to anti-caries effect.[595] Furthermore, fluoride has been shown to enhance the remineralisation and recovery of demineralised enamel.[596]

The issue with fluoride is how we use it. It is all well and good if applied topically, i.e., on the teeth, by using conventional toothpaste. But if ingested long-term, fluoride has been linked to neurotoxicity and lower IQ scores in children.

One review of many studies on this subject notes, "*Given the large number of studies showing cognitive deficits associated with elevated fluoride exposure under different settings, the general tendency of fluoride-associated neurotoxicity in children seems robust.*"[597]

This review goes on to conclude, *"The recent epidemiological results support the notion that elevated fluoride intake during early development can result in IQ deficits that may be considerable.*"[597]

Another study noted that fluoride concentrations of 3–11 parts per million (ppm) in drinking water were associated with noticeable cognitive impairment in children.[598]

The pathological effects of fluoride aren't restricted to neurocognitive decline. Fluoride is also linked to immunological dysfunction via a handful of mechanisms, including:

- Restricting the antioxidant activity of natural antioxidants glutathione and superoxide dismutase, and thus causing increased inflammation.[599,600]
- Damaging human lymphocyte chromosomes.[601]
- Reduce T-cell subset percentages and IL-2.[602,603]
- Being involved in cell death.[600]

Even though the link between fluoride and brain damage is clear, not much is known about how it affects our immune system. Much of the research we do have is based solely on animal models and/or is outdated. A 1991 paper titled "Is the ingestion of fluoride an immunosuppressive practice?" is a good example of this.[601]

Even so, you'd hope that the increased risk of neurocognitive impairment would be enough for the government to stop putting fluoride in our tap water or at least think about it. But no, in fact, *more* fluoride is planned to be added to UK drinking water in the very near future.[605]

Dentists haven't spoken up either, which is significant given that most commercial toothpaste contains 1,000 to 1,500 ppm of fluoride and mouthwash contains 230-900 ppm of fluoride.[606]

So, is the ingestion of fluoride an immunosuppressive practice? Well, this is what that 1991 paper concludes with, ***"...habitual ingestion of fluoridated drinking-water for a period of years, may damage some immune system cells and reduce the efficacy of others. Following on the recent string of about 40 in vitro studies which have found that fluoride is a mutagen even when in low concentrations this prospect raises further doubts about the safety of compelling whole populations to ingest daily, for the whole of their lives, uncontrollable and cumulative doses of fluoride through their drinking-water.***

This evidence that the ingestion of fluoride may damage the cells of the immune system certainly raises the question whether HIV + patients should be permitted to drink fluoridated water."[604]

$PM_{2.5}$ particles

"Air pollution is the leading environmental cause of premature reversible death and disability in the world today."[607]

Not the most promising start to a scientific study, but it doesn't get much better.

"A large body of evidence implicates the component of air pollution containing particulate matter smaller than 2.5 μm ($PM_{2.5}$) in size in the development of cardiovascular disease risk factors such as hypertension, insulin resistance (IR), and type 2 diabetes mellitus."[607]

So the air is contributing to disease too? It seems so.

"Contributing" is in fact an understatement, as the Global Burden of Disease (GBD) Study 2015 ranked $PM_{2.5}$ as the fifth leading risk factor for death, which caused 4.2 million deaths and 103.1 million disability-adjusted life-years (DALYs) loss, representing 7.6% of total global deaths and 4.2% of global DALYs.[608]

Out of the list of environmental toxins mentioned, $PM_{2.5}$ may be the environmental risk factor that poses the greatest public health hazard.

Unfortunately, if you live in a densely populated area, you are most likely currently affected. The WHO has claimed that nine out of every 10 people in urban areas are exposed to high levels of $PM_{2.5}$ from outdoor pollution.[609] As though some PM originates from natural sources such as dust, sea salt, and wildfires; most comes from emissions such as vehicles, household wood and coal burning and power plants.[610]

The components of PM are complex and vary greatly. They can include inorganic components such as heavy metals and sulfuric salts, organic components such as polycyclic aromatic hydrocarbons, and biological components such as fungi, spores, and viruses.[611]

All that pollution is thought to cause immunological havoc. A large number of epidemiological studies have shown that $PM_{2.5}$ exposure is closely related to a variety of respiratory diseases, especially in children, the elderly, and those with underlying medical conditions.[612]

There is also an interesting lag effect between being exposed to $PM_{2.5}$ and getting a respiratory illness. According to one study, there is a 7-13 day delay between $PM_{2.5}$ exposure and increased hospitalisation for acute respiratory infections.[613] Another study showed a 1-2 month delay, and another discovered that the association of $PM_{2.5}$ exposure with respiratory syncytial virus (RSV) infection occurred in 2–4 weeks.[614]

This may be due to the fact that monocytes and T helper cell types are impacted by acute exposure to air pollution, whereas B cells, CD8+ cells, and CD4+ cells are more sensitive to both acute and chronic exposure. Further studies are needed to confirm this.[615]

Regardless, it appears that breathing in pollutants on a daily basis is harmful to our health. *Who'd have thought it?* A number of mechanisms have been noted as to why $PM_{2.5}$ are immunotoxic, these include:

- Having the ability to suppress macrophage function and in turn, pulmonary pathogenic bacterial clearance.[616]

- Decreasing bacterial clearance by impairing the bronchial mucociliary system - a key part of the respiratory innate defence system.[617]
- Increasing the adhesion of certain bacterial strains to human airway epithelial cells.[618]
- Causing a decrease in phagocytic phagocytosis due to a decrease of NK cells.[619]
- Reducing the phagocytic capacity of macrophages that resided in air sacks via the shifting to a Th2-type immune response.[620]
- Increasing allergic responses by increasing IgE levels and Th2-related cytokines.[621]
- Reducing IL-1β and IFN-β production and in-turn increases susceptibility to viral infections.[622]
- Inducing inflammatory M1 pro-inflammatory macrophage polarisation over M2 anti-inflammatory polarisation.[623]
- Enhancing proinflammatory cytokine production, resulting in lung toxicity.[623]
- Causing methylation of immunoregulatory genes (DNA methylation is the transfer of one carbon atom and three hydrogen atoms from one area of the DNA to another - regulating gene expression)[615]
- Causing oxidative damage, inflammatory response and cell death - especially if $PM_{2.5}$ is composed of heavy metals.[625]

Overall, $PM_{2.5}$ is associated with inflammation and specific changes to genes related to inflammation, vessel wall dysfunction, and the production of inflammatory immune mediators. Worryingly too, due to their size, inhaled $PM_{2.5}$, especially nanoparticles, may also be able to translocate into blood circulation; passing through epithelial barriers; entering the bloodstream, causing organ dysfunction, insulin resistance and even cardiac damage.[625,626] *You may agree that this sounds like a little something else that has been injected into many of our bloodstreams too.*

With all that pollution, surely lockdowns and restrictions on travel helped reduce $PM_{2.5}$ levels? Shockingly, no. **One Chinese study noted that during the SARS period in 2003 and the COVID-19 pandemic period in 2020, there was an *increase* in $PM_{2.5}$ pollution, thought to be due to a redistribution of the air.**[627]

The Air Quality Life Index noted that, though the world's economy slowed during the pandemic, the global annual average $PM_{2.5}$ pollution was largely unchanged from 2019 levels.[628] The Guardian picked this up and recently released an article titled, "Air pollution got worse during lockdown in many countries, study finds."[629] But it's all a bit confusing, as other studies have noted the opposite.[630]

Higher or unchanged $PM_{2.5}$ levels are also a concern because viruses can piggyback on them, potentially worsening spread. According to one study, the **SARS-CoV-2 virus could have been carried by PM2.5 particles, as evidenced by the highest SARS-CoV-2 RNA on PM2.5 in a hospital ward with the number of occupants.**[631]

And as you have probably guessed, there have been significant associations found between the COVID-19 mortality rate and long-term exposure to air pollution.[632] **One study found that a 1 mcg/m3 increase in $PM_{2.5}$ led to a 9% increase in COVID-19-related excess mortality.**[633]

This is hardly shocking as the impact of average particulate pollution on life expectancy is quoted as being comparable to that of *"smoking, more than three times that of alcohol use and unsafe water, six times that of HIV/AIDS, and 89 times that of conflict and terrorism."*[628] Add COVID-19 to the mix, and it's hardly going to make things better.

We need to be making as much noise as possible to help fix this pollution crisis. $PM_{2.5}$ is just another example of how the world and all its inhabitants are all getting sicker day after day.

Other than wearing a respirator for the rest of your life, a more realistic option (other than moving to the woods) may be to improve one's own defences. In one study, it was found that adding N-acetylcysteine (NAC) stopped S. pneumoniae from sticking to human airway epithelial cells more when PM was present.[634] It has also been noted that autophagy confers a protective role against $PM_{2.5}$-induced cell death to promote cell survival.

Glyphosate

Glyphosate (N-phosphomethyl[glycine]) is the active ingredient in many of the world's most widely used herbicides. Discovered in 1970, it works by inhibiting an enzyme involved in the formation of certain proteins in plants and microorganisms.

Monsanto was an American agrochemical and agricultural biotechnology company that was bought by the German multinational pharmaceutical and biotechnology company Bayer in 2016. It was founded in 1901 and is best known for its herbicide Roundup®, which is made with glyphosate.

Other than introducing glyphosate to the world, Monsanto was one of the first businesses to implement the biotechnology industry's business model in agriculture.[636] It was also one of the first businesses to test out genetically modified crops in the field.[637]

First used as a drying agent and in the pretreatment of crops, Roundup® utilisation has shot through the roof since 1995 with the development of glyphosate-resistant plants. Glyphosate is now the most used herbicide globally, and its usage keeps increasing with the emergence of weed resistance, from 16 million kg spread in the world in 1994 to 79 million kg spread in 2014, including 15% in the United States alone.[638]

Glyphosate was introduced to the mainstream without question because it was regarded as harmless, allegedly, as it targets an enzyme that is nonexistent in animals. However, after more than 40 years of global use, glyphosate has been classified as *"probably carcinogenic"* in humans by the International Agency for Research on Cancer (IARC).[639]

Regardless, as of 2017, other national or international organisations, such as the European Commission or Health Canada, renewed their glyphosate use authorisations for 5 or 10 years, respectively, based on "scientific evidence."

The "scientific evidence" reviewed by international agencies must have been different from the emerging evidence indicating widespread cross-species biological glyphosate-related toxicity, as well as the evidence reviewed by the IARC. *Or maybe, as we have seen, corruption has taken place?*

In 2018, a set of 141 recently declassified documents with regards to the Roundup Products Liability Litigation were examined. The documents revealed *"Monsanto-sponsored ghostwriting of articles published in toxicology journals and the lay media, interference in the peer review process, behind-the-scenes influence on retraction and the creation of a so-called academic website as a front for the defense of Monsanto products."*[640]

Monsanto was found to have used third-party academics in its corporate defence of glyphosate. So it seems like both Big Pharma and Big Poison are likely heads of the same corrupt coin, involved in industry manipulation despite external efforts to enforce transparency.

Glyphosate and its metabolites can be found in soils, water, plants, food, and animals, as well as in human urine, blood, and maternal milk. Glyphosate most likely enters the body via the skin, mouth, and lungs. Once it gets into the body, it seems to build up mostly in the kidneys, liver, colon, and small intestine.[641]

As the list of its biological ills grows by the day, its omnipresence is a major safety concern. Various lab, animal, and human trials have shown that glyphosate imparts dose-dependent cytotoxic and genotoxic effects; increases oxidative stress; disrupts the oestrogen pathway; impairs some cerebral functions (including memory impairment and being linked with Parkinson's disease); induces cardiovascular toxicity; disrupts the gut microbiome; induces gut inflammation (possibly being linked with coeliac disease) and are allegedly correlated to the development of some cancers (multiple myeloma, large B-cell lymphoma and non-Hodgkin's lymphoma being the most linked with glyphosate exposure).[642,643]

Glyphosate is a multifaceted poison and has also shown to harm our and the immune systems of other species via direct and indirect mechanisms, including:

- Having an inhibitory effect on the complement system.[644]
- Reducing phagocytic activity.[645]
- Altering lymphocyte response.[646]
- Imparting genotoxic and oxidative stress on lymphocytes.[642]
- Increasing systeming inflammation.[642]
- Mimicking and disrupting oestrogen activity and reducing testosterone production, and thus in turn having downstream indirect negative effects on the gut microbiome and immunity.[643]
- Inducing gut microbiota dysbiosis.[642]
- Reducing Th1/Th2 ratio, mainly due to a decreasing Th1 cells.[647]

It must be understood that, though glyphosate was regarded as harmless to us as it targets an enzyme nonexistent in animals, this enzyme *is* present in several microorganisms, fungi, and parasites, some of which live in and on us.[648]

And by also satisfying many characteristics of an endocrine disruptor,[642] for example, having shown to inhibit progesterone synthesis *in vitro,* glyphosate may also be placed in the same hormone-disrupting category as BPA.[649]

It is becoming clearer that the health of our immune systems has a direct link to our overall health. And as we have learned, both our hormones and gut microbiome play a vital role in this too. It is increasingly looking like glyphosate disrupts them all and causes widespread immunological and biological harm. But unfortunately, at the time of writing this, there has been no research studying the effects of glyphosate exposure and COVID-19 risk.

If nothing else, think about the bees. Sad to say, a study from 2022 found that **glyphosate caused immune dysregulation in honey bees by reducing the expression of some antimicrobial peptides and the number of good gut bacteria**.[650] The downstream detrimental effects that this may have on global food supplies are chilling to think about.

Just like other environmental toxins, the best and most realistic approach to counteracting them in the short term is to improve one's own personal defences. Zinc, ginger, quercetin (a plant flavonoid), and the herb Ginkgo biloba are some potential supplements that may have protective roles against glyphosate toxicity.[651-654]

The longer-term strategy to save humanity is to save our planet. We are both inseparable.

Arsenic

Arsenic, a heavy metal, is one of the most dangerous natural pollutants on the planet because it is very toxic to all living things, including humans.[655] Arsenic is so toxic, in fact, that it ranks number one in the Agency for Toxic Substances and Disease Registry's Priority List of Hazardous Substances (ATSDR) of the USA.[656]

This is worrying considering arsenic occurs naturally in the environment and comes in a variety of different forms. We are exposed to arsenic through food, water, air, and skin contact with soil or arsenic-contaminated water.

It has been estimated that more than 200 million people, in at least 105 developing and developed countries, are at risk of contracting arsenic poisoning by consuming polluted drinking water.[657] Others are at risk of arsenic toxicity through cigarette smoking and eating foods like rice and fish that come from arsenic-contaminated sources.[658]

Though arsenic toxicity is usually thought of as solely a Third World problem, new countries and regions where the arsenic contamination problem was not previously reported are added every year, and consequently, the known number of affected people keeps increasing, demanding more stringent regulations.[659]

For example, arsenic is still a problem in many parts of the US, where over 2 million people get their drinking water from private wells with arsenic concentrations exceeding the regulatory limit.[660] Plus, rice grown in arsenic-contaminated areas is eaten by many people worldwide.[661]

Rice is of particular concern as it tends to take up more arsenic from the environment than other cereal crops. The arsenic in rice also tends to be in a more toxic form. This is especially concerning for baby food prepared from rice in many developed countries.[655]

In the industrial sector, arsenic is used to manufacture paints, fungicides, insecticides, pesticides, herbicides, wood preservatives, and cotton desiccants. In tech, forms like gallium arsenide or aluminium gallium arsenide crystals are components of semiconductors, light-emitting diodes, lasers, and a variety of transistors.[662]

Plus, beware that some herbal products might be doing more harm than good. The California Department of Health Services tested 251 products in retail herbal stores and found arsenic in 14% of them at concentrations ranging from 20.4 to 114 000 parts per million (ppm), with a mean of 145.53 ppm and a median of 180.5 ppm.[663] To put that in context, the Environment Protection Agency lowered the permissible level of arsenic in drinking water in the USA in 2001 from 50 ppb to 10 ppb.[662] **So some supplements may therefore contain 11400x the level of arsenic considered safe.**

Supplement-related arsenic poisoning is not uncommon. In a different study, it was noted that 82% of patients had toxicity due to arsenic in Chinese proprietary medicines.[664]

Arsenic is especially toxic as it inactivates up to 200 enzymes, especially those involved in cellular energy pathways and DNA synthesis and repair. Acute poisoning is known to cause bloody diarrhoea, abdominal pain, vomiting, blood disorders, bone marrow suppression, kidney failure, and even nerve damage that sometimes lasts for as long as two years.[662]

Chronic poisoning can cause skin disease; chronic diarrhoea and vomiting; cardiac injury, cardiac arrhythmias, and cardiomyopathy; peripheral neuropathy (mimicking Guillain-Barré syndrome); confusion and memory loss; kidney and lung inflammation; as well as a myriad of cancers.[662]

For those interested, levels between 0.1 and 0.5 mg/kg on a hair sample indicate chronic poisoning, while 1.0 to 3.0 mg/kg indicate acute poisoning.

Other than causing a whole host of illnesses, epidemiological and experimental evidence has shown that arsenic also impairs the activity of both the innate and adaptive immune systems. Specifically, arsenic has been shown to:

- Impair macrophage function and differential of peripheral blood monocytes into macrophages.[665]
- Cause oxidative stress and DNA damage.[665]
- Increase levels of cytokines, including TNFα, and IL-8.[666]
- Blocking dendritic cell differentiation and T cell function.[666,667]
- Decrease percentages of peripheral blood CD4+ T cells and CD4/CD8 ratios.[665]
- Inhibit the differentiation of T helper 17 cells.[668]
- Decreases the percentage of CD4+ T cells in the cord blood and alters the thymic function in newborns.[669]

- Affect the differentiation of T cell precursors in the thymus.[670]
- Regulate gene expression in white blood cells by modifying the epigenome.[665]
- Cause global DNA methylation.[671]

The consequences of arsenic-induced immunosuppression are thought to increase the incidence of lower respiratory tract infections and diarrhoea, which frequently develop in young, exposed children from low-income countries.[672]

In other human studies, arsenic exposure has been found to promote pulmonary tuberculosis and visceral leishmaniasis (a parasitic disease).[673,674] In mice, chronic exposure to low doses of arsenic has been linked to increased morbidity from influenza A.[675]

Arsenic-related immunosuppression and inflammation also contribute to cancer formation.[665] And epidemiological studies carried out in various countries demonstrate that arsenic significantly increases the risk of atherosclerosis too.[676]

At the time of writing this, the author is unaware of any studies looking into the risk of COVID-19 and arsenic exposure. Knowing what we know about arsenic and the fact that it can cause lung damage,[677] it may not be so crazy to say that an increased exposure to arsenic may predispose individuals to an increased risk of COVID-19.

As there is no official treatment for arsenic toxicity, the provision of safe drinking water, food, and supplements is a priority. Other than repairing societal infrastructure, NAC, curcumin, and quercetin have shown some potential in attenuating the harmful effects of arsenic.[678,679,680]

A summary of environmental toxins

2022 will go down as a catastrophic year for humanity. For it was the year that mRNA from COVID-19 shots and microplastics were independently discovered in human breast milk for the first time.[681,682] With regard to finding microplastics in breast milk, no significant relationship was found between the level of independent exposure and the presence of them in milk, which the study highlights by noting that *"the ubiquitous microplastic presence makes human exposure inevitable."*

This is the sad state of the world now, as we know it. Humanity's need for the next cheap, plastic-wrapped product and our total lack of care for the environment and the future will only lead to more disease and ecological damage.

This is the dark side of globalism, corporatism and crony capitalism; all made possible by printable money. In today's world whether it's Monsanto or Pfizer, the aim for global corporations is to make a profit and have a market monopoly. It seems like the health of our planet and its inhabitants doesn't even enter the picture.

Though many of the dangers of the environmental toxins mentioned have been known to the scientific community for years now, we continue to live in a world where their circulation continues to exist. I'd argue that in combination, these cause damage to global health many times worse than SARS-CoV-2 ever has or will. *We must ask why there was an international effort to control a virus but not environmental toxins.*

Also, keep in mind that the list provided is not exhaustive. I haven't even mentioned the many other herbicides, heavy metals, cosmetic products, electric and magnetic fields, and even light pollution that have been shown to harm human health and immunity.

You are literally what you consume, and it looks like most of us are made up of bits of plastic, heavy metals, car fumes, and other industrial waste products. Our biology was not evolved to handle the sheer onslaught of foreign materials that constantly bombard us. It is no wonder why so many of us are unwell.

Despite this, human beings still remain robust. In fact, this robustness may be why many of these toxins continue to be made. Plus, luckily, there are some mitigation measures that we might be able to take to lower the harm caused by these poisons.

The world is getting sicker by the minute, and so are we. Many of us are teetering on the edge of sickness and health, only an infection or mRNA-administered jab away from indefinite injury or death.

In order to heal ourselves, we must heal our planet.

MEDICINAL MUSHROOMS

If there is one thing that can get us both closer to better human and environmental health, it's mushrooms.

You've probably seen mushrooms sprouting from the grass, around trees, on decaying logs, and even on the trees themselves while walking through your local park or nearby forest. But I am willing to place a large bet on the fact that many of you are unaware of the sheer number and diversity, as well as the ecological and biological importance, that fungi possess.

Although more than 2,000 varieties of mushrooms are edible, those most familiar to western consumers (especially in the US and UK) are of the *Agaricus bisporus* species: the white button mushroom.[683]

Our ignorance of mushrooms is doing us and our world a great disservice. Especially since modern sequencing methods indicate that up to 5 million fungal species exist. And thus, at the rate of current discovery, it has been noted that it would take an additional 4000 years to discover all the fungi on this planet.[684]

If you didn't know, mushrooms are vital for all life on Earth. They are the great molecular decomposers in nature and grand recyclers of the dead, whether they are plants, animals, bacteria, or protozoa.

They, along with bacteria, help to make soil by converting hard-to-digest organic material into forms that other organisms can use, as well as forming threads of cells called *hyphae* that bind soil particles together, creating stable aggregates that help increase water infiltration and soil water holding capacity.[685] No fungi, no soil, no life on Earth as we know it.

Mushrooms have also been shown to help remove environmental pollutants such as polycyclic aromatic hydrocarbons (chemicals found naturally in coal, crude oil, and gasoline); eliminate heavy metal contamination from polluted sites; clean up agricultural wastes such as pesticides, herbicides, and cyanotoxins (toxins produced by blue-green algae); and even remediate areas affected by dyes and pharmaceutical drugs (a process known as "mycoremediation").[686]

The environmental benefits of fungi don't stop there. New forms of all-natural, non-toxic, mushroom-based insecticide have been invented that could make most other chemical pesticides obsolete in the very near future.[687] Aside from indirectly saving bees by reducing current toxic herbicide and pesticide use, the root-like structures of fungi called mycelia in certain mushrooms have also been shown to improve honey bee immunity.[688]

Mushrooms can not only heal nature, but man too. This is because, though usually alien-looking, we actually share about 50% of our genes with fungi.[689] Four hundred and sixty-five million years ago, we shared a common ancestry with them. We are cousins, and likely why us humans suffer from many of the disease organisms that also affect fungi, but in general, are not susceptible to those infecting plants.

Because we are so similar, certain mushrooms have the amazing ability to intricately activate certain biological systems within us to provide benefits without causing too many side effects. These benefits include antimicrobial, anti-inflammatory, immunomodulatory, antidiabetic, cytotoxic, antioxidant, hepatoprotective, anticancer, antioxidant, antiallergic, anti-fatigue, antihyperlipidemic, and prebiotic properties, among others.[690]

The benefits of medicinal mushrooms are thought to be due to several notable fungal medicinal compounds, and it is very likely that you've taken one in a more modern medical context already: antibiotics.

Penicillin was discovered in 1928 by Scottish scientist Alexander Fleming as a crude extract of the fungus *P. rubens*; it would later go on to be a key reason for the American and British victory in WWII and revolutionise healthcare forever.

Different antibiotics have been discovered in different mushrooms, but these aren't the only medicinal compounds to have been isolated. Other medicinally active compounds in mushrooms are primarily polysaccharides, glycoproteins, ergosterols, triterpenes, chitin, ergothioneines, lectins, trehalose, and statins.

Varying types and amounts of these compounds are found in different mushrooms. Out of the compounds mentioned above, polysaccharides—long chains of carbohydrate molecules with special shapes—have drawn the most attention for their immune-enhancing and/or tumour-reducing properties.

Polysaccharides, polysaccharide derivatives, and protein-bound polysaccharides can be viewed as precursor-nutrients, awakening the immune system and helping to bring about immunological balance. They do this by activating immune cells directly via receptors such as Dectin-1, Complement receptor 3 (CR3), Lactosylceramide (LacCer), and Toll-like receptor (TLR)2. For this reason and more, medicinal mushrooms are known as immunomodulators.[691]

Though I'd love to go through the various different types of medical mushrooms that we currently know of and the beneficial compounds they possess, I know that to include it all would involve writing an entirely separate book about the subject.

So instead, I will focus on the immunobeneficial properties of one of the most naturally occurring medicinal mushrooms, *Trametes versicolor*, also known as *Turkey Tail*, and the popularly quoted "King of Herbs,"[692] *Ganoderma lucidum*, also known as *Reishi*.

Turkey Tail

Trametes versicolor are non-edible, but safe to consume, bracket fungi with a history of use in Asia as a nonspecific immunomodulator.[693] They are called bracket fungi because they form thin structures in concentric circles and grow almost everywhere trees are found. Their colourful concentric rings look like the fan of a turkey's tail feathers, hence their name. They are small, growing up to four inches wide, and can be found on dead logs, stumps, tree trunks, and branches throughout the wooded temperate zones of Asia, Europe, and North America.[694]

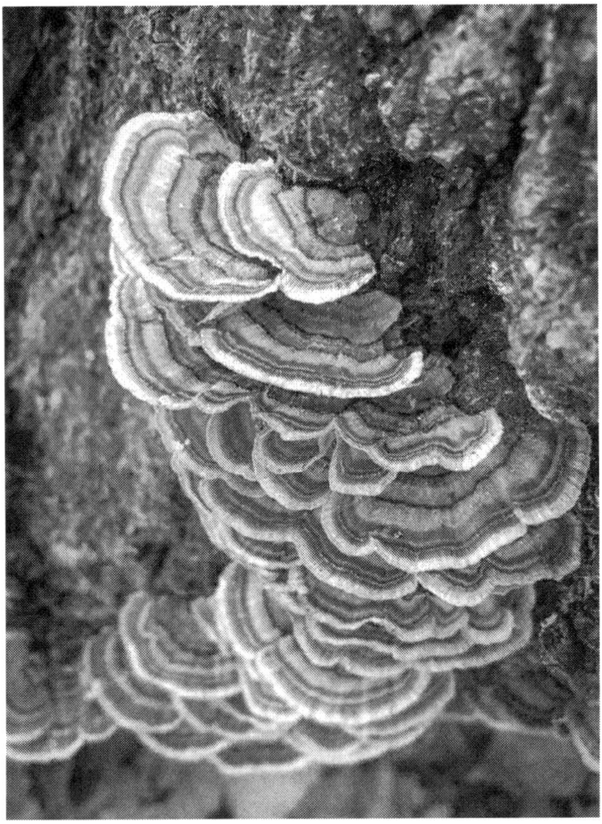

Turkey tail mushroom, from:
https://www.thesophisticatedcaveman.com/turkey-tail-mushrooms/

Traditionally, our ancestors boiled mushrooms in water to make a soothing tea. Boiling kills contaminants, softens the flesh, and extracts the fungi's rich soluble polysaccharides. In Turkey Tail's case, boiling releases, among many others, two well-studied and therapeutic polysaccharides: polysaccharide peptide (PSP) and polysaccharide K (PSK).

PSK has been used in Japanese medicine since the 1980s for treating several types of cancer, and it is the best-selling anti-cancer drug in Japan as a complement to surgery, chemotherapy, and radiotherapy.[694]

PSK, also known as Krestin, is highly bioactive and can be found in the bone marrow, salivary gland, brain, liver, spleen, and pancreas of mice and rabbits within 24 hours of administration. Once absorbed by the body, PSK induces immunomodulation, increasing certain inflammatory molecules like TNF-α, IFN-γ, IL-2, IL-12 and IL-8.[695]

The increase in IL-8 and IL-12 concentrations after PSK induction confirms the effect on certain white cells such as lymphocytes, monocytes and macrophages circulating in the blood. The immunomodulatory effect of PSK is associated with the IL-12-dependent increase in the CD4+ Th1 cell response to tumour cells.[696] PSK also stimulates a form of T cell called Tγδ lymphocytes, which are a small but significant population of T cells in the antitumor immune response. The higher the percentage of Tγδ cells, the better the prognosis, as these T cells infiltrate and help destroy tumour cells.[697] PSK also stimulates natural killer (NK) cells. NK cells increase tumour death through antibody-dependent activation.[697]

PSP was discovered more recently in China, and it is considered as a candidate with strong potential in drug development for treatment and prevention of human cancers because of its immunological properties as well as its ability to act selectively on cancerous cells.[694]

PSP is structurally similar to PSK and thus shows similar immunological activity. PSP has been shown to stimulate the expression of the toll-like receptor TLR4, which is an immunological protein in the innate immune system.[697] PSP also stimulates the immune messengers IL-1, IL-6, and TNF-α.[697]

Turkey Tail extracts have also been shown to contain the compounds baicalein and quercetin. Baicalein is a flavonoid with strong anti-inflammatory properties and has been shown to induce cell cycle arrest in cancer cells and suppress cancer cell colony formation and migration.[698]

Quercetin is known to help release interferon, an antiviral signalling molecule, and this in turn may help with cancer reduction.[698] Both these compounds have also been shown to inhibit acetylcholinesterase (AChE), the enzyme responsible for breaking down the neurotransmitter acetylcholine, and thus one study noted they may help with the treatment of cognitive impairment and dementia.[699]

Reishi

Ganoderma lucidum is a fan-shaped mushroom with a distinctive red to orange colour on top. It has a bright, white, outer growth margin while growing. As growth continues, the margin may begin to change colour and develop a tough skin that has a shiny lacquered appearance. *G. lucidum* grows on hardwoods (especially oaks) in warmer regions, such as Asia, the South Pacific, southern Europe, and the South-eastern United States.

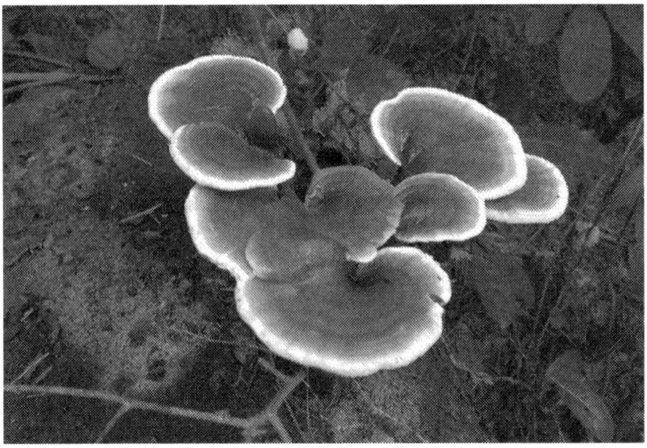

Reishi mushroom, from: https://www.freshnlean.com/blog/reishi-mushroom-benefits/

G. lucidum polysaccharides (GL-PSs) are reported to exhibit a broad range of bioactivities, including anti-inflammatory, hypoglycemic, antiulcer, antitumorigenic, and immunostimulating effects. *G. lucidum* proteoglycan (GLPG) is a peptidoglycan and has shown antiviral properties.[700]

Different components from *G. lucidum* have been shown to enhance the proliferation and maturation of T and B lymphocytes, splenic mononuclear cells, NK cells, and dendritic cells in culture *in vitro* and in animal studies *in vivo*.[701]

In one study, *G. lucidum* mycelia stimulated TNF- and IL-6 production in human and murine macrophages.[702] This was speculated to be due to increased synthesis of NO induced by β-D-glucan, a form of polysaccharide.[700]

Others have found a polysaccharide-enriched fraction from *G. lucidum* activated cultured macrophages and T lymphocytes *in vitro*, which led to an increase of IL-1β, TNF-α, and IL-6 in the culture medium.[703]

Only a few human clinical trials have been conducted using *G. lucidum* as a single agent on cancer patients. One recruited 134 patients with advanced cancers of different sites and supplemented them with *G. lucidum* capsules at a dosage of 1800 mg/day for 12 weeks. Cellular immunity was significantly improved in 80% of these patients, as measured by increased plasma IL-2, IL-6, and IFN- levels, as well as NK cell activity.[704]

In another study of lung cancer patients, immune parameters including total T cells, NK cells, and CD4/CD8 ratio were significantly enhanced in the Reishi-treated group. In addition, quality of life was improved in about 65% of these patients.[700]

A summary of medicinal mushrooms

Mushrooms have been used as medicines for thousands of years. The naturally mummified body of a man thought to have lived around 3300 BCE, referred to as "Ötzi", was discovered in the Ötztal Alp in 1991 and was found to have carried fragments of the Birch Polypore mushroom. It is believed that Ötzi might have used the fungus for medicinal and spiritual purposes, as well as a strop for finishing razor edges. This polypore is well-known in the field of folk medicine and was used for various medicinal purposes.

On the other side of the world, traditional Chinese and Indian medical systems have used medicinal mushrooms for over 2,000 years. And the Greek physician Hippocrates, circa 450 BCE, even knew about their anti-inflammatory properties.[705]

It seems like modern medicine is now catching up to what humanity once knew. I think that medicinal mushrooms will be a very important part of helping people get better. Even though I have only touched upon two mushrooms, I hope you can see why their immune-enhancing, immunomodulatory, and anti-cancer properties may be highly sought after by a vast number of people.

FREQUENT EXPOSURE TO PATHOGENS

I remember the night I encountered my first COVID-19 patient; this was *before* the introduction of mandatory mask wearing in healthcare. It was also before any isolation rules, PCR testing, or lockdowns. Good old times.

It was around 3 a.m., and I was managing around four other patients in the "resuscitation" section of the emergency department, a high-priority area of the department where patients need life-saving treatment urgently.

Ambulance staff wheeled in a disoriented woman in her early 70s who had been travelling recently and said that she had difficulty breathing and a fever. Her husband held her hand and comforted her as the nurses hooked up various leads to her body and hooked her up to oxygen.

She had lost her sense of smell and taste, was a little confused, and had a cough and diarrhoea. I took her blood, began fluids, and initiated the sepsis protocol.

I called for a portable x-ray, which revealed patchy areas of whiteness on areas of her lungs. As identification of the disease at that time relied on clinical evaluation and x-ray findings, I was pretty sure this lady had COVID-19.

Word got around quickly that night shift. This novel disease has made its way all the way from China to our hospital. Worried nurses covered their mouths with their hands when attending the patient. I didn't bother; the patient had already coughed a lot whilst I was examining her, and I had definitely breathed in whatever was in her lungs.

In the months that followed, and as more people arrived with COVID-19 and others died from it, including staff members, hospital rules changed, PPE and mask wearing were introduced, and other conditions came second to it.

A few months into the pandemic, a COVID-19 assessment area was built.

Anyone with respiratory symptoms and/or a fever was first checked out there and given a COVID-19 diagnosis or not before being moved to the right wards.

I'd spend hours there per shift in the final months of my time working in the emergency department. Most of the patients I saw did not have COVID-19 but other conditions like asthma, acute heart failure, bacterial chest infections, and pulmonary embolisms. Some did have positive PCR tests and were unwell with COVID-19, but this was the exception rather than the norm.

Understanding the importance of repeated mucosal exposure and T-cell immunity, I'd sometimes remove my mask and take deep breaths of whatever was in the air. We were meant to wear a new mask every time we entered that ward, and I did, but I knew deep down that this was all an act and not scientifically justified. We were being exposed anyway.

While the methods mentioned so far in this book to improve one's immunity are ways to improve overall health, repeated exposure to the pathogen is akin to stepping into the ring. But the trick to success is to stimulate the immune system without becoming ill.

I carried out my pathogen exposure self-experiment while making sure to keep the rest of my health as optimum as possible. I fasted regularly, ate a low-carbohydrate diet, slept well, exercised moderately, drank kefir, ate nutritious organ meats, and took certain supplements. It seemed to work.

Being able to properly handle frequent exposures to pathogens is, at the end of the day, one of the most important tasks that our immune system constantly deals with. But just like how our muscles are not *only* intended to help us move, but that movement itself makes our muscles stronger, it may not be too insane to think this sort of bidirectional relationship occurs with regards to our immune system too.

This is not a new way of thinking. You may know of the "Hygiene Hypothesis," which proposes that childhood exposure to certain microbes and infections helps the immune system develop healthily and reduces the risk of atopic diseases like asthma.[706]

Another similar theory, the "Old Friends Hypothesis," goes a step further, stating that infectious diseases have a long co-evolutionary history with human development and are thus *vital* for the proper development of our immune system.[707]

These theories, with supporting evidence, along with the growing understanding that we are more than just our own cells but made from millions of other microbes, are changing how we view immunology. We are slowly moving away from reductionist ideas and now fully appreciating that the diversity and the richness of an immune-stimulating microbial world in human habitats are crucial to establishing a competent, anti-autoimmune, and defensive immune system.

And now that we know this, we're starting to learn that a lack of these stimuli, which is common in post-modern environments, can cause the immune system to go off track and lead to immune dysregulation.

To make an immune system that is strong, flexible, and able to handle random events, one must, in a sense, train it. This is especially important because the world we live in now encourages a lack of training and, as a result, immunological atrophy.

It should also be noted that *when* our immune system is trained is just as important as how and by how much. It has been said that the window of opportunity for appropriate education of the immune system already starts in the mother's womb.[708] One study demonstrated that maternal exposure to a farm environment rich in microbial compounds was inversely associated with the development of allergic conditions and correlated with an upregulation of the innate immune system in the children at school age.[709]

Other evidence has shown that maternal farm activities during pregnancy were shown to alter allergen-specific immunoglobulin and cytokine responses in cord blood to a Th1 pattern.[710]

I understand that we cannot go back in time and change what our mothers did while carrying us, but it's never too late to make changes to one's current life that may prove beneficial in the future.

Firstly, as I have already noted in the chapter titled - "Why may an increased exposure to SARS-CoV-2 improve immunity?" - SARS-CoV-2 exposure increases both SIgA antibody secretion and TRM cell production, which properly primes and regulates a coordinated downstream immunological response.

Because lung TRMs are lost 4-5 months after an acute infection, frequent respiratory exposure is required because protection from reexposure is lost after this time.[711] This is especially true when dealing with a rapidly mutating respiratory virus.[712]

As I've also talked about in this book, people who have never been exposed to SARS-CoV-2 have been shown to have immunity to it already.[713] For example, one peer-reviewed study in the Journal of Clinical Investigation Insight notes, "*Majority of uninfected adults show pre-existing antibody reactivity against SARSCoV2.*" [714]

But one does not have to be exposed to the particular disease-causing virus (or even one similar to it) to be protected from it. Similar viruses help, as exemplified in those who recovered from the original SARS 17 years ago, having shown cross-immunity against COVID-19, indicating long-term immunity.[715]

Other viruses help form cross-immunity, As exemplified by another peer-reviewed study in Nature, where strong pre-existing T-cell immunity to SARS-CoV-2 was contributed by the engagement of cross-reactive T-cell receptors against other viruses like CMV & Flu antigens.[716]

And another showed pre-existing SARS-CoV-2–reactive antibodies in various B cell populations in the upper respiratory tract lymphoid tissue that may lead to limited COVID-19 disease progression.[717]

Going totally obscure, another study noted that **SARS-CoV-2-specific T-cells in unexposed adults had the ability to cross-react with *our own commensal antigens*, indicating that non-infectious exposure to common microbes from the gut and skin may be a key factor that shapes human pre-existing immunity to SARS-CoV-2**.[718] That's protection from a deadly virus by immune training using *our own* unrelated commensal bacteria.

At the end of the day, T cells that recognise SARS-CoV-2 are found in unexposed individuals; this fact makes me think that, just like sparring sessions, it might not be too wild to postulate that helping our immune system train using other, less deadly pathogens first before going in with the real thing may not be such a bad idea.

That's what I've been doing anyway. As well as exposing myself to the virus on multiple occasions during my time in healthcare and since then, I also consume homemade kefir daily and have been cold dipping in the stream of my local park once a week, every week, for more than a year now.

The cold dipping not only exposes my skin to various bugs and critters, but the water temperature is usually so cold that it shocks my system. The cold as well as the related short-term stress likely upregulates my immune system.[719,720] The short-term stress may also be helping me live longer by maintaining my cellular telomere length.[721]

My weekly dips into cold and dirty streams isn't so crazy now, ey?

OTHER SUPPLEMENTS

"A HEALTHY MAN WANTS A THOUSAND THINGS, A SICK MAN ONLY WANTS ONE."
CONFUCIUS

We are always looking for the quickest and easiest way to get well. *Can you blame us?* Most of us will get sick at some point, especially in this day and age. Nearly half of all Americans have at least one chronic disease,[1] which means that getting sick is becoming more common than not.

Last year, Nature published an article highlighting that there was an international team of researchers who want to find people who are genetically resistant to SARS-CoV-2, in the hope of "developing new drugs and treatments."[2] This, I thought, was the epitome of biological lunacy, establishing the precedent that the only reason certain people were able to avoid certain diseases *had* to be genetic reasons, reasons beyond our control.

This is not only extremely reductionist, fear-inducing, and promotes the need for the "other" for answers, but also opens the doors to the introduction of genetic therapies, which, in my humble opinion, is a futile and dangerous affair.

When we do eventually become unwell, a sign of biological imbalance, our physiology reacts in innumerably complex ways to find balance again. Some people are lucky and get back to good health quickly, while others sometimes live a life of suffering. This is only made worse by the fact that the world we live in is too fast-paced and too polluted to allow for proper healing.

We must also remember that the medical-industrial complex benefits from our physiological ailments, and the treatments provided, particularly for chronic diseases, are either out-dated, insufficient, or incorrect most of the time. Root causes are never addressed because doing so would result in less money being made.

If there's anything you take away from this book, I hope you appreciate the infinite biological and environmental complexity that makes you "you." You are not only your cells, the bugs that live in and on you, and everything else in between; you are also your environment, your family, the air you breathe, the food you eat, and the land you walk on. You are everything.

Good health thus exists in a time-dependent continuum that varies microsecond after microsecond, dancing with various aspects of nature and the many internal biological processes occurring within you at all times.

Immunity also exists in flux. It cannot be "boosted' nor helped with a rag covering the mouth. To suggest these things as protective measures is not only scientifically implausible (laughable, really), but a tactic used to sell products and promote fear.

I have only touched the surface of what we know about ourselves, but if you have been paying attention, the interconnectedness of it all is plain to see. All systems rely on each other.

For example, did you know that both fasting and exercise increase vitamin D production?[3,4] *Or that our immune system is inextricably linked to the levels and types of light we are exposed to throughout the day,*[5] *and that artificial light at night interferes with our immune function?*[6]

No one system is separate from another.

The state of the world now is inconducive to good public health, and the inoculation of mRNA technology into the arms of many millions of people multiple times has only added fuel to the fire, accelerating disease progression. Though we face catastrophic times, we must always remember that humans have an incredible ability to heal.

But to heal, we must approach health differently than we have so far. To begin, we must abandon the reductionist model of single cause and effect when considering disease and instead strive to implement lifestyle changes that address the individual as a whole.

We must also begin to realise that most chronic ailments are due to environmental toxins that are the lovechild of corrupt policy and globalism, all made possible by the use of printable money that is not backed by a commodity such as gold.

These toxins, whether they are mRNA in our bodies, microplastics in our food, or BPA in our water, are all evolutionary foreign substances that will have unanticipated consequences for us. We must therefore protect science and stand on the shoulders of giants to form new integrative models of disease prevention and treatment to help heal humanity.

The various methods mentioned in the book not only help improve and maintain a strong immune system, but are some of the ways to improve our overall health too. If integrated strictly and for a very long time, it is hard to argue that it will not result in an overall benefit.

Though the fundamentals are vital, we are all different, and emerging evidence continues to pile up indicating that we have all been differently affected by both

COVID-19 and mRNA shots. This is where the use of certain forms of therapy and supplements may be useful.

Due to the novelty of the virus and the underfunding of mRNA-related injuries, counteracting disease states that are related to both have been left in the dark. The data around specific supplements is lacking. Most of the research is just speculation.

Not all supplements are useful, safe, or even needed by everyone. And thus, an individualised approach must be taken when thinking about supplementing. Other supplements can lead to side effects as well as negatively interact with medications one may already be on, so the risk is yours.

Regardless, we must start somewhere. Throughout the last few years, I have been compiling a list of potential treatment aids for various jab-related injuries and post-COVID-19 sequelae. The list includes therapies that have a wide range of physiologically beneficial processes including anti-ageing, anti-inflammation, antioxidation, cardioprotection, neuroprotection, anti-cancer, immunomodulatory, anti-clotting, anti-toxin, anti-prion and pro-fertility. An individualised approach to introducing therapies on a background of the eleven foundational elements mentioned already looks like the most promising key to health optimisation. The list has been compiled strictly for educational purposes only.

Without further ado, in alphabetical order, these therapies include:

7,8-DIHYDROXYFLAVONE

Some possible benefits include: memory enhancement, mood boosting, and neuroprotection.

7,8-dihydroxyflavone (7,8-DHF) is also known as tropoflavin and is a naturally occurring molecule found in *Godmania aesculifolia*, *Tridax procumbens,* and primula tree leaves.[7,8]

7,8-DHF activates the same receptor as Brain-Derived Neurotrophic Factor (BDNF), a key molecule that helps the brain with learning and memory formation. The BDNF receptor is called the Tyrosine Kinase Factor B (TrkB) receptor. In fact, it has been shown that 7,8-DHF binds better to TrkB receptors than BDNF.[9]

7,8-DHF has proven therapeutically effective in animal models of a variety of CNS disorders, from depression and Alzheimer's disease to cognitive deficits in schizophrenia, and traumatic brain injury.[10-13]

7,8-DHF has shown to be effective in fear extinction, can promote the repair of damaged neurons and increase the production of brain cells in adult mice after brain injury. 7,8-DHF has also been shown to decrease the release of various proinflammatory factors in the brain.[7,14-17]

Dosage: There are currently no human studies on 7,8-DHF to take human doses from. Using rodent models, mathematically estimated doses include 1 mg/kg for subchronic or chronic usage in humans, with the acute dose correlating to approximately 2.5 mg/kg.[18]

ACETYL-L-CARNITINE

Some possible benefits include: mood-boosting and neuroprotection.

Also known as ALCAR, acetyl-L-carnitine is a form of L-carnitine, which is a derivative of the simple proteins lysine and methionine. ALCAR is both naturally produced in the body as well as available as a dietary supplement. For your body to produce it in sufficient amounts, you also need plenty of vitamin C.[19]

ALCAR has been shown to ameliorate neuroinflammation, increase concentrations of BDNF in the brain, and may have protective and therapeutic potential for inflammation-related neurodegenerative diseases.[20]

It has shown rapid-acting antidepressant-like effects on mice and has been shown to be at low levels in those with major depressive disorder.[21,22] Supplementation may also help with depression.[23]

Saying this, carnitine and ALCAR supplements carry warnings of a risk that they promote seizures in people with known epilepsy, but a 2016 review found this risk to be based only on animal trials.[24]

The supplementation of L-carnitine may also raise blood levels of trimethylamine-N-oxide (TMAO) over time. High levels of TMAO are linked to an increased risk of atherosclerosis.[25,26]

Dosage: ALCAR has most often been used by adults in doses of 1.5-3 grams orally daily, for up to 33 months. [27]

ALPHA GPC

Some possible benefits include: cognitive enhancement and energy-boosting.

Alpha-glycerylphosphorylcholine (Alpha-GPC) is a supplement thought to exert its effects by increasing the synthesis and release of the neurotransmitter acetylcholine in the brain, facilitating learning and memory.[28] Acetylcholine is also responsible for muscle contraction, so it is theorised that increases in acetylcholine may lead to stronger muscular force production.[29]

Alpha-GPC appears to easily cross the BBB and is said to be the best cholinergic for increasing blood and brain choline levels.[30] COVID-19 has been noted to cause dysregulation of the cholinergic system.[31]

In older adults with mild to moderate dementia, alpha-GPC has been shown to improve cognitive symptoms such as memory and attention impairment.[32,33] Those with Alzheimer's dementia are usually placed on medication called acetylcholinesterase inhibitors; alpha-GPC may also potentiate the effectiveness of these.[32]

Preliminary evidence suggests that alpha-GPC also increases vertical jump power as well as peak bench press force.[34,35]

Similar to ALCAR, there have been concerns raised about the potential of alpha-GPC to increase TMAO and thus increase the risk of adverse cardiovascular outcomes.[36]

One cohort study of more than 12 million participants, including 108,877 alpha-

GPC users, reported that alpha-GPC use for at least 12 months was associated with an increased risk of stroke over 10 years.[37]

Dosage: Alpha-GPC is generally well tolerated, serious side effects have not been reported in human trials at a dosage of 1,200 mg per day for six months.[38]

ANTHOCYANINS

Some possible benefits include: improving antioxidant levels, endothelial health, cardiovascular health, visual health, metabolic health, energy levels, DNA protection, gut microbiome modulation, antiviral defence, cognitive function, and reducing inflammation.

Anthocyanins are flavonoids responsible for the colours red, purple, and blue in fruits and vegetables.[39] Berries, currants, grapes, some tropical fruits, red to purplish blue-colored leafy vegetables (like red cabbage), grains, roots, and tubers all contain a high level of anthocyanins. The highest anthocyanin content, though, is found in elderberries and chokeberries, which can contain up to 1,4–1,8 g of anthocyanins per 100 g of product.[40]

In vivo and *in vitro* studies have shown that anthocyanins produce a whole host of health benefits, including antioxidative effects, endothelial protection, prevention of cardiovascular disease, anticancer, antidiabetes, improved visual health, anti-obesity, anti-microbial, and neuroprotective effects.[41]

Clinical studies on humans have shown cardioprotective effects, primarily through antioxidant effects. In one study of 150 participants with high cholesterol, those given an anthocyanin mixture of 320 mg/day showed reduced levels of C-reactive protein and IL-1β compared to the placebo group.[42]

Another study of older adults, this time with mild-to-moderate dementia, showed that the consumption of 200 mL of cherry juice per day led to improvements in verbal fluency, short-term memory, and long-term memory.[43]

And a 12-week supplementation with 80 mg/day or more of anthocyanins improved platelet function in individuals with high cholesterol.[44] Another study noted that a dose *"greater than 80 mg/d is an effective antioxidant and antiinflammatory agent in healthy young adults."* [45]

Anthocyanins may also influence the composition of the colonic microbiota, with consumption increasing beneficial bacteria such as *Bifidobacteria*, *Lactobacilli*, and *Actinobacteria*.[46]

Anthocyanins have also been shown to have potential robust binding affinities and inhibitory molecular interactions with SARS-CoV-2, and thus it has been speculated that they could be a potent antiviral in this regard too.[47]

Dosage: Anthocyanins are not considered essential nutrients, so no recommended daily intake has been established; however, China has recently suggested a daily intake of 50 mg.[48] **Other studies have used doses as high as 100 mg.**[49]

ARTEMISININ

Some possible benefits include: improving anti-viral defences, anti-cancer defences (blood and lung cancers specifically), anti-inflammatory activities and nerve protection.

Artemisinin is a compound isolated from the leaves of the shrub *Artemesia annua,* also known as sweet wormwood. Artemisinin has been widely used in modern medicine for the treatment of malaria for the past two decades and by traditional Chinese medicine practitioners for the same reason since 317 AD or longer.[50,51,52]

Artemisinin is thought to fight off malaria by being able to activate the iron inside the parasite to generate free radicals, which subsequently kill them.[53] Other than being an antimalarial, artemisin known to have antibacterial, antifungal, antiparastisitic, antioxidant, antitumor, and anti-inflammatory activities too.[54]

Artemisinin has been recently postulated to be possibly effective against blood-related cancers. Artemisinin has also been shown to inhibit the proliferation, inflammation, invasion, and metastasis of other cancers such as lung cancer, as well as to induce apoptosis and have multiple pharmacological actions against lung inflammation and viral infections.[55] And thus, it has also recently been postulated whether artemisinins could also be repurposed for the treatment of COVID-19 given its anti-viral and anti-inflammatory properties.[56]

This compound has also been shown to have nerve-protective properties, specifically acting as an anti-inflammatory agent and increasing motoneuronal survival to promote motor function recovery in rats after nerve damage.[57] Rats that were given artemisinin showed nerve protection, remyelination of axons, and good motor function recovery. Artemisinin has also shown therapeutic potential in neurodegeneration.[58]

Dosage: The People's Republic of China lists the daily dose of *Artemisia annua* for fever and malaria as 4.5 to 9 grams of dried herb prepared as an infusion.[59] Taking 300–1000 milligrams daily is often recommended for reducing inflammation, fighting fever and malaria, and combating infections.[60]

Those who are pregnant, breastfeeding, or on certain other medications should not take artemisinin. Higher doses (500 mg twice a day) for malaria are only used for short periods of time (5 days).

ASTRAGALUS

Some possible benefits include: improving overall health, immune-boosting, anti-cancer, protecting against heart damage and damage-related cardiac muscle changes, anti-aging, improving hair regrowth, promoting nerve growth, cognitive protection, reducing organ-specific inflammation, and improving male fertility.

Astragalus membranaceus is one of the fifty fundamental herbs in traditional Chinese medicine, and has been used as a medicine for more than 2000 years.

It has a plethora of reported benefits as well as improving overall health. *In vitro* and *in vivo* studies have shown that this medicinal root contains many compounds with health and protective properties, including antioxidant, anti-inflammatory, immunostimulant, anti-aging, neuroprotective, anti-cancer, and anti-diabetic effects.[61]

Astragalus membranaceus has been shown in studies to stimulate T and B lymphocytes and secrete lymphocyte cytokines such as IFN- and various interleukins to improve macrophage function and phagocytosis.[62]

Astragalus membranaceus has also been shown to help improve the mucosal immune system by increasing IgA secretion and proliferating intestinal mucosa, as well as protecting and proliferating the activity of NK to fight other disease cells.[63]

This root also contains a compound (TA-65) that increases telomerase activity and has age-reversal and protective effects in immune system cells.[64]

Interestingly, *Astragalus membranaceus* has been shown to protect the pancreas from autoimmune-linked cell death through the mechanisms of anti-oxidation, immunomodulation, anti-inflammation, and anti-apoptosis, as well as by helping to balance Th1 and Th2 responses.[65]

Various compounds of *Astragalus membranaceus* have also been shown to reduce various organ-specific inflammation, from bowel inflammation, kidney inflammation, and uterus inflammation to cardiac endothelial inflammation.[66-69]

Astragaloside IV (AST) is purified from the root of *Astragalus membranaceus*, and interestingly, one study of a mice model with myocarditis showed *AST* to have improved mouse survival times and improved cardiac scarring.[70] AST has also been shown to protect against ischemic and hypoxic myocardial cell injury, inhibit myocardial hypertrophy, enhance myocardial contractility, improve diastolic dysfunction, alleviate vascular endothelial dysfunction, and promote angiogenesis.[70]

With regards to neurology, AST and *Astragalus membranaceus* have been shown to improve neurological deficits and reduce the areas of cell death in stroke studies.[71]

Low-dose AST has been related to the growth and division of neural stem cells (NSCs).[72] In one study, rats were intragastrically administered AST (40 mg/4 ml/kg, once daily) for 14 days to investigate the effect of AST after stroke. The results showed that AST treatment reduced the tissue death volume, improved behaviour, increased body weight, and promoted the growth, migration, differentiation, and maturation of NSCs in the hippocampus (areas of the brain dedicated to learning and memory) by enhancing the BDNF pathways.[73]

Another study found that topical administration of AST in mice leads to hair regrowth and "may be used for treatment of hair diseases such as alopecia, effluvium and hirsutism."[74]

Animal and *in vitro* studies have also suggested that *Astragalus membranaceus* may also help male infertility by improving sperm parameters.[75,76]

Dosage: The daily dose recommended in China, 9–30g, is recognised as safe when used appropriately. The standard dose for AST is 5–10 mg.[77]

BACOPA

Some possible benefits include: improving cognition, memory, mood, and learning; neuroprotection; and anti-prion.

Bacopa monnieri, commonly known as water hyssop or Bacopa, is an herb that has been used in traditional Ayurvedic medicine for centuries primarily to tackle brain-related issues like improving memory, reducing anxiety, and treating epilepsy.[78]

Though there are only a handful of human trials, the recent scientific evidence that we do have seems to complement ancient knowledge.

Bacopa monnieri has various neuroprotective effects, such as reducing neural inflammation; up regulating neural antioxidant defences; improving mitochondrial dysfunction; stabilising levels of certain neurotransmitters; as well as reducing β-Amyloid plaque formation and protecting against prions.[79,80]

Bacopa monnieri has shown to upregulate the naturally reducing antioxidant T cell defences in ageing rats, as well as attenuate the effects of cigarette smoke exposure on brain cells.[79,81]

Bacopa monnieri is most popular nowadays as a nootropic and specifically as a memory booster. Lab studies have shown its ability to activate and help morph areas of the brain involved in learning and memorisation.[82] Clinical trials have been hit and miss so far, however.

Some studies have shown statistically significant improvements in memory in older people who complained of memory loss without any sign of Alzheimer's or dementia.[83] However, the improvements were modest, and only a few of the many neuropsychological tests showed statistically significant changes; furthermore, as with the healthy volunteers, no two studies have found significant differences in the use of Bacopa *monnieri* in the same cognitive tests.

One 12-week study in 46 healthy adults observed that taking 300 mg of *Bacopa monnieri* daily significantly improved the speed of processing visual information, learning rate, and memory, compared with the placebo treatment.[84] And another showed that taking 300 mg or 600 mg of *Bacopa monnieri* extract daily improved memory, attention, and the ability to process information compared with the placebo treatment.[85]

Dosage: The standard dose for Bacopa monnieri is 300 mg, assuming that the total bacoside content (the active compound) is 55% of the extract by weight. *Bacopa monnieri* is fat-soluble and requires a lipoid transporter to be absorbed; and thus it is traditionally consumed with ghee.[86]

It is not recommended for pregnant women due to a lack of safety trials.[87]

BAICALIN

Some possible benefits include: neuroprotection, anti-prion, anti-viral, anti-clotting, anti-inflammatory, and may aid with female fertility.

Baicalin is the main flavonoid glucoside of *Scutellaria baicalensis*, a medical plant also known as Baikal skullcap or Chinese skullcap that is native to China, Korea,

Mongolia, the Russian Far East, and Siberia. It is also one of the fifty fundamental herbs used in traditional Chinese medicine.

Research into baicalin has shown that it has antiviral, antibacterial, anti-oxidative, anti-inflammatory, anticancer, antidiabetic, antithrombotic, cardioprotective, hepatoprotective, and neuroprotective properties. But the majority of the studies carried out so far have been in cell lines and animal models.[88,89,90]

With regards to neurobiology, numerous studies have shown that baicalin may efficiently prevent various neurodegenerative diseases, such as Alzheimer's disease, Parkinson's disease, and strokes, by suppressing oxidative stress, reducing cell death, inhibiting the production of inflammatory cytokines, and promoting the growth of new brain cells.[89] Baicalin has also been shown to prevent human prion protein-induced neuronal cell death and reduce the "leakiness" of the BBB.[91,92]

Baicalin has shown early evidence of improving endothelial function and conferring cardiovascular-protective actions against oxidative stress-induced cell injury.[93] This flavonoid may also be of use to those suffering from inflammatory bowel diseases and/or other gastrointestinal disorders.[94,95]

In one mouse study, oral administration of *Scutellaria baicalensis* root effectively protected mice infected with influenza A virus, increased their survival rate, decreased the lung injury index, and improved their lung morphology.[96] Numerous other studies have claimed that baicalin could help to induce IFN-γ secreted by CD4+, CD8+ T-cells, and to NK cell activity.[97]

It is speculated that baicalin may be useful in combating COVID-19 by reducing cytokine-induced acute inflammation.[94]

With regards to female fertility, baicalin has shown to possibly help to improve degenerating ovarian function and delay ovarian ageing,[98] as well as promoting embryonic implantation.[99] But another study, again in mice, noted that prenatal baicalein exposure disrupted the menstrual cycle, which could negatively impact female fertility if exposed prenatally.[100]

Dosage: One study notes that, in the 200–800 mg dose range, multiple-dose oral baicalein administration was safe and well tolerated.[101] Another study, using similar dosages, also reflected this and noted that the most common adverse events were elevated CRP and high triglycerides.

CCR5 ANTAGONISTS

Some possible theoretical benefits include: helping with long COVID symptoms.

In one pre-print study comparing post-jabbed individuals with long COVID, healthy individuals, and individuals post-jabbed without long COVID, it was found that those with long COVID symptoms exhibited markers of platelet activation and pro-inflammatory cytokine production that the authors thought may be driven by the persistence of SARS-CoV-2 spike protein.[103]

Chemokine (C-C motif) ligand 5, also known as CCL5, is a proinflammatory immune messenger that helps recruit white blood cells to the site of inflammation and is presented on the surface of T cells, smooth muscle endothelial cells, epithelial cells, and other cell types. Though pro-inflammatory, some viruses like HIV use CCR5 as an entrance molecule to a cell, and thus CCL5 in high concentration has been thought to increase HIV replication.[104]

I introduce CCL5 because in the study mentioned above, researchers found that elevated post-jab long COVID symptoms were associated with an inflammatory profile with statistically significant elevations in CCL5, sCD40L (a protein member of the TNF family), IL-6, and IL-8.[104] Hence, theoretically, blocking the receptor for CCL5, C-C chemokine receptor type 5 (CCR5), may be useful for those suffering with long COVID.[105] Luckily, this has been researched.

In another study, a statistically significant correlation was found between decreased IL-8 and improvement in long-term COVID cardiac symptoms following treatment with a CCR5 antagonist and a statin. The CCR5 antagonist used here was Maraviroc, an antiretroviral.[106]

Long COVID sufferers have shown to have persistent spike protein in white cells called CD16+ monocytes up to fifteen months after infection. And CD16+ monocytes, which express CCR5, play a role in vascular health and endothelial immune surveillance, and thus microclot formation via the monocytic-endothelial-platelet axis has been postulated as one central aspect of the condition.

The two natural CCR5 antagonists I could find were anibamine and shikonin. Anibamine, from the plant *Aniba citrifolia*, is, as noted in one review, the "first and only natural product known as a chemokine receptor CCR5 antagonist."[107] There is some evidence that anibamine may be helpful against prostate cancer and certain parasitic infections, too.[108,109]

Shikonin, a pigment from the root of *Lithospermum erythrorhizon* (also known as the purple gromwell), has long been used as an ointment for wound healing in traditional oriental medicine and has been reported to have antibacterial, antitumor, and anti-inflammatory effects.[110] One 2003 study noted that Shikonin had the ability to down-regulate the surface expression of CCR5.[111]

Whether these natural products work to counteract long COVID in humans is yet to be studied. And in fact, not all studies note the relationship between CCR5 and long COVID. In another study, participants were given a drug called leronlimab, which *increased* cell surface CCR5 levels and led to related symptom improvement.[112]

The researchers of this study noted that an alternative mechanism for long COVID in some people might exist where there is abnormal immune downmodulation, possibly due to immune overshoot after the intense inflammation of acute COVID-19.[112]

More, and better quality studies are needed to further investigate the link between CCR5 and long COVID.

Dosage: There are no official dosage recommendations for anibamine or shikonin. Human trials assessing safety are also lacking for both.

CHAGA

Some possible benefits include: antiviral, antidiabetic, antioxidant, energy-boosting, anti-inflammatory, immunomodulatory, anticancer, and neuroprotective potential, and particularly high anti-oxidative capabilities.

The chaga (scientifically called *Inonotus obliquus)* mushroom has been a well-known source of traditional medicine since the time of Avicenna, also known as Ibn Sina, a Persian polymath who is regarded as one of the most significant scientists, philosophers, and writers of the Islamic Golden Age. He lived from 980 to 1037.

Word of its nutritional properties must have spread, as *I. obliquus* has also been used as a folk medicine in Russia, Siberia, and some Western countries as early as the 16th century. The name "Chaga" comes from the Russian word for mushroom, "czaga," and it is thought that a czar in 12th-century Russia credited the application of a chaga decoction with the disappearance of his lip tumours.

The pharmacological study of active substances in chaga was started in the middle of the 20th century. Recent *in vivo* and *in vitro* evidence has shown that Chaga has antiviral, antidiabetic, antioxidant, anti-fatigue, anti-inflammatory, immunomodulatory, anti-cancer, and neuroprotective potential.[113]

I. obliquus polysaccharides (IOPS) have particularly shown to have antitumor effects in both *in vitro* and *in vivo,* some think this property is due to the stimulation of the immune system, while others think antioxidative ability prevents the generation of cancer cells.[114]

Matrix metallopeptidases (MMPs) are enzymes involved with various physiological processes via the modification of the extracellular matrix. Its overexpression has been linked to cancer metastasis and tumour growth. IOPS have shown to decrease the expression of a handful of MMPs and increase the expression of metallopeptidase inhibitor 2 (TIMP-2).[115]

I.obliquus polysaccharides has shown to inhibit liver cancer cell lines;[116] the migration and invasion of non-small cell lung cancer;[117] kill ovarian cancer;[116] inhibit human cervical cancer cells as well as inhibiting bone marrow tumour cells and sarcoma cells.[118,119]

With regards to metabolic health, I.*obliquus* polysaccharides have been shown to ameliorate insulin resistance and metabolism disorders in streptozotocin-induced type 2 diabetic mice, as well as restoring the structure of the pancreas after diabetes-induced cellular damage.[120,121]

Oral administration of polysaccharides suppressed the in vivo growth of melanoma tumours in tumour-bearing mice.[119]

Another study showed that polysaccharides from I. obliquus affected the Th1/Th2 lymphocyte ratio and Th17/Treg in the colon and therefore could possibly treat inflammatory bowel disease.[122]

Other studies performed on mice showed that extracts from I. obliquus suppressed Th2 and Th17 immune responses.[123]

Some websites will claim that chaga has the highest known levels of antioxidants of any food. This claim is based on the oxygen radical absorbance capacity (ORAC) scale; however, ORAC values came under scrutiny in 2012, when the USDA removed its ORAC food database, citing that the test did not directly correlate to health benefits.[124]

Chaga is also claimed to have high antioxidant capabilities due to its high content of the antioxidant superoxide dismutase (SOD). These claims should be taken with a pinch of scepticism, as oral administration of SODs is not firmly believed to be effective as they are degraded before they can get absorbed into the bloodstream. Regardless, other studies *have* demonstrated the efficacy of oral SOD supplementation.[125]

Dosage: Chaga is most commonly sold as a dried extract, ranging in dose from 500 to 1,500 mg. There are no official, reliable guidelines regarding the appropriate dose of chaga to achieve a therapeutic effect.[126]

Be aware that chaga contains oxalate, a compound commonly found in plants that can cause kidney stones.

There have been case reports of oxalate-induced kidney disease due to long-term consumption of chaga.[127]

Vitamin C can increase the excretion of oxalates from the kidneys, and there have been case reports of oxalate-induced kidney disease due to vitamin C supplementation.[128]

Therefore, it would be wise to not oversupplement with both, both individually and separately, for a long period of time, especially if your risk of kidney disease is high.

COENZYME Q10

Some possible benefits include: antioxidant, energy-boosting, anti-inflammatory, immunomodulatory, neuroprotective, cardiovascular protection, anti-clotting, and fertility aid.

Coenzyme Q10, also known as CoQ10 or ubiquinol, is a fat-soluble compound that naturally occurs in all respiring animal cells and is primarily found in the mitochondria. Mitochondria, simply put, are the batteries found in most animal cells that help produce energy.

Other than being vital in cellular energy production, CoQ10 also functions as an antioxidant (mainly protecting cell membranes and plasma lipoproteins), working closely with vitamins C and E.[129,130,131]

The types of cholesterol that are normally referred to as "bad" may need a name change, as they are the ones that primarily carry CoQ10 in the blood, and it is believed that CoQ10 is capable of preventing them from oxidation.[132]

Statins, a drug used to treat high levels of "bad" cholesterol, also reduce levels of CoQ10, and CoQ10 has been considered a potential candidate for the treatment of statin-induced muscle disease.[132] *Counterintuitive if you ask me.*

CoQ10, and has been considered a potential candidate for the treatment of various other conditions, including cardiovascular, neurodegenerative, neuromuscular, mitochondrial, and fertility problems.[132]

Supplementing with CoQ10 has shown promise, helping to activate mechanisms controlling mitochondrial biogenesis and delay cellular ageing (senescence).[133,134]

Experimental studies in animal models suggest that CoQ10 may protect against neuronal damage caused by ischemia, atherosclerosis, and toxic injury.[135] CoQ10 supplementation has also been shown to decrease pro-inflammatory cytokines and inflammatory markers in the elderly with low CoQ10 levels.[136]

CoQ10 has also been shown to help patients with chronic heart failure, improving symptoms and reducing major cardiovascular events.[137]

CoQ10 deficiency syndrome is a spectrum of conditions where unfavourable mutations occur in genes and/or proteins indirectly or directly involved in the biosynthesis of CoQ10. Those afflicted with primary CoQ10 deficiency syndrome can suffer with a wide range of conditions including kidney diseases, strokes, cerebellar ataxia, spasticity, peripheral neuropathy, intellectual disability, movement disorders, exercise intolerance and muscular weakness.[129]

In individuals with primary CoQ10 deficiency, early treatment with high-dose oral CoQ10 supplementation has been shown to improve the pathological disease state, limit the progression of brain damage, and help recover kidney damage.[136]

The elderly (and especially the elderly that undergo low levels of physical activity - with related low muscle mass) have also shown more likely to have low levels of CoQ10.[137] Low plasma CoQ10 levels have been associated with acute influenza, viral papilloma infections, and sepsis; this is another reason why the elderly may be more susceptible to infection.[138]

SARS-CoV-2 also seems to damage mitochondrial health. In one study, COVID-19 pneumonia patients in Italy found that the infected monocytes displayed alterations in mitochondrial functions and disrupted bioenergetics.[139] Luckily, CoQ10 may come to our aid here.

In another small study it was shown that targeted mitochondrial therapy with CoQ10 supplementation and spa rehabilitation may improve mitochondrial health and accelerate the recovery of the patients after COVID-19.[140]

An *in vitro* study showed that CoQ10 attenuated platelet aggregation and thus clot formation induced by SARS-CoV-2 spike proteins, likely due to its strong antioxidative ability.[141]

CoQ10 levels in seminal fluid are considered an important biomarker of healthy sperm.[142] With regards to male fertility, it has been shown that CoQ10 improves semen parameters in the treatment of idiopathic male infertility.[143] Supplementation of CoQ10 (200–300 mg/day) in men with infertility has been shown to improve sperm concentration, density, motility, and morphology.[144] This has also been reflected when CoQ10 has been supplemented with vitamins C and E.[145]

A 2015 study showed that suboptimal levels of CoQ10 can lead to egg deficits and age-associated declines in fertility.[146] In women undergoing IVF, pretreatment with CoQ10 was shown to improve ovarian response to stimulation and embryological parameters.[147]

Dosage: The standard dose for CoQ10 is generally 90 mg for a low dose and

200 mg for the higher dose, but doses as high as 1200 mg daily and 3000 mg per day have been used in clinical trials.[148]

Since CoQ10 is mainly distributed in high-energy-demanding tissues, animal hearts and livers represent the richest source of this bioactive molecule, with a content between 30 and 200 mg/kg.[149]

Since the efficiency of absorption decreases as the dose increases, taking extremely high doses increases the treatment cost without having any impact on treatment efficacy. 90 mg tends to be the most cost-effective dose.[148] **But if you are thinking of taking higher doses, it is recommended that you split this into several doses throughout the day.**[149]

And as CoQ10 is a lipidic medium, it is recommended that you take it with meals containing fat.[149]

COLCHICINE

Some possible benefits include: anti-inflammatory, cardioprotective (helps treat cardiac inflammation), anti-amyloid, anti-cancer, anti-vascular inflammation, and "may interfere with the efficacy of the adenoviral vector–based vaccine for COVID-19."[150]

Colchicum autumnale is a flowering plant, of which the bulb-like corms contain colchicine, a historic medication for gout.[151] Colchicine is one of the oldest remedies still in use today. Its history as an herbal remedy for joint pain goes back at least to the 1500 BCE Egyptian manuscript, the *Ebers Papyrus*.[152]

Despite its use for thousands of years, colchicine's mechanism of action is still not fully known. Microtubules are polymers of proteins called tubulin that form part of the cytoskeleton and provide structure and shape to certain cells. Colchicine seems to induce microtubule destabilisation, thus affecting the cytoskeleton of certain cells.[153]

Colchicine also impairs neutrophil function by impacting inflammatory pathways and mediators of neutrophil activation; as well as being able to both decrease TNF-α receptor expression on macrophages (preventing activation).[151]

Mast cells are immune cells that play a key role in the inflammatory process. When activated, they release (in a process called "degranulation") mediators that drive inflammation. Mast cells are integral to allergic and anaphylactic reactions and are involved in conditions like autism and mast cell activation syndrome.[153] Colchicine is known to interrupt granule release in mast cells, thus preventing degranulation.[154]

Other than being used as a treatment for gout, colchicine has been the treatment of choice for Familial Mediterranean Fever (FMF) and the prophylactic treatment of choice for its most dreaded complication, secondary amyloidosis, a disorder in which abnormal proteins build up in tissues and organs (particularly the kidneys). It has been shown that colchicine not only prevents or considerably reduces the frequency of FMF attacks in 90–95% of patients when taken daily in doses of 1–2 mg, but almost always delays the onset of amyloidosis.[155]

Other than this, colchicine is looking promising at treating various other disorders, including acute and recurrent pericarditis, coronary artery disease, stroke, certain forms of vasculitis, and skin disorders, ranging from chronic urticaria to actinic keratosis.[151,152]

Colchicine use has also been associated with lower rates of cancer (especially prostate and colorectal cancers);[156] a significantly lower risk of cardiovascular events (especially in inflammatory cardiac conditions such as pericardial diseases, coronary artery disease, and atrial fibrillation);[151,157] and has even been shown to be associated with a 73% reduction in all-cause mortality.[158]

Due to its anti-inflammatory potential, colchicine has been researched as an agent to help target the cytokine storm post-SARS-CoV-2 invasion. One study showed that colchicine treatment decreased CRP levels and COVID-19 severity,[159] but others haven't been so promising.[160] More studies are needed.

Interestingly, it has been hypothesised that amyloidosis may be a factor causing systemic complications after coronavirus disease,[161] and another paper noted that the SARS-CoV-2 spike protein showed the ability to form amyloid proteins *in vitro*.[162] Colchicine's anti-amyloid properties haven't been researched in this regard, however.

Another researcher warned that colchicine may interfere with the efficacy of the adenoviral vector–based jabs for COVID-19 (ChAdOx1 nCoV-19 - Oxford, AstraZeneca vaccine).[150] This claim has not been followed up.

Dosage: Colchicine in the low doses used in most trials (≤ 1 mg/d) has been generally safe and well-tolerated.[163]

The most common side effect is diarrhoea (approximately 10%), which may be due to colchicine's ability to increase intestinal permeability and alter the gut microbiome.[164]

COLOSTRUM

Some possible benefits include: anti-inflammatory, immunomodulatory, antiviral, gut healing, neuroprotective, anti-cancer, immune-boosting post-exercise, anti-spike protein, and free iron chelating.

Colostrum is the first milk that mammals produce after giving birth; it has been known for centuries for its health benefits and has a very different composition from milk produced later in lactation.[165]

This milky fluid has evolved to optimise the care for mammalian neonates and is composed of various bioactive components that contribute significantly to the initial immunological defence in the baby as well as to the growth, development, maturation, and integrity of the neonatal gastrointestinal tract.

Research has shown that the bioactive components in bovine colostrum from cows are 100- to 1000-fold more concentrated than those in human colostrum; humans are also able to digest bovine colostrum; thus, it is emerging as a food supplement.[166]

Colostrum is rich in bioactive components such as immunoglobulins, lactoferrin, lactoperoxidase, oligosaccharides, vitamins, and various growth factors.

The available evidence suggests that bovine colostrum supplementation may reduce microbial translocation across the gut mucosa;[167,168] may suppress gut inflammation and thus a possible treatment aid in those with inflammatory bowel disease; helps maintain gut barriers; may improve overall immunological function (for e.g. increasing NK cell function); may improve post-exercise recovery as well as attenuate exercise-related immunosuppression; may help to reverse short-term memory lapses caused by neuronal cell death as well as attenuate the damage done by prions, just to name a few benefits.[169]

Lactoferrin, a glycoprotein found highly in colostrum, exerts antibacterial as well as antiviral, anti-inflammatory, immune-modulatory, neuroprotective, and anticarcinogenic effects. These activities are thought to be largely down to lactoferrin's capacity to bind to iron.[170] However, the potential molecular mechanisms by which lactoferrin exerts its multiple effects are still under investigation.

The other well studied component of colostrum is transforming growth factor beta (TGF-β), a cytokine with immunomodulatory and anti-inflammatory functions that has not only shown to balance and maintaining intestinal immunity, but also control or inhibit airway inflammation and the hyper-reactivity caused by effector Th2 cells.[171]

In one study of two hundred patients with COVID-19, the use of colostrum significantly reduced recovery time.[172] Another study showed that bovine colostrum-derived antibodies blocked the spike protein and ACE2 interaction in different *in vitro* assays.[173]

The use of lactoferrin in COVID-19 patients reduced the time it took to get a negative test.[174] Lactoferrin has also been shown to protect host cells from virus attachment as well as attaching to SARS-CoV-2 and the spike protein in particular.[175]

Dosage: The optimal dosage and duration of bovine colostrum supplementation have not been established. Most studies have been conducted in healthy adults using doses that range from 14 mg taken three times per day to 60 g daily. Some benefits are usually noticed after long-term use (>2 months).[167]

It is recommended that colostrum be produced organically and be free of adulterants like pesticides, herbicides, anabolic hormones, antibiotics, and other chemicals. It should also not be processed at high temperatures and pressures.[168]

Different breeds of cow, milking times, and various formulations change the composition of colostrum.

CORDYCEPS

Some possible benefits include: anti-inflammation, immunomodulation, antiviral, neuroprotection, anti-cancer, pro-insulin sensitivity, anti-fatigue, anti-spike, pro-mRNA degradation (theoretical), and pro-fertility.

Cordyceps is a genus of 750 identified species of fungi. *C. sinensis* and *C. militaris* are the two most prominent, widely explored, and most studied members of the genus, and though they differ with regards to the content of bioactive compounds and the way they are grown, they are both commonly known as "Cordyceps."

Though *Cordyceps* has been described as a therapeutic in ancient Chinese medical books and Tibetan medicine, *Cordyceps* did not come to the modern limelight until 1993, when Chinese long-distance runners who took the tonic of *C. sinensis* during their training periods broke world records.[176]

Cordyceps has shown a whole host of medical properties since then thought down to various compounds it contains including cordycepin, cordycepic acid, various polysaccharides and nucleotides.

Increasing evidence shows that *cordyceps* is a bidirectional modulator with both potentiating and suppressive effects on the immune system through regulating innate and adaptive immunity.[177]

Natural *C. sinensis* has a long history of use in the treatment of respiratory infections and cancer. It is thought this is down particularly by the promotion of innate immunity.

It has been shown that cultured *C. sinensis* induced production of inflammatory factors (IL-1β, IL-6, IL-10, and TNF-α); elevated phagocytosis of human peripheral blood mononuclear cells (HPBMC); and elevated macrophage phagocytosis and monocyte production of H2O2 but did not induce cytokine overdrive in mice.[178]

Other studies have shown *Cordyceps* stimulating IFN-gamma, cytokine production from macrophages, enhancing natural killer cells, promoting the adaptive immune system, helping with the maturation of dendritic cells, and upregulating T cells.[177]

This fungus has also been shown to have attenuated the severity of lupus in mice with increased survival, decreased protein in the urine, and reduced titers of anti-double-stranded DNA antibodies.[179]

Cordyceps has also been shown to help with autoimmune conditions by reducing inflammation, reducing T cell overstimulation, and protecting cartilage degeneration in conditions like inflammatory arthritis.[180]

Other than having immunomodulatory properties, research has revealed that *Cordyceps* also has anti-cancer, antioxidant, anti-diabetic, blood-pressure lowering, anti-fatigue, and possible pro-fertility properties.[181-185]

With regards to COVID-19, cordycepin has shown to be able to bind strongly with SARS-CoV-2 spike protein, and it has been postulated that this compound of *Cordyceps* may participate in other antiviral reactions such as mRNA destabilisation.[186]

You may be interested to know that *C. sinensis* has shown to stimulate oestrogen production in human granulosa-lutein cells by upregulating the expression of several key enzymes, especially StAR and aromatase, making it a possible brilliant candidate for increasing the fecundity of women.[186]

And with regards to male fertility, C. sinensis was shown to improve the function of reproduction and testis morphology in mice.[185]

C. militaris also remarkably protects testicles against oxidative damage caused by BPA, relieving degeneration of serum testosterone levels and improving the sperm count and motility in rats compared to the BPA-treated group.[187]

Dosage: The dosages of cordyceps that have been used in human trials range from 1,000 to 3,000 mg daily, either in one single dose or multiple doses with meals.[188] *Cordyceps* has been shown to be quite safe in the *in vivo* treatment of animals for up to 3 weeks.[177]

CORNUS OFFICINALIS

Some possible benefits include: anti-inflammation, immunomodulation, neuroprotection, anti-diabetic and pro-fertility.

Cornus officinalis, the Japanese cornelian cherry, is a herb and food plant in east Asia used in traditional Chinese medicine to primarily treat liver, kidney, and reproductive system diseases and low energy since ancient times.[189]

Recent pharmacological studies have found that *C. officinalis* extract has a variety of biological activities, such as anti-inflammatory, anti-oxidative, anti-apoptotic, anti-diabetic, neuroprotective, and cardiovascular protective activities.[189]

Animal studies have found that *C. officinalis* is particularly effective at reducing blood glucose levels,[190] promoting glucose uptake by cells,[191] reducing insulin levels in diabetic rats, and improving pancreatic function too.[192,193]

Other than having anti-diabetic properties, other research has shown that *C. officinalis* may have neuroprotective and pro-fertility properties. Experimental studies have confirmed that *C. officinalis* has therapeutic effects on neurodegenerative diseases such as Alzheimer's disease and depression.[194]

One study noted that a compound called iridoid glycosides from *Cornus officinalis* had a significant protective effect against glutamate (the most abundant excitatory neurotransmitter)-induced toxicity in the memory-forming cells.[195] And another study showed that *C. officinalis* could also treat neurodegenerative diseases through antioxidant effects.[195]

With regards to fertility, one study noted that some fractions of the aqueous extract of *C. officinalis* could enhance the motility of human sperm *in vitro*.[197] And a 2016 study noted that the iridoid glycosides of *C. officinalis* markedly protected against diabetes-induced testicular damage, increased the rate of live sperms, and upregulated the levels of testosterone and other hormones.[198]

Dosage: Dosages of *Cornus officinalis* are yet to be officialised. Safety data for short- and long-term use in humans is lacking.

CURCUMIN

Some possible benefits include: anti-inflammation; anti-oxidative; antimicrobial; anti-cancer; anti-amyloidogenic activity; anti-aging; iron-chelating; heavy mental binding; protecting against radiation; protecting against arsenic exposure; inhibiting alcohol-induced liver damage; promoting the growth of benefi-

cial gut bacteria; anti-spike protein; immunomodulation; energy-boosting; and recovery-aiding.

Turmeric, the yellow spice, comes from the plant *Curcuma longa* (and other *Curcuma* species) of the ginger family.

Its use is said to date back to 4000 years ago in the Vedic culture in India, where it was used as a culinary spice and had some religious significance. Since then, it has been traditionally used in Asian countries as a spice for its taste and colour and as a medical herb for its antioxidant, anti-inflammatory, antimicrobial, and anti-cancer properties.[199,200,201]

Curcumin is the bioactive polyphenol found in turmeric and has been shown to target many cellular pathways, conferring benefit to inflammatory conditions,[202] metabolic syndrome,[203] pain,[204] and the management of inflammatory and degenerative eye conditions,[205] as well as kidney diseases.[206]

Curcumin continues to show effectiveness in *in vitro*, *ex vivo*, *in vivo,* and even clinical trials. It has been shown to increase host antioxidant defences and enzymes,[207] have the ability to scavenge for different forms of free radicals,[208] and inhibit enzymes that are involved in making reactive oxygen species.[209]

Curcumin has also been shown to:[210] block NF-κB activation, which is increased by several different inflammatory stimuli; inhibit proinflammatory cytokines; have anti-amyloidogenic activity;[211] increase sirtuin activity;[212] chelate iron;[213] protect against radiation;[214] protect against arsenic exposure;[215] inhibit alcohol-induced liver damage;[216] and even promote the growth of beneficial gut bacteria.[217]

It seems like the benefits of curcumin are endless and wide-ranging. One study noted that working memory and mood were significantly better following long-term treatment with curcumin.[218] Another noted that the use of curcumin reduced the reported pain and markers of muscle damage in those after exercise.

In another study, children with recurrent respiratory tract infections were given both lactoferrin and curcumin. It was shown that this combination resulted in a significant skewing of CD8+ T cell maturation and upregulated other aspects of the innate immune system.[220]

Curcumin's ability to bind to toxins and metals and render them less harmful is known.[221] In fact, interestingly, metal–curcumin complexes may increase the solubility, cellular uptake, and bioavailability of curcumin and improve its antioxidant, anti-inflammatory, antimicrobial, and antiviral effects, too.

It's not just metals and toxins curcumin can bind on too. Studies have noted that curcumin can bind strongly to the spike protein,[222,223] the host receptor ACE2, *and* also to their complex. In a lab study, curcumin has also been shown to inhibit the spike protein of the Omicron variant.[224]

This, as well as curcumin's antioxidant and anti-inflammatory properties, may be why various studies have shown curcumin supplementation led to a significant decrease in common symptoms, duration of hospitalisation, and deaths in those with COVID-19.[225]

The "problem" with curcumin is that it has poor bioavailability—only a tiny amount of curcumin ingested leads to any biological benefit. However, the addition of piperine, the major active component of black pepper, when combined in a complex with curcumin, has been shown to increase bioavailability by 2000%.[210]

In one study of 46 outpatients with COVID-19 disease, the supplementation of a curcumin-piperine combination for 14 days showed to significantly help reduce weakness.[226]

Dosage: The Allowable Daily Intake of curcumin is 0–3 mg/kg body weight.[227] **It has been noted that to supplement curcumin with piperine, take 500 mg of the former with 5–6.7 mg of the latter, three times a day (i.e., 1,500 mg of curcumin and 15-20 mg of piperine per day).**[228] **Tumeric has been considered safe at a dosage of 6 grams a day for four to seven weeks.**[229]

Pure turmeric powder has a curcumin concentration of 3.14%.[230]

As curcumin can bind to iron to form ferric-curcumin complexes, long-term use has the potential to cause iron deficiency anaemia.[231]

Curcumin has also been shown to modulate oestrogen activity, even blocking oestrogen's effect on oestrogen-positive breast cancer.[232] **However, one study noted that tumeric use reduced the thickness of the womb lining, and though this property may be beneficial for those suffering with a condition called endometriosis, high doses (>3000 mg a day) of turmeric consumption may disrupt female fertility in this regard.**[232]

FIASMA ACTIVITY DRUGS

Some possible benefits include: anti-inflammation, anti-viral, anti-cancer, anti-aging, cardioprotection, and neuroprotection.

Acid sphingomyelinase (ASM) is an important enzyme that breaks down sphingomyelin, a type of fat predominantly found wrapped around nerve cells, into a molecule called ceramide.

Ceramides are a family of waxy fat molecules found in cell membranes that were once purely thought to support cellular structural elements; however, recent evidence has suggested that they are involved in a variety of other biological activities, mainly regulating the differentiation, growth, movement, and death of cells.[234]

A proper balance between regulation of normal cell growth and cell death is the basis of life, and it is said that dysregulation of this feature is the basis of nearly all diseases and ageing. Ceramide holds a vital role in regulating biological development and lifespan, and a deregulation in ceramide metabolism has been shown to increase the risk and progression of age-related diseases.[235]

A compelling and growing body of evidence is showing that ceramides account for much of the tissue damage seen in various diseases. Ceramides have been shown to build up in many tissues, including blood vessels and the heart, in individuals with cardiovascular disease.[236] They have also shown to increase in those with cancer;[237] and high ceramide levels are thought responsible for the increased susceptibility of brain cells to cell death.[238]

Ceramides have been shown to induce senescence and activate genetic and biochemical pathways involved with ageing.[239] And certain viruses, like the rhinovirus, also activate ASM and induce ceramide for their use. The ceramides clump together and serve as entrances for the virus.[240]

Inhibiting the production of ceramides in mice and rats has been shown to prevent the development of hypertension, atherosclerosis, diabetes mellitus, and heart failure.[236] It has also been shown that drugs that reduce levels of ceramides may have a protective role against SARS-CoV-2 infection.[241]

Functional Inhibitors of Acid Sphingomyelinase (FIASMA) are drugs that inhibit ASM and thus the downstream production of ceramides and related metabolites. This influences the balance between cell death and cell growth and has shown promise in ceramide-related diseases and ageing.[242]

A recent spotlight has been placed on high-FIASMA activity drugs within the scientific community as a handful of studies have shown that their use may have protected individuals from severe COVID-19.

Many commonly prescribed antidepressants have high FIASMA activity. One study noted that the *"use of antidepressant use was significantly less prevalent in inpatients with COVID-19 than in a matched control group of inpatients without COVID-19; and that antidepressant use was significantly associated with reduced 28-day mortality among COVID-19 inpatients."*[241]

Another noted that *"despite being significantly and substantially associated with older age and greater medical severity, FIASMA medication use was significantly associated with reduced likelihood of intubation or death."*[243]

High-FIASMA-activity drugs, like certain antidepressants, are thought to act as disease modulators with regards to COVID-19 in two main ways.[241] Firstly, these drugs may reduce the ceramide-enriched membranes that help SARS-CoV-2 enter cells, and secondly, via an anti-inflammatory response.

Though promising, it must be noted that high-FIASMA activity drugs vary in their primary effects and side-effect profiles. Though these medications may have benefits with regards to the ceramide pathway, long-term use may cause other unwarranted ramifications.

Interestingly, a quick search revealed that both curcumin and cordyceps have the potential to reduce the formation of ceramides too.[244,245]

Dosage: As the list of high-FIASMA-activity drugs is large, no one dosage can be presented.

FISETIN

Some possible benefits include: anti-inflammation, anti-oxidative, anti-aging, anti-allergic, immunomodulation, cardioprotection, neuroprotection, and anti-cancer.

Fisetin is a bioactive flavonoid found in small concentrations in fruits and vegetables such as strawberry, apple, persimmon, grape, onion, and cucumber. In one study, the highest concentration of fisetin was found in strawberries (160 mcg/g), followed by apples (26.9 mcg/g), and persimmons (10.5 mcg/g).[246]

Flavonoids in general are known to have a range of positive biological effects, mainly due to their ability to scavenge free radicals.[247] Their regular consumption is associated with a reduced risk of a number of chronic diseases, including cancer, cardiovascular disease, and neurodegenerative disorders.[248] They have also been shown to have anti-cancer, antioxidant, anti-inflammatory, and antiviral properties.[249]

Fisetin is no different from other flavonoids in this regard. Feinstein has been shown to inhibit oxidation, activate antioxidant defences, inhibit the growth of various types of cancer, inhibit MMP activity (similar to Chaga), inhibit mast cell activation, act as a neuroprotective agent, reduce the impact of age and disease-related brain function, as well as have immunomodulatory effects.[250-257]

Fisetin has also shown great cardiovascular protective potential. One study showed that fisetin protected against cardiac cell death, and another showed it stopped cardiac hypertrophy in mice.[258,259]

Senolytics are a class of drugs that selectively clear senescent cells. Senescent cells (as we have already discussed) are cells that cannot divide or die and are associated with ageing and inflammation (as well as COVID-19).[260]

Fisetin has recently been a lot more talked about in certain scientific circles after a 2018 study demonstrated that, when tested against a panel of other flavonoids, fisetin had the most potent senolytic activity in several cell types *in vitro*.[261] And when given to mice, fisetin showed a significant reduction in the percentage of senescent cells. Most interestingly, the study also showed that fisetin reduced the fraction of senescent T and NK cells, in other words, revitalising the immune system.[261] The authors of the study note that *"Chronic exposure to fisetin improves healthspan and extends the median and maximum lifespan of mice."*[261]

In another study comparing four flavonoids, only fisetin was shown to significantly help the induction of memory formation in certain areas of the brain. Fisetin was also shown in another study to be very effective at inducing nerve growth, giving results almost indistinguishable from those obtained with nerve growth factor.[262]

Dosage: There have been no trials on the use of fisetin on humans as of yet, and thus no established recommended dosage. Most fisetin supplements range from 100 to 500 mg a day. In clinical trials, the equivalent human daily doses of 100–1400 mg of fisetin were used[263] (the 2018 study gave mice 100 mg/kg of fisetin for 5 consecutive days,[261] which comes out to be approximately 8 mg/kg in human adults).[264]

GINKGO BILOBA EXTRACTS

Some possible benefits include antiapoptotic, antioxidant, and anti-inflammation actions that may translate to better cognition in the cognitively impaired. May help with tinnitus.

Ginkgo biloba extracts are a classic and popular herbal product isolated from *Ginkgo biloba,* a medicinal tree native to China and one of the oldest living tree species in the world. It outlived the dinosaurs.[265]

Ginkgo biloba has been used for medicinal purposes for centuries. In traditional Chinese medicine, it is used for treating pulmonary issues, bladder infections, and alcohol abuse. But as a modern supplement, *Ginkgo biloba* extract is quoted as the most commonly ingested herb taken for cognitive health.[266]

Though commonly used by people of all backgrounds, its neuroprotective benefits seem to predominantly help those with cognitive impairment.[267] *Ginkgo biloba* extracts have shown several health benefits for memory, cognition, Alzheimer's disease, Parkinson's disease, and dementia.[268] These pharmacological effects are thought to be thanks to the antiapoptotic, antioxidant, and anti-inflammatory actions that it has.[269]

Ginkgo biloba extracts have also been shown to improve cognitive function via increasing BDNF levels in aged female rats.[270] Another study, again in rats, showed that those pre-treated with *Ginkgo biloba* extracts induced an antidepressant role through its modulation effect on the hippocampal BDNF expression.[271]

And one cell culture study noted that *Ginkgo biloba* extracts induced neurite outgrowth after 3 days of treatment with a comparable effect to that of nerve growth factor.[272]

One systematic review of studies on humans noted that the *Ginkgo biloba* extract called EGb 761® was an evidence-based treatment option for tinnitus.[273]

Ginkgo biloba extract has also been shown to inhibit platelet activation and platelet aggregation.[274,275] Combining *Ginkgo biloba* extract with aspirin has also shown both synergistic and additive effects in restraining platelet aggregation.[276] One review noted that human trials have not noticed an overall bleeding risk or significant interaction with anticoagulants or antiplatelet agents in *Ginkgo biloba*.[267]

Human trials using *Ginkgo biloba* extracts on healthy people haven't been so promising, however. A review of clinical studies of the health effects of *Ginkgo biloba* extracts from 1984 to 2018 alluded to the fact that in many studies where a negative or no significant result was found, smaller doses than therapeutically needed were used.[267] The review notes that *"treatment can achieve better therapeutic effect when the dosage of EGb was more than 240 mg/day."* (EGb stands for *Ginkgo biloba* leaf extracts).[267]

Dosage: It is recommended to take 120–240 mg of *Ginkgo biloba* extracts, one to four hours before performance, and 40–120 mg, three times a day, to alleviate cognitive decline in older adults. The supplement form of Ginkgo biloba is also called EGb-761 extract. It should be a 50:1 concentrated extract. Ginkgo biloba should be taken with meals.[268]

GINSENOSIDE RG1

Some possible benefits include: anti-inflammation, anti-oxidation, neuroprotection, pro-cognition, and gut microbiome modulation.

Ginsenoside Rg1 (G-Rg1) is the most abundant component isolated from Panax notoginseng saponins (PNS), the major bioactive components extracted from the root of *Panax notoginseng,* commonly known as Chinese ginseng.

Chinese ginseng has been used in East Asian countries for more than 2,000 years for the treatment of ageing, inflammation, stress, diabetes mellitus, hepatic diseases, cancer, and memory impairment.[278] Numerous studies, mostly on animal models, have shown that G-Rg1 can cross the BBB and exert potential neuroprotective effects, improving the cognitive functions of animals with Alzheimer's disease.[279]

G-Rg1 has a structure similar to steroid hormones and has been shown to reduce inflammation due to this.[280,281] G-Rg1 has also shown anti-oxidation and anti-inflammatory effects, as well as the ability to upregulate nerve cells, reduce nerve cell death, and ameliorate Alzheimer's disease-related pathology.[282,283,284]

One study showed that Rg1 extracts from Chinese ginseng significantly reduced areas of cell death and alleviated neurological deficits caused by stroke.[285]

G-Rg1 has also been demonstrated to dose-dependently promote the neural cell adhesion molecules (NCAMs) and synapsin-1 (SYN-1). NCAM is involved in nerve growth, while SYN-1 is involved with the molecular machinery in nerves that regulates neurotransmitter release.[286]

Though potentially useful, G-Rg1 has limited scientific evidence in humans and also has a low bioavailability when taken orally.[287] This low bioavailability may actually be a feature and not a bug, however, as one study noted that the use of G-Rg1 improved the cognitive capability and affected the microbiota of the large intestine in a tree shrew model.[288]

The abundance of the gut bacteria *Bacteroidetes* is increased in patients with Alzheimer's disease, whereas the number of the bacteria *Firmicutes* is decreased in the condition.[289] And thus, a low *Firmicutes/Bacteroidetes* ratio has been shown to be indicative of Alzheimer's disease as well as other conditions.[290] It is thought that the *Firmicutes/Bacteroidetes* ratio is one of the energy output indicators of microbial fermentation; the higher the ratio, the higher the energy output.[291]

In the shrew study mentioned above, shrews that were given G-Rg1 had a reduced abundance of *Bacteroidetes* and an increased *Firmicutes/Bacteroidetes* ratio.[288] G-Rg1 also increased *Lactobacillus salivarius,* a gut bacteria associated with improved cognition.[292]

Dosage: Human trials on G-Rg1 are limited. Converting from mice dosages corresponds to 2-3 g of ginseng/day in a 60 kg adult human.[283]

Panax ginseng tends to be taken in doses of 200 to 400 mg daily.

GOTU KOLA

Some possible benefits include: anti-inflammation, antioxidation, neuroprotection, memory enhancement, pro-cognition, wound healing, anti-aging, helping with varicose veins and vein disease-related swollen legs, and preventing visual impairment.

Gotu kola is a plant in the flowering plant family *Apiaceae*. It is scientifically known as *Centella asiatica* and is also commonly known as Indian pennywort.

Gotu kola has been used as a medicine in the Ayurvedic tradition of India for thousands of years, in traditional Chinese medicine for over 2000 years, and by the people of Java and other Indonesian islands.[295]

Throughout this time and in various cultures, Gotu kola has been used as a blood purifier, for treating high blood pressure, for memory enhancement, for promoting longevity, and for treating emotional disorders like depression.[295]

The primary bioactive components of Gotu Kola are various triterpenoids and carotenoids. These, along with other bioactive constituents, have shown antioxidant, antidiabetic, anticancer, neuroprotective, cardioprotective, anti-inflammatory, antimicrobial, and memory-enhancing activities.[296]

Various animal studies have shown gotu kola to improve oxidative stress in the nervous system, thereby alleviating brain and nervous system damage and increasing attention span and concentration.[297] Another study showed protective effects of Gotu Kola compounds in inhibiting beta-amyloid- and free radical-induced cell death.[298]

Gotu kola has also been shown to upregulate BDNF levels as well as increase the length and branches of nerve cells,[299,300] which is useful for repairing damaged neurons. Gotu kola has also been shown to increase the availability of the neurotransmitter acetylcholine in the brain and thus may help with memory formation and have anticonvulsant potential.[301]

Gotu kola has been shown to increase the working memory of elderly participants in one study as well as improve the function of stroke patients in another.[302,303]

People most commonly use Gotu Kola for its cognition-enhancing benefits, but its benefits do not end there. Gotu kola also has good evidence as a wound healing agent as well as helping the skin to tighten and helping with other skin conditions when applied topically.[304,305]

Gotu kola has also been postulated to help with venous insufficiency conditions like varicose veins,[306,307] prevent visual impairment,[306] and act as an anti-aging agent by activating the enzyme telomerase.[308]

Dosage: Gotu kola extract has most often been used by adults in doses of 60–450 mg by mouth daily for 4–12 months.[309]

Dosages differ with the conditions intended to be treated; for example, it has been recommended that, for anxiety, one should take 500 mg of gotu kola extract twice a day for up to 14 days at a time. One may take up to 2,000 mg per day in cases of extreme anxiety.[310]

Whilst to boost cognition it is recommended to take 750 to 1,000 mg of gotu kola per day for up to 14 days at a time.[310]

GREEN TEA EPIGALLOCATECHIN-3-GALLATE

Some possible benefits include: anti-inflammatory, antioxidant, cardioprotective, neuroprotection, and anti-prion.

Tea comes from the leaves of *Camellia sinensis* and is primarily produced in four varieties, i.e., white, green, oolong, and black, depending on the oxidation and fermentation technique applied.[311]

Out of all tea produced, only 20% is green tea.[312] Green tea is made from unfermented leaves and reportedly contains the highest concentration of powerful flavonoids. The main flavonoid in green tea is called catechins, which make up 30–

40% of the solid components of the tea. And out of the various catechins in green tea, epigallocatechin-3-gallate (EGCG) is the most abundant.[313]

It is thought that the various beneficial effects of green tea, including anti-inflammatory, anti-carcinogenic, antimicrobial, and anti-oxidative effects, are mainly due to EGCG.[313]

In vitro and *in vivo* studies have shown the ability of EGCG to counteract various cancer cells via down regulating the MMPs and induce cancer cell death by inactivating NFκB.[314.315] With regards to metabolic and cardiovascular health, EGCG has been shown to exhibit a wide range of therapeutic properties, including anti-atherosclerosis, anti-cardiac hypertrophy, anti-myocardial infarction, and anti-diabetic effects.[316]

Interestingly, in one study of twenty-five male patients with wild-type transthyretin amyloid cardiomyopathy, a disease primarily affecting the heart caused by accumulation of a protein called transthyretin, 12 months of daily consumption of 1,200 mg green tea extract containing 600 mg EGCG was shown to reduce the pathological growth of part of the heart.[317]

ECGC has also been shown to inhibit the aggregation of other proteins in the brain that are linked to various disease states.[318] ECGC seems to have preventative effects on prion disease too, in part due to autophagic pathways.[319] EGCG is known to promote autophagy.[320]

With regards to COVID-19, ECGC has shown in lab studies that it inhibits the interaction between the RBD of spike proteins and the ACE2 receptor.[321]

Dosage: There is currently no clear dosage recommendation for ECGC. A single cup of brewed green tea typically contains about 50–100 mg of EGCG.[322] **One group of researchers suggested a safe intake level of 338 mg of EGCG per day when ingested in solid supplemental form.**[323]

High levels (800 mg of EGCG or more) have been linked to liver damage.[324] **EGCG may not be safe if you are pregnant and/or breastfeeding.**[325]

GYNOSTEMMA PENTAPHYLLUM

Some possible benefits include: anti-inflammation, antioxidation, cardioprotection, neuroprotection, anti-cancer, anti-diabetes, and anti-obesity.

Gynostemma pentaphyllum is a herb that belongs to the family Cucurbitaceae. It is a well-known edible medical plant that has been used since the Ming dynasty.[326] The earliest record of *Gynostemma pentaphyllum* use as a drug comes from the herbalist Li Shizhen's book *Compendium of Materia Medica,* published in 1578, which identified the herb for treating various diseases, from swelling of the pharynx and blood in the urine to neck tumours and trauma. The Chinese call *Gynostemma pentaphyllum* an "immortality" herb, claiming it has rejuvenating properties and the ability to extend life.[327]

Gynostemma pentaphyllum contains a variety of active compounds, but the gypenosides isolated from the herb are believed to be the major active constituents responsible for its various biological activities and reported clinical effects. Many gypenosides have been noted to be ginsenosides. Ginsenosides make up around 25% of the total gypenosides in *Gynostemma pentaphyllum*, and thus this plant was identified as the first plant containing ginseng saponins outside of the Araliaceae family. For this reason, *Gynostemma pentaphyllum* is also known as "southern ginseng."[328]

Various lab studies have shown that *Gynostemma pentaphyllum* has anti-cancer, anti-atherogenic, neuroprotective, anti-diabetic, and immunomodulatory effects.[326]

The anti-cancer properties of *Gynostemma pentaphyllum* are thought to be due to its ability to modulate the immune system (increasing lymphocytes and the activity of NK cells);[329] induce cancer cell death;[330] inhibit the migration of metastases;[331] regulate the gut microbiome;[332] and cause cancer cells to stop dividing.[333]

Gynostemma pentaphyllum's antioxidant properties are thought to help prevent amyloid-related brain cell death.[329] *Gynostemma pentaphyllum* may also help with a type of dementia called vascular dementia, where there are neurological defects caused by reduced blood flow to the brain. *Gynostemma pentaphyllum* treatment of rats in one study noted that the oxidative neuronal damage was ameliorated, and the activation of inflammatory certain brain cells was reduced after blood flow was reduced in the brain.[334]

Gynostemma pentaphyllum has also shown anti-fatigue, anti-platelet, anti-depressant, and antiviral potential.[326,335,336]

All evidence mentioned so far have been lab and studies on animal models. Clinical trials on humans are severely lacking. There are only a small handful of studies on humans, and they specifically look at *Gynostemma pentaphyllum*'s effect on diabetes and weight.

One study noted that *Gynostemma pentaphyllum* tea improved insulin sensitivity and reduced fasting plasma glucose in patients receiving 6 g of the tea herb for two weeks.[337] Another researcher noted that the use of *Gynostemma pentaphyllum* alongside a regular antidiabetic medication decreased HbA1C (a marker of long term blood sugar control) levels by 2%.[338] Supplementing with *Gynostemma pentaphyllum* has also been shown to reduce fat around the organs and BMI in obese participants.[339,340]

Dosage: There is currently no clear dosage recommendation for *Gynostemma pentaphyllum*. As mentioned above, some clinical trials have used 6 g of leaves (dry weight) and made tea from that.[341]

INFRARED LIGHT

Some possible benefits include: anti-inflammation, wound-healing, improving vascular health, immunomodulating, neuroprotection, nerve growth, and aiding with overall recovery.

The use of light in treating illness has been reported since Ancient Greece; initially called "heliotherapy," it involved leaving the sick exposed to the sun to cure their ailments.[342] In the 1918 Spanish Flu pandemic, the use of light as therapy, termed "phototherapy," was pointed out as one of the most significant factors in reducing mortality.[343] Since then, several studies have been carried out to better understand the beneficial effects of light on our health.

All light is electromagnetic radiation, with only a portion in the middle termed "visible light" that our eyes are able to perceive. Visible light is usually defined as having wavelengths in the range of 400–700 nanometres (nm), but other forms of light exist on opposite ends of this spectrum.

Infrared (IR) and ultraviolet (UV) light are forms of light that our eyes cannot perceive. IR includes wavelengths between 780 nm and 1000 µm. IR can be further split into near-infrared, mid-infrared, and far-infrared, while UV light has a wavelength of 10 nm to 400 nm.

UV light is used to treat various skin disorders and is the primary type of light that helps us form vitamin D.[344,345] Though vitamin D from sunlight has been shown to be associated with various health benefits, a vast body of studies has failed to confirm any major health benefits from vitamin D supplementation. This may be because red and near-infrared light, both of which are present in sunlight, could explain the associations between sunlight exposure and better health status.[346] And thus, there has been a particular interest in understanding the effects of red and IR light on our health.

Photobiomodulation (PBM) therapy is "*a form of light therapy that utilizes non-ionizing forms of light sources, including lasers, LEDs, and broadband light, in the visible and infrared spectrum.*"[347] It is now understood that PRM works by the absorption of energy by molecules that accept the light called chromophores. There are two main types of chromophores: cytochrome c oxidase (CCO) and intracellular water.

The theory goes that CCO enzyme activity may be inhibited by NO, especially in hypoxic or damaged cells, and that the dissociation of NO by IR light causes improved energy production by the mitochondria.[348]

There is also a brief increase in ROS produced in the mitochondria when they absorb light delivered during PBM.[348] It is thought that this short burst of ROS triggers mitochondrial signalling pathways, leading to cell-protective, antioxidant, and anti-apoptotic effects in the cells.[348]

We also possess light-sensitive ion channels, which are types of receptors that are activated by light. These have been mainly studied in algae and insects.[349]

When IR light gets absorbed by the skin, it activates these molecules and receptors, stimulating various biological processes.[347] This facilitates events such as mitochondrial respiration, calcium transport—which results in more significant cell proliferation—repairing, and regenerating tissues.[350] NO is also released, which helps to increase blood flow and can activate a number of beneficial cellular pathways downstream.[348]

Via these biological processes and more, PBM has been shown to assist in the recovery of wounds, nerve, bone, respiratory tract disease and other injuries.[351,352,353]

Near-IR can also penetrate the head and reach the brain.[348] The effects of this were possibly illustrated in one study of a 23-year-old professional hockey player with a history of concussions who treated himself at home with commercially available, low-risk PBM devices that used light-emitting diodes (LEDs) to emit 810-nm light pulsing at 10 or 40 Hz. After 8 weeks of PBM treatments, increased brain volumes, improved functional connectivity, increased blood flow around the brain, and improvements on neuropsychological test scores were observed. Though there was no placebo control in this study, results look promising for those with traumatic brain injury.[354]

In a small placebo-controlled clinical trial with dementia patients, PBM with a near-IR helmet showed that light therapy could improve various neurological factors including memory, visual attention, task switching, brain wave patterns, the ability to learn, and mitochondrial enhancement.[355]

Other than wearing light-emitting helmets, IR saunas are another modality that has shown benefit. It has been demonstrated that IR sauna therapy improves vascular endothelial dysfunction in hamsters with experimental cardiomyopathy. Hamsters were treated daily with an experimental far-IR sauna system for 15 minutes, and after 4 weeks, NO production had increased significantly compared with normal controls.[356]

PBM has also shown anti-cancer activity via immunomodulation.[357] PBM has also been shown to alter the gut microbiome in a favourable way, which in turn improves overall immune function.[358] *In vitro* and lab experiments have shown the effect of PBM on the prevention of thrombosis and positive results in wound healing during viral infection.[350] Another lab study showed that PBM was able to relieve hyperinflammation of the type induced by COVID-19. And though more human trials are needed, case reports have shown PBM to improve the respiratory indices, radiological findings, and inflammatory markers in severe COVID-19 patients.[350]

In one trial of 300 patients with COVID-19, methylene blue and 660 nm red light was applied in the oral and nasal cavity, compared to placebos, and showed to lead to significant decreases in morbidity and reduced mortality rates.[359]

Dosage: As we are dealing with energy in the form of light, dosing is not as straightforward as when ingesting a supplement. Things are further complicated by the fact that there are no official guidelines on how to use PBM, plus light comes in various forms and via various devices, and "doses" depend on power density and time.

Online sources state that most clinical literature suggests that light in the mid-600 nm range and low-to mid-800 nm range is the most effective,[360] with a dose in the range of 0.1J/cm² to 6J/cm² being optimal for cells.[361]

It may be best to follow the instructions of trusted PBM manufacturers if you do decide to use PBM.

IVERMECTIN

Some possible benefits include: anti-inflammation, anti-parasitic, antiviral, antibacterial, anti-cancer, and it may help with motor neuron disease.

Other than mRNA and DNA vector agents themselves, there has been no other medication in the last three years that has been as politically controversial as ivermectin.

Ivermectin is an antiparasitic drug that was originally made from a fermented metabolite made by the bacterium *Streptomyces avermitilis*.[362] Ivermectin was introduced for medical use in 1982 and is effective against parasites such as *Onchocerca volvulus*, the cause of Onchocerciasis (river blindness), and other parasitic worms, as well as mites and lice.

Ivermectins' impacts in controlling tropical diseases like Onchocerciasis and Lymphatic filariasis, diseases which blighted the lives of billions of the poor and disadvantaged throughout the tropics,[363] is why its discoverers were awarded the Nobel Prize in Medicine in 2015 and the reason for its inclusion on the WHO's "List of Essential Medicines."

Ivermectin is not only an effective anti-parasitic but is generally well tolerated, has a broad-spectrum effect, is safe, easily administered, and is cheap. With regards to having anti-viral properties, ivermectin has been shown in *in vitro* studies to have properties against an increasing number of RNA viruses, including influenza, Zika, HIV, Dengue, and SARS-CoV-2.[363] It has also shown promise as an antibacterial and anticancer agent and may even help with motor neuron disease.[364]

Ivermectin gained much interest as a promising treatment option against SARS-CoV-2 in 2020 when researchers published their study results showing that it inhibited the replication of SARS-CoV-2 in cell culture.[365]

Other studies since then have shown that ivermectin can bind to the host receptor-binding region of the SARS-CoV-2 spike protein.[363] In fact, ivermectin has been identified as having the highest or among the highest binding affinities to spike protein S1 binding domains of SARS-CoV-2 among hundreds of molecules collectively examined, with ivermectin not being the particular focus of these studies.[366] Ivermectin has also been shown to bind to or interfere with multiple essential proteins required by the virus in order to replicate, inhibiting viral replication.[367] Ivermectin has also shown anti-inflammatory properties *in vitro*.[368]

Lab studies do not always reflect human trials. And this is where the controversy begins. Firstly, it is undeniable that various trials *have* found that the use of ivermectin in those with COVID-19 helped with recovery. In one study of four hundred patients, the use of 0.4 mg/kg ivermectin was associated with a statistically significant lower rate of progression of COVID-19.[369] In another study of 280 hospitalised patients, a statistically significant lower mortality rate was found among ivermectin-treated patients.[370] And a meta-analysis of 15 trials found that ivermectin reduced the risk of death in COVID-19 patients compared with no ivermectin use.[371]

Other than trial data, real-life evidence seems to support ivermectin use too. In Peru, one of the worst-hit nations in terms of COVID-19 disease and death, the government approved the use of ivermectin by decree on May 8, 2020. After its introduction, a decrease in total case incidences and total deaths/population due to COVID-19 was noted.[369] This was also seen similarly in Paraguay.[369]

However, though it has been noted in various studies that ivermectin hastens recovery and helps avoid ICU admission and death in hospitalised patients, this fact has not been shared by everyone.[369]

Cochrane is a highly prestigious group that conducts systematic reviews of health-care interventions and diagnostic tests. In their review of 11 trials with a total of 3409 participants, they note, *"Based on the very low-certainty evidence for inpatients, we are still uncertain whether ivermectin prevents death or clinical worsening or increases serious adverse events, while there is low-certainty evidence that it has no beneficial effect regarding clinical improvement, viral clearance and adverse events."*[372] There are other meta-analyses that have reached similar conclusions too.[373]

Meta-analysis and reviews depend on the studies and the quality of each study included in the overall review. Though Cochrane did not come out with a definitive "no," totally disproving the effectiveness of using ivermectin in COVID-19, this and other studies showing no benefit caused great confusion and division online and within society.

The differences in study outcomes may be due to differences in study design, biases, and differences in drug dosage and when it was used. Regardless, we still don't have a clear-cut answer as to whether or not it helps. What certainly didn't help was the labelling of ivermectin, a medication placed on the WHO "List of Essential Medicines" and described in the scientific literature as a "wonder drug"[364] by the mainstream media as "horse and cow dewormer."[374] The FDA, referring to ivermectin, also tweeted *"You are not a horse. You are not a cow. Seriously, y'all. Stop it."*[375]

Understanding the close ties between the government, pharmaceutical companies, and the mainstream media, it may not be too outlandish to assume that the heavy vilification of ivermectin, a safe, cheap, and possibly anti-COVID-19 drug, was actually a reflection of its effectiveness and thus its position as a direct competitor to the thing they wanted to flog.

It is all the more worrying when these entities have already shown a track record of lying to the public over and over again. Only recently has a Pfizer executive admitted that the company did not test whether its COVID-19 jabs stopped transmission of the virus before its launch.[376] And yet ivermectin has shown repeatedly to prevent transmission and development of COVID-19 disease in those exposed to infected patients.[369]

And the real kicker is that the NIH has included ivermectin as being evaluated to treat COVID-19 in their COVID-19 Treatment Guidelines.[377]

Who and what do we trust?

For now, eyes are on whether ivermectin may be able to treat long COVID. In one study of 33 patients with the condition, a protocol using ivermectin was given, and it was found that in 87.9% of the patients, resolution of all symptoms was observed after 2 doses, with an additional 7% reporting complete resolution after additional doses.[378]

The protocol is as follows: *"in cases with mild symptoms, Ivermectin was administered at a dose of 0.2 mg per kilogram of body weight per day for 2 days. If patients still had symptoms after the 2 doses, 2 additional days of Ivermectin treatment were given at the same dose. For cases with moderate symptoms, a dose of 0.4 mg per kilogram of body weight was prescribed for 2 days, followed by 0.2 mg per kilogram of body weight for 2 additional days. If a patient continued to have symptoms after the fourth day of treatment, more doses of Ivermectin were indicated. Treatment then continued for additional days until either clinical improvement was observed, or there was no longer further clinical improvement with treatment."*[378]

Dosage: It is not officially advised to use ivermectin to treat COVID-19 and/or long COVID.

The Front Line COVID-19 Critical Care Alliance (FLCCC) recommends 0.2mg/kg per dose of ivermectin as a prophylaxis for high-risk individuals, noting to use *"one dose today, 2nd dose in 48 hours, then one dose every 2 weeks."*[363]

Ivermectin is also recommended at a dose of 0.2 mg/kg per dose as part of the Early Outpatient Treatment Protocol by the FLCCC. They note *"one dose daily for minimum of 2 days, continue daily until recovered (max 5 days)."* [363]

LION'S MANE

Some possible benefits include: antimicrobial, anticancer, anti-inflammation, anti-fatigue, liver protection, cardioprotection, improved wound healing, immunomodulation, and pro-cognition.

Hericium erinaceus, commonly known as "Lion's Mane," is an edible fungus that has a long history of usage in traditional Chinese medicine. It is mainly naturally distributed throughout the northern hemisphere in Europe, Asia, and the southern states of America.

The Lion's Mane mushroom isn't just exceptionally spectacular-looking; it is also known for its plethora of health benefits, which are thought to be due to its large amount of structurally novel bioactive compounds.

This mushroom can biosynthesize about 70 different secondary metabolites, which is astonishingly high compared to other mushroom species. The two most researched of these secondary metabolites are hericerins and erinacines. These, along with other metabolites and polysaccharides, have been shown to have promising antimicrobial, anticancer, anti-inflammatory, anti-fatigue, liver-protective, pro-cardiovascular, improved-wound healing, and pro-cognitive effects.[379]

Lion's Mane is most popularly known for its neuroprotective and nerve-growing abilities. The bioactive compounds erinacine A, B, and C from the mushroom mycelium have been shown to stimulate nerve growth factor (NGF) synthesis. Hericenone E has been shown to stimulate NGF secretion too.[380,381] This may be particularly useful in those with cognitive decline, as NGF is involved in organising the function of cholinergic neurons in certain areas of the brain, areas that degenerate during the progression of Alzheimer's disease.

Oral administration of Lion's Mane powder added to the diet of mice with amyloid dysfunction over a 23 day experimental period showed that mushroom powder improved the cognitive deficits induced by the amyloid protein, further suggesting that the powder might be a promising treatment for cognitive dysfunction.[382]

In humans, a randomised, double-blind, placebo-control trial of 30 women over 4 weeks showed orally consumed Lion's Mane had the potential to reduce depression and anxiety.[383]

And a study examining the efficacy of oral administration of 250 mg tablets containing Lion's Mane mushrooms on patients with mild cognitive impairment showed those in the mushroom group scoring significantly higher on the cognitive function scale compared with the placebo group.[384]

Other than pro-cognitive effects, Lion's Mane has shown anti-cancer potential in both *in vitro* and *in vivo* experiments. For example, in one study, Lion's Mane showed antimetastatic activity, reducing the spread of murine colon carcinoma to the lungs by up to 69%. The same extracts reduced the expression of matrix metalloproteinase cells and their activities in culture media.[385]

Daily oral administration of three amounts (50, 100, and 200 mg/kg/day for 10 days) of Lion's Mane polysaccharides to 50 mice with sarcoma solid tumours reduced the increase in tumour weight from 100% for the control group to 68.5, 32.1, and 43.2% in the treated groups, respectively, as compared to 18.5% for treatment with the cancer drug cyclophosphamide.[386]

Like other medicinal mushrooms, Lion's Mane has also shown immunomodulatory properties. Lion's Mane has been shown to increase T cells (CD4+) and macrophages in mouse models. In one study, this mushroom also showed significant anti-tumour effects against pulmonary metastatic tumours, suggesting that the anti-tumour effects might be associated with the immune-enhancing activities of the polysaccharides.[387]

Dendritic cells are immune cells that process antigen material and present it on the cell surface to T cells. *H. erinaceus* mushrooms on murine dendritic cells induced activation and promoted morphological changes, increased the expression of surface molecules that are important for antigen presentation, and stimulated the secretion of cytokines that promote immune responses.[388]

Some of you may also be interested to hear that Hericenone B isolated from Lion's Mane exhibited strong antiplatelet aggregation activity, suggesting that it had the potential to be used in antiplatelet therapy to prevent cardiovascular disease and stroke.[389]

Dosage: Currently, one human study has used an oral dose of 1,000 mg Lion's Mane (96% purity extract) three times a day for a cumulative total of 3,000 mg extract.[384]

And the only other human trial used 2 g a day of the fruiting body for four weeks.[383]

LUTEOLIN

Some possible benefits include: anti-inflammation, anti-oxidation, antimicrobial, antiviral, anti-cancer, cardioprotection, mast cell stabilisation, heavy-metal protection, neuroprotection, alleviation of "brain fog," and immunomodulation.

Luteolin is a flavone, a type of flavonoid, present in many medicinal plants, fruits, and vegetables, including broccoli, onion leaves, carrots, peppers, cabbages, apple skins, Indian chrysanthemum flowers (*Chrysanthemum indicum)*, telegraph plants (*Codariocalyx motorius),* and *Artemisia asiatica*.[390] High luteolin content has also been reported in oregano, parsley, thyme, peppermint, basil, celery, and artichokes.

Plants with high luteolin content have been used across various cultures and for a long time to treat inflammation-related diseases. Examples include lemongrass (*Cymbopogon citratus)*, Alumã (*Vernonia condensata*), common sage (*Salvia plebeia),* and dandelion (*Taraxacum officinale)*. Traditional uses of these plants range from treating arthritis to reducing the redness of the skin, and they have been used across the world, from Southeast Asia to Latin America.

In silico, *in vitro,* and *in vivo* clinical studies suggest that luteolin is a powerful anti-inflammatory,[390] as well as having been reported to have antioxidant, anti-microbial, anti-cancer, cardioprotective, anti-diabetic, neuroprotective, and anti-allergic properties.[391-397]

The anti-inflammatory activity of luteolin has been attributed to inhibition of nitric oxygen synthase (iNOS), and NO production; scavenging of ROS; inhibition of ROS production and activation of antioxidant enzymes; inhibition of inflammatory mediator production and release; suppression of pro-inflammatory cytokine expression; inhibition of the NF-κB pathway, protein kinase B (AKT), and the mitogen-activated protein kinase (MAPK) pathway; inhibition of adhesion molecule membrane binding, hyaluronidase activity, and elastase activity; stabilisation of mast cells; reduction of vascular permeability; and modulation of cell membrane fluidity.[390]

Various animal studies, done primarily on mice and rats, have demonstrated the wide-ranging benefits of luteolin. In one study on rats, luteolin was shown to have a protective role in chronic pancreatitis (inflammation of the pancreas) via various mechanisms.[398] In another study, luteolin was able to suppress the early-stage growth of prostate cancer in rats by inducing cell death.[399]

Luteolin could also be used against the negative health effects elicited by toxic heavy metals. Various studies have shown luteolin has the ability to protect our biology and DNA from damage from various metals such as copper, zinc, nickel, cobalt, and lead.[400-404]

With regards to the cardiovascular system, in a study performed on male mice, luteolin administration was found to improve cardiac function, attenuate the inflammatory response, alleviate mitochondrial injury, decrease oxidative stress, inhibit cardiac apoptosis, and enhance autophagy.[405]

Luteolin's anti-inflammatory and anti-oxidative properties have also translated to better cognitive outcomes in various studies.[405] This is no better demonstrated in studies using luteolin on children with Autism Spectrum Disorder (ASD).

In one case series study, capsules containing luteolin (100 mg, from chamomile, >95% pure), quercetin (70 mg, from Sophora, >95% pure), and quercetin glycoside rutin (30 mg, from Sophora, >95% pure) formulated in microspheres (liposomes) mixed in olive kernel oil were given (at least 2 capsules/20 kg weight) to 37 children with ASD for at least four weeks who had not obtained any benefit from multiple other regimens. Results showed that GI and allergy symptoms improved in about 75% of children, eye contact and attention improved in 50%, social interaction improved in 25%, and speech resumed in about 10% of children.[407]

In another study, children with ASD were given one softgel capsule containing luteolin with food for 26 weeks. Among the 50 children, 40 completed the protocol and showed significant improvement in adaptive functioning and overall behaviour.[408]

Many children with ASDs have been reported to have "allergic-like" symptoms implicating mast cell activation.[409] To understand if the benefits of luteolin in children with ASD had anything to do with modulating the immune system, blood was drawn in children before and after luteolin administration. Results showed that serum IL-6 and TNF levels were significantly lower in children with ASDs after treatment with luteolin in comparison to their levels before the beginning of treatment. And as expected, the children with ASDs in whom the elevated serum IL-6 and TNF levels decreased by the end of the treatment period were the ones whose behaviour improved the most.[410]

Mast cells can be triggered by viruses, and a recent report correlated coronavirus infection with the activation of mast cells and subsequent cytokine storms in the lungs.[411] Luteolin inhibits mast cells, and thus the use of luteolin has been speculated to attenuate COVID-19-related lung damage.[412,412]

Luteolin has also been shown to reduce viral genome replication,[414] be a potential modulator of the spike protein,[415] and bind to the RBD of the virus.[416] Moreover, the world's most powerful supercomputer, SUMMIT, ranked the luteolin structural analogue eriodictyol (5,7,3′,4′-tetrahydroxyflavanone) among the best potential inhibitors of COVID-19.[417]

One review noted that these properties, as well as the fact that luteolin can inhibit the serine protease required for spike protein processing, may make it a good supplement for those with long COVID.[405]

Luteolin has also been shown to improve the symptoms of "brain fog" in children with ASD and brain "fog" in mastocytosis (a rare condition caused by an excess number of mast cells gathering in the body's tissues) patients.[418]

Dosage: There are no official dosages for luteolin in humans. Supplementation is generally considered safe, but one review noted that luteolin intake should not exceed a cumulative dose of 1–2 g/day because it can reduce liver metabolism.[413,418]

The review also notes that it is *"important to avoid the cheapest source of peanut shells that may affect persons allergic to peanuts, or fava beans, consumption of which could cause hemolytic anemia to Mediterranean extraction persons who lack the enzyme G6PD."* [413]

MACA

Some possible benefits include: neuroprotection, memory enhancement, pro-fertility, antidepressant, antioxidant, anti-cancer, anti-inflammatory, and skin protection activities.

Peruvian maca (*Lepidium meyenii*) is a root native to the Andean region that has been cultivated for at least 2000 years. It grows in areas of high altitude characterised by rocky formations, intense sunlight, strong winds, and extreme weather conditions, making them unsuitable for the growth of many other species.[419]

Maca roots come in three main colours. Yellow maca corresponds to about 60% of all maca in Peru.[419] Yellow is the most widely used and researched form among all maca products followed by red maca and then black maca. All forms are consumed traditionally by the indigenous population.

Yellow maca is said to help increase energy, improve concentration, and balance hormones.[420] Red is the sweetest and is said to aid women with hormonal balance and bone health.[420] Black maca may be the most effective form for men, especially for muscle gain, endurance, mental focus, and libido.[420]

Besides containing essential nutrients, maca also contains unique bioactive compounds that have shown medicinal promise. Of these, macamides are believed to be the major bioactive compounds in the root.[421]

Recent scientific findings suggest that this root may aid in sexual dysfunction regulation, have neuroprotective effects, help with memory enhancement, as well as have antidepressant, antioxidant, anti-cancer, anti-inflammatory, and skin protection activities.[419]

Though different colours of maca are traditionally thought to have different properties, this rule is not set in stone. In one study, extracts of black Maca showed to improve memory impairment brought on by the removal of ovaries in mice. In animal studies, the removal of ovaries is done to mimic post-menopausal pathophysiological changes in women related to learning and memory.[422] And thus, black maca may be a potential aid for women with menopause-related cognitive decline.[422]

A decrease in mitochondrial function and a decline in autophagy are thought to participate in the process of age-related cognitive decline; maca may help alleviate these changes. This was shown in another study where mice given maca showed improvements in cognitive function, motor coordination, and endurance capacity, accompanied by increased mitochondrial respiratory function and upregulation of autophagy-related proteins in the brain.[423]

The indigenous population of certain parts of South America believed that maca was able to increase vitality and treat infertility. These beliefs have been analysed in several studies with mixed results. In one study, men aged 21–56 years received black maca in one of two doses: 1500 mg, 3000 mg, or a placebo. The study evaluated the groups after 4, 8, and 12 weeks of treatment. An improvement in sexual desire was observed with Maca at 8 weeks of treatment, with no change in testosterone and/or mood.[424]

In a study on horses treated with 20 g a day of maca over 60 days, maca improved sperm concentration and total sperm count. The total sperm count was almost two times higher at the end than at the beginning of the trial with the use of maca.[425] Increased seminal volume, sperm count per ejaculum, motile sperm count, and sperm motility were also seen in men given maca for 4 months.[426]

Dosage: The standard dose for maca is said to be 1,500–3,000 mg. It should be taken daily alongside food.[427]

MELATONIN

Some possible benefits include: potent antioxidation, anti-inflammation, anti-cancer, anti-coagulation neuroprotection, anti-prion, cardioprotection, pro-fertility, anti-viral, mitochondria-healing, anti-venom, anti-ageing and pro-synergistic effects of other antioxidants.

Melatonin is an ancient molecule that can be traced back to the origin of life. It is a hormone that exists in all living organisms, including bacteria, yeasts, fungi, animals, and plants, and is most widely known for regulating sleep and modulating circadian rhythms; however, growing evidence indicates that melatonin may be the most potent lipophilic antioxidant around.[428,429]

In fact, melatonin's initial evolutionary function has been speculated to be a free radical scavenger.[428] In plants, melatonin continues to function in reducing oxidative stress as well as in promoting seed germination and growth, improving stress resistance, stimulating the immune system, modulating circadian rhythms, and controlling the closure of the "breathing" pores on leaves.[428]

In animals including humans, other than regulating sleep and our circadian rhythms, melatonin has shown to enhance immunity; act as an antioxidant; anti-inflammatory agent; suppress cancer growth; have anti-pathogenic properties; help with fertility; have neuroprotective properties and may even prevent ageing.[429]

On a cellular level, melatonin is made in, taken up by, and concentrated in mitochondria. Mitochondria are also the major source of ROS, which is a byproduct of mitochondrial energy production. Melatonin protects against mitochondrial DNA damage induced by mitochondrial-produced ROS, and given mitochondria's role in the production of ROS, it makes sense that the highest concentration of melatonin would be in the mitochondria, the greatest site of ROS production and where oxidative stress occurs the most.[430,431]

The pineal gland was described as the "Seat of the Soul" by René Descartes and is commonly referred to as the "third eye" in many spiritual traditions. Reptiles, birds, and some fish have an area of light-sensitive cells usually on top of their heads called the third parietal eye that produces melatonin.[432] There is evidence that this primitive third eye evolved into the pineal gland in mammals.[433]

The main function of the pineal gland is to receive information about the state of the light-dark cycle from the environment and convey this information through the production and secretion of melatonin.[434]

Melatonin production is not exclusive to the pineal gland, however. There is evidence that melatonin can be synthesised in other sites of the body, including (but not exclusive to) the skin, gastrointestinal tract, retina, bone marrow, placenta, and immune system.[435] But except for the pineal gland, other structures contribute little to blood circulating concentrations in mammals, since after the pineal gland is surgically removed, melatonin levels in the blood become mostly undetectable.[436]

However, removing the pineal gland does not reduce tissue levels of melatonin, suggesting that there are two separate pools of melatonin in the body.[436] One is made in the pineal gland; the other is present in virtually every body tissue. And in fact, the total amount of melatonin found in other areas of the body is far greater (10–400 times) than that derived from the pineal gland.[437]

With regards to our sleep-wake cycle, melatonin secretion reaches a maximum peak between 2:00 and 4:00 a.m. and then gradually decreases with exposure to early morning bright light. Excessive brightness just before bedtime, being subjected to stressful situations or shift work, and undergoing jet lag can disrupt melatonin production. In one study, two hours of continuous use of a tablet or smartphone in the evening reduced melatonin production by 22% in 20-year-old subjects, resulting in poorer sleep length and quality.[438]

Melatonin disruption in a light-filled world is increasingly being recognised as a great problem in our modern world, so much so that nighttime shift work is now considered a potential carcinogen as a result of decreased melatonin levels caused by light exposure at night.[439]

Other than being a result of sleep disruption, altered melatonin secretion has been associated with significant reduction in sleep efficiency and continuity typical of the elderly.[440] Some studies even suggest that ageing is actually a syndrome resulting from melatonin deficiency.[441]

Melatonin is currently only prescribed as a medication or used as a supplement to treat insomnia and/or jet lag.[442] But due to its potent antioxidant abilities (thought twice as active as vitamin E);[429] other greatly beneficial physiological actions; good safety profile and ability to freely cross the cell, nuclear membranes and the BBB;[437] it's looking promising at being able to help with a vast range of diseases.

Melatonin is not only great at mopping up ROS, but these reactions also lead to the formation of other metabolites, which in turn exhibit further antioxidant function with a consequently amplified effect.[443] The activation of melatonin receptors MT1 and MT2 also stimulates the activity of other antioxidant enzymes, and melatonin helps protect these enzymes from oxidative damage too.

Melatonin exerts anti-inflammatory action through inhibiting the proinflammatory protein complex NF-κB, as well as being able to blunt inflammation by lowering the levels of various other inflammatory mediators.[444] A recent meta-analysis concluded that melatonin supplementation could be effective in reducing inflammatory biomarkers, particularly the pro-inflammatory cytokines TNF-α and IL-6.[445]

Melatonin is an ingenious hormone that is able to modulate cell death by differentiating its action on the basis of cell type. Melatonin acts as an antioxidant on normal cells by enhancing DNA repair enzymes, thus slowing down cell death and toxicity induced by radio and chemotherapy;[446] however, on most cancer cells it exerts a pro-oxidant action stimulating ROS production with consequent DNA damage and cell death of cancer cells.[447]

Melatonin's anti-cancer properties have been demonstrated in a variety of different cancer types.[429] Another way melatonin acts as an anti-cancer agent is by modulating the release of exosomes derived from tumour cells, which are responsible for tumour progression;[448] altering the immune system positively;[449] and influencing the production of oestrogens, which has shown benefit in oestrogen receptor (ER)-positive breast cancer.[450]

With regards to the heart, rat studies have shown that melatonin is able to protect the heart via fixing mitochondrial damage, reducing heart-damaging proinflammatory proteins, reducing cardiac scarring, blood pressure, platelet aggregation, and circulating catecholamines, reducing the number and area of atheromatous plaques, reducing the occurrence of abnormal heart rhythms, and reducing heart tissue damage after a heart attack.[451-456]

Melatonin is able to freely cross the BBB and exert various neuroprotective roles. Melatonin has shown to protect animal models against stroke;[457] counteract nerve cell damage;[458] inhibit amyloid-β synthesis and fibril formation;[459] inhibit the production of other proteins involved with cognitive decline;[460] alleviates nerve damage in prion disease and improves the cognitive function in mice with Alzheimer's disease through the reduction of mitochondrial damage.[460,461,462]

In one study of those with mild cognitive impairment, the dietary supplementation of melatonin (0.15 mg/kg for 6 months) increased various areas of the brain as well as reduced concentrations of pathogenic proteins compared with a placebo.[463]

Another study, this time of patients with Parkinson's disease, showed that melatonin supplementation (10 mg/day for 12 weeks) significantly improved markers of conditions and mental function, as well as ameliorating inflammatory and oxidative features together with insulin resistance.[464]

As a hormone, melatonin regulates various other hormones involved with puberty and reproduction.[465] It also regulates embryonic implantation and has been shown to block the production of oestradiol.[466,467] Melatonin has positive effects on gynaecological disorders such as PCOS, premature ovarian failure, and ovarian inflammation. It is thought it does this by reducing follicular cell death due to its anti-apoptotic activity.[468]

In women with PCOS, melatonin treatment has been shown to restore menstrual cyclicity,[469] improve markers of inflammation, and help normalise hormone levels.[470] PCOS is also associated with high levels of insulin, and interestingly, melatonin has shown beneficial effects on insulin levels and insulin resistance, as well as cholesterol levels and improvements in mental health parameters in those with PCOS in another study.[471]

Melatonin has been shown to improve egg development, egg quality, and consequently the fertility and probability of pregnancy.[472,429] Notably, the intake of melatonin along with myo-inositol (another supplement we will get to later on) has been shown to synergistically improve egg and embryo quality, clinical pregnancy, and implantation rates.[473]

Melatonin also regulates male fertility by modulating the endocrine function of Leydig cells (the primary source of testosterone or androgens in males) and Sertoli cells (one of the most important cells necessary for sperm production in males). Low concentrations of melatonin have been shown to induce a reduction in testicular size.[474]

Treatment with melatonin improves endothelial health, which in turn may help with erectile dysfunction.[475] In a study of rabbits, melatonin improved the motility, integrity of the membrane, and potency of sperm.[476] And the supplementation of melatonin either alone or in combination with myo-inositol has been shown to improve male semen quality.[477,478] The daily supplementation of 6mg of melatonin for 45 days of treatment in men enhanced both urinary and seminal total antioxidant capacity, and consequently reduced oxidative damage caused in sperm DNA.[479]

Melatonin also plays an important role in various immune disorders, such as infections, autoimmunity, and immune senescence; plus, emerging evidence is showing that the immune system is not only affected by melatonin but also able to produce the hormone too.[480]

Melatonin has shown the ability to influence the differentiation and trafficking of immune cells, to activate Th1 lymphocytes, to enhance NK activity, to modulate the gut microbiome, to act as an antiviral and antibacterial agent, and reduce the damage done by pathogens. [448,480,481]

Due to its potent antioxidant and anti-inflammatory effects, melatonin has frequently been proposed for use to overcome the cytokine storm in virus-related infections, including that caused by SARS-CoV-2.[482] Melatonin has been put forward as a potential treatment aid for COVID-19 and long COVID for a number of other reasons too, including:

- **Shifting cellular energy production by quelling HIF-1α.** When unwell with an infection, immune cells need higher energy demands more immediately and thus switch from getting energy from mitochondrial oxidative phosphorylation to cytosolic glycolysis. Glycolysis is an oxygen-independent and relatively inefficient way to generate energy compared to oxidative phosphorylation but found to be the dominant metabolic pathway in pro-inflammatory cells. One of many regulators that help this switch is hypoxia-inducible factor-1α (HIF-1α).[482] Increased mortality is observed in patients with elevated HIF-1α and is associated with severe cytokine release.[483] Melatonin is able to quell HIF-1α and switch cellular energy production back to the healthier mitochondrial oxidative phosphorylation.[484]
- **Increasing energy production.** Adenosine triphosphate (ATP) is the source of energy for use and storage at the cellular level, and melatonin is well recognised for its ability to protect and enhance ATP production in mitochondria.[485] ATP is capable of completely dissolving viral factories in cells but only if it outnumbers viral proteins by many folds. One study showed ATP was capable of completely dissolving viral condensates

formed by SARS-CoV-2 N protein, but only at ratios of 1:500 (N-protein:ATP).[486] Higher ATP may thus reduce viral replication, which may explain why severe COVID-19 in children is rare. Children have higher plasma levels of ATP that are negatively correlated with the frequency of regulatory T cells but positively correlated with the frequency of CD4+ T cells.[487] Melatonin may upregulate ATP production and thus help with viral protection.[488]

- **Changing the pathological shape of mitochondria.** Mitochondria infected by SARS-CoV-2 display swollen inner folds, this causes mitochondria to not work effectively preventing higher ATP production via oxidative phosphorylation in favour of glycolysis.[489,490] The mitochondria of white blood cells in those recovered from COVID-19 have also shown dysfunction even at 11 months post-infection.[491] Damaged mitochondria continue to produce more ROS. Melatonin and its metabolites are able to attenuate mitochondrial damage and are extremely effective at scavenging different types of ROS.[492,493]
- **Suppressing LINE1 derepression.** As discussed near the start of this book, one way in which external genetic material can be integrated into our DNA is via a molecule called long interspersed element-1 (LINE-1 or L1) retrotransposons. And so various mRNAs in humans could be reverse-transcribed and integrated into the genome via L1 retroelements, with negative health consequences. Though coronavirus RNAs are not supposed to reverse-transcribe and integrate into host DNA, recent research found that, via LINE1, SARS-CoV-2 and other human coronaviruses could insert into the host genome.[494] Repression is a mechanism often used to decrease or inhibit the expression of a gene, and in healthy states, LINE-1 is repressed. Removal of repression is called derepression, and LINE-1 derepression is linked to ageing, diabetes, cardiac abnormalities, mitochondrial dysfunction and cancer. Melatonin may inhibit LINE1 expression via antioxidant-dependent and independent mechanisms.[488,495,496,497]

The anti-viral, mitochondrial healing, and genetic stabilising properties of melatonin go beyond what this book covers. Research on melatonin's effect on COVID-19 patients is lacking, but what we do have looks promising. For example, in a recent case series of 10 patients with COVID-19 pneumonia, melatonin supplementation (36–72 mg per day given in four divided doses) was associated with a reduction in hospital stay, mortality, and mechanical ventilation.[498] Another study showed that the addition of melatonin may have helped to reduce thrombosis, sepsis, and mortality in COVID-19 patients.[499]

But its applications do not end there. Melatonin has shown to prevent conformational changes that can result in aggregation and/or conversion to pathological prions;[500] reduce blood coagulation activity;[501] can help with neurodegenerative disorders;[502] potentially prevent the heart damage done by the spike protein;[503] help with eye conditions like glaucoma and macular oedema;[504,505] potentially increase lifespan (up to 20 extra days in melatonin-fed flies);[506] help with over oxygen exposure (like in newborns given oxygen therapies);[507] possibly help with mitochondrial damage associated with electromagnetic fields (EMF) exposure and even inhibits snake venom and antivenom induced oxidative stress.[508,509]

Melatonin also works hand-in-hand with other antioxidants like fisetin and vitamin C.[510,511,512] It also helps stop other antioxidants, like vitamin C, from turning into pro-oxidants, as well as reducing the toxicity of noxious prescription drugs.[513]

A lot of the recent research around this area has been done by published independent researcher Doris Loh.[514] She has written extensively about melatonin as well as ascorbic acid and the positive relationship they both have together on our health.

Melatonin, put forward as the "Cornucopia of the 21st Century" by one set of researchers,[429] may be the most powerful tool we have against COVID-19, long COVID, and mRNA agent-related injuries.

The world, with its ever-increasing light pollution, hormone disruptors, EMF exposure, fluoride in tap water, viral illnesses, and proposed "treatments," takes us away from optimum mitochondrial health.[515,516] Thus, it is paramount that sleep is not disturbed and other factors are improved as much as possible to maximise melatonin production.

Dosage: Doses of melatonin to treat insomnia and jet lag range from 2 mg to 6 mg once a day. [517]

There is no official dosage information regarding the use of melatonin in other diseases. Doris Loh has infographics on her website with regards to the use of melatonin and COVID-19, but this does not constitute medical advice.[514]

There has been some speculation that exogenous melatonin supplementation may result in long-term suppression of endogenous production or pineal gland atrophy. One old study reported possible suppression of endogenous melatonin in two subjects after twelve weeks.[518]

A more recent systematic review found little to no evidence for adverse events associated with melatonin in this regard,[519] **and a 2018 study reported recovery to normal circadian melatonin rhythms within three days after discontinuation of exogenous melatonin supplementation in two subjects.**[520]

Melatonin for the treatment of insomnia in the UK can only be prescribed for use in adults 55 years of age and older for up to 13 weeks.

METHYLENE BLUE

Some possible benefits include: antioxidation, neuroprotection, memory enhancement, anti-prion, anti-amyloid, anti-viral, mitochondrial healing, and anti-ageing.

Methylene blue (MB) has a colourful history, having been the first synthetic drug used in medicine as well as being used as a dye in the textile industry.[521] In medicine, it was used to treat malaria more than one century ago, as well as being one of the first drugs used to treat patients with psychosis at the end of the 19th century.

Its discovery led to the development of other antimalarials and antipsychotics.[521] It is now used primarily to treat certain haematological conditions, and since the 1980s, interest in it being able to treat bipolar disorder and neurodegenerative disorders has been the primary focus of research.

MB is currently FDA-approved to treat methemoglobinemia, a condition when one type of iron (Fe2+) in haemoglobin gets oxidised to another (Fe3+), reducing the oxygen-carrying capacity of haemoglobin.[522] Patients with methemoglobinemia typically present with blue discoloration of the lips and fingertips and have reduced oxygen levels; the use of MB reverses this.

Other non-FDA approved indications of MD include treating vasoplegic syndrome, a condition of sudden low pressure that occurs during procedures done on the small vessels of the heart;[523] to map out lymph nodes and to note if any have signs of cancer during operations where they are removed;[524] to treat certain chemotherapy-related brain toxicity by preventing neurotoxic metabolites that cause the brain toxicity;[525] and as the treatment of drug-resistant malaria.[523]

Other than in medicine, it is now more commonly found in aquariums to clean fish tanks, in lab settings as a staining agent in histology, or on the tongues of so-called "bio-hackers" who use it as a nootropic.

It is used as a nootropic because MB has a selective affinity for the nervous system, increasing brain activity and mitochondrial energy efficiency.[526] This drug has also been shown to inhibit the activity of various enzymes like monoamine oxidase, nitric oxide synthase, and guanylyl cyclase and thus increase certain circulating neurotransmitters like serotonin and norepinephrine.

Furthermore, MB has shown to reduce pathological protein build-up within the brain, like tau protein, which is linked to dementia;[526] as well as reducing amyloid-β levels and prion-related protein aggregation.[527] For these reasons and more, there has been significant interest in the repurposing of MB for brain-related conditions.

At low doses (0.5 to 4 mg/kg in most studies), MB concentrates in tissues with the most mitochondria (e.g., the brain, where it readily crosses the BBB, the heart, the liver, and the kidneys).[528]

In the mitochondria, MB acts like oxygen, helping to increase the production of ATP, but MB also bypasses certain mitochondrial reactions and thus reduces the production of ROS.[529,530] MB has the unique ability to quickly both accept and hand out electrons, which in turn means that MB also acts as a catalytic redox cycler in mitochondria, promoting cytochrome oxidase activity (a bit like IR light) and ATP production, as well as acting as a powerful antioxidant.[531,532] MB also stimulates glucose metabolism in conditions without oxygen and increases the amount of NAD+ produced by mitochondria.[528]

NAD+ (nicotinamide adenine dinucleotide) is a crucial coenzyme found in every cell in our body. It is involved in hundreds of metabolic processes, like cellular energy and mitochondrial health. NAD+ is also needed for sirtuins to work. Sirtuins are a family of proteins that regulate cellular health, promote DNA repair, and promote longevity. Thus, MB may potentially aid in anti-aging; in fact, MB has shown the ability to delay skin ageing as well as protect skin from UV exposure, and accelerate and help with the wound healing process.[531]

Improved mitochondrial efficiency, increased ATP production, reduced ROS production, reducing pathogenic protein aggregation, changes in levels of certain neurotransmitters, and its ability to aid in stopping nerve cell death have been reflected in real-life research.[533]

Several studies on rats with low blood flow to the brain showed MB had the ability to prevent neurodegeneration and memory impairment.[534,535] Other animal studies have shown that low-dose MB reduces neurobehavioral impairment in animal models of optic neuropathy, Parkinson's disease, and Alzheimer's disease and reduces functional deficit and MRI lesion volume in rodent models of ischemic stroke.[532,536,537,538]

In humans, MB has shown the ability to improve memory and fear extinction.[539] Another study showed that a single oral dose of 4 mg/kg of MB increased resting-state functional connectivity in multiple regions of the brain, linking perception and memory functions.[540] Long-term use of MB in bipolar disorder has also shown to lead to better stabilisation and a reduction in residual symptoms of the illness.[541]

Interestingly, both MB and low-level near-IR light share various similarities. Firstly, both interventions increase the expression of brain cytochrome oxidase *in vivo* and thus enhance mitochondrial respiration.[542] Both are also highly bioavailable, and both produce non-beneficial effects at high doses. It has been noted that anything above the dose of 10 mg/kg of MB can cause negative effects.[543]

MB, other than the benefits mentioned above, also has anti-pathogenic and specifically anti-viral properties.[544] One study showed MB has potent antiviral activity against SARS-CoV-2 and H1N1 influenza viruses *in vitro*.[544] And another study of 80 hospitalised people showed that the addition of MB to the treatment protocols of those with COVID-19 significantly improved oxygen levels and respiratory distress in patients.[545]

MB is also a photosensitizer, being able to absorb light in the 550–700 nm region, and thus the combination of photodynamic therapy has also been researched and has shown anti-wart, anti-viral, and anti-cancer activities.[546,547,578] There is an ongoing trial to assess whether the combination of both would help people with COVID-19 too.[579]

Vitamin C is also another treatment option for methemoglobinemia, suggesting similarities between it and MB. A combination of MB, vitamin C, and N-acetyl cysteine (NAC) has shown some promise against COVID-19.[550,551]

It is also important to note that MB has shown protective activities, such as against heavy metal toxicity.[552]

Dosage: MB is only FDA-approved to treat methemoglobinemia. Low dosages (0.5 to 4 mg/kg) have been shown to be safe and effective in studies. The most common side effect is blue or green urine.

It is not advised to take MB if you are already on certain antidepressants, as the combination of the two increases one's risk of a life-threatening condition called serotonin syndrome.

MYO-INOSITOL AND OTHER INOSITOLS

Some possible benefits include: anti-inflammation, insulin-sensitisation, pro-fertility, anti-autoimmune, and pro-thyroid health.

Inositols are types of sugar alcohols that make up a component of the outer membrane of cells and thus help control what goes in and out of them.[553] They also act as second messengers involved in the binding of extracellular signalling molecules to receptors located on the cell surface or inside the cell that trigger events inside the cell.[554] Inositols also participate in gene expression and facilitate mRNA export from the nucleus.[555,556]

There are various forms of inositols, of which *myo*-inositol (MI) is the most common and found in a variety of food products,[557] with the greatest amounts of myo-inositol being present in fruits, beans, grains, and nuts.[558]

Other than in food, MI is also produced in the human body from glucose and is present in all living cells as other forms such as phosphatidylinositol, D-chiro-inositol (DCI) and phytic acid (also known as Inositol hexaphosphate or IP6).[559] Our gut microbiome, with its bacterial phytases and phosphatases, is primarily responsible for digesting dietary IP6 in the body and for releasing myo-inositol and phosphate.[560]

Though not classed as an essential nutrient because it is formed from glucose, it is very likely that a great majority of us are living with inositol deficiency and imbalance. Firstly, caffeine (particularly coffee) increases the need for MI.[561] MI also concentrates in tissues such as kidneys, brain, and blood cells, which are typically no longer consumed by us. MI requirements rise with age, usage of antibiotics, consumption of sugar and refined carbohydrates, salt deficiency, insulin resistance, and both type I and type II diabetes.[562] Plus, the biosynthesis of myo-inositol requires NAD+ and magnesium. Thus, a deficiency in either may lead to a deficiency in MI.[563]

Altered ratios of certain inositols have been linked to certain disease states. For example, high foetal inositol concentrations in the fluid that surrounds the brain has been attributed to the pathogenesis of Down's syndrome;[563] and high MI levels has also been observed in diseases like Alzheimer's disease, diabetes mellitus, systemic lupus erythematosus and multiple sclerosis.[564]

Low MI levels have been seen in chronic liver disease, stroke, certain thyroid diseases, lymphoma, and various other diseases.[564] The presence of free-floating MI in the blood seems to deter the formation of fatty liver, and so it makes sense why MI deficiency causes the accumulation of fat in and around the liver.[565]

MI is also important for insulin signalling as it makes up many secondary messengers in response to insulin.[566] Elevated blood sugar levels (via insulin) decrease the absorption and biosynthesis of MI and increase its degradation and excretion via urine. MI levels are higher in tissues that use large amounts of glucose, such as the brain, heart, and ovaries. DCI is higher in tissues requiring glucose storage, such as the liver and muscles. Insulin resistance impairs this balance and the conversion of MI to DCI in muscles, fat, and liver.[560] All in all, this translates to individuals with type 2 diabetes having a decreased urinary excretion of chiro-inositol and a 10-fold higher urinary excretion of MI compared with healthy people.[567]

MI supplementation, especially in those with diabetes, has been shown to improve insulin sensitivity and is speculated to improve diabetes-related diseases such as eye and nerve damage.[568,569] One study on diabetics used a supplement containing MI and DCI at a ratio of 40:1 (550 mg of MI and 13.8 mg of DCI twice a day for three months), stating that it was the physiological ratio found in the blood. The combination of both in this study led to better overall blood sugar levels.[570]

The benefits of supplementing with inositol are not restricted to diabetes. Animal studies have shown that the administration of MI and IP6 independently has anti-cancer effects, and a combination of IP6 and MI has been shown to be significantly better at fighting certain cancers than either of the two acting alone.[571,572] MI administration has been shown to remove fat accumulation from the heart and improve heart muscle stiffness, whereas IP6 has shown the ability to reduce the calcification of coronary arteries.[564,573] Plus, inositol may be beneficial for depressed patients (especially those related to premenstrual changes) and as a mood stabiliser.[574,575]

A lot of recent research on inositol has been carried out in women with PCOS, a condition where the ovaries are inflicted with multiple cysts and symptoms including irregular menstrual periods, excess hair growth, and fertility issues. Insulin resistance is a frequent finding in patients with PCOS, but the underlying issue may be a deficiency in MI or an impairment in the function or expression of the enzyme that converts myo-inositol to DCI, which can in turn lead to insulin resistance, causing the ovaries to produce more androgens.[560]

Supplementing MI and/or DCI in women with PCOS has shown to improve insulin resistance, helped normalised menstrual periods, improve egg maturation, pregnancy rates, delivery rates and fertility hormone profiles.[577-580] Clinical evidence has demonstrated that the 40:1 ratio between MI and DCI is the optimal combination to restore ovulation in PCOS women.[581]

Regardless of whether someone has PCOS or not, an inositol imbalance has been postulated to lead to reduced fertility or pregnancy complications;[582] thus, its administration may be useful in the prevention and treatment of several pregnancy-related pathologies.[583]

Dietary supplementation of inositol in men with fertility issues is looking promising too. In one study of men with reduced sperm motility and metabolic syndrome, the use of a supplement containing MI and other antioxidants resulted in increased testosterone levels and improved semen characteristics.[584] In another study, MI improved sperm motility and improved pregnancy rates.[585]

With regards to immunity, mice with deletions of genes encoding members of the inositol phospholipid signalling pathway cascade showed defects in NK cell expression and function.[586] Disruption of inositol pathways in other animal studies lead to autoimmunity.[587] MI seems to be vital for the proper running of the thyroid gland, and in one study, people with autoimmune thyroid disease were given MI and selenium (600 mg MI plus 83 mcg selenium in the form of L-selenomethionine for 6 months), resulting in lower auto-immune thyroid antibodies, enhanced thyroid hormones, and better personal wellbeing.[588]

There has been no research so far studying the use of inositol and COVID-19 outcomes specifically, but one scientific review did hypothesise that inositol and vitamin D may naturally protect human reproduction and women undergoing assisted reproduction from COVID-19 risk.[589]

Dosage: For the treatment of PCOS, MI is taken in the range of 200–4,000 mg once daily before breakfast; higher doses seem to be used more often and to be more effective.[590]

Antidepressant effects of MI have been noted when supplementing it at doses as low as 6 g, with the standard dose being between 14 and 18 g daily.

NAC

Some possible benefits include: anti-inflammation, anti-oxidation, anti-viral, immunomodulation, neuroprotection, pro-fertility, metal chelating, and preventing oxidative damage caused by nanoparticles.

N-acetylcysteine (NAC) was introduced in the 1960s as a drug to break down the mucus in those suffering from chronic respiratory diseases. It is also prescribed in hospital settings as an antidote for paracetamol overdoses (intravenously and at high doses).[591]

Acetylcysteine is a derivative of the natural amino acid cysteine, which is used to make glutathione, one of the most important agents of the antioxidant defence system. Glutathione is similar to glutathione peroxidase, but it does not contain selenium; instead, it is made up of the amino acids cysteine, glutamic acid, and glycine. At higher doses, NAC acts as an antioxidant by increasing the intracellular concentration of glutathione. Glutathione reduces proinflammatory cytokines such as IL-9 and TNF alpha as well as having vasodilating properties.[592,593]

The oral administration of NAC has been shown to significantly improve cell-mediated immunity and increase the reaction from immune cells to foreign substances in the elderly.[594] NAC treatment has also been shown to significantly decrease the frequency of influenza as well as the severity and duration of most symptoms.[595]

NF-κB is a protein complex responsible for copying parts of gene sequences, producing cytokines, and regulating the immune response to infection.[596,597] It is involved in cellular responses to stress stimuli, and the incorrect regulation of NF-κB has been linked to cancer, inflammatory and autoimmune diseases, septic shock, viral infection, and improper immune development.[598-603]

RNA viruses (e.g., coronaviruses) need an active NF-κB pathway within host cells to replicate.[604] The suppression of NF-κB significantly reduced the replication rate of these viruses, and therefore, drugs that inhibit NF-κB activation could potentially reduce viral replication. Curcumin, ketones, and melatonin are all able to inhibit NF-κB, and NAC can do this too.

NAC has been demonstrated to inhibit NF-κB, as well as the replication of human influenza virus, human immunodeficiency virus (HIV), and respiratory syncytial virus (RSV).[605,606] In SARS-Cov-2, the main protease (Mpro) is required for viral replication. NAC has been theorised to be able to bind to an active site of Mpro, which could potentially inhibit its protease activity and then inhibit viral replication.[607] Thus, NAC could have served as a first-line drug specifically for SARS-Cov-2 due to its structural characteristics, but further studies are needed to confirm this.

Other than reducing viral replication, NAC has other useful properties, such as reducing the production of proinflammatory cytokines and effectively reducing ROS production without compromising the phagocytosis of viruses in neutrophils.[608,609] The administration of high dose NAC has been shown to increase the antioxidant properties of T cells as well as block virally-induced T cell death.[610] NAC has also been demonstrated to reduce the occurrence of pneumonia in those ventilated,[611] and *in vitro* studies have shown NAC to block ACE.[612] There are a handful of case studies demonstrating the usefulness of NAC in patients with COVID-19 in combination with other therapeutic agents.[594]

Due to its potent anti-inflammatory and anti-oxidative properties, NAC has been shown, as well as postulated, to be useful in treating various medical conditions, including PCOS, sleep apnea, Alzheimer's disease, Parkinson's disease, multiple sclerosis, peripheral neuropathy, stroke outcomes, diabetic neuropathy, Crohn's disease, and ulcerative colitis.[613,614]

NAC has also shown to improve the mental health symptoms of various serious psychiatric conditions including schizophrenia, obsessive compulsive disorder, bipolar affective disorder and addictive behaviour (even decreasing marijuana and nicotine use and cravings.)[615-621]

NAC has shown some effectiveness with regards to male fertility too. In one randomised controlled trial, NAC of dose 600 mg twice a day showed to improve oxidative status along with semen quality (improved motility, viscosity, and volume).[622] In another study, NAC along with selenium significantly improved semen quality.[623]

Another beneficial characteristic of NAC is its ability to chelate heavy metals and thus reduce related toxicity,[624,625] as well as its ability to reverse and prevent the oxidative damage caused by engineered metal nanoparticles.[626]

Dosage: NAC is most commonly taken orally in doses of 600–1200 mg daily.[627]

Long-term use of NAC *may* increase one's likelihood of having pulmonary arterial hypertension, a serious condition characterised by high blood pressure in the arteries that carry blood to the lungs.[628] **NAC also carries a theoretical risk of mineral depletion.**

NATTOKINASE

Some possible benefits include: anti-clotting, fibrin-dissolving, blood-pressure lowering, anti-atherosclerotic, cholesterol-improving, antiplatelet, and neuroprotection.

Natto is a food that has been consumed in Asian countries for more than 2000 years. It is made of soybeans fermented with *Bacillus subtilis* and is particularly popular in Japan. Natto consumption is believed to be one significant contributor to the longevity and reduced cardiovascular disease of the Japanese people.[629]

Fibrinolytics are agents able to dissolve fibrin, a fibrous protein involved in the clotting of blood. And thus, they are used to disintegrate blood clots clogging up arteries or veins, helping to improve blood flow and prevent damage to affected organs. In 1987, it was found that natto contained a potent fibrinolytic enzyme called nattokinase.[630] Since then, research has confirmed that nattokinase has both fibrinolytic *and* clot-preventing (antithrombotic) activities.[631,632]

Plasmin is a naturally occurring fibrinolytic enzyme that we all possess, and nattokinase has been found to be four times more potent than that.[633] Tissue plasminogen activator (tPA) is another naturally-occurring enzyme found on endothelial cells involved in the breakdown of blood clots, and it is now known that nattokinase not only degrades fibrin directly but also increases the release of tPA with a subsequent increase in the formation of plasmin.[633] Nattokinase also enhances the production of other clot-dissolving agents as well as inhibiting a molecule called thromboxane, which is normally involved in sticking platelets together.[634] Thus, nattokinase inhibits platelet aggregation, and it looks like it does this without the side effect of causing bleeding.[635]

Research has shown that nattokinase has other beneficial activities including blood-pressure lowering, anti-atherosclerotic, cholesterol-improving, antiplatelet and neuroprotective properties too.[635-639]

Although nattokinase has recently gained popularity as a candidate drug for cardiovascular disease, clinical investigations of NK in humans are relatively limited. The studies that *have* been carried out have been promising, though. For example, in one study of 24 participants with an acute stroke, the use of nattokinase showed a clear neuroprotective effect without causing clinical signs of bleeding.[640] And in another study, the daily use of nattokinase at 6000 fibrinolytic units (FU), or 300 mg/day, improved the cholesterol profiles of participants as well as reducing vessel narrowing and plaque size in the carotid artery.[637] This property of nattokinase was further shown in a 2022 study involving over 1,000 participants. Higher doses of 10800 FU/day were shown to be effective and safe, with regular exercise and the co-administration of vitamin K2 and aspirin working synergistically too.[641]

As nattokinase modulates our clotting systems, there is always a worry that it increases our risk of bleeding disorders. These worries may be unwarranted, however. There is a long history of the use of natto and purified nattokinase in the diet in Asian countries, especially Japan, and it has been shown that there is no concern for toxicity when adults take 1,000–14,000 FU daily.[642] Plus, no toxic side effects have been observed in rats using significantly higher doses of 22,000 FU/kg/day, equivalent to 1.43 million FU daily in humans.[642] And in human volunteers, no adverse effects were observed following 4 weeks of nattokinase consumption at a daily dose of 10 mg/kg for 28 days.[642]

An increased risk of bleeding events may occur if nattokinase is taken with aspirin or if the person is already prone to bleeding. There is one report of a patient who was concurrently using aspirin and nattokinase (400 mg daily) and experienced an acute brain bleed.[643] And not using enough nattokinase may increase one's risk of clots. In another report, one person developed a clot in a mechanical valve after nearly a year of nattokinase use without warfarin and underwent a successful repeat valve replacement.[644]

Evidence of nattokinase combating COVID-19 or its side effects is lacking. The one study that does exist shows nattokinase having the ability to degrade spike proteins in a lab setting.[645] But the use of nattokinase in COVID-19 may be beneficial.

Dense fibrin clots are observed in the lungs of patients with severe COVID-19.[646] Plus, the high incidence of venous thromboembolism, pulmonary embolism, deep vein thrombosis, and cardiovascular disease experienced by those with severe COVID-19 and/or gene-therapy-related side-effects points towards a clotting disorder in the disease. Clots generated in COVID-19 blood have been shown to exhibit higher density and are more resistant to breakdown compared with clots formed in severe influenza patients.[646] Plus, as we have already noted, long COVID is looking like a condition with an underlying pathophysiology of endothelial inflammation and micro-clot formation.

It is known that the SARS-CoV-2 spike protein causes substantial impairment of fibrinolysis as well as binding platelets and forming clots.[647,648] The use of nattokinase may theoretically aid with this in a multi step manner. More studies are needed.

Dosage: Clinical studies to guide safe and effective nattokinase dosing are lacking. Nattokinase 100 mg/day (equivalent to 2,000 FU) for 8 weeks have been used in some studies. But it has been shown that there is no concern for toxicity when adults take 1,000–14,000 FU daily. Plus, no toxic side effects have been observed in rats using significantly higher doses of 22,000 FU/kg/day, equivalent to 1.43 million FU daily in humans.[649]

An increased risk of bleeding events may occur if nattokinase is taken with aspirin or if the person is already prone to bleeding.

Some may opt to eat natto, not only for its specific flavour and aroma but also due to the fact it contains a range of essential nutrients and bioactive compounds other than just nattokinase. These include vitamin K2, soybean isoflavone, γ-polyglutamic acid and biogenic amines. Some of these may potentiate nattokinase's activities.[650]

NIACIN

Some possible benefits: anti-ageing, cardioprotective, DNA stabilising, improving mitochondrial function, and neuroprotection.

Niacin (also known as nicotinic acid) is a form of vitamin B3. It is usually obtained through the diet, with the highest contents found in fortified packaged foods, meat, poultry, and redfish such as tuna and salmon. Nicotinamide (also called niacinamide) is a "nicotinic acid amide" and is also a form of vitamin B3, derived from niacin.

Though structurally similar, they vary with regards to the effect they have on the body when supplemented. Niacin has been shown to decrease LDL (colloquially termed "bad cholesterol"), increase HDL ("good cholesterol"), and reduce triglycerides.[651] Niacin also has the added side effect of causing a "flush," where those who supplement experience redness of the skin, which may be accompanied by an itching or burning sensation. Though harmless, it can be uncomfortable and is thought to be due to its vasodilatory capabilities, which increase the flow of blood to the skin's surface.[652]

Nicotinamide, on the other hand, does not cause a flush and does not have cholesterol-lowering properties. Nicotinamide has been shown to improve acne when applied to the skin and have potential anti-skin cancer effects when supplemented.[653,654]

As noted earlier, NAD+ is involved in hundreds of metabolic processes, like cellular energy and mitochondrial health. NAD+ is also needed for sirtuins to work and regulate telomere length. As well as a declining telomere length, NAD+ levels also decline with age, and this decline is believed to be a tremendous risk for diseases and/or disabilities, like hearing and vision loss, cognitive dysfunction, autoimmunity, and dysregulation of the immune response.[655] The aim is then to maintain adequate NAD+ levels, which in turn increase sirtuin activity and stabilise telomeres. This reduces DNA damage and improves telomere-dependent diseases. And thus, to put it simply, an inadequate level of NAD+ is associated with ageing, so maintaining an adequate amount of it is vital.

Both niacin and nicotinamide help form NAD+, and supplementing with either or both has been shown to increase NAD+ supplies.[656] Administration of NAD+ is associated with an increase in sirtuin activity, stabilising telomeres, and beneficially impacting immune cell functions. And so niacin and nicotinamide may have anti-ageing or age-slowing effects.[655]

We all know that COVID-19 disproportionately affects the elderly (the average age of death due to COVID-19 is 80.4 years).[657] Ageing not only affects the efficiency of organs but also impairs immune function too. Our ability to protect ourselves against infectious diseases declines with age. But your birth certificate doesn't solely determine your age.[658] A 70-year-old may have the body and cellular function of a 50-year-old, and vice versa.

Your biological age depends on the lifestyle you lead, which in turn affects one's telomere length. I point this out because those with short leukocyte (white blood cell) telomere lengths were associated with a high risk of pneumonia and a significant risk of death related to infections.[659]

Shorter leukocyte telomere length is associated with increasing age, obesity, male gender, diabetes, alcoholism, atherosclerosis, and cardiovascular disease, and these are all linked with a higher risk of both suffering from symptomatic COVID-19 and subsequently dying from it too.[660] The biologically older you are, the more at risk you are of suffering and potentially dying from COVID-19.

NAD+ is also released during the early stages of inflammation, has immunomodulatory properties, and is known to decrease pro-inflammatory cytokines such as IL-6.[656] This may be useful, as recent evidence indicates that targeting IL-6 could help control the inflammatory storm in patients with COVID-19.[661] Niacin has also been shown to have anti-inflammatory properties in animal studies with sepsis, and nicotinamide has been shown to reduce viral replication.[662,663] The use of niacin and/or nicotinamide may then have a beneficial role with regards to COVID-19 treatment by acting as an immunomodulator, especially in those who are biologically older and thus at higher risk.[664] Niacin has shown to reduce lung tissue damage in animal models with chemo-induced lung injury.[664] And as researchers from a paper in Nature note, "It might be a wise approach to supply this food supplement to the COVID-19 patients."[665]

Other beneficial properties of niacin include its ability to help with DNA stabilisation, as a potential AIDS preventative factor, improving mitochondrial function, as a neuroprotective agent, preventing prion-related neuronal death, and even treating schizophrenia.[666-671]

Interestingly, it has been noted that those with schizophrenia are less likely to experience a skin flush from niacin than those who do not have the condition.[672] The skin flush response to niacin is caused by prostaglandins made from AA (arachidonic acid) molecules, and a blunted skin flush response to niacin in those with schizophrenia might be due to a reduced level of membrane AA.

A vitamin B3 deficiency, called pellagra, can cause many symptoms similar to what those with COVID-19 and long COVID suffer with, including diarrhoea, skin inflammation, loss of smell and taste, and mental confusion. SARS-CoV-2 is also known to induce NAD+ depletion. Other journals have highlighted the possible link between long COVID and NAD+ depletion.[673,674]

Though niacin supplementation seemingly may fix these issues, one 2022 review on this topic noted that may not be the case and may in fact worsen an acute infection. It goes on further to note, *"The robustness of the host's NAD+ salvage pathway, prior to the SARS-CoV-2 infection, is an important determinant of COVID-19 severity and persistence of certain symptoms upon resolution of infection."* In other words, our body's natural ability to produce NAD+ *before* we become infected may likely be more important in determining infection outcomes than acute administration of niacin and other NAD+ precursors whilst unwell.[675] One way to do this is via regular exercise and possible top-ups with niacin. More studies are needed.

Dosage: Most of the benefits from niacin supplementation have been reported to occur after doses of at least one gram. This is approximately 5,000% of the recommended daily intake.[678]

Using niacin alongside selective serotonin reuptake inhibitors and/or non-steroidal anti-inflammatory drugs can increase one's risk of bleeding events.[679]

The use of niacin alongside statin use can increase the risk of rhabdomyolysis (a pathological muscle breakdown that can be fatal or result in permanent disability).[679]

Long-term use may increase one's risk of developing diabetes, especially if one's risk of diabetes is elevated before use (e.g., raised BMI).[680]

NIGELLA SATIVA

Some possible benefits include: antioxidation, anti-inflammation, immunomodulation, anticancer, neuroprotection, antimicrobial, antihypertensive, cardioprotection, antidiabetic, organ-protective, metal and toxin chelating, pro-fertility, and anti-COVID-19.

Nigella sativa, also called black cumin or black seeds, is a plant famous for its culinary uses and medicinal properties. It is native to a vast region of the eastern Mediterranean, northern Africa, the Indian subcontinent, and Southwest Asia, and is cultivated in many countries, including Egypt, Iran, Greece, Syria, Albania, Turkey, Saudi Arabia, India, and Pakistan.[681]

N. sativa has been used in traditional medicine to treat a variety of ailments and conditions, including asthma, bronchitis, rheumatism, headache, back pain, anorexia, amenorrhea, paralysis, inflammation, mental debility, dermatitis, and hypertension, to mention a few.[682] Topical application is also used in various cultures to aid nasal abscesses, orchitis, swollen joints, and to treat skin conditions, such as blisters and eczema.[681]

Ancient herbalists considered *N. sativa* to be "The herb from heaven."[683] It is also known as "Prophetic medicine" in the Muslim community because the Prophet Mohammad (PBUH) once stated, "This black cumin is healing for all diseases except death."[684] The Holy Bible mentions black cumin for its curative properties and designates it as "melanthion" by Hippocrates and Dioscorides.[685] Avicenna (Ibn Sina), the same renowned physician of the 10th century who first described the medicinal properties of chaga, also highlighted several health-beneficial properties of black cumin, such as enhancement of the body's energy and recovery from tiredness and the feeling of hopelessness.[686]

N. sativa has even been found in the tomb of the Egyptian Pharaoh Tutankhamun. Ancient Egyptians are thought to have used black cumin as a preservative in the process of mummification, probably due to its antibacterial and insect repellent properties. [687,688]

The traditional use of *N. sativa* seeds is largely due to their wide range of medicinal properties, including antioxidant, anti-inflammatory, immunomodulatory, anticancer, neuroprotective, antimicrobial, antihypertensive, cardioprotective, antidiabetic, and organ-protective properties.[681] These properties are due to containing a variety of bioactive compounds such as thymoquinone (TQ), thymohydroquinone, thymol, carvacrol, nigellidine, nigellicine, and α-hederin. TQ, a terpene, is the most studied bioactive component of *N. sativa*.[689]

The health benefits of *N. sativa* cover almost every physiological system; this is largely due to its antioxidant properties. *N. sativa* has shown to lower ROS, whilst upregulating antioxidant enzymes like SOD in several studies.[690] In one meta-analysis of five studies using 293 human subjects, *N. sativa* supplementation was shown to have a beneficial role as an antioxidant by improving SOD levels and improving total antioxidant capacity.[691]

As well as having antioxidant capabilities, *N. sativa* (and especially *N. sativa* oil) has shown anti-inflammatory properties too.[692] In one study, *N. sativa* oil was shown to reduce IL-6 and IL-1β levels in inflamed fat cells.[692] Rats with inflammatory paw swelling given *N. sativa* oil showed significant improvement in the pro-inflammatory cytokines IL-6, IL-12 and TNF-α in another.[693] *N. sativa* has also been shown to inhibit proinflammatory NO in cell studies.[694]

With regards to the brain, *N. sativa* has shown neuroprotective properties against neuroinflammation and promising results against animal models with a wide range of neurodegenerative diseases.[681] *N. sativa* and TQ have shown to restore neuronal intracellular antioxidant levels; inhibit ROS generation and associated cell death; decrease brain amyloid-β fragment length; decrease amyloid-β formation and accumulation by downregulating the NF-κB pathway; improve memory; increase BDNF; attenuate convulsions as well as protecting against neurotoxicity induced by various chemicals, such as chlorpyrifos (an organophosphate pesticide); dichlorvos (an insecticide); acrylamide and arsenic.[695-703]

N. sativa and its constituents are well known for their anticancer properties. A growing body of research demonstrates that the chemical contents of black cumin seeds are chemopreventive and effective at suppressing unwanted cell growth and inducing cell death.[681] *N. sativa*'s anti-cancer properties have been demonstrated in various cell lines from human breast cancer to kidney cancer and more.[704,705] TQ has shown to also synergize anticancer activity of several standard chemotherapeutic drugs as well as natural chemopreventive molecules such as paclitaxel, 5-fluorouracil, resveratrol and piperine.[706-709]

N. sativa has also shown the ability to improve cholesterol and blood sugar levels in various human trials.[710,711] Following *N. sativa* oil treatment, one randomised clinical trial on patients with diabetic kidney disease showed a significant reduction in blood glucose, serum creatinine, blood urea, and 24 h total urinary protein levels and improved kidney function, 24 h total urinary volume, and haemoglobin levels.[712] And *N. sativa* oil supplementation was associated with a reduction in lipid profile, glycemia, C-reactive protein level, and lipid peroxidation in another double-blind randomised clinical trial on T2D patients.[713]

The cardiovascular system may also benefit from the use of *N. sativa,* both pre-treatment as protection and post-conditioning, improving cardiac function by reducing cardiac injury.[714,715] Plus, a clinical study on patients with mild-to-moderately raised blood pressure using black cumin virgin oil demonstrated positive outcomes on lipid profiles and blood pressure.[716]

Other than the heart, studies have shown *N. sativa* to have liver-protective, stomach-protective, and lung-protective properties.[681,717] In several preclinical investigations *N. Sativa* oil and TQ have shown to protect against lung damage induced by various chemicals such as lipopolysaccharide (LPS), bleomycin, cigarette smoke, or nicotine, and cadmium, via anti-inflammatory and antihistamine effects that attenuate inflammation, oxidative stress, and apoptosis that accompany chemical-induced lung injury or fibrosis.[718-721] *N. sativa* extract has also been shown to improve asthma symptoms, lung function, and asthma biomarkers in several human trials.[722]

With regards to fertility, *N. sativa* oil has been shown to significantly improve testicular sperm production, semen parameters, and seminal vesicle development in rats; as well as mediate certain toxin- (insecticide) related effects on reproduction.[723] With regards to humans, so far, just one clinical investigation has verified black cumin's impact on male reproductive health.[724] The study found that *N. sativa* oil (2.5 mL twice daily p.o. for 60 days) significantly increased sperm quality (e.g., volume and pH) and functional characteristics of spermatozoa (e.g., sperm concentration, motility, and morphology) in infertile Iranian males when compared to the placebo control group (liquid paraffin).[724]

When it comes to female reproductive health, *N. sativa* has been shown to improve menopausal symptoms and reduce postpartum pain in humans.[725,726] In animal models, the herb has been shown to improve ovarian function in rats with polycystic ovaries, as well as several reproductive hormones and overall reproductive performance in female rats in another study.[727,728]

N. sativa's therapeutic properties do not end there; research has also shown that this herb is capable of helping with wound healing, skin disorders, bone regeneration, kidney protection, chelating heavy metals, and even reducing venom-induced acute toxic shock.[729-734]

The use of *N. sativa* aids immune function, too. *N. sativa* has shown to increase macrophage population;[735] stimulate phagocytic activities of three types of macrophages;[736] enhance antibody production;[737] and stimulate certain subsets of white cells.[738] A 46-year-old HIV patient treated with a black cumin mixture recovered entirely and remained seronegative for six months.[739] In another case report, HIV infection in a 27-year-old woman was entirely sero-reverted after a year of black cumin and honey therapy (60:40, 10 mL thrice day), and three children born after the woman was HIV positive were uninfected.[740]

With regards to COVID-19, the use of *N. sativa* has been extremely promising. So far, of the 11 studies carried out, statistically significant improvements have been seen for mortality, hospitalisation, recovery, cases, and viral clearance with its use, with a pooled analysis improvement of 53%.[741] In one randomised-controlled trial of 358 hospitalised patients in Iran, 184 who received treatment with a combination of *N. sativa* and several other herbal medicines, showed shorter hospitalisation time and improved recovery with treatment.[742] An open-label study with 419 patients in Iraq, 160 of whom were treated with Nigella sativa, showed lower mortality and fewer severe cases with treatment. In this study black seeds were given 40 mg/kg orally once daily for 14 days.[743] And *N. sativa* may even be beneficial in reducing the risk of infection, as shown by another study of 376 mostly high-risk patients, of whom 188 were treated with *N. sativa*, showing significantly fewer cases with treatment.[744] Black seeds were again given 40 mg/kg orally once daily. And the use of honey and *N. sativa* in combination in another study showed improved symptoms, viral clearance, and mortality in COVID-19 patients.[745]

Dosage: There is no official dosage information for *N. sativa.* The most common dosage is 1–3 g per day, with studies ranging from using 40 mg/kg orally once daily to a dessert spoon amount of *N. sativa* oil applied to affected limbs three times a week.[746,747]

The FLCCC has recommended the use of 40 mg/kg daily of *N. sativa* if ivermectin is not available or added to ivermectin for optimal prevention.[748]

OLEUROPEIN AND OLIVE LEAF EXTRACT

Some possible benefits include: antioxidation, anti-inflammation, anti-atherogenic, cardioprotective, anti-cancer, antimicrobial, antiviral activities, immunomodulation, and antithrombotic.

The "Mediterranean diet" is a diet popularly known for its association with a reduced risk of most age-related diseases, including metabolic syndrome and neurodegenerative disorders.[749] It is composed of various plant-based foods, fish, goat milk, sunshine, and olive oil. The last on that list, olive oil, not only tastes objectively wonderful, but has gained increasing scientific attention in recent years due to containing the health-promoting compound, oleuropein.

Oleuropein is a bitter polyphenolic compound enriched in olive oil and the leaves of the olive tree. It is found most often in the early stages of olive fruit growth and declines as the fruit matures. Black olives have higher levels of anthocyanins but lower levels of oleuropein than green olives.[750] But shop-bought olives of both varieties have likely had most of the harsh-tasting oleuropein leached out through the process of curing.[751] If you can, go fresh, one study noted that 10 g of freshly olive stoning includes approximately 20 mg oleuropein.[752]

Oleuropein is best known for its blood pressure-lowering and high blood pressure-preventing effects, which are now thought to be due to improving mitochondrial function and reducing oxidative stress in certain parts of the brain.[753]

Beyond high blood pressure, *in vivo* and *in vitro* studies have shown that oleuropein has several pharmacological properties, including antioxidant, anti-inflammatory, anti-atherogenic, anti-cancer, anti-microbial, and antiviral activities.[754-760]

Of interest, oleuropein has been shown to reduce oxidative damage to the region of the brain that is most affected by neurodegeneration in Parkinson's disease, as well as prevent the toxic aggregation of both amyloid beta and tau proteins that are involved in Alzheimer's disease.[761-763]

Oleuropein has also shown anti-cancer abilities, especially with regards to breast cancer. Oleuropein is a potent inhibitor of human epidermal growth factor receptor 2, a protein that is frequently overexpressed in breast cancer cells.[764] Other lab studies have shown oleuropein having the ability to decrease breast cancer cell viability and triggering high levels of cell death in breast cancer too.[765,766]

With regards to COVID-19, one molecular dynamic simulation study showed the potential of oleuropein at alleviating COVID-19 neurological complications. Oleuropein has also been shown to be able to target the surface glycoprotein HIV-1 gp41, which blocks HIV entry and replication.[767,768]

The most common form of oleuropein in supplement form is olive leaf extract. Other than oleuropein, olive leaf extract contains other medically beneficial metabolites like hydroxytyrosol, verbascoside, apigenin-7-O-glucoside, and luteolin-7-O-glucoside, too.[769]

Olive leaf extract, as well as demonstrating similar effects to oleuropein alone, has shown antiatherogenic (via improving cholesterol quality), immunomodulatory, and antithrombotic activities.[770] In one *in vivo* study using the mucosal explant cultures of Crohn's disease patients and healthy volunteers, the ethanolic extract of olive leaves (0.1–100 mcg/ml) reduced the expression of pro-inflammatory mediators such as IL-1β, IL-6, IL-8, TNF-α, and iNOS and improved the integrity of the epithelial barrier.[771]

Hydroxytyrosol and hydroxytyrosol acetate are two compounds found in olive leaf extract. Oral administration of both of these compounds for seven days in rats inhibited platelet aggregation with similar effectiveness as aspirin.[772] And maslinic acid, another compound found in olive leaf extract, was reported to regulate platelet aggregation and exhibit antithrombotic activity by various mechanisms.[773]

Dosage: Though there are no official dosing recommendations, supplemental olive leaf is taken in the 500–1000 mg range daily.[774]

OROXYLIN A

Some possible benefits include: antioxidant, anti-inflammation, anti-bacterial, anti-viral, anti-cancer, neuroprotective, hepatoprotective, eye-protective, immunomodulatory, memory-boosting, and potentially anti-COVID-19.

Oroxylin A is a flavone found mainly in the plants *Oroxylum indicum* (Indian Trumpet tree), *Scutellaria baicalensis* (Chinese skullcap), *S. lateriflora* (blue skullcap), *Anchietea pyrifolia, and Aster himalaicus* (Himalayan Aster).[775]

O. indicum has been used in various ancient Ayurvedic preparations for the treatment of various disorders including arthritic and rheumatic problems, diabetes, diarrhoea, dysentery, gastric ulcers, jaundice, respiratory diseases, tumours, anorexia, asthma, bronchitis, cough, dysentery, dyspepsia, fever, gout, leucoderma, neuralgia, rheumatoid arthritis, vomiting, and wounds.[776]

S. baicalensis and *S. lateriflora* are and have been widely used in traditional Chinese medicine for treating an array of diseases, including diarrhoea, dysentery, hepatitis, high blood pressure, and vomiting.[777]

Though these plants contain an array of bioactive compounds, oroxylin A found in these plants is thought to be the major flavonoid with potential alleviatory effects against several life-threatening chronic diseases.[778]

Modern science is seemingly catching up to ancient wisdom with studies revealing that oroxylin A has a variety of possible health benefits, including anti-bacterial, anti-viral, anti-oxidant, anti-inflammatory, anti-cancer, neuroprotective, hepatoprotective, and pro-apoptotic properties.[779-784]

As well as having direct antioxidant properties, oroxylin A has shown to downregulate the NF-κB pathway, and other pro-inflammatory pathways that have been implicated in the growth of cancers; as well as being able to inhibit the expression of several pro-inflammatory cytokines, such as TNF-α and other inflammatory cytokines.[775,779,785]

The majority of the studies performed on oroxylin A have shown anti-cancer properties *in vivo* and *in vitro* on various cancer types, including breast, cervical, colon, blood, gliomas, liver, lung, and skin cancers.[786-793]

Other than the benefits already mentioned, oroxylin A has also shown potential in treating various eye disorders, allergic illnesses and as a neuroprotective agent. In one study of rats with anterior ischemic optic neuropathy, a disease causes irreversible vision loss through damage of the optic nerve caused by a blockage of its blood supply, oroxylin A was shown to be protective on eye cells from injury, by reducing optic disc swelling, the apoptotic death of retinal ganglion cells, and the infiltration of inflammatory cells.[794]

In another study of mice with asthma, oroxylin A was shown to attenuated pro-inflammatory lung histopathologic changes, airway hyperresponsiveness, the number of inflammatory cells, as well as inhibited the levels of IL-4, IL-5, IL-13 and allergy related IgE.[795]

Oroxylin A has also been shown to enhance the cognition of unimpaired mice as well as improve the memory of impaired mice. Oroxylin A administered on memory centres of mice brain showed nerve growth potential. Plus, oroxylin A has been shown to increase the production of BDNF.[796]

With regards to COVID-19, one lab study noted that oroxylin A could be a "potential candidate in the treatment for COVID-19 by virtue of its blocking the entrance of SARS-CoV-2 into ACE2 cells by specifically binding to the ACE2 receptor."[797]

Dosage: Dose standardisation for different diseases and safe and toxic doses of oroxylin A for humans are currently unknown due to a lack of clinical studies.

One website notes, "*Sabroxy, which is a standardized extract prepared from the Indian trumpet tree (Oroxylum indicum), containing a minimum of 10% Oroxylin A, is typically taken at a dose of 100mg.*"[798]

Using rat and mouse studies, as there is a lack of human evidence to support the optimal dosage of *S. baicalensis* for supplementation purposes, doses of "*of around 500mg of the root extract should be efficacious*", notes another.[799]

PINE NEEDLE TEA

Some possible benefits of suramin and shikimic acid include: anti-inflammation, anti-bacterial, anti-viral, anti-cancer, cardioprotection, and potentially anti-COVID-19 and anti-spike protein.

Pine-needle tea is an herbal tea made from pine needles, or the leaves of pine trees. It gained popular attention throughout social and mainstream media during the pandemic as it was claimed that "*White pine tea contained suramin and shikimic acid, which could prevent COVID-19 vaccinated people from "shedding" the spike protein.*"[800]

One news outlet batted away this claim, noting, *"But white pine tea doesn't prevent vaccine shedding among people who have received the COVID-19 shot because vaccine shedding caused by that injection isn't an actual phenomenon, experts say. And while some research has found suramin might be potentially helpful against COVID-19 infection, it doesn't come from pine needles, and both it and shikimic acid may actually be more harmful than beneficial."*[800]

As I have noted earlier in this book, spike proteins have been found to be released from cells via the creation of exosomes for up to four months.[801] Combine this with the fact that exosomes can be exhaled out, then theoretically adding two together would mean that there is a likelihood that shedding in those who are jabbed could occur.[802]

Prolonged viral shedding is known to occur in patients with mild to moderate COVID-19 disease, and if you combine this with the fact that those who have taken the shot are more likely to contract COVID-19, then one could argue that over a long enough time, those who have taken the shot *will* in fact shed.[803] Plus, one recent study showed aerosol transfer of antibodies between immune and non-immune hosts was possible.[804] Thus, the first statement by the news outlet may be false.

Their second statement might not be so false, however. I could not find evidence stated in scientific journals confirming that suramin came from pine needles. Surmain is in fact one of the first anti-infective agents that had been developed in a modern medicine, synthesised in 1916 with the help of Bayer from the dye trypan blue.[805] There are websites online stating that suramin can be naturally sourced from pine needles, but these claims don't seem to be backed by scientific evidence or references.[806]

Since its discovery, suramin has been used as an antiparasitic to primarily treat African sleeping sickness caused by the single-celled parasite *Trypanosomiasis*. Other than this, suramin was used to treat river blindness, caused by the parasite *Onchocerca volvulus*, but it was subsequently replaced by the less toxic and more bioavailable ivermectin.[807,808]

Suramin has been shown to help against other parasitic infections too, but it is not used for Chagas' disease as studies in mice have even suggested that suramin would exacerbate the disease.[809] Suramin has also been studied as an anti-cancer agent with mixed results;[805] initial clinical tests did not warrant the further development of suramin as an anti-cancer monotherapy, but suramin does seem to potentiate other chemotherapeutics and has shown some success in this regard.[810]

Suramin has also shown the ability to block a variety of inflammatory proteins, like phospholipase A2, as well as gene sequences from snake and bee venom, suggesting that it can act as an antidote.[811,812,813] The venom from some snakes also contains toxins that mimic thrombin, a protein involved in clotting that has the role of converting fibrinogen into insoluble strands of fibrin.[814] Suramin not only inhibits thrombin itself, but also the thrombin-like proteases of snake venom, and was therefore proposed as an antidote for snakebite.[815,816]

Other than venom, due to its large molecular size and unique shape, suramin has been shown to bind to and thereby inhibit various proteins. For example, suramin has been shown to decrease the activities of a large number of enzymes involved in DNA and RNA synthesis and modification, as well as enzymes involved in the winding and unwinding of DNA.[805,817]

With regards to COVID-19, suramin was shown to be a potent inhibitor of SARS-CoV-2 RNA-dependent RNA polymerase, an enzyme that helps with viral replication.[818] More specifically, suramin was shown to act by blocking the binding of RNA to the enzyme, an activity shown in biochemical assays to be at least 20-fold more potent than remdesivir, the currently approved nucleotide drug for treatment of COVID-19.[818]

Its anti-COVID-19 potential was further demonstrated in another study that showed suramin having the ability to inhibit SARS-CoV-2 replication and decrease viral load in cell culture, as well as demonstrating potent antiviral efficacy against SARS-CoV-2 in a primary human epithelial airway cell infection model.[819] This should not come as a surprise, as suramin's antiviral activities have been known since the mid-20th century.[820]

Though useful, suramin is not totally safe. There are many side effects of using suramin including nephrotoxicity, hypersensitivity reactions, dermatitis, anaemia, peripheral neuropathy, and bone marrow toxicity. But the dose makes the poison.[805] Concerns about the toxicity of high-dose suramin arose when the cumulative antiparasitic dose was increased five times or more over several months to treat AIDS or kill cancer cells during chemotherapy. In a recent study where low-dose suramin (given intravenously to achieve blood levels of 1.5–15 μmol/L for 6 weeks) was given to children with ASD, the only side effect noted was a self-limited asymptomatic rash.[821]

Unlike suramin, shikimic acid *has* been confirmed in the scientific literature to be found in pine needles.[822] It is also found in star anise, as well as being the key ingredient in the formulation of the drug Oseltamivir phosphate (also known as Tamiflu) for the treatment of swine or avian flu.[823,824]

Tamifu works by inhibiting the action of the viral neuraminidase enzyme on sialic acid. Sialic acid is a carbohydrate occurring on the surfaces of cells in humans, and by hindering the relationship between the neuraminidase enzyme and sialic acid, Tamiflu stops new viral particles from being formed in infected cells.[825]

Given that SARS-CoV-2 does not encode any neuraminidase proteins, neuraminidase inhibitors such as oseltamivir and others were not thought to be effective for treating patients with COVID-19.[826] Interestingly, though, a recent retrospective analysis showed that neuraminidase inhibitor treatment was associated with decreased mortality in COVID-19 patients.[827] The study also found that the use of neuraminidase inhibitors led to a decreased incidence of acute heart injury but not liver or kidney injury in patients. Other research has indicated that neuraminidase inhibitor treatment has a beneficial effect on myocarditis to prevent cardiac damage and cytokine storm by the released neuraminidase.[828] The effect of shikimic acid on SARS-CoV-2 has yet to be studied.

Shikimic acid has shown other biological properties such as antibacterial, antifungal, anti-inflammatory, anti-aging, anti-dandruff, deodorising, anti-acne, and stimulating hair growth.[829,830,831]

Dosage: There are no official dosages for pine needle tea.

POLYGALA TENUIFOLIA

Some possible benefits: neuroprotection, anti-amyloid-β aggregation, anti-Tau protein, anti-inflammation, antioxidation, enhancing central cholinergic system, anti-neuronal cell death and promoting neuronal proliferation.

Polygala tenuifolia is among the most frequently used herbs in 3000 years of history of Chinese medicine for the treatment of neuronal problems. Recent evidence suggest that *P. tenuifolia* extract and many active components exert neuroprotective effects including anti-amyloid-β aggregation, anti-Tau, anti-inflammation, antioxidant, enhancing central cholinergic system, anti-neuronal apoptosis and promote neuronal proliferation.[832]

In one rat model, tenuifolin - a compound from the root, showed to inhibit the aggregation of amyloid-β and activation of Tau proteins.[833] *P. tenuifolia* also has a therapeutic effect on amyloid-β -induced neurotoxicity.[834] This was evidenced in another study that showed that crude extract from the root of *P. tenuifolia* inhibited oxidative stress and amyloid-β-induced nerve cell death in rats.[834]

Tenuigenin, a natural extract from *P. tenuifolia*, has also been shown to inhibit inflammatory cytokines, inhibit inflammatory NO production, and protect the memory centres of the brain against oxidative stress, neuronal damage, and cognitive dysfunction by increasing natural antioxidants and inhibiting ROS generation.[833,835,836] This has led to increased BDNF expression and further suppression of amyloid plaques within the brain.[837]

P. tenuifolia has also shown to improve the learning and memory ability of mice, via reducing the activity of acetylcholinesterase, an enzyme involved in breaking down the neurotransmitter acetylcholine.[838] Acetylcholine is essential for processing memory and learning, and is decreased in both concentration and function in patients with Alzheimer's disease.[839]

Human trials are sparse but promising. In otherwise healthy middle-aged adults, 100 mg of *P. tenuifolia taken* three times a day over four weeks improved immediate word recall relative to a placebo, although long term recall improvements were not significant. The group treated also showed improved working and strategic memory.[840]

In elderly adults, the same dose of *P. tenuifolia* extract given for eight weeks showed improvement in mental test scores and word list learning.[841] But in contrast, benefits to other parameters such as Mini Mental State Examination scores, verbal fluency, and recognition did not reach significance, and word list recall failed to improve with supplementation. This study concludes that the extract (BT-11) *"could enhance some cognitive functions, including memory, in elderly humans and therefore may be used as nutraceuticals that provide health benefits, including disease prevention and/or treatment."* [841]

Dosage: The only human studies on *Polygala tenuifolia* have used 100 mg of an ethanolic extract called BT-11, three times a day, for a total daily dose of 300 mg.[842]

Traditional Chinese medicine suggests taking 3–9 g (dry weight) of Polygala

tenuifolia root through a water decoction, like tea or soup, to reduce forgetfulness.[842]

PROGESTERONE

Some possible benefits include: anti-viral; anti-COVID-19; blood-pressure lowering; improving lung ventilation; maintaining balanced levels of iron; improving taste and smell; neuroprotection; and immunomodulation.

Progesterone is one of three major sex hormones, the other two being oestrogen and testosterone. Though it is found in both men and women, it is most commonly associated with women for its involvement in the menstrual cycle, pregnancy, and the growth and functioning of embryos. Progesterone is also combined with oestrogen to form the combined contraceptive pill.

In men, progesterone influences the production of sperm cells and testosterone biosynthesis. But its physiological influence does not end with fertility-related functions. Progesterone is a precursor to both oestrogen and testosterone, and affects nearly all other aspects of our health including sleep, immunological function, blood clotting, kidney function, behaviour and even appetite.[843-849]

One study noted that progesterone promoted faster recovery following influenza A virus infection in mice.[850] And another study concluded that progesterone is anti-inflammatory and has analgesic effects.[851] Due to progesterone's wide array and seemingly pro-recovery effects, it has been put forward in recent times as a potential therapeutic agent against SARS-CoV-2.

SARS-CoV-2 enters cells by binding its spike protein to ACE2, and in order to do this successfully, the virus needs to prime its spike protein using an enzyme called transmembrane protease, serine 2 (TMPRSS2).[852] It has been found that androgens, like testosterone, upregulate TMPRSS2 and help develop COVID-19.[853] Progesterone is anti-androgenic and can block the upregulation of TMPRSS2 by androgens.[854] Other than TMPRSS2, progesterone also blocks sigma receptors,[855] which are again involved in the infectivity of SARS-CoV-2.[856] These reasons may be why COVID-19 infections have been shown to be significantly more severe in males than in females.[857]

Other than directly inhibiting viral infectivity, progesterone has shown to help with lung ventilation in part by relaxing airway muscles;[858,859] help open blood vessels and reduce blood pressure and thus may protect the cardiovascular system;[860,861] help form hepcidin, a regulator of iron levels, and thus maintain balanced levels of iron;[862] be linked with better taste and smell;[863] enhance brain mitochondrial energy metabolism, and decrease oxidative stress and reverse the decrease of mitochondrial respiration rate following brain injury;[853,864] help with cellular debris accumulation and clearance;[853] inducing the vitamin D receptor in T cells and regulation of Th1/Th2 balance.[853.865]

Human platelets possess receptors for progesterone metabolites, and thus get activated when these bind to platelet receptors. This may be efficacious in those with lower than normal platelet numbers, but may increase the risk of clots in others.[853]

At the moment, though seemingly efficacious, the use of progesterone is understudied. But the data we do have is promising. One study of hospitalised men with COVID-19 did show that the addition of 100 mg of progesterone injected under the skin twice daily for five days improved clinical status on day 7, reduced the need for supplemental oxygen, and reduced the hospital length of stay with no significant adverse effects.[866]

Dosage: The only study using progesterone in COVID-19 patients used progesterone at a dose of 100 mg twice daily by subcutaneous injection. Patients in the study were also given prophylactic-dose anticoagulation to reduce the potential risk of progesterone-induced blood clots.[866]

QUERCETIN

Some possible benefits include: antioxidation, anti-inflammation, anti-cancer, anti-ageing, anti-diabetic, immunomodulation, antihypertensive, anti-allergy, neuroprotection, anti-viral, cardioprotection, anti-prion, anti-COVID-19, pro-autophagy, iron-chelator, enhances the effects of other molecules like zinc, resveratrol, genistein, and green tea catechins when used in combination.

Quercetin is a flavonoid found abundantly in nature. It shows a relatively higher bioavailability than other phytochemicals and exists in a variety of plant-based foods such as grapes, berries, cherries, apples, citrus fruits, buckwheat, kale, tomatoes, and black tea.[867] Quercetin is also known to be present in herbs such as dill, certain varieties of tea, and wine, as well as in various medicinal plants such as ginkgo, American elderberry, and Hypericum species.[868,869] Of all vegetables, onions are known to possess the highest quantity of quercetin.[870]

Quercetin is considered to be one of the most studied flavonoids, and research has shown that it has antioxidant, anti-inflammatory, anti-cancer, anti-diabetic, immunomodulatory, antihypertensive, anti-allergy, neuroprotective, and antimicrobial properties.[871,872,873]

Many studies have shown quercetin to be a promising drug for treating diabetes. Quercetin possesses the ability to increase insulin sensitivity, reduce insulin resistance, promote the proliferation of pancreatic cells, maintain the mass and function of diabetic pancreatic cells, as well as inhibit certain enzymes that lead to a lowering of the rate of glucose absorption within the intestine.[874-877] Quercetin has also shown potential in alleviating and/or protecting against diabetic-related diseases such as liver, kidney and eye disorders.[878,879,880]

Most research studying quercetin's effect on diabetes has been done on animal models. There are very few human trials in this regard. One trial of 24 diabetics taking a single dose of 400 mg of quercetin showed that this flavonoid has the ability to reduce the spike in blood sugar levels after consuming sugar.[881] But another study, where the study group took 250 mg of quercetin four times a day for eight weeks, showed improved antioxidant status in patients but no other significant effect on blood sugar control or lipid profile.[882]

Quercetin has shown some cardioprotective potential. In one study, quercetin and its derivative epicatechin were shown to improve endothelial function through modulation of the blood nitric oxide concentration and enhance vascular activity.[883] Quercetin has also shown the ability to prevent abnormal enlargement of the heart, reduce blood pressure in patients with high blood pressure, and reduce markers of inflammation in heart disease patients.[884,885,886]

Quercetin has also shown neuroprotective potential, being able to inhibit amyloid-β aggregation;[887] reduce the formation of tau proteins and inhibit acetyl-cholinesterase.[888] It is thought that the structural shape of quercetin may play an important role in amyloid-β aggregation inhibition and disrupt the mature protein fibrils by forming bonds with Aβ.[889]

There have also been a plethora of *in vitro* studies on various cancer cell lines, including lung, ovarian, nasopharyngeal, breast, leukaemia, prostate, bone, colon, and skin, that show some anti-cancer potential of quercetin.[890-898]

Quercetin and its derivatives have also shown antiviral potential against various viruses, including hepatitis B and C, various herpesviruses, orthomyxoviruses like influenza viruses, retroviruses like HIV, coronaviruses, and more.[899-903] Its promising antiviral effects are due to its ability to inhibit various enzymes such as polymerases, reverse transcriptases, and proteases, suppress DNA gyrase, and bind viral capsid proteins.[904] And with regards to SARS-CoV-2, the literature reveals that quercetin may exhibit anti-COVID-19 activity via its inhibitory effect on the expression of the human ACE2 receptors and certain enzymes of the virus.[905]

In one study of 429 patients with COVID-19, the use of quercetin, vitamin C, and bromelain in combination showed improvements in the recovery rate and blood parameters of those who took the combination.[906] And a smaller study revealed that supplementing with quercetin at the start of illness shortened the timing of molecular test conversion from positive to negative, reducing at the same time symptoms severity and negative predictors of COVID-19.[907] This was similarly seen in a study of 25 participants given a daily oral co-supplementation of 168 mg curcumin, 260 mg quercetin, and 9 mcg (360 IU) of vitamin D3. This study concludes with, *"The co-supplementation of CQC may possibly have a therapeutic role in the early stage of COVID-19 infection including speedy negativization of the SARS-CoV-2 RT-PCR test, resolution of acute symptoms, and modulation of the hyperinflammatory response. In combination with routine care, the adjuvant co-supplementation of CQC may possibly help in the speedy recovery from early-stage mild to moderate symptoms of COVID-19. Further research is warranted."*[908]

As we have already discovered in this book, quercetin has shown other useful properties such as attenuating the harmful effects of arsenic, protecting against glyphosate toxicity, and helping with post-exercise immunodeficiency.[909,910,911] Quercetin's impressive range of biological potential doesn't end there. Research has also shown this flavonoid to have anti-parasitic properties,[887] be able to promote autophagy,[912] be able to chelate iron,[913] have the ability to inhibit the formation of prion amyloid fibrils,[914] as well as turning them into protease-sensitive,[915] structurally loose, and non-cytotoxic forms; have the ability to clear senescent cells (similar to fisetin);[916] and enhance the effects of other molecules like zinc and resveratrol when used in combination.[917,918]

Dosage: The dosages of quercetin used are in the range of 12.5 to 25 mg per kg body weight, which translates to a range of 1,136-2,272 mg daily consumption of quercetin when taken alone.[919]

One may theoretically gain benefits at lower dosages if quercetin is supplemented with other flavonoids such as resveratrol, genistein, or green tea catechins, as these increase the potency synergistically.

RAPAMYCIN

Some possible benefits include: anti-inflammation, anti-cancer, anti-ageing, anti-diabetic, immunomodulation, immune-enhancing, cardioprotection, neuroprotection, antiviral, and anti- prion.

Rapamycin was first isolated as an antibiotic in 1975 by researchers in the soil of the South Pacific island of Rapa Nui, where the islanders never wore shoes and were rarely infected with tetanus.[920] It later became known as an antifungal agent, and in addition to its anti-inflammatory effects, it was found that rapamycin also suppressed the immune system. It was later approved as an oral immune inhibitor in 1999. Rapamycin is now primarily used in clinical settings to suppress tissue rejection after organ transplantation and as an adjuvant in therapy for certain cancers.[921]

In 2009, though, it was found that rapamycin extended the maximal lifespan of both male and female mice by 9% and 14%, respectively.[922] And ever since then, research on the role of rapamycin in anti-aging has increased tremendously. Animal studies since 2009 have shown that rapamycin has powerful pharmacological effects on delaying ageing, extending healthspan, and attenuating age-related diseases by inducing autophagy (similar to what happens when fasting).[923,924]

More specifically, rapamycin increases the lifespan of multiple species by inhibiting the mammalian target of rapamycin (mTOR), a master regulator of cell growth, metabolism, and ageing.[925,926] And it's not just mice; evidence exists showing that rapamycin-induced mTOR inhibition prolongs the lifespan of many other species, ranging from yeast to flies.[927,928] The longest documented lifespan extension by rapamycin was 26%; this was in mice. Unfortunately, there has been no study of rapamycin in the lifespan extension of humans and primates so far.[929]

As biological function declines with and also contributes to ageing, it has been put forward that rapamycin might not only result in longer lifespans but better overall health by delaying the ageing of multiple organs systematically.

With regards to the nervous system, rapamycin has shown great potential in targeting and reversing many aspects of ageing and disease progression found in age-related neurodegenerative disorders like dementia and Parkinson's disease. In animal models rapamycin has been shown to induce autophagy and activate various signalling pathways to reverse amyloid β-induced oxidative stress and synaptic dysfunction in areas of the brain linked to memory formation.[930] Rapamycin has also been shown to protect against age-related oxidative stress, cell death, and neuroinflammation, as well as improving mitochondrial function and acting as an anti-inflammatory agent within the brain.[931,932,933] Rapamycin has also been shown to extend the survival of prion-infected mice when administered orally, starting at day 100 post-infection.[934]

Rapamycin has continued to show promise for reversing age-related diseases in other parts of the body. Though related to an increased risk of menstrual disturbances in women, in animal models rapamycin has shown to improve ovarian reserve, as well as improve ovarian lifespan, increase egg cell quality, and improve the ovarian microenvironment.[935,936] Similarly, in male mice, rapamycin was shown to protect against age-caused testicular shrinking and improve markers of sperm production.[937]

With regards to the cardiovascular system, rapamycin has shown to prevent age-related pathogenic heart muscle growth, whilst improving overall pump function.[938] It has also shown to attenuate cardiac scarring that is usually linked with myocardial dysfunction, increased stiffness, decreased cardiac compliance, decreased myocardial systolic function, and increased incidence of arrhythmia.[939] Importantly, rapamycin has also been shown to reduce myocarditis associated with *Trypanosoma cruzi*, the causative agent of Chagas disease, as well as experimental autoimmune myocarditis.[940,941]

Usually, mTOR signalling activation leads to impaired endothelial function and foam cell formation, which is the initial process of atherosclerosis formation.[942] And thus, rapamycin has been hypothesised to, and later shown to, reduce vascular inflammation and alleviate atherosclerosis progression.[943] Apart from artery disease, rapamycin also exerts effects on venous disease. In aged mice (16 months old) with experimental deep vein thrombosis (DVT), 2-month rapamycin (1.5 mg/kg/d intragastrically) treatment resulted in a significant reduction in susceptibility to DVT as compared to the aged controls. This was thought to be done by rapamycin's effect of significantly decreasing platelet size and activation.[944]

As we have already touched upon earlier in the book, SASP (senescence-associated secretory phenotype) are pro-inflammatory, tissue-destructive molecules that are expressed by senescent cells, having deleterious effects on the tissue microenvironment, as well as promoting tumour progression.[945] One study noted that SARS-CoV-2 induced senescence in human non-senescent cells and exacerbated the SASP in human senescent cells.[260] Another study noted that the spike protein amplifies SASP in senescent, cultured human cells.[946] Well in a clinical trial involving older adults with coronary artery disease, 12-week daily oral low-dose rapamycin had some positive effects on alleviating SASP.[947] This has also been demonstrated in mice.[948]

The immune system is also negatively impacted by ageing. Clinically, rapamycin is used as an immunosuppressant for preventing rejection in transplant patients, and there have been queries about whether it may have a potential negative effect on immunity. However, rapamycin is now recognised as an optimal immunomodulator rather than an immunosuppressant.[949] In fact, rapamycin has immunostimulatory effects on the generation of memory CD8 T cells, and in one study, treatment of mice with rapamycin following a viral infection increased not only the quantity but also the quality of virus-specific CD8 T cells.[949] And in humans rapamycin has shown to enhance the ability of vaccine response in the elderly.[950] Rapamycin has also been shown to inhibit the replication of the 1918 flu virus by 100-fold.[951] Though no specific studies have been performed evaluating the effectiveness of rapamycin in treating COVID-19, one review did note that it may *"represent a better candidate for COVID-19 therapy than commonly tested antivirals"* and also *"that its efficiency will not be reduced by the high rate of viral RNA mutation."*[952]

The beneficial effects of rapamycin do not stop there. This drug has shown anti-aging potential in nearly all biological areas, from helping with alopecia to helping with age-related frailty.[953,954] But the use of rapamycin does not come without the risk of side effects. Side effects reported using rapamycin in clinical studies include low white blood count levels, low platelets, raised triglycerides, hypercholesterolemia, aphthous ulcers, oedema, joint pain, pneumonia, acne, delayed wound healing, sinus tachycardia, decreased renal function, gastrointestinal toxicity, rash, menstrual cycle disturbance, ovarian cyst, and infection.[923]

It must be noted that most of these side effects are not reported by healthy participants. Furthermore, an increasing amount of evidence continues to suggest that most of these adverse reactions are due to rapamycin-related dose dependence and are reversible after ending treatment.[923]

Plus, other studies show more side effects in the placebo group than in the rapamycin group. Take this study of healthy male participants given a single dose of rapamycin. Complaints about fatigue were reported by 23% in the rapamycin group and by 40% in the placebo group.[955]

The other commonly stated "side effect" of rapamycin, usually when taken for a prolonged period of time, is insulin resistance.[956] Confusingly, rapamycin can actually induce insulin sensitivity as well as insulin resistance. This in fact mirrors the effect of fasting which improves insulin sensitivity and reverse type 2 diabetes, but also can cause a form of glucose intolerance known as benevolent pseudo-diabetes. One research paper noted that this was not to worry about as the raised blood sugar levels in some who take rapamycin are reversible and suggested that for anti-aging purposes, rapamycin *"can be administrated intermittently (e.g., once a week) in combination with intermittent carbohydrate restriction, physical exercise, and metformin."*[957]

It has been said that *"rapamycin is not much more dangerous than ordinary drugs"*, and that *"if used properly, rapamycin is not much more dangerous than ordinary aspirin."*[958] This was no better demonstrated than in a case series of a failed suicide attempt involving an 18-year-old woman who ingested 103 rapamycin tablets (103 mg). The only detected effect was an elevation in total blood cholesterol.[959]

The benefits of rapamycin seem near endless, and given that rapamycin is a fasting- and ketogenic diet-mimicking medication, the benefits and potential side-effects of the three have considerable crossover.

Dosage: There is no official dosage of rapamycin for age prolongation. Anecdotally, one researcher is noted to take 20 mg once every two weeks

(noting that high peak levels theoretically may cross the BBB, and should be given under doctor supervision).[960]

Everyday treatment in the elderly (1 mg/day for several weeks) was not associated with side effects and has been shown to be safe. But, as one research paper puts it, *"to avoid side effects and maximize anti-aging effects, a feasible approach would be to prolong intervals between rapamycin administrations while keeping the total dose constant. For example, instead of daily administration, a weekly administration of a higher dose can be suggested to achieve a high peak blood level, followed by drug-free period to avoid undesirable effects."*[961]

RESVERATROL

Some possible benefits: anti-inflammation, anti-cancer, anti-ageing, anti-diabetic, immunomodulation, immune-enhancing, cardioprotection, neuroprotection, antiviral, and anti-prion.

Resveratrol is a naturally occurring non-flavonoid polyphenol that is produced by several plants in response to injury. It naturally occurs in numerous foods, such as blueberries and peanuts, as well as grapes and their derived products like red wine.[962]

Resveratrol was first isolated in 1939 from the roots of the white hellebore (*Veratrum grandiflorum*), a poisonous medicinal plant mainly found in China and Japan. In traditional Chinese medicine, the dried roots and the part of the hellebore that runs underground horizontally are known as "li lu" and are indicated for jaundice, malaria, diarrhoea, and headache. The highest concentrations of resveratrol are found in the Japanese knotweed, *Polygonum japonicum,* which is also used in traditional Chinese medicine in diverse tea products.[962]

Resveratrol became popular within the scientific community after it was found to have radical-scavenging, antioxidant, and anti-cancer properties.[963] And as it was found in red wine, it was thought that resveratrol may have a role to play in the so-called "French paradox," originally formulated in 1981 by French epidemiologists who observed a lower mortality incidence of coronary heart disease in France despite high levels of dietary saturated fat and cigarette smoking. But recent evidence suggests that the amount of resveratrol in red wine is so low that you'd have to consume 505–2762 litres of it to attain 1 g of it, the estimated therapeutic dose.[962] You'd agree that the harms of drinking that much outweigh any potential benefits.

Regardless, since 1997, scientific research has revealed that resveratrol possesses a plethora of beneficial biological properties, including anticancer, cardioprotective, antidiabetic, neuroprotective, anti-aging, anti-oxidative, anti-inflammatory, immunomodulating, and liver-protective properties.[964-967]

Like many other plant-derived molecules mentioned already, resveratrol protects against oxidative stress in numerous ways, including by reducing ROS generation, directly scavenging free radicals, improving our own natural antioxidant defences, promoting antioxidant molecules, helping to express genes involved in mitochondrial energy production, and inducing autophagy.[964]

With regards to inflammation, resveratrol has been shown to regulate the pro- and anti-inflammatory cytokines mainly by upregulating SIRT1, suppressing NF-κB, as well as inhibiting NLRP3 inflammasome activation.[964] NLRP3 is a component of the immune system that detects damaged parts of cells and triggers immune inflammation as a result. Mutations in the NLRP3 gene are associated with a number of organ-specific autoimmune diseases.[968]

These properties and more have shown to translate to various health protective effects. Focusing on the cardiovascular system, resveratrol has shown to aid with endothelial health;[969] reduce vessel thickness inflammation, fibrosis, and oxidative stress in aged mice;[970] have antithrombotic effects via decreasing the tissue factors like TNF-α;[971] be able to reduce the 'rusting' of red blood cells;[972] and mitigate toxin-related heart reshaping and dysfunctions in pumping.[973]

Neurologically, resveratrol has been shown to inhibit the aggregation of amyloid β, remove prion accumulation, and has been shown in animal studies to improve learning, memory, and mood functions via increasing the growth of brain cells and the blood vessel network in the brain.[994,995,996] Animal studies have also reported that resveratrol reversed an age-dependent decline in cognitive functions through enhancing the secretion of neurotransmitters, including serotonin, noradrenaline, and dopamine.[977]

Many studies have also shown resveratrol to be effective in the prevention and treatment of cancers, mainly through inhibition of cell proliferation, induction of cell apoptosis, and suppression of cell migration.[967] These have all been *in vitro* and *in vivo* studies, however.

Resveratrol has exerted immunomodulating effects in various studies. In one study, resveratrol upregulated immune responses, reduced the death of immune cells, and improved the growth of young chickens receiving conventional vaccinations.[978] The polyphenol has also shown to reduced the activity of respiratory syncytial virus;[979] reduce the virus-induced elevated IL-6 and TNF-α secretion;[980] enhance immune activity in immunosuppressive mice;[981] and reverse the imbalanced Th17/Treg, the main characteristic of immune thrombocytopenic purpura.[982] For these reasons and more, resveratrol has been put forward as a potential therapeutic against SARS-CoV-2.[983] But in a very small study of those with mild COVID-19, the use of resveratrol did not show a significant benefit compared to controls.[984]

With regards to fertility, resveratrol has shown some promise in improving ovarian function as well as having a positive effect on sperm motility.[985,986] However, while resveratrol has been advanced as a potential fertility drug, it has also been shown to negatively interfere with the process of embryo implantation.[987] Furthermore, it is structurally similar to various forms of oestrogen and modulates oestrogen-response systems, which has led to it being classified as a phytoestrogen.[988] Whether this trait positively or negatively affects male and female fertility is yet to be known.

Other than having antioxidant and anti-inflammatory properties, resveratrol is popular in the anti-aging scientific community as it is the most potent natural compound activator of sirtuin 1.[988] This may account for its metabolic benefits in humans. Though promising on paper, human trials using resveratrol are limited and have shown mixed results.

In 23 healthy overweight older adults who took 200mg/day, resveratrol was shown enhanced memory performance accompanied with improved glucose metabolism and improved functional connectivity in areas of the brain related to memory formation.[989] In another study, where participants took 350 mg of resveratrol-enriched grape extract for 6 months, those who supplemented it showed improvements in cholesterol quality.[990] Plus, resveratrol prevented bone density loss (500 mg/day for 6 months) in type-2 diabetic patients in another study.[991]

But not all studies have shown effectiveness and have, in fact, shown various negative effects. For instance, resveratrol intake (250 mg/day for 8 weeks) did not increase SIRT1 nor improve many cardiovascular risk factors in healthy aged men, and supplementation actually *reduced* the positive effect of exercise training on blood pressure, blood cholesterol, and maximal oxygen uptake and did not affect the reduction of atherosclerosis.[992] Other studies have documented that resveratrol may also behave as a pro-oxidizing agent, increase DNA damage, and interact with several other drugs.[993,994] Additionally, long-term intake of resveratrol may act as a thyroid disruptor and even induce cancer growth.[994,995]

The background health of the individual, when it is taken, the dose taken, and for how long all play a part in resveratrol's risk and effectiveness. It has been suggested that in lower doses, resveratrol acts as a potent antioxidant, while at higher doses, it acts as a pro-oxidant.[996] This has also been described for melatonin, quercetin, and epigallocatechin.[997,998,999] Furthermore, in a rat study, it was documented that resveratrol behaved as an antioxidant during the dark period and as a pro-oxidant during the light period, possibly reflecting the putative changing ratio between pro- and antioxidant activities in various organs during the 24-h cycle.[1000] In another study authors found that resveratrol improved insulin sensitivity in old mice fed standard diet, while did not improve insulin resistance status in old mice receiving high-protein diets. Healthy mice given resveratrol in fact exhibited increased inflammation, demonstrating that resveratrol seemed to be beneficial to malnourished states of physiological ageing.[1001]

Dosage: There is no official dosage for resveratrol. The lower end of supplementation in those who are otherwise unhealthy is 5–10 mg daily, while dosages between 150–445 mg have been used in those who are otherwise healthy.[1002]

Doses greater than 1000 mg per day may increase the likelihood of side-effects and drug interactions.[994]

RHODIOLA

Some possible benefits: anti-inflammation, anti-cancer, anti-ageing, immunomodulation, immune-enhancing, cardioprotection, neuroprotection, anti-stress, mood-improving, anti-fatigue, and pro-fertility.

Rhodiola rosea is a rare and highly valued medicinal plant that grows at high altitudes, up to 2280 m, in the arctic and mountainous regions throughout Europe, Asia, and North America.[1003] It has been a part of traditional medicine systems in parts of Europe, Asia, and Russia for centuries.[1004] The Mongolians use *R. rosea* to help treat cancer and tuberculosis;[1005] it is given to newlyweds in efforts to boost fertility in Siberia and used as a food and cosmetic in Norway.[1004,1005] The Vikings used *R. rosea* to increase endurance and physical strength, too.[1005]

More recently, *R. rosea* has received attention from the scientific community for its potential therapeutic capacity as an "adaptogen."[1006] The term "adaptogen" was coined in 1947 by Russian scientist Nikolai Lazarev as an agent that permits an organism to fight severe physical, chemical, or biological stressors by creating non-specific resistance.[1007] As a result, adaptogens are regarded as having the ability to direct physiological processes in order to initiate generalised adaptation and deal with stressful situations more resourcefully. Medicinal mushrooms are another example of adaptogens.

Results from recent studies have revealed *R. rosea* to have a wide variety of medicinal properties, including anti-ageing, anti-inflammation, anti-stress (both psychological and physical), antioxidant, anti-viral, and anti-cancer effects, as well as immunomodulating, enhancing DNA repair, and modulating adaptation to low levels of oxygen.[1008-1015]

Chronic stress can lead to psychological turmoil, immune dysfunction, sleep problems, and even premature ageing by negatively impacting cellular processes like mitochondrial function, cell senescence, and DNA damage.[1016-1021] And thus, it is promising to know that *R. rosea* has shown the ability to protect the organism from stress. In one study, *R. rosea* showed to reduce circulating levels of stress hormones in rats subjected to stress.[1022] In another instance, *R. rosea* enhanced the stress resistance in the silkworm against heat stress (37 °C) and starvation.[1023]

With regards to mental resilience in humans, a statistically significant improvement in the Fatigue Index was observed in the *R. rosea* treatment group given 170 mg of the plant for 14 days a night in one study.[1024] Another study in over a hundred adults showed significant, consistent, and steady improvements in stress symptoms, fatigue, quality of life, mood, concentration, disability, functional impairment, and an overall therapeutic effect when given *R. rosea* root extract 200 mg twice daily.[1025] *R. rosea* has also been shown to exert a notable anti-fatigue effect that increases mental performance, particularly the ability to concentrate in those with fatigue syndrome.[1026] This was also shown in another study of patients with chronic fatigue syndrome. The researchers in this study recommend a daily dosage of 400 mg of a dry ethanolic extract of *R. rosea*.[1027]

R. rosea has also shown to help with symptoms of anxiety and depression. In one study of participants with diagnosed anxiety who took 340 mg *R. rosea* extract for 10 weeks showed significant reduction in their anxiety.[1028] And in another study of 91 patients with mild to moderate depression, supplementing with *R. rosea* showed overall improvement in depression, together with insomnia and emotional instability.[1029]

Like animal studies, the use of *R. rosea* has also been shown to help attenuate physical fatigue. In one small study, the use of *R. rosea* was shown to enhance explosive resistance training performance.[1030] And with regards to endurance exercise, the use of *R. rosea* in another study was shown to decrease the heart-rate response to submaximal exercise and improve endurance exercise performance by decreasing the perception of effort.[1031] Other studies have shown *R. rosea* to have the ability to improve both aerobic and anaerobic fitness.[1006]

R. rosea has also shown to improve the electric stability of the heart, as well as possibly having a positive effect on treating ischemic heart disease alone and in combination with routine western medicine.[1032]

Other than improvements in psychological and physical stress resistance, the use of *R. rosea* in animal models has shown to improve egg quality and fertility, as well as attenuating stress-induced reproductive dysfunction.[1006] *R. rosea* has also been shown to help start periods in women suffering from the absence of menstruation;[1006] help with menopausal quality of life;[1033] and help men with erectile dysfunction and/or premature ejaculation substantially improve sexual function.[1006]

R. rosea extracts have been documented with immunostimulating activity both *in vitro* in human peripheral blood cells and *in vivo* in animals. More specifically *R. rosea* has shown to increase total CD3+ and memory CD4+ T cell pools;[1034] as well as increase production of Th1 cytokines.[1035] In one recent study, researchers supplemented participants with long COVID with a fixed combination of adaptogens—Rhodiola, Eleutherococcus, and Schisandra—for two weeks.[1036] The supplemented group had a lower number of patients with a lack of fatigue and pain symptoms, significantly better daily walk time, and significantly decreased blood creatinine compared to the placebo group, suggesting prevention of renal failure progression in long COVID.

Dosage: Rhodiola rosea supplementation often refers to either the SHR-5 extract in specific or an analogous extract, any extract that provides both 3% rosavins and 1% salidroside.[1037]

Rhodiola has been shown to be beneficial as a daily fatigue preventive in doses as low as 50 mg.

Short-term rhodiola use for fatigue and anti-stress has been seen to be in the 288–680 mg range.

ROYAL JELLY

Some possible benefits: anti-inflammation, anti-oxidation, anti-ageing; immunomodulation, cardioprotection, neuroprotection, mood-improving, anti-fatigue, and pro-fertility.

Royal jelly (RJ) is a yellowish-white, creamy, acidic secretion produced by the mouth area (mandibular and hypopharyngeal glands) of immature *Apis mellifera* nurse bees.[1038] During the first three days, nursing bees offer two different larval meals for the queen and workers: RJ and worker jelly. The RJ given to the larvae in the queen cells causes the larvae to make large amounts of juvenile hormone at 3 days old, leading to the development of the queen bee.

RJ has a pungent smell, a distinct sweet-sour taste, and is thought to be a powerful promoter of healthy ageing and longevity since it improves the overall health and fertility of queen bees, which may lay up to 3000 eggs per day and live for up to five years compared to infertile workers, who only live up to 45 days.[1039]

Though human trials are significantly lacking, many people take it as a supplement for it has shown to possess a wide range of health-promoting activities like antioxidant, anti-inflammatory, neurotrophic, blood-pressure reducing, antidiabetic, cholesterol-improving, anti-cancer, anti-fatigue, antimicrobial, and anti-ageing.[1038,1040]

RJ is composed of a variety of sugars, fats, proteins, flavonoids, vitamins, minerals, and bioactive substances. 90% of the fats found in RJ are rare and small in structural length, one of the most prominent being 10-hydroxydecanoic acid (10-HDA). It has now been shown that 10-HDA may be used to treat age-related neurodegenerative disorders, as it induces neuronal development by imitating BDNF.[1041] 10-HDA has also been shown to have neuroprotective effects as well as anti-cancer effects, specifically on melanoma cells.[1042]

Proteins are the dominant component of RJ, and 80% of total RJ proteins are composed of nine major RJ proteins (MRJPs). Research has shown that MRJPs have anti-senescence activity *in vitro* and anticancer effects.[1043,1044]

The most abundant vitamin in RJ is pantothenic acid (vitamin B5), followed by niacin. RJ also contains small amounts of various B-group vitamins (B1, B2, B6, B8, B9, and B12), ascorbic acid (vitamin C), vitamin E, and vitamin A. Pantothenic acid has been shown to increase the lifespan of mice.[1045]

Pantothenic acid, specifically from RJ, has been postulated to have anti-aging effects by itself or by synergizing the action of other vitamins.[1046] In a recent study, RJ given to flies extended their lifespan; this has also been evidenced in other insects and animals like crickets, silkworms, nematodes, and mice.[1039] In terms of increasing the lifespan of mice, research has shown that long-term intragastric administration of royal jelly avoided age-related weight loss, increased memory, and delayed age-related thymus shrinkage.[1047] The treated mice also had better physical performance and lower age-related muscle loss.

RJ has also been shown to improve the cognitive function of various animal models with different forms of toxin-related Alzheimer's disease. RJ dramatically increased spatial learning and memory retention in typically aged rats by up to 48.5%, as well as correcting cognitive deficits in copper and cholesterol-fed rabbits and ameliorating nerve death and BBB dysfunction.[1048,1049,1050]

RJ is thought to help neuronal health by enhancing our antioxidant capabilities, inhibiting the "leakiness" of the BBB induced by toxins, decreasing the formation and enhancing the clearance of amyloid β, activating autophagy genes, helping to repair DNA, enhancing brain neurotransmission, contributing to the production of ketone bodies, and alleviating hormonal and metabolic abnormalities underlying cognitive impairment.[1038,1051-1056]

RJ has also shown immunomodulatory potential. In one study of 20 children with systemic lupus erythematosus, the addition of 2 g of freshly prepared RJ daily for 12 weeks showed increases in CD4+ and CD8+ regulatory T cells and improvements with regard to the clinical severity score and laboratory markers for the disease.[1057] Various components of RJ have shown anti-allergic potential, an ability to increase and decrease certain subsets of T cells (depending on the concentration of the water extract), and an ability to encourage Th1 polarisation.[1058,1059,1060]

It is interesting to note that crude RJ has been shown to stop cellular damage caused by BPA, which in turn causes the enlargement of human breast cancer.[1061] Another thing to note is that some studies have shown that RJ has a beneficial effect on sperm count and motility and improves the fertilising ability of sperm cells, as well as increasing testosterone production.[1062,1063] But despite the fact that RJ is extensively used in assisted reproductive processes, no clear clinical data supports its fertility-improving impact on women, though evidence suggests that it may increase oestrogen in post-menopausal women.[1064]

Dosage: There is no official recommended or optimal dosage for RJ. Researchers have observed benefits when using 50-300 mg doses. Dosages as high as 6 g a day have also been shown to provide benefits.[1065]

The MRJPs in RJ have been reported to cause several allergic reactions such as asthma, dermatitis, skin rashes, eczemas, oral allergy syndrome, bronchospasm, anaphylaxis, hemorrhagic colitis, or even anaphylactic shock and death in some situations.[1064,1066-1068]

One case study involved an 87-year-old man with long-term warfarin therapy who was also supplemented with royal jelly capsules and was referred to the hospital for blood in his urine. The most probable explanation for his symptoms was a possible interaction between warfarin and royal jelly.[1069]

SALVIANOLIC ACIDS

Some possible benefits include: anti-inflammation, anti-oxidation, anti-fibrosis, anti-vascular dysfunction, and anti-cancer.

Salvia miltiorrhiza, also called red sage or Danshen, is a commonly used medicinal plant in traditional Chinese medicine, belonging to the category of promoting blood circulation and removing blood stasis. It has been used for thousands of years in Asian countries to treat vascular disorder-related diseases, including coronary heart disease, myocardial infarction, angina, and atherosclerosis.[1070]

Salvianolic acids are the most water-soluble compounds in *S. miltiorrhiza*. Among salvianolic acids, salvianolic acid A (Sal A) and salvianolic acid B (Sal B) are the most abundant components.

Fibrosis, also known as scarring, is a chronic stage of many diseases that affects millions of people around the world. It is characterised by the excessive deposition of a meshwork of cells called extracellular matrix, which is brought on by long-term inflammation and then leads to structural damage and organ dysfunction.[1071] Fibrosis can be caused by a variety of factors, including chemical insults, autoimmune reactions, radiation, tissue injury, allergic responses, and persistent infections.[1072]

COVID-19 has shown to cause lung fibrosis lasting 4 months after the initial infection, and the incidence rate of post-COVID lung fibrosis is estimated at 2-6%

after moderate illness.[1073,1074] But it's not just the lungs; COVID-19 has also been linked to cardiac fibrosis and even pancreatic fibrosis associated with multiple vascular thrombi.[1075,1076]

The problem with fibrosis is not only organ dysfunction but also its propensity to increase the development of cancer. For instance, most lung cancer cases are found in the outer areas of the lung tissue and lower lobes, and changes in lung fibrosis also occur mainly in these areas.[1077]

Although the beneficial effects of salvianolic acids on cardiovascular and neurological protection have been demonstrated in recent years (mainly through their antioxidative properties), the most important impacts of salvianolic acids seem to be cancer treatment and alleviation of fibrotic diseases.[1070,1078,1079]

Animal studies have shown the ability of salvianolic acids to attenuate lung scarring by reducing the thickness of small air sacs and collagen deposition;[1080] reducing lung fibroblast numbers (cells that contribute to the formation of connective tissue);[1081] and inhibiting downstream scar signalling pathways.[1082]

Salvianolic acids have also been shown to attenuate cardiac fibrosis by inhibiting the NF-κB pathway, inhibiting the movement of fibroblasts to sites of injury, and improving vascular inflammation and dysfunction.[1083,1084,1085] In one study, Sal B was shown to reverse the impaired endothelial function of mice with high blood pressure in 11 days. Sal B has also been shown to attenuate platelet-triggered inflammation in endothelial cells mediated by NF-κB activation.[1086,1087]

Other than helping with fibrosis, a large number of cell studies have shown that salvianolic acids have a good effect in treating various types of cancer, including breast, head and neck, lung, squamous cell, eye, ovarian, melanoma, colorectal, and liver cancers.[1088-1096] One major way salvianolic acids have shown anti-cancer potential is via the inhibition of a process called epithelial-mesenchymal transition, where one type of cell loses its characteristics and acquires other characteristics.[1071]

Dosage: Due to the lack of human trials on specific salvianolic acids, there are no official recommended dosages or safety data on them.

S. Militorrhiza **is commonly sold in China as dripping pills (to be absorbed under the tongue) or as oral tablets. The Fufang Danshen Dripping pill is most frequently taken as 30 tablets spread over three times a day (10 each), sublingually or orally.**[1097]

Fufang Danshen tablets are taken three times a day, with three taken each time. The standard therapeutic dose of Danshen is 6.56 mg per kg of body weight.

SAUNA

Some possible benefits include: anti-inflammation, cardioprotection, anti-vascular dysfunction, anti-prion, pain-reduction, neuroprotection, and mood-boosting.

Sauna bathing is a form of whole-body thermotherapy that has been used in various forms and in various cultures across thousands of years for hygiene, health, social, and spiritual purposes. Generally speaking, there are two main types of saunas: wet saunas and dry saunas. Wet saunas (70-100 °C; humidity 50%) are specifically designed to raise an individual's thermal load by maintaining a high internal humidity to reduce evaporative cooling, whereas dry saunas (temperature = 80-90 °C; humidity = 10-20%) are often built of wood and heated by an electric heater and are the focus of the majority of clinical research.[1097,1098]

Traditional Finnish saunas are the most popular example of dry saunas and are the most researched.[1100] They involve short (5–20 minute) exposures in dry air (relative humidity of 10%–20%) interspersed with intervals of high humidity caused by the throwing of water over heated rocks. Infrared sauna cabins have become increasingly popular of late. These saunas use infrared emitters of various wavelengths without the use of water or additional humidity and generally operate at lower temperatures (45–60 °C) than Finnish saunas with comparable exposure times.[1101]

Sauna use has profound physiological effects. Short-term heat exposure elevates skin and core body temperatures, which in turn activates thermoregulatory pathways leading to the activation of the autonomic nervous system. This, along with the activation of other hormonal systems, leads to well-documented cardiovascular effects with increased heart rate, skin blood flow, cardiac output, and sweating.[1102,1103]

Heat also activates other desirable physiological processes, one of which is the activation of heat shock proteins (HSPs). HSPs are a group of proteins that cells create in response to stressful situations. They were first described in relation to heat shock, hence their name, but are now known to be expressed during other stresses such as cold exposure, UV light exposure, and wound healing.[1104-1107,] Many members of this group serve as chaperones, either by stabilising proteins to ensure proper folding or by assisting in the refolding of proteins damaged by cell stress.

HSPs also aim to remove abnormal proteins, dissociate protein aggregates, stabilise misfolded proteins, and help sequester misfolded protein species in a way that prevents harmful interactions with the rest of the cellular environment, and thus they are involved in keeping proteins like prions in check.[1108]

It has been noted that people who suffer from diabetes and/or obesity have an increased risk of a severe outcome from COVID-19, and one explanation put forward for this observation is that these conditions disrupt the heat shock response (HSR), a natural response to a fever that normally leads to resolution of the inflammatory response.[1109] Thus, HSP activation may aid these individuals too.

Other than activating HSPs, sauna use increases NO bioavailability, increases insulin sensitivity, improves endothelial health, improves cardiac function markers, reduces epinephrine and/or norepinephrine, improves cholesterol markers, and decreases fasting blood glucose levels.[1110-1114]

Hormesis is defined as an adaptive response of cells and organisms to a moderate (usually intermittent) stress, and it has been suggested that sauna bathing may induce a general stress-adaptation response that leads to "hormetic adaptation,"[1115] inducing adaptive hormesis mechanisms similar to exercise.[1116]

The ability for saunas to provide a "good type of stress," as you will, was demonstrated by analysis methods that suggested sauna bathing increased the generation of free radicals and ROS along with enhanced antioxidant activities and upregulated specific HSPs in semen.[1116,1117]

This sauna stress also works physiologically. Dynorphin is an opioid that is commonly associated with a psychological sense of uneasiness or discomfort.[1118] Dynorphin may also serve to moderate the body's response to heat, allowing it to cool down. Heat activates dynorphin-expressing neurons in the brain. When this thermosensory pathway is activated, it causes heat-defence responses in which the binding of dynorphin to kappa opioid receptors causes cellular processes that enhance discomfort and misery. Heat stress from sauna use may boost dynorphin release, which may be responsible for the general feeling of discomfort during heat exposure. Interestingly, once dynorphin attaches to the kappa-opioid receptor, other opioid receptors that are linked to euphoria (mu) become more sensitive to beta-endorphins in a biological feedback reaction, meaning that the discomfort felt in the sauna can help improve one's mood afterwards.

Saunas also make you sweat. Many industrial poisons, heavy metals, hormone disruptors, and immunotoxins may be excreted in sweat, leading to an enhancement of metabolic pathways and processes that these toxic agents inhibit.[1119] The loss of toxic metals such as arsenic, cadmium, lead, and mercury via sweat has been reported with rates of excretion matching or exceeding urinary routes.[1120] Plus, there is evidence that organochlorine pesticides, BPA, and phthalates may be excreted via induced sweating at rates that exceed urinary excretion.[1121,1122,1123]

Most of the human research on saunas has focused on cardiometabolic outcomes. According to one study, increased duration and frequency of sauna bathing decreased the risk of fatal cardiovascular disease incidences. The more sauna activity translated to better cardiovascular protection, participants who attended one, two to three, or greater than four sauna sessions a week had a reduced cardiovascular mortality rate of 10.1, 7.6, and 2.7 per 1000 person-years, respectively.[1124]

In another study, it was found that men who attended a sauna bathing session two–three times per week reduced their cardiovascular mortality rates by ~30% and men who attended a sauna session four or more times per week reduced their risk by ~50%.[1125]

Those with underlying cardiological conditions may benefit from sauna use too. In the largest and most recent prospective multicenter randomised controlled trial involving 149 patients with advanced heart failure, sauna use was linked with 6-minute walking distances and beneficially reduced heart size.[1126] The use of sauna bathing for 5 minutes daily for 4 weeks demonstrated improved cardiac structure in 12 infants with ventricular septal defects, which averted the need for surgical repair in 9 infants.[1127] And a randomised controlled trial noted a reduction of premature ventricular arrhythmias after 2 weeks of repeated sauna sessions.[1112]

And it's not just the heart. Two studies of patients diagnosed with chronic fatigue syndrome or myalgic encephalomyelitis reported subjective improvements after repeated sauna sessions, with improvements in mood and fatigue levels being noted.[1116,1128] And Finnish studies have noted that after adjusting for various confounding factors (such as blood pressure, resting heart rate, smoking status, Type 2 diabetes, previous myocardial infarction, LDL levels, and alcohol consumption), those who frequently sauna bathed had a 66% reduction in the risk of dementia, a 65% reduction in the risk of Alzheimer's disease, a 63% reduction in the risk of sudden cardiac death, and a 40% reduction in the risk of all-cause mortality.[1125,1129]

Though seemingly greatly beneficial for various biological processes, like all things, regular sauna use does come with safety warnings. Firstly, although observational data have found a negligible association between sauna use and birth defects, in pregnant women, heat exposure has been found to induce some birth defects in the foetus, such as spina bifida.[1130] And thus, avoiding sauna use during pregnancy is currently considered the best practice.

Heat exposure and repeated sauna use in men have been linked to reduced sperm counts, fewer motile sperm, and abnormal sperm parameters. However, 6 months after quitting sauna practice, all indicated abnormalities returned to normal, and no significant changes in plasma sex hormones from baseline were identified immediately after sauna or after 3 or 6 months.[1117]

And although regular sauna usage has been shown to improve heart disease indicators and lessen depression symptoms, both medication and alcohol use can have serious and potentially deadly side effects when mixed with sauna use.[1131] As a result, alcohol should be avoided whenever possible when using a sauna, and anyone on medication should consult with their main physician before introducing sauna bathing into their regular regimen.

Dosage: One 2021 review on sauna use noted:

"For individuals interested in implementing sauna bathing into their daily routine, observational data suggest sessions initially lasting at least 10 min that should be prolonged to 15 min two–three times a week, to induce the process of acclimation and begin seeing benefits such as a reduced risk of sudden cardiac death, lowered blood pressure and resting heart rate, and an improvement of arterial compliance.

Following six–seven sauna bathing sessions, the duration of each session can increase in increments of 5 min every 2–3 days, until a timeframe of 45 min is reached, as research shows no meaningful health benefits beyond this duration.

Studies incorporating dry saunas have used a range of temperatures (70–95 °C) to induce adaptations; however, in general, the American College of Sports Medicine recommends a temperature range between 70 and 77 °C to achieve the cardiometabolic benefits of sauna bathing. It is assumed that temperatures less than 70 °C may not be sufficient to induce a hormetic effect, while temperatures greater than 100 °C would likely cause cellular damage and premature protein denaturation."[1131]

SEAWEED

Some possible benefits include: anti-inflammation, anti-oxidation, anti-cancer, anti-viral, immunomodulation, cardioprotection, mood-boosting, and neuroprotective.

Seaweed has been used and is continuing to be used traditionally as food in China, Japan, and Korea, as well as in some Latin American countries such as Mexico, for several centuries. In 600 BCE, the Chinese writer Sze Teu wrote, "Some algae are a delicacy fit for the most honoured guests, even for the King himself." a statement that is now being appreciated in other countries that haven't typically eaten them.[1132]

The use of seaweed for medicinal purposes has also been common since ancient times, especially in traditional medicine in Asian countries.[1133] Documented evidence of this has been found in Chinese medical books called "The Compendium of Materia Medica," written by Shizhen Li in 1578. In these books, certain seaweeds were noted to treat thyroid-related diseases such as goitre, whilst others were said to have the ability to soften hard lumps, dispel nodes, eliminate phlegm, and induce urination in humans.[1134]

Seaweed are aquatic plant-like algae of simple structure with little or no cellular differentiation nor complex tissues. They are classified taxonomically into three groups: Chlorophyta, Phaeophyceae, and Rhodophyta, which correspond to green, brown, and red algae, respectively.[1135] Seaweeds are frequently subjected to harsh environmental conditions with no visible damage; as a result, they produce a wide range of metabolites (xanthophylls, tocopherols, and polysaccharides) in order to defend themselves from living and non-living factors. These metabolites, as well as other nutritional components, are beginning to be recognised as a source of great pharmacological promise in modern medicine.[1135]

The chemical composition of seaweed depends on the species, place of cultivation, atmospheric conditions, and harvesting period. Overall, seaweed have a high protein content (higher in green and red seaweed compared to brown);[1135] are a good source of omega fatty acids; and have an abundance of essential minerals such as sodium, calcium, magnesium, potassium, chloride, sulphate, phosphorus, and micronutrients such as iodine, iron, zinc, copper, selenium, molybdenum, fluoride, manganese, boron, nickel, cobalt, etc.[1136]

They are also an excellent source of vitamins A, B1, B12, C, D, and E; riboflavin; niacin; pantothenic acid; and folic acid, as well as containing other health-promoting bioactive compounds.[1137]

The differences in colour between the three main types of seaweed correspond to differences in their structural makeup and, thus, biological properties. The typical brown colour of Phaeophyceae is due to the presence of a particular pigment called fucoxanthin. Studies showed that fucoxanthin has anticancer, antioxidant, and anti-obesity properties.[1138,1139,1140] Phlorotannins are also very specific polyphenols present in brown algae and function to protect seaweeds from UV radiation, stress, and herbivory but also contribute to cell wall resistance.[1138] Phlorotannins have shown antiviral, antioxidant, anti-inflammatory, anti-diabetic, and neuroprotective activities.[1138,1141,1142,1143]

Brown seaweed also contains fucoidan, and fucoidan has been shown to possess anti-bacterial, antiviral, anti-inflammatory, antithrombotic, antidiabetic, anti-cancer, and procoagulant effects.[1144-1149] The structural size of fucoidan plays a part in its effect, with low- and high-molecular-weight fucoidan having different properties in clotting, for example.

Secondary metabolites such as sesquiterpenes, diterpenes, triterpenes, and many others are abundant in marine red algae and have a variety of biological activities such as antifungal, antibacterial, and anticancer properties.[1150] Carrageenans are sulfated polysaccharides present only in red algae and have shown antioxidant and antiviral characteristics, as well as strong cholesterol-lowering capabilities.[1151,1152]

Green algae are green due to the presence of chlorophyll and carotenoids, owing to their antioxidant activities.[1153] The most important sulfated polysaccharide from the cell wall of green seaweeds is ulvan. Ulvan has shown antioxidant and cholesterol-lowering properties.[1154]

The majority of research studying the benefits of seaweed has been done in cell cultures or on animal models. Epidemiological evidence indicates that seaweed-containing diets are inversely associated with all-cause mortality and cardiovascular disease mortality in Japanese adults.[1155] And case control studies have shown an inverse relationship between seaweed consumption and stomach and colon cancer.[1156,1157]

Interestingly, one randomised placebo-controlled clinical trial showed the use of the edible algal extract (Ulva Lactuca) daily for three months significantly improving the feeling of reduced ability to experience pleasure as well as sleep scores in those depressed.[1158]

With regards to COVID-19, one cell study showed sulfated polysaccharides having better SARS-CoV-2 blocking abilities than Remdesivir.[1159] Another *in vitro* study of iota-, lambda-, and kappa-carrageenan sulfated polysaccharides extracted from red seaweed on SARS-CoV-2 Wuhan type and variants Alpha, Beta, Gamma, and Delta showed that all three carrageenan types had antiviral activity, with authors concluding that iota-carrageenan might be effective for prophylaxis and treatment of SARS-CoV-2 for existing and potentially future variants.[1160] Plus, another review hypothesised that orally ingested seaweeds might exert direct antiviral effects against SARS-CoV-2 within the intestine through fucoidan and other components.[1161]

Nasal sprays may be the way forward, though. A meta-analysis of individual patient data from two randomised controlled trials found that nasal iota-carrageenan enhanced recovery rates and decreased the duration of protracted colds.[1162] Long colds (lasting more than 20 days) were reduced by 71%. For coronavirus infections, the recovery rate increased by 139%, for influenza A infections by 119%, and for rhinovirus infections by 70%. And an *in vitro* study showed that carrageenan-containing nose spray and mouth spray inhibit SARS-CoV-2 in human airway epithelial cells.[1163]

Though a non-toxic food, the overconsumption of seaweed, especially if sourced from polluted areas, is a concern. Firstly, seaweed is known for its high iodine levels. Iodine intake in Japan, known for their love of seaweed, varies from 0.1 to 20 mg/day, which can greatly exceed the official RDA of 150 mcg/day.[1164,1165] The epidemiology research on the risks and benefits of consuming iodine from seaweeds is ambiguous. Seaweed consumption was linked to an increased risk of papillary thyroid carcinoma in Japanese postmenopausal women but not in premenopausal women.[1166] However, another study found no link between seaweed consumption and total thyroid cancer risk or papillary thyroid carcinoma in premenopausal or postmenopausal women.[1167]

Sufficient iodine levels are paramount to the proper functioning of the thyroid, but overconsumption has been linked to both overactive and underactive thyroid function.[1168,1169] Due to the unpredictability and excessive iodine concentration of seaweeds, the use of seaweed supplements is not suggested for pregnant women, with kelp-based products being of particular concern.[1170] Plus, the interaction of iodine supplementation and exposure to heavy metals in seaweed, such as mercury, may further compromise thyroid function by lowering total T3.[1171]

The consumption of anti-thyroid compounds called goitrogens, such as soybeans, broccoli, and bok choy, may protect against high iodine levels, and intriguingly, many traditional Japanese dishes (such as soups) that contain seaweed also contain foods with a known goitrogen content.[1172]

This brings us to the second point. Another concern about seaweed consumption is exposure to heavy metals such as arsenic, aluminium, cadmium, lead, rubidium, silicon, strontium, and tin.[1173] The majority of edible seaweeds have been shown to contain trace quantities of heavy metals. Cooking, boiling, and food processing operations may help minimise the amount of heavy metals in edible seaweeds; however, more studies are needed in this area.[1164,1174]

Dosage: Due to the variety of seaweed and lack of scientific guidance, there is no recommended daily consumption of seaweed.

9 g of Nori (the lowest source of iodine from seaweed) is estimated to be enough to meet your daily requirements of iodine when consumed.

A daily dosage of 2.4–8 mg of fucoxanthin has shown benefit in some human studies over a prolonged period of time.[1175]

SERRAPEPTASE

Some possible benefits include: anti-inflammation, anti-oxidation, anti-cancer, anti-bacterial, anti-amyloidogenic, and anti-mucus.

Serrapeptase is a zinc-containing enzyme originally obtained from the bacteria *Serratia marcescens,* isolated from the intestine of the silkworm *Bombyx mori* L.[1176] It is a proteolytic enzyme, meaning it breaks down proteins. It has also been shown to have anti-inflammatory, fibrinolytic, and other beneficial properties against breast disease, atherosclerosis, Alzheimer's disease, sinusitis, hepatitis, lung disorders, and uterine fibroids.[1176,1177]

Serrapeptase is most commonly used as an anti-inflammatory agent, but though this is the case, there is very little evidence about the molecular mechanism of how serrapeptase actually works. It has been alluded to that serrapeptase reduces the leakiness of small blood vessels caused by a variety of hormones, breaks down abnormal exudates and proteins, and facilitates the absorption of decomposed products through the blood and lymphatics.[1178] It is also thought to be different from other conventional anti-inflammatory drugs by working to regulate immune cell migration from lymph nodes to inflamed and injured tissues.[1179]

In one study of 24 individuals undergoing the surgical removal of impacted molars, it was noted that those in the serrapeptase group had a significant reduction in the extent of cheek swelling and pain intensity compared to controls.[1180] And a clinical trial on 70 patients with breast engorgement demonstrated that serratiopeptidase treatment resulted in moderate to marked improvement in breast pain, swelling, and induration with no adverse events reported.[1181]

Serrapeptase has properties other than acting as an anti-inflammatory agent. The use of this enzyme has been shown to reduce the thickness and viscosity of mucus and improve the elimination of bronchopulmonary secretions in allergic conditions, as well as having wound-healing properties by dissolving dead tissue surrounding the injured area without harming living tissue.[1182,1183]

Bacterial biofilms are clusters of bacteria that are attached to a surface and/or to each other and embedded in a self-produced matrix.[1184] Biofilms have great resilience to the adaptive and innate immune systems, as well as tolerance to high doses of antibiotics/antimicrobial drugs. They are associated with a variety of infections like urinary tract infections, chronic lung infections, endocarditis, osteomyelitis, and chronic and acute otitis media, and are nearly 100 times more resistant to antimicrobial agents as compared to individual bacterial colonies, thus leading to antibiotic treatment failure.[1184,1176]

Serrapeptase has shown to be effective against bacterial biofilms, as well as enhancing the effects of antibiotics against bacterial biofilms.[1185,1186] Colonisation of bacteria occurs at the surface of the implants. In one study of 64 adults, serrapeptase in combination with antibiotics was shown to significantly improve clinical, microbiological, and inflammatory parameters as compared to the control group. The authors concluded that serrapeptase enhanced the efficacy of antibiotics by increasing their tissue concentration.[1186]

Another novel and intriguing application of serrapeptase is in the therapy of Alzheimer's disease by lowering amyloidosis. In a rat model, serratiopeptidase was found to be equally effective as nattokinase in alleviating Alzheimer's disease pathogenesis. These results were confirmed by histological examination of brain tissue and showed that serrapeptase can down-regulate the amyloidogenic pathway due to its proteolytic, anti-oxidant, and anti-amyloidogenic effects.[639]

Most interestingly, one 2020 review on serrapeptase notes, *"Because the enzyme digests non-living tissue and leaves live tissue alone; it may be effective in removing the deposits of fatty substances, cholesterol, cellular waste products, calcium and fibrin on the inside of the arteries. The fibrinolytic (clot removal) activity of serratiopeptidase may also be able to help with thickened blood, increased risk of stroke, and phlebitis/thrombophlebitis."*[1182]

Though used for a decade and with high safety evidence supported by various studies, side effects are not unheard of. In the literature, Stevens-Johnson syndrome and buccal space abscess have been reported as side effects of this molecule.[1176,1187,1188] To further investigate the safety profile, detailed, professionally designed controlled clinical investigations must be done.

Dosage: In the majority of human trials, the common doses of serrapeptase vary from 10 to 60 mg/day in divided doses, with the most desired amount of 10 mg, thrice daily for up to 4 weeks on an empty stomach.

10 mg is considered equal to 20,000 units of enzyme activity.

Due to its anti-inflammatory, fibrinolytic, and mucus-breaking effects, one review proposed that *"the dose of 10 mg thrice daily could be examined as an adjuvant in COVID-19."*[1189]

SHILAJIT

Some possible benefits include: anti-inflammation, anti-oxidation, neuroprotection, immune-boosting, testosterone-boosting, connective-tissue strengthening, anti-fatigue, anti-viral, anti-COVID-19, graphene oxide-removing, glyphosate-removing, and oxygen level-increasing.

Shilajit is a Sanskrit word meaning "conqueror of mountains and destroyer of weakness" and "winner of rocks."[1190] It is a natural blackish-brown powder or resin-like substance found in high mountain rocks, especially in the Himalayas, although it has also been found in Russia, Tibet, Afghanistan, and now in the north of Chile, where it is named Andean Shilajit.[1191]

Shilajit is produced by the decomposition of plant material from a variety of species and has been known and used for centuries by Ayurvedic medicine as a rejuvenator and an anti-aging compound.[1192]

Shilajit is composed mainly of humic substances, including fulvic acid (which accounts for around 60% to 80% of the total nutraceutical compound), humic acid, and other minerals, including selenium.[1193] In total, it is said to contain more than 84 types of minerals, providing most of the body's essential minerals.[1190]

Though few in number, investigations on shilajit have been promising and show a variety of physiologically beneficial properties, including antioxidant; cognition and mood enhancing; antidiabetic; anxiety-reducing; antiallergic; immunomodulatory; anti-inflammatory; analgesic; antifungal; neuroprotective; energy-increasing; testosterone increasing; connective-tissue strengthening; and properties useful for protection at high altitudes.[1190,1991,1194-1199]

Shilajit is also said to help with the absorption of iron into the body, making it bioavailable to bone marrow stem cells for blood formation and thus helpful in coping with hypoxia-like conditions as well as helping the body eliminate toxins.[1190] Most interestingly, fulvic acid has been shown to inhibit the aggregation and promote the disassembly of tau fibrils associated with Alzeimer's disease.[1191]

Other than in shilajit, large amounts of humic substances are generated in forests and peat, originating from decayed plants in the soil that are decomposed by microbes. Humic substances have been used in other ancient medical practices and have since been clinically trialled and found to confer numerous beneficial features, e.g., possibly protecting the human body against blood coagulation or fibrinolysis as well as decreasing the effects of ionising radiation.[1200,1201]

Both fulvic and humic acids have shown further benefits, including antiviral, immunomodulatory, and heavy metal chelating properties.[1202] In one study, mice and rats given fulvic acid substantially increased their total T cell and antibody production.[1202] Another source speculated that the use of humic substances may prove effective at preventing HIV transmission.[1203] Plus, there has been some evidence suggesting that fulvic acid may be able to interact with and remove graphene oxide; however, these tests have not been carried out on animals or humans.[1204,1205] Fulvic and humic acidsweres also shown to reduce glyphosate in adult humans over a two-week course.[1206]

With regards to COVID-19, one 2020 study showed that fulvic acid had a strong binding affinity to spike proteins and ACE2 receptors.[1207] And more recently, *in vitro* humic acid complexes containing vitamin C, selenium, and zinc ions, even at tiny concentrations, were enough to achieve 50% viral replication inhibition in the applied SARS-CoV-2 virus inhibition test.[1208]

Dosage: There is no official recommended dosage for shilajit.

One trial gave participants 500 mg of shilajit for eight weeks with no reported related adverse effects.[1197]

In another study, participants received 250 mg/capsule orally, twice a day, for 90 days.[1198]

And one review on the subject noted, *"The recommended dose of Shilajit for maintenance of optimal health is 300–500 mg/day." Shilajit powder taken with milk twice a day will ensure optimal blood levels and therapeutic efficacy."*[1190]

TAURINE

Some possible benefits include: anti-inflammation, anti-oxidation, mitochondrial healing, neuroprotection, anti-prion, cardioprotection, anti-diabetes, blood pressure reduction, and anti-muscle wasting.

Taurine is an amino acid found in very high concentration in most cells. In some species, such as cats and foxes, taurine is an essential nutrient, whose deficiency not only causes pathology in those animals but also shortens their lifespan.[1209,1210,1211] By contrast, taurine is classified as a conditionally essential nutrient or a functional nutrient in humans.[1212] Although humans are incapable of producing huge amounts of taurine, human tissues retain more taurine than those of cats or foxes. Thus, unlike cats, people do not typically develop overt indications of taurine deficiency.

The rate of taurine biosynthesis by the liver, heart, and brain is low in humans; therefore, the major source of taurine in humans is the diet, with the primary sources being seafood, eggs, and meat.[1213] Thus, a lack of taurine consumption may contribute to taurine deficiency.

Taurine deficiency has been reported to induce several diseases in animal models, including retinal degeneration, dilated cardiomyopathy, immune dysfunction, raised blood pressure, and ageing.[1215-1218]

In humans, higher incidences of the development of hypertension as well as cardiac diseases have been reported in populations with low-taurine diets,[1213] whereas elevated taurine consumption has been associated with a decreased risk of high blood pressure and high cholesterol.[1219,1220] Taurine supplementation is also linked to diminished BMI and reduced levels of inflammation markers in obese women.[1217,1221]

Taurine transporter knockout mice were recently employed to study the effects of taurine tissue depletion. These mice developed multiorgan dysfunction. This likely happened because taurine is involved in a multitude of vital biologically protective processes.[1222]

It has been found that taurine acts as an antioxidant via three mechanisms. Firstly, it neutralises the neutrophil oxidant, hypochlorous acid.[1223,1224] Second, it diminishes the generation of superoxide by the mitochondria.[1225] Third, ROS produced by mitochondria can harm antioxidant enzymes that protect against oxidative stress.[1217] Because the function of some antioxidant enzymes is vulnerable to oxidative damage, taurine may minimise oxidative stress by avoiding enzyme damage.

Mitochondrial oxidative stress not only negatively impacts surrounding cellular components but is capable of triggering mitochondrial death itself.[1226] The antioxidant and especially mitochondrial-protective properties of taurine are no better highlighted in mitochondrial disease, mitochondrial encephalopathy (brain disease), lactic acidosis, and stroke-like episodes (MELAS), where the formation of the taurine conjugate is impaired. Taurine treatment in MELAS acts as a substrate for the taurine conjugation reaction, restoring mitochondrial protein production, enhancing mitochondrial activity, and decreasing superoxide formation.[1227,1228] Toxins also promoting mitochondrial oxidative stress, including ozone, nitrogen dioxide, bleomycin, amiodarone, arsenic, iron, Adriamycin, and catecholamine (to name a few), also respond favourably to taurine therapy.[1229]

Taurine also improves cellular energy metabolism by aiding mitochondrial function. This is demonstrated when those with heart failure are given the protein. Taurine is deficient in the hearts of patients suffering from heart failure. Restoration of taurine levels in these patients through supplementation leads to improved contractile function.[1230]

The endoplasmic reticulum (ER) is the transportation system of the cell; it also has many other important functions, such as protein folding. When exposed to damaging stimuli, like the accumulation of defective proteins, the ER becomes dysfunctional. These stressors can trigger the ER stress response, which causes cell death by altering ER protein levels. According to current research, ER stress is linked to the occurrence and progression of neurodegenerative disorders such as prion diseases.[1231] Taurine deficiency is associated with ER stress, and it has been proposed that taurine might alter protein folding, either by reducing oxidative stress or by providing a better environment for protein folding.[1232] Thus, taurine may aid in the treatment of neurodegenerative diseases, including Alzheimer's, Huntington's, and Parkinson's diseases.

Taurine may also aid as a neuroprotective agent as it can substitute for gamma-aminobutyric acid (GABA), the major inhibitory neurotransmitter that reduces neuronal excitability.[1233] Glutamate works oppositely and is the most abundant excitatory neurotransmitter, produced in massive amounts in neurodegenerative conditions like stroke. Toxicity in the CNS commonly occurs when an imbalance develops between excitatory and inhibitory neurotransmitters. As taurine has shown to activate GABA receptors, it may be one way it aids in conditions like stroke.[1234]

Another thing that happens during a stroke and/or heart attack is the excess accumulation of calcium ions (Ca2+) in the affected organ.[1217] This, in turn, kills surrounding tissue. Taurine protects the cell by diminishing Ca2+ overload via a variety of mechanisms.[1235] There is abundant evidence that taurine is effective in treating stroke in animals, however only a few in humans.[1234] In one observational study, the analysis of five diet-related factors revealed that both magnesium and taurine concentrations were negatively associated with ischemic heart disease mortality, while taurine was also negatively associated with stroke mortality.

The use of taurine has also been seen as beneficial in other conditions, including Parkinson's disease, epilepsy, retinal degeneration, heart failure, high blood pressure, atherosclerosis, cardiac arrhythmias, mitochondrial diseases, diabetic-associated conditions, arthritis, age-related muscle loss, and muscular dystrophy. [1217,1228, 1236-1244]

Interestingly, taurine is effective in reducing the adverse actions of norepinephrine through its ability to both decrease catecholamine overflow and diminish cell signalling.[1217] Excess catecholamine release being the working theory of recent spike related cardiac death.

The use of magnesium and taurine together has shown improvements in endothelial function and diminished risk of atherogenesis.[1241] Plus, according to a clinical report, oral taurine plus L-arginine treatment significantly reduced ventricular arrhythmias in three individuals.[1242]

With regards to COVID-19, the use of taurine has been recommended by researchers *"as a promising available therapeutic approach in COVID-19 patient management, for which minimal to no side effects are known."*[1245]

Raised circulating blood sugar levels down regulate the human taurine transporter, and as we know, increased glucose concentration has shown to significantly promote viral proliferation and inflammatory cytokine production.[1246] During the severe and critical phases, taurine levels could be depleted by SARS-CoV-2-induced hyperglycemia, thus explaining the decreased taurine levels found in several studies.[1247] During the recovery phase, inflammation is controlled and taurine levels gradually increase, except in long COVID-19 patients.[1247] Potentially, this means that those with long-term sequelae may need extra taurine for support. But evidence with regards to this has been mixed.[1248]

Dosage: A range of 1–6 grams per day has been used in studies. The most

common protocol to reduce blood pressure is 1.5 grams per day, divided into three doses of 0.5 grams.[1249]

TULSI

Some possible benefits include: adaptogenic, immunomodulation, anticancer, anti-inflammation, antioxidant, hepatoprotection, radioprotection, heavy metal and toxin protection, antimicrobial, anti-viral, antidiabetic effects, mood-boosting, anti-spike protein, testosterone-boosting, and anti-male fertility.

Tulsi, also known as holy basil, is an aromatic herb native to India and has been highly valued for its medicinal properties in the Ayurvedic and Siddha medical systems for thousands of years. It is thought to have originated in north central India and now grows native throughout the eastern world tropics.[1250] Tulsi is known as "The Incomparable One," "Mother Medicine of Nature," and "The Queen of Herbs" in Ayurveda and is treasured as an "elixir of life", unparalleled in both medical and spiritual virtues.[1251]

Tulsi is treasured in Hinduism, and every part of the tulsi plant is revered and considered sacred, including the leaves, stem, blossom, root, seeds, and oil.[1251] Even the surrounding soil, which has lately been discovered to carry beneficial endophytic fungi, is seen as divine.[1252] Many households in India are regarded as incomplete without a tulsi plant, which is generally housed in an elegant earthen pot in a courtyard where tulsi serves both utilitarian and ceremonial purposes. The clove-like aroma from its high eugenol content serves to link the householder to the divine while also repelling mosquitoes, flies, and other harmful insects. Tulsi is also incorporated into daily life through nightly and morning rituals, as well as various spiritual and purifying acts that may include ingesting its leaves or drinking tulsi tea.[1251]

Three types of tulsi are commonly described. *Ocimum tenuiflorum* (or *Ocimum sanctum* L.), which includes two types, Rama or Sri tulsi (green leaves) and Krishna or Shyama tulsi (purplish leaves);[1253] and *Ocimum gratissimum*, also known as Vana or wild or forest tulsi (dark green leaves).[1254] The different kinds of tulsi vary greatly in shape and phytochemical composition, including secondary metabolites, but they are used in the same way to treat similar ailments.[1255] The three may be differentiated from other *Ocimum* species by the colour of their yellow pollen, which contains significant levels of eugenol.

Traditionally, tulsi is said to help prevent sickness, increase general health, wellbeing, and longevity, and aid in dealing with daily pressures.[1251] It is credited with "giving lustre to the complexion, sweetness to the voice and fostering beauty, intelligence, stamina and a calm emotional disposition."[1251] It is also used to treat a variety of conditions, including anxiety, cough, asthma, diarrhoea, fever, dysentery, arthritis, eye diseases, otalgia, indigestion, hiccups, vomiting, gastric, cardiac, and genitourinary disorders, back pain, skin diseases, ringworm, insect, snake, and scorpion bites, and malaria.

Tulsi is increasingly being recognised as a potent adaptogen with a unique combination of pharmacological actions that promote wellbeing and resilience.

Numerous *in vitro* and animal studies attest to tulsi leaf having potent pharmacological actions that include adaptogenic, metabolic, immunomodulatory, anticancer, anti-inflammatory, antioxidant, hepatoprotective, radioprotective, antimicrobial, and antidiabetic effects.[1256-1265]

Like many other herbs described in this book, it is thought that many of the physiological benefits of tulsi can be attributed to its ability to assist with the body's internal housekeeping and protection of the body from toxin-induced damage via increasing levels of antioxidant molecules such as glutathione and enhancing the activity of antioxidant enzymes such as superoxide dismutase and catalase.[1266,1267]

This ability to protect the body from external toxins is further demonstrated by its ability to help prevent cancer by reducing DNA damage.[1268] Lab studies have shown that extracts are able to induce the killing of unwanted cancerous cells, thereby reducing the growth of experimental tumours and enhancing survival.[1269,1270] Furthermore, tulsi not only protects against the damage caused by toxic compounds but also helps the body transform and eliminate them more effectively by increasing the activity of liver detoxification enzymes such as the cytochrome P450 enzymes, which deactivate toxic chemicals and allow them to be safely excreted.[1271]

Numerous experimental studies have documented the ability of tulsi to protect against the damaging effects of various toxicants including butylparaben (food, pharmaceutical and cosmetic preservative);[1272] carbon tetrachloride (an industrial solvent);[1273] copper sulphate (a fungicide, algaecide, root killer, and herbicide);[1274] ethanol;[1275] rogor (an insecticide);[1276] chlorpyrifos;[1277] endosulfan (an insecticide);[1278] lindane (a neurotoxin antiparasitic);[1279] meloxicam (an antiarthritic NSAID);[1280] paracetamol;[1281] haloperidol (an antipsychotic);[1282] various anti-tubercular drugs;[1283] lead;[1284] arsenic;[1285] iodine;[1286] mercury[1287] and radiation.[1288]

Other than protecting against the toxic effects of chemicals, heavy metals, and radiation, tulsi may also protect against mental and physical stress-related pathology. Tulsi has been shown in preclinical tests to increase swimming survival times in mice and to prevent stress-induced ulcers in rats, with antistress benefits comparable to those of antidepressant medications.[1289,1290] Similarly, recent research has shown that ethanolic and aqueous tulsi leaf extracts protect rats against stress-induced cardiovascular alterations.[1291,1292] Similarly, experimental investigations have demonstrated that tulsi can lessen the effects of acute and chronic noise-induced stress in rats, with increased neurotransmitter and oxidative stress levels in certain brain regions, as well as enhanced immunological, ECG, and corticosteroid responses.[1293,1294,1295]

Neurologically, tulsi has been shown to improve memory and cognitive function in animals and protect against age-related memory losses.[1296,1297] Tulsi has also been shown in human research to reduce stress, anxiety, and depression, with a 6-week, randomised, double-blind, placebo-controlled study finding that it considerably reduces general stress levels, sexual and sleep issues, and symptoms such as forgetfulness and weariness.[1298,1299] The two studies mentioned reported reductions of 31.6%–39% in overall stress-related symptoms in patients with psychosomatic problems compared to a control group.[1298,1299]

Tulsi has also shown anti-diabetic, metabolically improving, and thus cardioprotective properties. Tulsi has been demonstrated in animal studies to lower blood glucose levels, rectify aberrant lipid profiles, and protect the liver and kidneys from the metabolic damage caused by high glucose levels.[1300,1301,1302] Tulsi has also been proven in laboratory animals fed high-fat diets to enhance lipid profiles, prevent weight gain, hyperglycemia, hyperinsulinemia, hypertriglyceridemia, and insulin resistance, as well as protect organs and blood vessels from atherosclerosis.[1303,1304,1305] In humans, one randomised placebo-controlled clinical trial reported daily ingestion of 2.5g of tulsi leaves led to significant improvements blood and urine glucose levels in type 2 diabetes patients after 4 weeks.[1306] In comparable trials with longer durations, FBG and PPG improved by 1.2–2.2 and 1.5–6.0 folds, respectively, while HbA1c improved by 1.5 and 3.2 folds after 12–13 weeks.[1307,1308] In a separate 12-week randomised experiment of diabetic patients, 2 g of tulsi leaf extract alone or in combination with neem leaf extract reduced diabetes symptoms significantly, with the combination having the highest benefit.[1309]

Other than blood sugar levels, trials have found that giving those with high blood pressure 30 mL of fresh tulsi leaf juice once a day or twice daily for 10 and 12 days improved their blood pressure significantly.[1310] Another study reported improvement in serum cholesterol numbers with no difference in blood pressure in healthy adults who administered 300mg per day of tulsi leaf ethanolic extract for 4 weeks.[1311] A more recent study found that obese participants who took 250mg capsules of tulsi leaf extract twice day for 8 weeks improved their lipid profiles and BMI.[1308]

With regards to immunology, tulsi has also been shown to boost defences against infective threats by enhancing immune responses in non-stressed and stressed animals and healthy humans.[1251] There is also evidence showing its ability to help in the treatment of various bacterial, fungal, parasitic, and viral illnesses.[1312-1315] Tulsi has also been shown to be effective against many animal pathogens, which has led to its use in animal husbandry to reduce infections;[1251,1316] and tulsi's activity against water-borne and food-borne pathogens suggests that it can be used in food preservation, herbal raw materials, water purification, and as a hand sanitiser.[1317,1318,1319]

Human trials assessing tulsi's immunomodulatory activities have been promising. After 4 weeks of taking 300 mg of ethanolic tulsi leaf extract daily before food, one small randomised double-blind, placebo-controlled trial demonstrated improved immune response with increased NK and T-helper cells in healthy adult participants compared to placebo volunteers.[1311] Another 2-week study in which young adult volunteers were given nutrition bars fortified with 1 g of ethanolic tulsi leaf extract discovered that the intervention group had significantly improved exercise capacity, less fatigue, and an improved immune response to viral infection, as indicated by a lower load of human herpesvirus 6 in their saliva compared to the control group.[1320]

Another clinical trial investigated the effect of daily administration of 10 g of an aqueous extract of fresh tulsi leaves in patients with acute viral encephalitis, reporting increased survival after 4 weeks in the tulsi group compared to a dexamethasone-treated group.[1321] And a further trial of asthmatic patients discovered that taking

500mg of dried tulsi leaves three times daily enhanced lung function and relieved asthmatic symptoms within three days.[1255]

With regards to COVID-19, eugenol, the aromatic compound in tulsi, was found to inhibit the interaction between SARS-CoV-2 spike S1 and ACE2 to induce therapeutic responses.[1322] Eugenol also inhibited the activation of NF-B by SARS-CoV-2 spike S1 and the production of IL-6, IL-1, and TNF in human A549 lung cells.[1322] Furthermore, in SARS-CoV-2 spike S1-intoxicated mice, oral eugenol treatment reduced pulmonary inflammation and fever, improved heart function, and increased locomotor activities; with authors stating, *"Therefore, selective targeting of SARS-CoV-2 spike S1, but not ACE2, by eugenol may be beneficial for COVID-19 treatment."*[1322]

Eugenol has been reported to be present in several other plant families not excluded only to tulsi leaves, including Eugenia caryophyllata (clove), *Zingiber officinale* (ginger), bark and leaves of *Cinnamomum verum* (cinnamon), *Curcuma longa* (turmeric), and peppers (*Solanaceae*) as well as various aromatic plants such as *Cinnamomum* verum (true cinnamon), *Ocimum basilicum* (basil), *Myristica fragrans* Houtt. (nutmeg), and *Cinnamomum loureirii* Nees. (Saigon cinnamon).[1323] The major natural source of eugenol is *Eugenia caryophyllata* (syn. *Syzygiumaromaticum)*, which comprises 45-90%.[1324]

Eugenol has shown remarkable anti-inflammatory, antioxidant, analgesic, and antimicrobial properties, has a significant effect on human health, and may be the major bioactive component of tulsi.[1323]

The other researched bioactive compound in tulsi is ursolic acid, which is also found in apple peels. Ursolic acid may have *anti*-fertility properties. In one study 2g fresh tulsi was given to male albino rabbits for 30 days and showed a significant decrease in sperm count but significant increase in testosterone levels.[1325] Ursolic acid was shown in another study to aggravate metabolic syndrome related negative impact on male fertility in rats.[1326] However, results are mixed, with another study showing that ursolic acid protecting LPS-induced reduced sperm motility by increasing sperm density and motility.[1327]

Dosage: There are no official dosages for tulsi. 250 mg taken twice daily to 14 g once a day of the leaf extract appears to be the range of dosages used in studies.[1328]

VITAMIN K2 (MENAQUINONES)

Some possible benefits include: antioxidation, bone health improvement, endothelial health improvement, immunomodulation, anti-diabetic, neuroprotection, anti-cancer, and pro-fertility.

The original term "vitamin K" comes from the K in the Germanic word "Koagulation", meaning the ability to clot blood or prevent haemorrhage, which is why drugs like warfarin, which work by blocking the function of vitamin K, are given to patients with clotting disorders.[1329]

However, in recent years other forms of vitamin K have been discovered, and thus the term "vitamin K" refers to not just one, but a group of fat-soluble vitamins regarded as crucial cofactors for the creation of numerous proteins involved in coagulation *and* calcium homeostasis.

Vitamin K1 (phylloquinone) participates in blood clotting, serving as a cofactor for proteins found in clotting factors. It is naturally sourced in green leafy vegetables and some plant oils. Vitamin K2 (menaquinones) acts on organs other than the liver (bone, brain, vasculature, testis, pancreas, kidneys, and lungs) to activate K2-dependent proteins such as osteocalcin and matrix gla protein (MGP). The most common forms of vitamin K2 in the human diet are menaquinone-4 (MK-4) and menaquinone-7 (MK-7), short- and long-chained molecules, respectively.[1329]

Menaquinones, which are mainly bacterial in origin, are found in small amounts in various dairy and fermented products. MK-4 is found naturally in butter, egg yolks, lard, and animal-based foods, as well as being synthesised by bacteria in the intestinal tract (however, synthesised MK-4 is bound to the membranes of bacteria in the gut and very little is absorbed in humans).[1330] While the main sources of MK-7 are hard cheeses in the Western diet and natto in Asian cuisine, Natto contains the highest content of K2, in particular MK-7 (321 ng/g of K1 and 10,985 ng/g of K2).[1331,1332]

There is also menadione, or vitamin K3—a synthetic form of the vitamin—but it's also formed in the body as a result of the metabolic conversion of phylloquinone. Menadione has been banned by the FDA due to potential toxicity (hemolytic anaemia), but is being studied as a potential aid in cancer and cosmetic therapies.[1333,1334]

Osteocalcin, a protein activated by vitamin K2, also referred to as bone γ-carboxyglutamic acid (Gla) protein, is a protein that binds to calcium ions in hydroxyapatite found in teeth and bone.[1335] It functions to regulate bone mineralisation as well as prevent bone damage by external forces by improving fracture toughness.[1336,1337] Osteocalcin also acts as a hormone helping to regulate glucose metabolism by increasing insulin sensitivity, insulin secretion and promoting pancreatic β-cell proliferation.[1338] In fact, insulin receptor signalling in the bone-forming cells is required for osteocalcin production. This has been shown with mice lacking osteocalcin, which accumulate body fat and exhibit dramatic impairments in glucose metabolism.[1339] Mice without osteocalcin were also revealed to have low testosterone levels, low sperm counts, cognitive deficiencies, and features of anxiety and depression.[1340,1341] In this sense, osteocalcin is also likely involved in cognition and fertility. This was later confirmed with work indicating that insulin favours male fertility by stimulating bone turnover and bone cell-mediated activation of osteocalcin;[1342] osteocalcin has also been shown to cross the BBB and influence the production of many neurotransmitters that promote learning and memory formation.[1341] Other beneficial actions of osteocalcin appear to involve its ability to reverse autophagic dysfunction and endoplasmic reticulum stress resulting from diet-induced obesity.[1343,1344]

MPG is another vitamin K-dependent protein and is involved in the inhibition of vascular calcification.[1345] Upon activation by vitamin K2, MGP binds calcium salts with high affinity, thereby affecting the calcification processes. Mice without MPG die within two months after birth due to severe arterial calcification and rupture of the aorta.[1346] The activation of MGP by vitamin K2 also dampens inflammation-induced vascular and pulmonary tissue damage and is protective against atherosclerosis.[1347,1348]

Vitamin K may also suppress IL-6 production as well as inhibit the activation of proteins that are required for NF-kB activation.[1349,1350] Plus, vitamin K1 and especially vitamin K2 act as antioxidants with effects against the oxidative degradation of lipids and a 10- to 100-fold higher activity than other radical scavengers, such as alpha-tocopherol (vitamin E) and ubiquinone (coenzyme Q).[1351,1352] Both vitamin K1 and K2 prevent oxidative stress in neuronal cells, and K2 has shown to help facilitate the generation of ATP, rescuing mitochondrial dysfunction.[1353,1354]

K2 has also been shown to decrease the proliferation of T cells.[1355] T cells are known to play a critical role in promoting bone loss in postmenopausal osteoporosis as well as bone cancers and rheumatoid arthritis.[1356,1357] And thus, its T-cell-suppressing effects in this regard may be another mechanism by which vitamin K2 promotes healthy bone turnover.

The physiological importance of vitamin K2 has been noted in various studies. MK-7 has been proven in numerous trials with healthy and diseased patient cohorts to have a long-term protective effect on the development of calcification, reduce the overall risk of cardiovascular disease development, and even regress arterial stiffening and improve vascular elasticity in healthy population cohorts following supplementation.[1358-1361] It is important to note that in a study investigating all vitamin K1 and K2 isoforms, only K2 was effective and beneficial for cardiovascular health and not K1.[1361] It is also important to note that vascular calcification is one component of ageing.[1362]

Vitamin K2 supplementation has also been shown to reduce fracture risk in studies of population groups over 50, as well as the risk of diabetes development.[1363,1364] In one study of 38,000 men and women, aged 20–70, just 10 mcg/day of K2 was shown to decrease diabetes risk by 7%.[1365]

The status of dephosphorylated-uncarboxylated-MGP (dp-ucMGP) is a recognised research marker for vitamin K deficiency that was initially identified in individuals with chronic kidney disease (CKD).[1366] Those with CKD commonly suffer from vascular calcification, and in fact, circulating dp-ucMGP in one study was associated with mortality and decreased renal function in diabetic CKD.[1367,1368] Fortunately, vitamin K2 supplementation has been shown to improve renal artery function and prevent further development of renal artery calcification.[1369]

Other than this, vitamin K2 has been shown to prevent the growth and metastasis of multiple cell lines in lab studies.[1370,1371,1372] It is thought vitamin K2 has anti-cancer effects by promoting programmed cell death and inhibiting NF-kB pathways, as well as having chemosensitizing effects on cancer cells by working synergistically with other chemotherapeutic agents.[1372-1375] A study evaluating the effect of the K2 analogue menatetrenone on the recurrence rate of hepatocellular carcinoma (HCC) recurrence suggests that it may increase survival among surgically treated patients.[1376] Plus, a meta-analysis of randomised controlled trials and cohort studies on the efficacy of K2 therapy in HCC patients revealed that K2 can reduce the frequency of relapses and enhance overall survival in HCC patients as early as one year following surgery.[1377]

Other than these benefits, K2 supplementation has been shown to aid with PCOS symptoms and the related hormone profile,[1338] as well as showing the ability to improve body weight, waist circumference, body composition, and visceral fat levels.[1378,1348]

With regards to COVID-19, one study showed significantly lower levels of MK-7 in COVID-19 patients compared to healthy controls.[1350] They speculated that the disease itself may have in fact led to depleted levels of this protective vitamin, which in turn further led to pulmonary and vascular damage.[1350] Those with severe SARS-CoV-2 infections also often have comorbidities that are associated with reduced vitamin K status, such as hypertension, diabetes, and cardiovascular diseases.[1379] Another study showed elevated dp-ucMGP levels in COVID-19 patients compared to controls, indicating extrahepatic vitamin K insufficiency, leading to accelerated elastic fibre damage and thrombosis.[1380] Thrombosis because vitamin K is also known to activate the anticoagulant protein S which is made in endothelial cells and thought to play an important role in the local prevention of thrombosis.[1347]

Remember too that COVID-19 has been speculated to cause vascular calcification via oxidative stress and endothelial dysfunction, as well as being linked to worsened disease states.[1381] This was highlighted by one study that showed those with coronary artery calcification were more likely to require intubation and die than those without calcification.[1382]

The importance of vitamin K2 is further highlighted by the fact that it works closely with vitamin D. One common argument against vitamin D3 supplementation is that increasing intake could result in vitamin D toxicity, in turn causing a buildup of calcium in the blood and leading to vascular calcification, osteoporosis, and kidney stones.[1383] However, it has been reported that the reason for high calcium levels rather lies in a vitamin K2 deficiency.[1384] As osteocalcin synthesis rate is increased by higher vitamin D levels, K2 is thought to be required as a natural antagonist.[1385] Plus, it has been shown that high-dose vitamin D administration depletes extrahepatic vitamin K stores in rats by strongly up-regulating MGP synthesis and hastening elastic fibre calcification and degradation.[1386] Vitamin D administration in a state of vitamin K deficiency may thereby endanger pulmonary and vascular health, and so, as one group of researchers notes, *"It may therefore be prudent to first supplement vitamin K in invariably vitamin K-insufficient Covid-19 hospitalised patients and to start vitamin D supplementation in those who are vitamin D-deficient only when extrahepatic vitamin K status has been restored."*[1347]

MK-4 is more used in trials with bone outcomes, while MK-7 is more in trials with cardiovascular outcomes with dosages between 90–360 mcg.[1387] Of all the menaquinones, MK-7 is absorbed most efficiently and exhibits the greatest bioavailability.[1388] For this reason, MK-7 is rapidly becoming popular as a supplement and is available over the counter, usually at a dose of 100–120 mcg/day.[1329] It is critical to be aware that MK-7, when administered in excess of 50 mcg/day, can interact with anticoagulant medication.[1332]

Dosage: The minimum effective dose for MK-4 is 1,500 mcg. Doses of up to 45 mg (45,000 mcg) have been safely used in a superloading dosing protocol.

The minimum effective dose for MK-7 is between 90 and 360 mcg. Further research is needed to determine the maximum effective dose for MK-7.[1389]

It is critical to be aware that MK-7, when administered in excess of 50 mcg/day, can interact with anticoagulant medication.

VNS

Some possible benefits include: anti-inflammation, cardioprotection, autonomic dysfunction regulation, brain plasticity-inducing, sensory-boosting, memory-boosting, nerve growth, analgesic, anti-epileptic, fear-diminishing, and motor and sensory rehab-aiding.

As explained in the "Reduce Stress" section, the vagus nerve is the autonomic nervous system's longest nerve. It sends parasympathetic fibres to all of our organs (except the adrenal glands), from the neck down to a portion of our small intestine, allowing us to "rest and digest." It also helps regulate our heartbeat and is involved in other biological processes such as sweating and speaking. One way to activate the vagus nerve is via deep breathing; another way is to electrically stimulate it.

Vagus nerve stimulation (VNS) has been used as a treatment since 1997 to control seizures in epilepsy patients. Here, a neurostimulator is implanted in the chest to stimulate the vagus nerve. It has now been accepted that non-invasive VNS of the vagus nerve branch running around the left external ear (described as transcutaneous VNS) produces similar effects to invasive VNS.[1390] This highlights the potential benefits of using non-invasive VNS, similar to the application of invasive VNS in previous studies. And the benefits of VNS seem to be manyfold.

A 2019 study involving rats with severed nerves demonstrated that those who received rehabilitation *and* bursts of closed-loop vagus nerve stimulation (CL-VNS) had significantly larger areas of the brain related to movement (motor cortex) that evoked specific movements than those that didn't have vagus nerve stimulation. The rats that received rehabilitation *and CL-VNS* together also performed better than their counterparts who had vagus nerve stimulation after rehab.[1391] This study demonstrates that CL-VNS reverses the maladaptive central reorganisation resulting from nerve injury.[1391]

Furthermore, the study goes on to note that CL-VNS, when (and only when) coupled with rehab, reversed long-lasting pathological alterations in the cortical motor maps and improved motor function. In addition to reversing the maladaptive changes in the structure and function of the brain (a term called "plasticity") arising from nerve injury, the rats also displayed enhanced recovery of motor *and* sensory function without any observable changes in the peripheral nerves or muscles, as well as a reduction in pain.

Dopamine is typically said to play a key role in mediating motor cortex synaptic plasticity and is critical for motor skill acquisition; however, the VNS is thought to engage a different, unique set of neuromodulatory signalling pathways to promote plasticity.[1392]

These neuromodulatory signalling pathways are in two areas of the brain run by two different neuromodulators: the basal forebrain (the area of the brain responsible for wakefulness and the production of acetylcholine) and the locus coeruleus (an area in the brainstem responsible for stress and panic and a major producer of noradrenaline). The stimulation of these centres results in the subsequent release of neuromodulators throughout the cortex. Both of these neuromodulatory systems are key substrates in the expression of plasticity within the brain.[1393]

The rat study mentioned above goes on to state, *"These findings provide direct evidence that insufficient central plasticity can interfere with functional recovery after nerve damage and demonstrate that techniques that reverse maladaptive plasticity that occurs after nerve damage hold promise for improving function in the chronic phase of injury. Importantly, this strategy acts in conjunction with target reinnervation, and thus could be employed synergistically with therapeutics that aim to promote peripheral regeneration."*[1391]

Pairing VNS with rehabilitation may prove useful in treating a wide range of neurological disorders. In fact, a 2018 study that delivered cyclical VNS every 10 seconds for 30 minutes to stroke patients alongside rehab showed a sustained improvement in upper-limb impairment and functional measures at 1 year.[1394] This has similarly been shown in mice.[1395]

VNS paired with sounds have shown to drive the reorganisation in the auditory cortex (this has shown to help with tinnitus);[1396,1397] delivery of VNS after behavioural experience can enhance memory retention;[1398] and VNS paired with extinction training was effective at reducing a specific fear memory (and may be helpful in those who suffer with conditions like PTSD).[1398,1400] High-frequency (80 Hz) non-invasive VNS has also been shown to improve the sense of smell (olfactory function) in healthy adults.[1401]

In one study, memory was enhanced using VNS *after* the activity was performed.[1398] Here, the participants received one 30 second (30 Hz, 0.50 ms pulse width) shock after reading a paragraph of text. The study highlights the importance of shock strength with regards to memory consolidation; either too low or too high an intensity was found, but no significant changes were noted. Only 0.5 mA showed a benefit. This just highlights the fact that we need more studies in this area of research.

The benefits of VNS are not only restricted to the neurological realm, either. The most common autonomic mechanism behind numerous arrhythmias and conditions like postural orthostatic tachycardia syndrome (POTS) is likely an imbalance of the sympathetic and parasympathetic nervous systems, and VNS here may bring about balance.[1402] In one study of patients with an arrhythmia called atrial fibrillation (AF), low-level transcutaneous VNS (20 Hz) was shown to suppress AF and decrease levels of inflammatory cytokines.[1402] Another study showed that low-level transcutaneous VNS (20 Hz) for one hour a day for six months reduced the median AF burden by 85% in the active arm compared to the control arm.[1403] TNF-α levels were significantly decreased by 23% in the active relative to the control group too.[1403] In a study of dogs with heart attacks, researchers discovered that persistent transcutaneous low-level VNS (for 2 hours per day for 2 months) reduced the inducibility of another form of arrhythmia called ventricular tachycardias, as well as improving how the heart remodelled after injury.[1403] It must be noted however that other studies have shown VNS enhancing arrhythmias like AF depending on the strength of stimulation.[1404]

With regards to POTS, one case study presented a 29-year-old lady with intractable epilepsy and POTS who was treated for seizures with an implanted VNS device, and her POTS symptoms subsided and her tilt table test became normal with VNS therapy.[1405]

Other than helping with arrhythmias, VNS has shown to mitigate intrinsic cardiac nerve damage and adverse cardiac remodelling after a heart attack;[1406] as well as helping to preserve cardiac function in animal models with heart failure.[1407] One meta-analysis of 1,263 patients showed that there was a high grade of evidence indicating that VNS improved the functionality and quality of life of those with severe heart failure too.[1408]

Communication between the immune system and the brain is critical for inflammation regulation. The vagus nerve plays a major role in both sensing and acting on inflammation, acting as a highway between the brain and the immune system. For example, peripheral administration of endotoxin or IL-1β causes afferent vagus nerve activation, and in mice with endotoxemia, VNS reduces local and serum proinflammatory cytokine levels, and acetylcholine inhibits the release of TNF, IL-1, and IL-18 from endotoxin-stimulated macrophages.[1409,1410]

Interestingly, vagus nerve fibres sending information to the brain appear to be important for relaying information about immune status to the brain when proinflammatory cytokines are present at fairly low levels.[1411] In addition to this, the vagus nerve may also work directly to regulate immune function by releasing acetylcholine, without the requirement for either signalling along the other nerves or T cells.[1409]

Vagus nerve activity is reduced in chronic inflammatory disorders, including obesity, and vagus nerve signalling has been linked to attaining and maintaining weight loss after bariatric surgery.[1412] Unpublished also indicate that vagus nerve stimulation suppresses insulin resistance in rodents.[1409] But it's not just obesity. Data from the clinical trials that used VNS in treatment of rheumatoid arthritis and Crohn's disease suggest that there was a therapeutic potential of electrical VNS in diseases characterised by excessive inflammation.[1413] In one study of 110 participants with COVID-19, the use of non-invasive VNS (25 Hz) showed to lead to significant reductions in levels of inflammatory markers, "specifically CRP and procalcitonin.". The authors go on to state, *"Because nVNS has multiple mechanisms of action that may be relevant to COVID-19, additional research into its potential use earlier in the course of COVID-19 and its potential to mitigate some of the symptoms associated with post-acute sequelae of COVID-19 is warranted."*[1413]

Other than acute COVID-19 infection, VNS has also shown potential in helping with symptoms of long COVID, this may be because long COVID possesses an element of autonomic dysfunction.[1414,1415] In one small study, self-administered transcutaneous VNS on settings 25Hz, 500us pulse width, tonically on for 1 hour, twice per day, 6 days per week for 4 weeks, showed to have mild to moderate effect in reducing mental fatigue symptoms in a subset of individuals.[1417] Though not long COVID, similar results were also seen in a small study of Primary Sjögren's syndrome (an autoimmune condition) sufferers with chronic fatigue.[1418] In this study, the use of non-invasive VNS was shown to reduce feelings of sleepiness, IL-6, IL-1β, IP-10, MIP-1α, and TNFα levels and significantly altered patterns of NK- and T-cell subsets.[1418]

Dosage: Just like UV light, as we are dealing with energy, dosing is not as straightforward as when taking a supplement. Things are further complicated by the fact that there are no official guidelines on how to use VNS, plus a wide range of modes/frequencies have been used in studies, sometimes with contradictory results.

One review noted that with regards to transcutaneous VNS, various studies used a range of pulse widths of 20–500 μs; frequencies of 1–30 Hz; on/off times of 0.5 s - 30 min ON/30–270 s OFF; times administered ranging from 6 min - 9 months; and a current of 0.13–50 mA.[1419]

B-CARYOPHYLLENE

Some possible benefits include: anti-inflammation, antioxidation, immunomodulation, anti-viral, cardioprotection, neuroprotection, kidney-protection, lung-protection, analgesic, and anti-cancer.

The endocannabinoid system is a biological system that consists of endocannabinoids, which are types of neurotransmitters that bind to cannabinoid receptors (CBRs), and cannabinoid receptor proteins, which are found throughout the CNS (including the brain) and nerves throughout the body.

The endocannabinoid system is linked to all aspects of human physiology and is activated externally by the hemp plant *Cannabis sativa,* and internally by endocannabinoids formed naturally in our body. Cannabis (containing tetrahydrocannabinol (THC) and cannabidiol (CBD)) as well as arachidonic acid (the polyunsaturated omega-6 fatty acid) are common endocannabinoids that bind non-selectively to both CB1 and CB2 receptors.

Both cannabinoid receptor types 1 and 2 (CB1 and CB2) have been demonstrated to be expressed throughout the CNS.[1420] CB1 is expressed mainly in brain cells and is primarily responsible for the psycho-modulatory effects of cannabis, whereas CB2 receptors are expressed throughout the body, mainly in peripheral immune cells, and moderately expressed in certain brain areas.[1421,1422]

The activation of CB2 has been shown to inhibit acute, inflammatory, and neuropathic pain, as well as having antioxidant, anti-inflammatory, immunomodulatory, and organ-protective effects that can be achieved without causing psychotropic effects (a "high").[1423,1424] Due to this, CB2 has recently received attention from the scientific community.

Among the many plant-derived chemicals studied for bioactivities, β-caryophyllene (BCP) has piqued the interest of researchers for its pharmacological properties and therapeutic potential due to its strong ability to activate CB2 and lack of ability to activate CB1. Other than in cannabis, BCP is found in large amounts in the essential oils of many different spices and food plants, such as oregano (*Origanum vulgare* L.), cinnamon (*Cinnamomum* spp.), black pepper (*Piper nigrum* L.), basil (Ocimum spp.), rosemary (*Rosmarinus officinalis* L.), and cloves (*Syzygium aromaticum*(L.), among others.[1425]

Accumulating experimental studies have demonstrated that CB2R activation by BCP helps to attenuate inflammation, oxidative stress, apoptosis, fibrosis, and initiate immune modulation.[1425] The protective effects of BCP-mediated CB2 activation have been demonstrated in various preclinical models of various diseases, including rheumatoid arthritis, ischaemic stroke, Parksinon's disease, liver fibrosis, colitis, oral mucositis, glioblastoma, neuropathic pain, bipolar disorders, wound healing, interstitial cystitis, autoimmune encephalomyelitis/multiple sclerosis, metabolic and neurobehavioral alterations, insulin resistance and vascular inflammation, raised blood sugar levels, neuropathy, atherosclerosis, cardiotoxicity, osteoporosis, lung inflammation, intestinal inflammation, heart attacks, acute kidney injury, and addictions.[1246-1424]

On the molecular level, β-caryophyllene via the activation of CB2 is thought able to help with a wide range of pathological disorders due to the inhibition of pro-inflammatory cytokines, NF-κB, adhesion molecules, and chemokines, followed by the modulation of signalling pathways, primarily involving toll-like receptors, opioid receptors, SIRT1 and the activation of nuclear peroxisome proliferator-activated receptors (PPARs).[1425]

PPARs are a group of receptors with three subtypes that are involved in fat and glucose homeostasis and inflammatory responses.[1445] The three subtypes include: PPAR-α, PPAR-β/δ, and PPAR-γ. Activation of PPAR-α reduces triglyceride level, is involved in regulation of energy homeostasis and activates SIRT1.[1446,1447] Activation of PPAR-γ causes insulin sensitisation, enhances glucose metabolism, as well as being involved in attenuating cytokine storms and inhibiting viral replication.[1425,1448,1449] Activation of PPAR-β/δ enhances fatty acid metabolism.

CB2 receptors are well expressed in several organs, including the liver, spleen, thymus, brain, lungs, kidneys, tonsils, nasal epithelium, pancreas, uterus, and reproductive tissues, and play a vital role in modulating the immune system.[1450] This is no better demonstrated than in one study showing that mice lacking CB2R were more susceptible and vulnerable to influenza infection, indicating that CB2R are critical in immunoregulation in respiratory viral infections.[1451] Further studies have shown that CB2R activation induces effective immunomodulation by mediating cell death induction, cytokine suppression, and cell proliferation inhibition, as well as the induction of regulatory T cells and anti-inflammatory cytokines.[1452,1453]

The use of BCP as a CB2 activator has shown promise in this regard. In one study, the activation of CB2R was reported to suppress lung pathology in infants infected with acute respiratory syncytial virus by reducing the levels of cytokines and chemokines.[1454] In HIV patients, the activation of CB2R was shown to impair a productive infection and viral transmission.[1455]

Independent of CB2, various plants with high BCP content have shown antiviral activities against various viruses, including influenza A, human herpes virus types 1 and 2, and dengue viruses. Plants containing high BCP content include *Glechon marifolia, Buddleja cordobensis, Mosla dianthera,* and *Melissa officinalis* (lemon balm).[1425]

PPlus, BCP has also shown to act as an antioxidant by decreasing ROS production, inhibiting lipid peroxidation and glutathione depletion, free radical scavenging, and enhancing our natural antioxidant defence in tissues of several organs.[1425] One study showed that BCP had higher antioxidant capacity than vitamin E (α-tocopherol).[1428]

The multifaceted and widespread benefits of BCP are due to its independent antioxidant and anti-pathogenic effects, as well as its ability to activate CB2 receptors that are involved in processes of disease inhibition and are found all throughout the body. I will go into a few studies that may interest the reader about the various disease states that BCP may help, as mentioned above.

In one mouse study BCP was found to inhibit age-dependent cognitive decline which correlated with lower β-amyloid deposition within the brain and a decreased expression of inflammatory mediators too.[1456]

Another study showed that BCP protected rats with doxorubicin (a chemotherapy drug) against long-term heart damage by reducing cardiomyocyte enzymes, preserving histology, and restoring heart function.[1457]

One study reported that BCP improved sociability and reduced anxiety- and depression-like behaviours in mice.[1458]

And another of mice showed BCP therapeutically aiding with autoimmune encephalomyelitis.[1432] This was similarly seen in another study using a CB2 receptor agonist.[1459]

With regards to COVID-19, various *in silico* studies have noted BCP as a potential phytocompound out of many to have anti-COVID-19 efficacy.[1460,1461] And due to BCP's pharmacological mechanisms and therapeutic properties, one group of researchers noted, *"we speculate that BCP has potential to be investigated against COVID-19 and will inspire further preclinical and clinical studies."* in their review. So far, the use of BCP in COVID-19 and other disease states remains theoretical.[1425]

Dosage: To my knowledge, there aren't any β-caryophyllene supplements on the market as of yet. Due to this and the fact that human trials using β-caryophyllene are lacking, there are no recommended dosages for this compound. Remember that it is widely distributed in the plant kingdom, however.

A SUMMARY OF SUPPLEMENTS

The next several pages include a table summarising all the therapeutics from the "Other Supplements" section of this book.

Side-effects; possible drug interactions; and quality of evidence are not included.

	CARDIO	NEURO	IMMUNE	CANCER	CLOT	FERTILITY	INFLAM-MATION	OTHER
7,8-DHF		●						
ALCAR		●						
Alpha-GPC		●						●
Anthocyanins	●	●	●				●	
Artemisinin			●	●			●	
Astragalus	●	●	●	●		●	●	●
Bacopa		●						
Baicalin		●			●	●	●	

	CARDIO	NEURO	IMMUNE	CANCER	CLOT	FERTILITY	INFLAM-MATION	OTHER
CCR5 antagonists							●	●
Chaga		●	●	●			●	●
CoQ10	●	●	●		●	●	●	●
Colchicine	●			●			●	●
Cordyceps		●	●	●		●	●	●
Cornus officinalis		●				●	●	●
Curcumin		●	●	●			●	●
FIASMA activity drugs	●	●	●	●			●	●

	CARDIO	NEURO	IMMUNE	CANCER	CLOT	FERTILITY	INFLAM-MATION	OTHER
Fisetin	●	●	●	●			●	
Ginkgo biloba extracts		●					●	
G-Rg1		●					●	
Gotu Kola		●					●	●
EGCG	●	●					●	
G. pentaphyllum	●	●					●	●
IF light		●	●				●	●
Ivermectin		●	●	●			●	●

	CARDIO	NEURO	IMMUNE	CANCER	CLOT	FERTILITY	INFLAM-MATION	OTHER
Lion's Mane	●	●	●	●			●	●
Luteolin	●	●	●	●			●	●
Maca		●				●	●	●
Melatonin	●	●	●	●	●	●	●	●
Methylene Blue		●	●					●
Inositols			●			●	●	●
NAC		●	●			●	●	●
Nattokinase	●	●			●			

	CARDIO	NEURO	IMMUNE	CANCER	CLOT	FERTILITY	INFLAM-MATION	OTHER
Niacin	●	●						●
Nigella sativa	●	●	●	●		●	●	●
Oleuropein	●		●		●		●	●
Oroxylin A		●	●	●			●	●
Suramin			●	●				●
Shikimic acid	●		●					●
Polygala tenuifolia		●					●	●
Progesterone		●	●					●

	CARDIO	NEURO	IMMUNE	CANCER	CLOT	FERTILITY	INFLAM-MATION	OTHER
Quercetin	●	●	●	●			●	●
Rapamycin	●	●	●		●		●	●
Resveratrol	●	●	●	●			●	●
Rhodiola	●	●	●	●			●	●
Royal Jelly	●	●				●	●	●
Salvianolic acids	●			●			●	●
Sauna	●	●					●	●
Seaweed	●	●	●	●			●	●

	CARDIO	NEURO	IMMUNE	CANCER	CLOT	FERTILITY	INFLAM-MATION	OTHER
Serrapeptase	●			●			●	●
Shilajit		●	●				●	●
Taurine	●	●					●	●
Tulsi		●	●				●	●
Vitamin K2	●	●	●	●		●		●
VNS	●	●	●			●		●
β-Caryophyllene	●	●		●		●		●

ALI'S STORY

Unhappy Anniversary.

A year ago today, I had my one and only covid 19 injection. It was under duress to keep my job and two months after my older brother died after having 1 dose of the AZ injection.

I never wanted this injection, it was rushed through too quickly and anything you have to bribe or force people to get is always a massive red flag. I had spent nearly a year watching and reading what censored Drs were saying about these injections, read medical papers, watched videos and saw what was happening to people around the world after taking this new gene therapy. I knew it was unlike other vaccines and was causing people lots of harm that was being covered up. My brother had his on 1st Sept 2021 and within a week he had a headache he could not shift. Then he started falling over and lost control of his legs. By the time he went to hospital on the 13 of September, he was also losing control of his arms and then his speech. He was in a coma a week later and was dead by mid October. Not of the "vaccine" though, it was attributed to pneumonia, undiagnosed GBS, cardiac events and a mild reaction to the AZ "vaccine". He had no health issues and had been off sick once since starting his job two years previously.

So, I had mine and as it was being done I felt

violated. I did not want this stuff in my body but hoped I would fare better than my brother. For two weeks I was fine, full of my usual energy and able to run up to 7 miles at a time or cycle 10-20 miles on my days off work. Then the shit hit the fan. I started getting nerve pains and lower back pain and immediately knew what was happening so called my Dr. He ran the usual tests, all normal, nothing to see here and he wiped his hands of me stating " I have injected thousands of people, no one has ever had a reaction like yours."

This pain in my back continued, followed by electric shocks all over my lower body and then I started getting numb between my legs. The lower back pain spread to my entire back and then my ribs. I now have tinnitus in both ears and hearing loss when previously I had excellent hearing. I had fatigue and brain fog, the latter affecting my mood and how I did my job. I cannot run anymore and have had to massively scale back my exercise and anything else I want to do. At times, I could not even get out of bed, I had no energy and would wake up feeling like I had not slept for a week. In October this year I was taken to hospital with tachycardia and low BP and after this I took 6 weeks off work. My Drs were useless at best and I had to do my own research to try to get well again. My gp referred me to a neurologist and gave me pain killers for the nerve pain but that was it.

I had to pay to see an osteopath, a private neurologist, get an MRI scan, see a private GP and get private meds that my Gp would not prescribe for me. I have worked out that I have had an inflammatory response to this injection and my immune system has gone into overdrive. I found a list of anti-inflammatory supplements on a website called realnotrare and they helped my back pain go within a week but at a cost of £250 per month. I take over 60 pills a day. Pre injection I took a handful of vitamins. I then found a support group and got the name of a UK based Dr who would prescribe me with things that would help me to heal and hopefully negate any further damage from this injection. It has taken at least three months but I am now taking a drug that has helped me no end. My brain fog has gone and I have energy again. I am regaining sensation between my legs and the electric shocks in my legs are far less painful.

I have been able to reduce my pain meds and I can do my job, albeit with reduced hours.

As I look back over the last year, it seems like a bloody nightmare. I have been injected with a toxic gene therapy against my will and when I became ill I had next to no help from the NHS. If I had not gone out and found things to calm this inflammation down, my injuries could have been far worse. I have had to do my own research on the mechanisms of action of this injection and figure out what it has done to my body. I have spent hours trawling thorough medical papers, videos and lectures to try and work out what I need to read next, where I need to go for some answers to this bloody mystery. I have met others who are injured by this injection and now have irreparable heart damage or autoimmune disorders. Others have nerve damage or vision loss and some are now in wheelchairs. The injuries suffered are wide ranging and non exhaustive but we all share one thing in common, the utter lack of care and compassion by the NHS. We have been lied to, gaslit, told it is down to anxiety, ignored and demeaned, refused referrals and left to get worse with a few painkillers thrown in for good measure. We have had to fight for basic healthcare and on top of being injured, this is really tiring. Some have gone to their Gp after an adverse reaction to one injection and told a second one will make things better....

Long covid clinics are promoting boosters to its members and do not recognise injection injury. Others who are not even aware they have had an adverse reaction to the injection but have suddenly developed a new illness are also being told to get another of these injections.

This is sheer madness. It needs to stop. If I can pass one thing along to anyone who reads my story it is this, DO NOT GET ANOTHER MRNA INJECTION. EVER AGAIN. This is a new technology and it can cause irreparable damage. It can cause cancers, infertility, heart issues, take your pick. If you do become ill you will get sod all help from the NHS and will be left to figure things out on your own. Do not throw away your health, do not throw away your children's health.

THIS IS ALL THAT WE'VE GOT

Supplements may work, they may not, and they may even make things worse. Some may interact with others beneficially; some may not. Some may cause side effects, while others may be completely fine. Some may need to be taken at specific times and in specific ways, whereas others can simply be popped in. There is a lot we, and the scientific community as a whole, simply do not know.

Take uridine, for example. Uridine is one of four repeating units that make up RNA and DNA. It is also a supplement that has it all: positive effects, side effects, reduced bioavailability when consumed via the diet, and synergistic effects when taken with other substances.

As a supplement, it has possible neuroprotective effects, as evidenced by reducing amyloid-β production, plaque formation, and neurodegeneration.[1,2,3] It is also an antidote for 5-fluorouracil (a chemotherapeutic drug) poisoning.[4]

One study of gerbils showed that using uridine with DHA and choline improved the acquisition and retention of spatial memory, and its memory-improving and neuroprotective qualities are why uridine is taken as a nootropic by some.[5]

But real-life studies have been mixed. When a uridine-, choline-, and DHA-enriched multinutrient was used in patients with moderate Alzheimer's disease, no significant cognitive improvements were seen over a 24-week intervention period.[6] The authors hypothesised that patients with mild Alzheimer's disease had progressed to the point where neuronal loss and synaptic dysfunction were irreversible and unresponsive to pharmacologic or non-pharmacologic therapies, proposing that the potential impact of multi-nutritional therapies to enhance the formation of synapses may be limited in intermediate Alzheimer's disease compared to mild disease due to higher levels of neurodegeneration.[6] And lo and behold, two further clinical trials showed that the multinutrient was associated with a statistically significant improvement in memory in patients with mild and very mild Alzheimer's disease dementia.[7,8]

Uridine *can* be obtained from dietary sources, but it's unavailable to the brain as it is degraded by the liver.[9] Plus, food substances proposed to increase uridine levels, such as beer, are impractical and harmful to drink in high quantities.[10] The long-term use of uridine may not be so safe either, being associated with both insulin resistance and possible cancer formation.[11,12]

I've used uridine to show how complicated it is to take supplements and how important it is to know everything about a therapy before using it. This is becoming ever more vital as the world turns to alternative forms of treatment as trust in the pharmaceutical industry and existing healthcare models diminishes day after day.

Though the number and variety of therapeutics available to us appear to be limitless, the ones highlighted in this book have been chosen with care. Uridine, like many others, has not been included due to a combination of reasons, including, but not limited to, a negative safety profile, a lack of data, and limited benefits.

Other examples that didn't make the cut include bile acids (which have shown mixed results in terms of reducing prion formation);[13,14] thiamine (with a belief that many features of long COVID mimic thiamine deficiency);[15] low-dose naltrexone (a drug primarily used to manage alcohol or opioid use disorder, which also has immunomodulatory effects showing to help with symptoms of long COVID);[16] boron (a chemical element with the ability to improve cardiac contractility and fibrotic remodelling following myocardial infarction injury in rats);[17] and *Uncaria tomentosa*, also known as Cat's Claw (with some evidence of helping with protection against glyphosate toxicity;[18] reducing fatigue in patients with solid tumours;[19] increasing white blood cells;[20] working as an antiplatelet agent;[21] and having the ability to reduce brain plaques and tangles).[22] Though *U. tomentosa* was most promising, it lacked overall data.

The therapeutics included were carefully selected for having optimal effectiveness across a wide range of disease states, ample scientific and real-life evidence, as well as being fairly safe to use. That being said, there are many known unknowns and many more unknown unknowns in the field of natural medicine.

Some argue that antioxidants should not be used in people who are predisposed to cancer. Large trials have had to be abandoned because the patients receiving antioxidants had a higher incidence of cancer than patients who did not receive them. In one study, researchers found that adding NAC or vitamin E to the diet of mice with small lung tumours substantially increased the number, size, and stage of the tumours.[23] In another study, vitamin B3 showed a significant increase in the prevalence and spread of brain cancer.[24] And in mouse models of melanoma, the researchers found that levels of oxidative stress were higher in circulating cancer cells than in cancer cells in primary tumours.[25] The growth and spread of certain cancers seem to be controlled by oxidative stress, so antioxidants may promote cancer spread in some.

The other major problem is that we have no real idea what we are treating as we still do not have anonymised participant-level data from the jab trials, as highlighted in a recently published editorial by the senior editor of the BMJ, Peter Doshi.[26] In this editorial, he also explains that the underlying data for COVID-19 therapeutics are similarly hard to find, and when shared, the datasets offered are limited.[26]

He goes on to note, *"We are left with publications but no access to the underlying data on reasonable request. This is worrying for trial participants, researchers, clinicians, journal editors, policy makers, and the public. The journals that have published these primary studies may argue that they faced an awkward dilemma, caught between making the summary findings available quickly and upholding the best ethical values that support timely access to underlying data. In our view, there is no dilemma; the anonymised individual participant data from clinical trials must be made available for independent scrutiny."*[26] I agree with him.

Transparency is vital. And if we had the raw data at hand, regulators and public health organisations could reveal why jab trials were not designed to assess efficacy against SARS-CoV-2 infection and transmission. Joshi says that if the government had insisted on this outcome, it would have learned about how the jabs affect transmission sooner and could have made plans based on that information.

Without raw data and transparency from the trials, we are left swinging in the dark, not knowing not only how bad the current situation is but also having no idea how to treat jab-related injuries. We must also remind ourselves that we are playing with never-before-seen genetic technologies that did not undergo thorough pharmacokinetic studies for the determination of drug biodistribution, dosage, and efficacy without toxicity; technologies that in fact need to undergo *more* scientific scrutiny due to their multi-phased mode of action.[27]

To make matters worse, it has been suggested that findings for most research designs in most scientific fields, COVID-19 or not, are likely false and that claimed research findings are frequently simply accurate measures of the prevailing biases.[28] The greater the financial and other interests, the greater the flexibility in designs, definitions, outcomes, and analytical mode, and the smaller the effect sizes in a scientific field, the less likely the research findings are to be true.[28] And, with an estimated 50% of research being published, it leaves us wondering,[29] "Why not share all findings?" and "Can we trust anything published at all?"

Though scientific corruption has been going on for a long time, the recent COVID-19 pandemic debacle is likely the greatest example of science being used to fit narratives that has garnered the most attention. As we have noted, government policies throughout the pandemic were made using poorly done studies with small numbers of people and animals, arbitrary endpoints like antibody levels, and hiding data that went against them. Those who funded the research were involved in the outcomes too.

Science is the process of starting with "I don't know" and asking questions until some answers are found. What's happening is the reverse. It appears that "scientists" now begin with an end goal in mind and tailor their study design to meet that goal. This is scientism, not science.

This extends to other areas of research too. We don't know if various therapies and supplements will help with jab-related injuries.

Also, if I were a betting man, I'd say that many people will argue that supplements and other alternative therapies don't work by pointing out that there isn't enough high-quality data to show that they do. This has already happened in the case of examples like vitamin D and ivermectin. To them I say, "What about the rollout of Pfizer's new booster shot that had only been tested on eight mice before mass rollout?"[30] *Is that sufficient evidence?*

What we *can* all agree on is that the human body is remarkably exceptional at being able to heal itself; this is especially true when it is given the right level and type of stimuli at the right time. The first step towards better health is to minimise toxic stress and optimise underlying physiological processes. Certain supplements may then aid with the healing process, or they may not.

Strengthening of our current biological systems and symptomatic relief are currently all we can hope for using lifestyle modifications and natural therapeutics. For some, this may be enough, but with no way to effectively clear the spike protein and some evidence even suggesting that the injected genetic material has a potential to embed itself into our own DNA, for others, these natural therapeutics may never be enough.

Regardless, for now, they're all that we've got.

THE FUTURE OF HUMANITY.

WHAT WILL OUR FUTURE LOOK LIKE?

We have been conditioned over the last three years to regard COVID-19 as the deadliest disease ever known to man. Constant reminders, such as daily death rates on the news and mandatory mask wearing, were pushed in front of us month after month and did not help anyone. There is no wonder why I remember regularly speaking to patients who were too worried to go to the hospital for what I deemed more urgent medical matters, such as receiving a cancer diagnosis or treating chest pain.

To this day, I see the odd person wearing a face mask while driving. Fear scrambles logical and lateral thinking, paralysing any proper progress. Some people were tormented so badly that a diagnosis called "COVID-19 anxiety syndrome" has been recently formulated to describe their severe angst.[1]

Because of the worldwide focus on COVID-19, other conditions fell by the wayside, both in our minds and in reality. Cheap and effective medications and supplements that may have proven useful for prevention were vilified and banned. Gyms were closed, and fast-food restaurants were left open. *Was it ever about our health?* Well, seemingly not.

Lockdowns will go down as the second-most disastrous public health policy of all time. A nearsighted approach to reduce the transmission of a rapidly spreading pathogen that did not care if you were hiding in your home or not. Getting infected, whether asymptomatically or symptomatically, was an inevitability. Lockdowns caused economic turmoil and an international mental health crisis, as well as forcing others to fester with illnesses that were deemed too late to cure once the world opened up again.

Instead of encouraging preventive approaches like weight loss, hospitals began selling donuts, and healthcare workers became TikTok stars overnight for their uncoordinated moves. I was there and refused both the junk food and pleas from my former colleagues to join ward dances. To me, it all felt nightmarishly surreal. I knew lockdowns, whether they were introduced to "curb the spread" or "reduce the burden on the healthcare system," would eventually end, and at that point we'd face a health crisis many times worse than the pandemic.

It has now been estimated that lockdowns may claim 20 times more life years than they save.[2] Plus, the other real kicker is that lockdowns may have inadvertently made everyone less immunologically prepared and more at risk of symptomatic infection due to understimulating resident memory T and B cells of the lungs.

There are now more than 400 studies on the failure of compulsory COVID-19 interventions like masks and school closures.[3] In other words, all government-recommended anti-viral interventions have been repeatedly shown to be useless and harmful. Well, useless and harmful for us, the civilians, anyway.

For governments and major pharmaceutical companies alike, the last three years or so have been a massive success. Apart from the colossal profits that have been generated by mandating their products, governments and corporations have viscerally understood the amount of power they possess. They were able, using behavioural and psychological tactics, to control many billions of people overnight, setting the foundations for a bleak future for humanity.

In less than three years, massive amounts of money and power have been transferred to those who do not have our best interests at heart. Pillars of medical bioethics have been crumbled, immunology has been rewritten, and intersocietal division has been encouraged. Scientism, a new religion, took its place on the throne and continues to do so to this day. Anyone or anything that goes against it is now labelled as spreading "misinformation" and deemed by some as mentally unstable.

Logic, human decency, and scientific debates vanished in a matter of weeks and have only begun to return slowly again. Still, many people are stuck in the dark spell of mass formation psychosis, a type of mass hysteria. And many healthcare workers live a double life, unable to speak out against the mandates due to the painfully hypocritical feelings that even merely considering a different narrative evokes.

Above all, the most dangerous thing to have come out in the last few years has been genetic technology and the mass celebration of it. Though praised and pushed heavily by everyone from politicians to healthcare workers to celebrities, the introduction of mRNA technology and all new forms of genetic "vaccines" will go down as the number one most disastrous public health policy of all time.

The only placebo-controlled trial (if you can even call it that) comparing the unjabbed and jabbed told us everything that we needed to know from the very start. It was us that didn't want to see. In the original Pfizer trial, though COVID-19 numbers were seemingly better, there were more adverse events and deaths in the jabbed group.[4] Billions were injected from data gathered from only 170 cases of COVID-19 in this trial.[5] Many swapped their risk of attaining a commonly non-fatal infection for an increased risk of side effects *and* an increased likelihood of attaining COVID-19 in the future.

These genetic shots cause harm and death. They have ruined families, put an end to the athletic careers of many, caused others to be on lifelong medication, and continue to kill many thousands of others of all ages and backgrounds.

They are harmful literally beyond comprehension, preying on underlying individual biological weaknesses to accelerate disease processes like cancer and autoimmunity. Some will run into problems quicker than others, and there is not one organ that this technology seems to spare.

The most vital and vulnerable organ, the heart, of many thousands of people has been compromised due to these jabs, and every other day we hear of someone "suddenly dying" due to "unknown reasons."

There is no such thing as "death of an unknown cause." This is a misnomer; there is *always* a reason, regardless of whether or not we are ready to address and investigate it.

We only feared, and many still continue to fear COVID-19 because the media repeatedly told us to do so. And, while COVID-19 is a dangerous condition for some, we must remember that it is not the only disease that plagues mankind. Whilst we were glued to our screens, distracted by the pandemic, wars, and current affairs, other, more worrying, unreported trends continued to silently progress without receiving the attention they deserved. *But out of sight, out of mind, right?*

Well, maybe, but you can only avoid the truth for so long. Excess deaths are rising, and yet no one wants to report on them. And this alone speaks volumes. The relationship between governments, cooperation, and mass media is extremely chummy. Reporting on rising death figures, arguably the most important news currently, *would* happen in an ideal world where we are given information untainted by biases and conflicts of interest. But we live in a world far from ideal.

It's not just the mainstream media. From the way pro-genetic studies have been conducted to the way data is collected, drawn on graphs, and presented, there has been an overwhelming push and manipulation of figures to place mRNA and DNA technology in a positive light. Heck, it's extremely difficult to get science papers criticising mRNA technology published in the first place due to publishing biases and flaws with the whole system of peer-reviewing.

The corruption runs deep and at all levels. Deaths and mRNA-related injuries are becoming normalised. We are entering a new normal. But not all hope is lost. Many have begun to understand what is truly going on, and the mass corruption only gets clearer if one is willing to see.

But just because one has woken from the mass formation nightmare and appreciated the colossal humanitarian pickle we are in doesn't mean that reality will magically get back on track. For that to happen, we must work together and take action.

The link between genetic technology and the rise in excess deaths and disease must be shared and accepted publicly. Then only can legal proceedings take place, severing the grip that Big Pharma currently has on the market. Only when this occurs will the breadth and depth of government, mass media, and cooperative corruption be exposed. And only when people acknowledge this mass deception can we mitigate errors and build ethical, philosophical, and institutional structures that will protect humanity in the future.

This is why I began writing this book as a means of accumulating the most pertinent pieces of information in one place that have been hidden from most of us in the last few years. And thus you may appreciate that every single person that has been inoculated and continues to get inoculated with these new forms of "vaccine" has not been appropriately consented, *"a process by which the treating health care provider discloses appropriate information to a competent patient so that the patient may make a voluntary choice to accept or refuse treatment."*[6]

Whether prescribing paracetamol or preparing for surgery, the doctor must inform the patient of the risks involved. This conversation is called "shared decision making" (SDM) and is a patient-centred approach in which clinicians and patients work together to find and choose the best course of action for each patient's particular situation.[7]

In a nutshell, the six main parts of SDM are: figuring out the situation, being aware of the choices, making sure the options are clear, talking about the risks and benefits, thinking about what the patient wants, and making a decision.

Were alternatives addressed before you were jabbed? Did your healthcare professional discuss the various risks and benefits of these shots? Did they ask you about your understanding of mRNA technology? Were you given the option to talk about it?

If these things weren't done, then your choice was put aside. And the frightening truth is revealed: **every jab given around the world has ended up in people's arms through mass coercion, corruption, and the use of half-truths and full lies**.

The Nuremberg Code requires comprehensive and absolute requirements of informed consent and the right of the subject to withdraw from participation in an experiment.[8] It was formulated after the atrocities of World War II to protect us against human experimentation. But this has fallen by the wayside as of recently. **What has happened over the last three years is a crime against humanity.**

Would you have gotten inoculated if you knew what you know now?

You were tricked and harmed.

The health of many millions has been damaged in efforts to further monopolise the power of all parties involved in the medical-industrial complex. And via the creation and mandating of genetic bioweapons, the pharmaceutical industry has tactically secured a colossal income stream for many decades to come.

With current information at hand, I predict a future plagued with heart disease, sudden deaths, infections, cancers, blood clots, and cognitive impairments. We are entering an age where rare conditions will no longer remain rare, where the young succumb to diseases that were once only common to the elderly, and where human death becomes normalised.

This future is a certainty, especially if the medical field fails to recognise the link between genetic technology and disease progression. Regardless, we have no time to wait for them to show their appreciation. There is a lot that must be done now to help secure a better future. We must begin rebuilding society again, and to do this successfully, we must first help those injured by mRNA and DNA technology.

MASKING DEATH

During a night shift months into the pandemic, I remember looking out of the staff room window at the hospital morgue across the road in deep contemplation. With a lot of the population already likely immune via cross-reactivity and the virus seemingly targeting only those at risk, I did not get the state's incessant need for everyone to get the shot. Yes, seemingly healthy people have died and continue to die as a result of the virus, but on the grand scale of things, this was and is extremely rare.

At the start, everything done by authorities was allegedly to prevent deaths that would not otherwise have occurred. Later, the goal became preventing serious illness and then stopping the virus from spreading. Three years later, these claims have all turned out to be lies. Only recently, Janine Small, president of international markets at Pfizer, confirmed that the COVID-19 shots were not tested for their impact on transmission prior to their release,[1] and yet many people begrudgingly rolled up their sleeves as they were told it would help protect grandma.

In those early two years, it seemed as if the world was designed to care for nothing else. Big killers like cancer, depression, loneliness, and heart disease were put to the wayside to make way for the big C. If you weren't affected or murdered by the virus, it didn't count.

Non-virus news stories were ignored, and presenters instead focused on ingenious alternative ways to announce just how terribly infected the world was becoming. Daily death figures were on repeat 24/7, and if not in number form, other ways like elaborate graphs were used instead to highlight humanity's supposed decline.

I was always sceptical of the news, knowing from a young age that they only told us what they wanted us to know, but my scepticism was solidified after witnessing so-called journalists interviewing hospital staff members in full hazmat suits, masks, and visors—far more overdressed than the medical workers themselves.

Still looking out the window, my thoughts turned to a project I did during university. In this project, I studied the town I was living in at the time and noted that the areas that were financially worse off were also more likely to have individuals with lower quality of life, shorter life expectancies, and higher rates of disease. I didn't discover anything extraordinary; deprivation and its impact on health are common knowledge in medicine and especially public health, and yet lockdowns were introduced internationally.

I did not understand how halting social human interaction and worldwide economic movement would benefit humanity, pandemic or not. Viruses spread; it's what they do. Sitting at home or stopping air travel wasn't going to change this fact. And yet we were told it would.

The quality-adjusted life year (QALY) is a broad measure of disease burden that takes into account both the quality and quantity of life lived. One QALY equates to one year in perfect health. It is thought that so far, light or severe restrictions have cost the world a total of 3,259 million QALYs.[2] And I will repeat what I said earlier in this book: it has also been estimated that lockdowns claim 20 times more life years than they save.[3] More lives would be saved if we stayed at home, they said. They lied.

At work, I was being pestered by my consultants to shave my beard so I could have an n95 facemask fitted as per hospital infectious disease control policy. Not only did I like my beard and did not appreciate people telling me what to do with my body, but I also knew that the recommendations were baseless, as exemplified by the fact that those who had religious reasons were exempt from beard-shaving.

Masks are useless at preventing infection at best and psychologically, physiologically, socially, and environmentally catastrophic at worst. Neither institutions such as the WHO or the European Centre for Disease Prevention and Control (ECDC) nor national ones such as the CDC have substantiated a positive effect of masks in public with scientifically sound data in terms of a reduced rate of COVID-19 spread in the population.[4]

In fact, when studied, masks have shown no effect at all. For example, in a Danish prospective study on wearing masks that included about 6,000 people and was published in 2020, scientists found no statistically significant difference in the rates of SARS-CoV-2 infection between the group of 3030 people who wore masks and the group of 2994 people who didn't.[5]

Masks provide a deceptive sense of safety, acting as a form of psychological support for those who are anxious.[4] Ironically, too, seeing others wear masks reinforces the fear of infection, creating a vicious cycle that I see some people to this day still finding difficult to get out of.

The recommendation to use masks has no scientific basis and instead creates a fearful environment, encouraging the stigmatisation of non-mask wearers while fueling groupthink and a feeling of altruism among those who do.[4] It is also a reminder to adhere to other measures. For these reasons, it might be why Professor Susan Michie, a member of the Scientific Advisory Group for Emergencies (SAGE) committee and a known Communist, felt that face coverings and social distancing should continue "forever."[6]

Face masks not only perpetuate Communist ideologies but have also been scientifically shown to: increase the risk of self-contamination by the wearer; increase the risk of eczema, skin damage, and overall impairment of the skin barrier function; worsen breathing ability; increase the feeling of exhaustion, drowsiness, and anxiety; and even decrease the ability to perceive empathy.[4] All these things, you could argue, *increase* one's risk of infection and perpetuate fear.

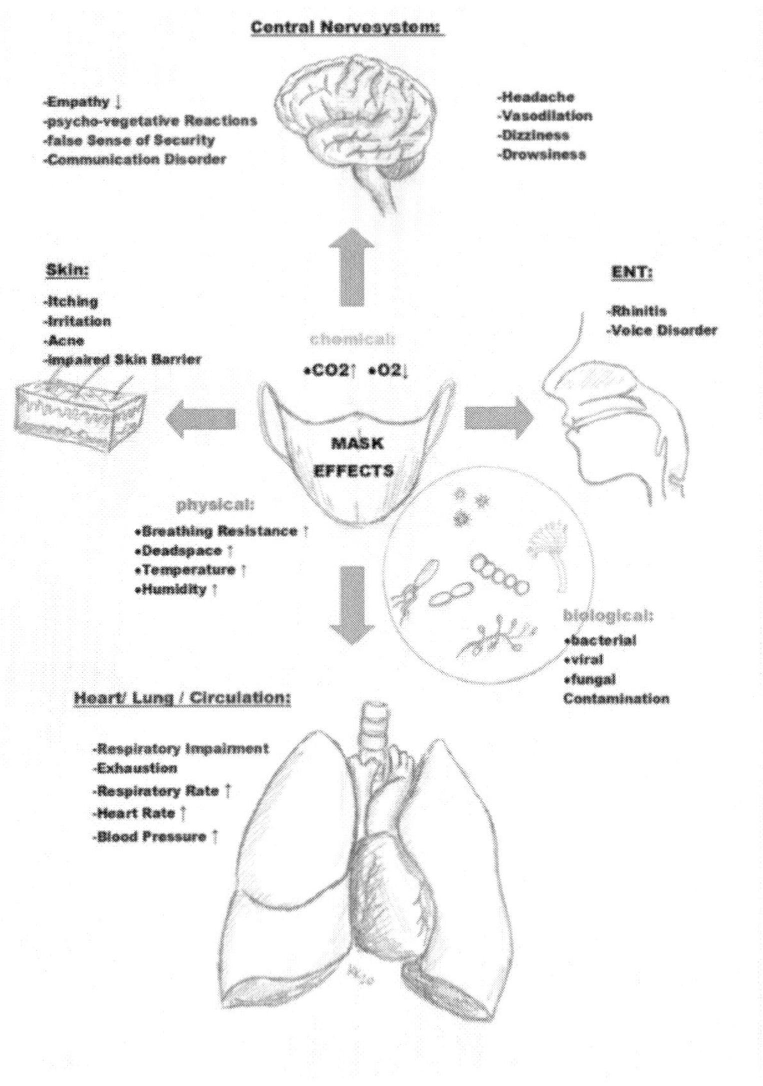

Unfavorable mask effects as components of Mask-Induced Exhaustion Syndrome (MIES), from: https://www.mdpi.com/1660-4601/18/8/4344/

It seems nothing about this pandemic was natural or eco-friendly. Disposable face masks and plastic gloves pose an ongoing risk to wildlife for tens, if not hundreds, of years.[7] Animals have and will continue to die in entanglements and by swallowing PPE. And these microplastics will contaminate our food and environmental systems, causing immunological and other health issues in us as well.

Whenever I see a muddied face mask on my walks in the forest, I am reminded of the time where a medical error occurred in the emergency department that I worked at due to their use. The story goes that an incorrectly high dose of a drug was given to a patient due to miscommunication between the nurse and doctor due to words being muffled under masks. The story ends with a loss of patient life, a doctor who had to take extended time off work, and a disheartened nurse. Regardless of this, mask-wearing continued to be encouraged in that department after this happened. I wonder how many incidents like this one continue to happen in healthcare to this day.

The problem throughout the pandemic was that real-life data was ignored. If it wasn't noted in a scientific journal, peer-reviewed, or modelled on a graph in the news, it wasn't taken seriously. Not only did this delay treatment and cause chaos amongst scientists bickering over insignificantly minor details, but it also meant that anyone who controlled the "science" controlled the narrative.

The clattering of trolley wheels on the unevenly paved road outside jolted me back to reality while I was deep in thought looking at the morgue. Two men were wheeling a recently deceased patient into the cold building. A life had been lost, a family was left in mourning, and a heart had stopped beating. This was the reality, and I wondered how many more would succumb prematurely to this fate in the coming future?

Jabs, lockdowns, and masks introduced by authorities during the pandemic were allegedly implemented to prevent deaths that would not otherwise have occurred. And yet, non-COVID excess deaths have been higher now, in most places, than at any point during the pandemic. In spite of this, our media and government are almost universally complicit in their silence.

At the end of the day, mortality is the only important measure of health outcomes, and it is a fact that more people are dying now than there should be.

We urgently require answers to why.

It's time we stopped hiding from the truth.

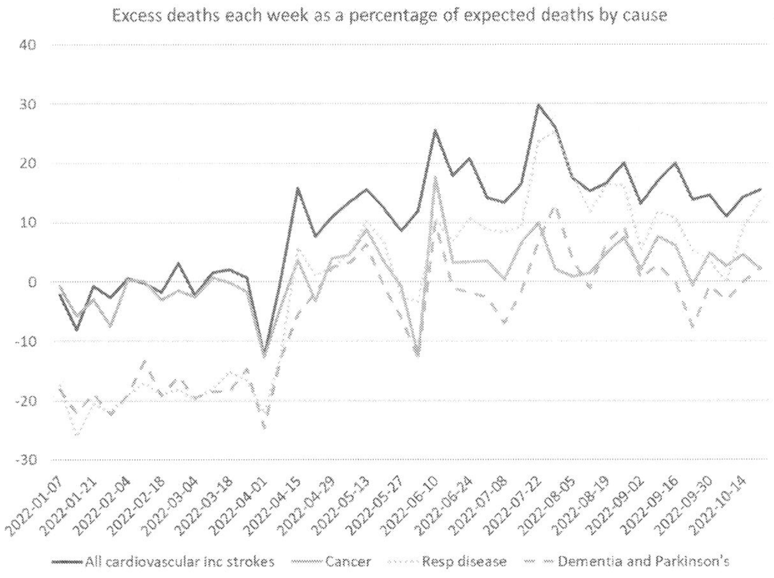

Rising excess deaths England, from: https://www.ons.gov.uk/

WHY DID WE HAVE A PANDEMIC?

In 2015, Bill Gates confidently proclaimed to the audience in his TED talk that *"if anything kills over 10 million people in the next few decades, it's most likely to be a highly infectious virus rather than a war."* [1]

Skip seven years (and a pandemic later) and leaked declassified emails from early 2020 have revealed that the authors of one of the first peer-reviewed papers shutting down the COVID-19 lab leak theory knew that there was a potential that the virus may have been developed in a lab,[2] and yet they fail to mention any of this in their pivotal paper titled "The proximal origin of SARS-CoV-2," which has been accessed more than 5 million times to this day.[2] This not only invalidates the peer-reviewing process but also altered subsequent scientific thinking as well as the direction in which humanity was led.

More recently, a major Lancet paper noted that the pathways of natural transmission and research-related transmission were both feasible.[3] The lead author of this report, Dr. Jeffrey Sachs, who chaired the commission for the Lancet for two years on COVID-19, further noted in an interview, ***"I'm pretty convinced it came out of U.S. lab biotechnology, not out of nature, just to mention. After two years of intensive work on this. So it's a blunder in my view of biotech, not an accident of a natural spillover. We don't know for sure, I should be absolutely clear. But there's enough evidence that it should be looked into. And it's not being investigated, not in the United States, not anywhere. And I think for real reasons that they don't want to look underneath the rug."***[4]

The US government, in their interim report titled "An Analysis of the Origins of the COVID-19 Pandemic," also alluded to the fact that **"the emergence of SARS-CoV-2 that resulted in the COVID-19 pandemic was most likely the result of a research-related incident."**[5]

With the lab leak theory becoming more fact than theory with every passing day,

Bill Gates' 2015 predictions seem more problematic than prophetic, knowing his heavy involvement with vaccine development and the surveillance industry.[6]

Gates denied that a global war would be a threat to humanity in the future, and though he is likely correct that a world war using archetypal military equipment is improbable due to multinational nuclear deterrents, I believe we are in a war of another kind. Let me explain.

Over the last 20 years, technology has become ever more sophisticated, interconnected, and widely used. Even while volunteering in rural Cambodia before the pandemic, I noticed that many of the village leaders owned smartphones yet had no access to clean drinking water. At the time, this baffled me, but I later understood that the internet was fast becoming a necessary commodity just as vital as food.

Digital technology was the last nail in the coffin of the Industrial Revolution, and its arrival marked the beginning of the Information Age. And things don't seem to be slowing down. Factory work is now increasingly carried out by automated machines. The new Amazon stores don't even have cashiers. Tesla will soon successfully bring out self-driving cars. Artificial Intelligence (AI) is able to diagnose skin cancers, illustrate images from text, and even write blog posts. The world is rapidly changing.

Though many have lost their jobs to machines and will continue to do so, if used correctly, digital technology is able to make individuals more powerful than ever before. On the internet, there are no rules. Historically, the key to societal success was controlling territory and people by force. Kings had empires and armies. Now all you need to be successful is a desk, an internet connection, and a good idea. Jeff Bezos, one of the richest people in the *world*, started off with just these three things.

The internet can allow anyone to share their ideas with the world; there are no jurisdictions. The internet also rewards individuals quickly and fairly. There are no middlemen (art gallery owners, music managers, book publishers, etc.) taking a large chunk out of the creatives' pocket. Now, what if the middlemen were the government?

The advent of cryptocurrency, AI, and the ability for people to earn a decent living anywhere in the world is destabilising international politics and traditional infrastructures. If an individual has the freedom to move and earn a good salary sitting on a beach in Barbados, why would he stay in Wolverhampton where his cost of living is high, his quality of life is low, and taxes are super high? He would move. Politicians don't want this.

In the Information Age, power doesn't reside with those who are born into wealth or those who are able to coerce others for personal gains, like in times gone by. In this new information-centric era, the power lies with those who are information-rich. Those who *know* more and can be trusted will be better off. Politicians don't want this.

The blockchain technology on which crypto is run is also self-governing and fully transparent, making it undesirable to those who have things to hide. Politicians don't want this either.

Governments run nations through mass coercion and taxation. The fact is, we are all free—free to move and start again. But the cost of living, the daily 9–5, and other aspects of modern living, like materialism and eating ultra-processed foods, keep us dependent on government aid and healthcare. We die in wars started by those sitting comfortably in parliament. And when we're upset, we demonstrate our rights, usually without success.

The war you are told is happening is the war between the digital age and traditional governments. As technology further develops, more people are noticing the hamster wheel and the outline of the cage they are trapped within. But governments will not back down without a fight. In fact, it may be getting harder to escape.

Now that the average person has more power over the world than at any other time in history, industries that currently have a monopoly over our attention feel threatened. A power shift is occurring in real time, and seeing this, world leaders are fighting back by trying to implement a global communistic regime via a technocratic, pharmaceutical biosurveillance approach.

Yet many still remain unconvinced and think the last three years were just an elaborate way for those involved to make more money, and though a massive shift in wealth to the world's top 1% *has* occurred in recent years, one must ask oneself why take the elaborate approach of possibly accidentally leaking a genetically altered virus and then later inoculating a large proportion of the globe with a previously untested agent to secure cash? something they can just print more of. Surely there are easier ways to make money?

To those with a lot of money, control over others becomes the primary objective, even at the expense of human life. In a world where immoral behaviour is more profitable, those who rise to the top of traditional systems are more likely to have sociopathic tendencies and thus more money and power. With the advent of AI and the transparent blockchain, these individuals are likely feeling more threatened.

Those with power have a tendency to want more power, as John Emerich Edward Dalberg-Acton famously quotes, *"Power tends to corrupt, and absolute power corrupts absolutely. Great men are almost always bad men, even when they exercise influence and not authority."* But those with power who *also* feel positionally threatened are even more dangerous. This is because man will always fight harder to keep what he has rather than putting that same amount of energy into acquiring newer and better things.

It is a hard pill to swallow to even consider that those that we once trusted are capable of evil, but there are countless examples throughout history where this has been the case. Genocide and public control over others go hand in hand.

In essence, the world is becoming more decentralised, i.e., distributed or delegated away from a central, authoritative location or group. Feeling intimidated that these traditional pillars of society are crumbling, the "elites" of the old system are inventing ways to maintain power and control.

One of these is the creation of the Central Bank Digital Currency (CBDC), which is a type of currency that is issued and controlled by a country's central bank. This has been invented to counteract decentralised forms of currency like Bitcoin that eliminate the need for banks. Bitcoin also fundamentally removes governmental financial control, as more of it can never be made and thus manipulated by the state.

In essence, Bitcoin is a stronger form of currency than gold and gives power back to the people. The invention of CBDC is to counteract this.

The other invention is vaccine passports and related forms of biosurveillance that were tried to be implemented during the pandemic under the guise of reducing transmission. However, the clear evidence that these shots did not stop transmission has prevented its widespread implementation thus far.

Vaccine passports are the equivalent of identity documents that perpetrators of genocides have historically used to discriminate, dehumanise, and then carry out mass violence against certain groups.[7] Groups at great risk if vaccine passports are ever introduced include those who are not up-to-date with their shots and/or anyone else the state deems unfit to travel. Vaccine passports are the best way to stop people from moving around in a world where travel is currently unrestricted.

It seems like those in power and running centralised institutions worldwide will not stop until these countermeasures to human freedom are implemented. Emergencies provide the perfect opportunities for power grabs, and thus it is not illogical to think that emergencies may even be cultivated for future power-grabbing purposes. Along this line of thinking, another pandemic or other global threats are likely on the cards in the near future

Well, Gates thinks so anyway, and he's written about a possible global future pathogenic threat and what we may be doing about it in his recent book titled, "How to Prevent the Next Pandemic."

What are his proposed solutions? A centralised global infection control task force, QR codes, endless jabbing, and other dystopic measures like digital ID systems.

The G20, an intergovernmental forum comprising 19 countries and the European Union, also thinks a future pandemic is possible and has recently outlined their plans in their G20 Bali Leader's Declaration document, stating,[8]

"We recognize the need for strengthening local and regional health product manufacturing capacities and cooperation as well as sustainable global and regional research and development networks to facilitate better access to VTDs *(vaccines, therapeutics and diagnostics)* globally, especially in developing countries, and underscore the importance of public-private partnership, and technology transfer and knowledge sharing on voluntary and mutually agreed terms. **We support the WHO mRNA Vaccine Technology Transfer hub** as well as all as the spokes in all regions of the world with the objective of sharing technology and technical know-how on voluntary and mutually agreed terms. We welcome joint research and joint production of vaccines, including enhanced cooperation among developing countries. **We acknowledge the importance of shared technical standards and verification methods, under the framework of the IHR (2005), to facilitate seamless international travel, interoperability, and recognizing digital solutions and non-digital solutions, including proof of vaccinations.** We support continued international dialogue and collaboration on the establishment of trusted global digital health networks as part of the efforts to strengthen prevention and **response to**

future pandemics, that should capitalize and build on the success of the existing standards and digital COVID-19 certificates."

The Defense Advanced Research Projects Agency (DARPA) is a United States Department of Defense research and development agency responsible for the development of emerging military technology.[9] Three years before Gates' 2015 TED Talks speech, DARPA began investing in the development of gene-encoded vaccines based on DNA or RNA.[10] And so it seems like the US military has been toying with genetic agents for at least 10 years now, which really questions the authenticity of Operation Warp Speed, "a federal effort that supported multiple COVID-19 vaccine candidates to speed up development."[11]

With more reading and understanding, it seems like where we are today as a human race was always inevitable.

I will leave you with this excerpt from ***The Sovereign Individual: Mastering The Transition To The Information Age, by James Dale Davidson and Lord William Rees-Mogg***, published in 1999.[12]

> **"THOSE WITH THE EARNING ABILITY AND CAPITAL TO MEET THE COMPETITIVE CHALLENGES OF THE INFORMATION AGE WILL BE ABLE TO LOCATE ANYWHERE AND DO BUSINESS ANYWHERE. WITH A CHOICE OF DOMICILES, ONLY THE MOST PATRIOTIC OR STUPID WILL CONTINUE TO RESIDE IN HIGH-TAX COUNTRIES.**
>
> **FOR THIS REASON, IT IS TO BE EXPECTED THAT ONE OR MORE NATION-STATES WILL UNDERTAKE COVERT ACTION TO SUBVERT THE APPEAL OF TRANSIENCE. TRAVEL COULD BE EFFECTIVELY DISCOURAGED BY BIOLOGICAL WARFARE, SUCH AS THE OUTBREAK OF A DEADLY EPIDEMIC. THIS COULD NOT ONLY DISCOURAGE THE DESIRE TO TRAVEL, IT COULD ALSO GIVE JURISDICTIONS THROUGHOUT THE GLOBE AN EXCUSE TO SEAL THEIR BORDERS AND LIMIT IMMIGRATION".**

Though you may not see it, we are all amidst the greatest war humankind has ever faced.

A war on all of our freedoms.

CHARLET'S STORY

After having a reaction to the Astrazeneca vaccine, at the start of 2021 and going from not taking any medication, being fit and healthy to being bedbound with over 35 symptoms, I set up UK CV Family. We started off as just a small group of 20, all having had ongoing adverse reactions to now over 900 people affected by this in the uk. We have around 15 volunteers and we are completely run by those affected by an adverse reaction to a Covid vaccine.

We have been in two documentaries, we have written to over 200 MPs on behalf of their vaccine injured constituents, are part of the Covid 19 public inquiry and we provide mutual support to our members

The stigma both medically and socially that surrounds our illness is a barrier to timely and appropriate treatment and support and this is what we would like to see change in the future

Charlet, founder of UK CV Family.
www.ukcvfamily.org
enquiries@ukcvfamily.org

THE PANDEMIC OF FEAR

"FEAR IS THE DESTRUCTIVE ENERGY IN MAN. IT WITHERS THE MIND, IT DISTORTS THOUGHT, IT LEADS TO ALL KINDS OF EXTRAORDINARILY CLEVER AND SUBTLE THEORIES, ABSURD SUPERSTITIONS, DOGMAS, AND BELIEFS."
J. KRISHNAMURTI

A few months into the pandemic, and not so long after fully appreciating the wonders of natural immunity in protecting us specifically against SARS-CoV-2, I made a conscious decision to never wear a mask in public ever again. Wearing a mask symbolised scientific ignorance and fear, two things I did not want to associate myself with.

Though I was not bothered publicly on most occasions, there was one time I was refused entry to a charity furniture store for not wearing one. On this occasion, the staff at the store asked me to wear a mask. I respectfully refused and said I had a medical exemption. I could see real fear in their eyes when I said "no," and since they had probably never dealt with a person without a mask, they called their manager for help.

I was told again, this time by the manager, that I was not allowed entry unless I wore a mask. And again, I repeated that I wasn't going to due to having a medical exemption. At this point, the manager asks me what the exemption was. In reply to this discriminatory question, I ask them on what grounds it is ethical or fair to disallow an individual service due to medical reasons. I also reminded them that asking an individual about their medical exemption was not only not their business but also wouldn't hold up in court, and encouraged them to read the government guidelines with regards to face coverings.

I remained calm and polite throughout this exchange, and having had enough at this point, I headed out of the store, genuinely disappointed at what the world had become. As I was walking out, a customer passing by exclaimed, "It's only a mask, for goodness sake; it's not hard to just wear one."

But it's not *only* a mask, is it?

Fear comes in various shapes and sizes, ruling most people and turning them into subservient slaves. Most people are scared of death, of rejection, of confrontation, of being different, of saying the wrong thing, of authority, of being maskless; the list goes on endlessly.

Those who are fearful act selfishly, ignorantly, angrily, and enviously, and are willing to go to any extent to quell the feeling quickly. People who are afraid stay willfully ignorant when they see wrongdoing. They gaslight, ostracise, and discriminate. They follow inhumane rules. They become puppets, unable to think intelligently. They tell others how to think and act. They pull triggers and inject poisons.

For three years and counting, for reasons ultimately leading to fear, we, the many billions of individuals who make up society, have kept quiet and been willfully ignorant. The world is burning, and everyone knows it, but no one wants to say anything because we are scared, not because of the facts.

The manipulation of scientific data to fit an agenda is real. Jab-related injuries are real. Excess deaths corresponding to jab roll-outs are real. The harms caused by lockdowns are real. The ineffectiveness of masks is real. Natural immunity is real.

And yet doctors, nurses, lawyers, researchers, public health officials, psychologists, lab assistants, ambulance staff, care home workers, politicians, military personnel, journalists, your boss, your friends, your family, every single thinking person on this planet, and you yourself likely continue to lead a double life full of hypocrisy due to fear.

Keep in mind that silence is also a choice.

To all those who value their status and supposed mental prowess, it is no use being intelligent if you are also fearful. In fact, I'd go to the extent of saying that those who are afraid cannot act intelligently.

The harsh truth is that we're where we are now as a human race because we collectively let it happen. People are dying and suffering because we all individually let it happen. We must take responsibility for this.

Though it may be true that there is an authority-led master plan aiming to create one global communistic state using a technocratic pharmaceutical biosurveillance approach, the only reason we have gotten this far, and the only reason so many have died and continue to die, is not because of a virus but because so many people were and continue to be fearful.

We are amidst a pandemic of cowardice; a pandemic of fear.

HOW DO WE FIX THE BROKEN SYSTEM?

Every day, the level and depth of fraud across various industries that we once trusted wholeheartedly continue to be exposed. *Well, online anyway*. Journalism, healthcare, the pharmaceutical industry, the justice system, and governments have all failed us in astronomical ways, and since the mainstream media continues to hide the truth, I can only say that they are still working together as we speak.

The thing that has worried me the most about the last three years is that science, which is based on fighting against false stories and made-up beliefs, has been taken hostage and used to trick the general public. And with science falling, medical ethics, a cornerstone of human rights, also crumbled in many parts of the world.

I understand the human tendency to wield anything for the control of power, but I was deeply disappointed that no one stood up or said anything.

The ease and pace at which this all happened also scared me. To control an airborne virus, we were all placed under house arrest with no additional advice on how to keep healthy or immunologically robust. Instead, local parks were taped up, hospitals were discouraged from hosting visitors, and schools closed. Only one thing was dangled in front of our faces, promising freedom.

We went from old normalcy to fear-stricken society in an instant. New cultures, new rules, and new fashions were created. And all of them were unscientific, wasteful, environmentally detrimental, and narrative-promoting.

People still continue to wear facemasks outdoors, and the fact that unscientific rules and regulations continue to take place in various parts of the world tells me that we are not living in an age of scientific enlightenment but a stronghold of Big Pharma corruption.

Who do we trust now?

Can you put your trust in your sweet family doctor, who believes information tainted by pharmaceutical misanthropy and is complicit in medical tyranny?

Can you trust the nurses who injected genetic agents into the arms of millions of people without asking any questions?

What about those involved in the production of the medicine we take, who appear to have been involved in possibly leaking the virus in the first place and then conveniently developing an agent before the pandemic?

What about governments that have locked us down, ruined the lives of children, the elderly, the economy, and the health of all?

Can you trust social media companies that shut down the voices of many highly qualified doctors and scientists, ending scientific debate when it was most needed?

What about the journalists who have remained silent on the issue of excess deaths and jab harms?

We are by ourselves.

This is the truth, especially since those in power will never admit to committing crimes against humanity. This is only made worse by the fact that they have considerable leverage over the justice system too. The hands that administered the poison will not be the same ones that will help. *And even if they did lend a helping hand, could we trust it?*

Corporations do not have our health or wellbeing at the forefront of their minds. Pharmaceutical industries rely on our sickness for their profits. The pesticides and plastics used to grow and package our foods are killing us. Healthcare services are abysmal at treating chronic health problems. Research opposing the effectiveness of the shots or highlighting their dangers is difficult to publish due to bureaucratic gatekeeping. Big Tech frequently works with government bodies to distract us and manipulate online algorithms, controlling the public consciousness. At the end of the day, people we call "elite" will always put money, power, and the dominion of others before the betterment of humanity.

Answers to deaths, solutions to jab-related injuries, and justice will have to come from ourselves and certain societal figureheads that have proven to be worthy of being trusted.

Though this may all sound devastating in the short term, I'd argue that this is a good thing in the long term for humanity as a whole. The pandemic has only revealed the tip of the iceberg in terms of global scandal and corruption. Many of us are beginning to wake up.

Since the beginning of reductionist biological science, big companies have always been able to obscure data to make more money, but the pandemic was an example of overreach that led to one of the biggest wealth transfers to the top 1%.

But the overreach has not gone unnoticed. Trust in criminal organisations and institutions is dwindling, and rightly so. These systems will fall.

It is important to remember that, though traditional authoritative systems are falling and at times it might feel like we are alone, we should not feel lonely. Always keep in mind that we are 7 billion people. We are more.

We must also remember that, like in war, though the state may use some human life as cannon fodder, they ultimately require the majority of the population to be alive and well to run the system that they rely upon. So, threats are very unlikely to be as dangerous as they are made out to be, especially if we plan ahead, work smart, and work together.

To make sure that humanity has a better future, we must all work together to find justice and heal. The only way meaningful and lasting changes can be made is if we put our differences aside and make our voices heard as one. There must be a cultural shift impactful enough to change legal policies in our favour. I think that for that to happen, we need to win some smaller battles, such as (not in any particular order):

- The halting of the development of all mRNA and DNA pharmaceutical technology.
- Publicly funded independent analysis of raw trial data, excess deaths, and investigation into the extent of jab-related injuries and multi-corporation corruption.
- A formal apology from major pharmaceutical companies, international governments, mainstream media companies, major medical institutions and medical practices for the harms they have caused.
- Incarceration of those involved in the potential development of the virus and/or cover-up of lab leak concerns.
- Incarceration of those involved in the development of genetic agents and roll-out.
- Full compensation to those jab-injured and bereaved families.
- Helpline and mental health support dedicated to the emotional support of the jab-injured.
- Open conversations on public platforms of those with jab-related injuries and/or bereaved families.
- The removal of all forms of censorship on social media platforms.
- A boycotting of centralised forms of media and news outlets.
- New updated international rules of medical ethics drawn up in law.
- Removal of the word “vaccine” to describe these genetic agents.
- Full transparency using blockchain technology of all new research, grants and scientific endeavours especially when it concerns human life.
- The wide use of decentralised secure cryptocurrencies in opposition to CBDC.
- Re-education of the public and especially children about immunology, natural immunity and how to look after themselves properly.
- Population-wide cardiac and genetic screening programmes.
- Research into jab-related pathophysiology and treatment options, with special emphasis on finding ways to clear the spike protein.
- The introduction of jab-related injuries into the medical literature.

- International campaign aimed at raising awareness of and removing the stigma toward adverse reactions to genetic agents.

It will now be necessary for us to construct new systems based on truth, openness, and proper values. No one else is coming to save us.

We must do this together.

WE ARE ONE

It's been a year since I stopped working in healthcare and deregistered myself from the GMC records. I cannot give medical advice or prescribe medications now. I have no comfortable office, no steady income, no job security, and yet I wouldn't change a thing.

Before my exit, my former supervisors asked me if there was anything they could do to change my mind. Their questions only continued to highlight their ignorance of the problem at hand, further cementing my decision to leave.

Thinking back, the only aspect of working in healthcare I truly miss is looking after patients and using what I know to improve people's lives. I take great pleasure in helping others heal. I love people. And though this book is not meant to constitute medical advice, I hope you, the reader, have found it helpful educationally.

I hope you have learned that the COVID-19 genetic shots work by hiding from our natural defences and then tricking our own cells to produce bundles of harmful toxins that trigger our immune system to attack ourselves. I hope you have learned, in a similar vein, that we were lied to on a societal scale and tricked into harming our own.

I hope you have learned about possible ways to mitigate jab-related injuries, but also that the scientific community still has no idea about the long-term effects of these shots.

To find out, we must begin to practise science again—the study of the world through observation, experimentation, discussion, and debate. And through this, we will learn and appreciate that both we and the world are not only infinitely complicated but intimately connected.

We are the world, and the world is us.

Currently, the world is sick, but I know that we have all the resources and knowledge necessary for every single person on this planet to live happily and healthily. The world can only heal if we heal.

In a land of lies, the truth must be protected at all costs. Freedom of speech, freedom of movement, and freedom of thought are our birthrights. Discussions and debates must openly take place. Knowledge must not be hidden or used for control.

We must collectively come together and demand answers. We must ask why governments continue to ignore those jab-injured and the reason for excess deaths? We must pester our politicians, doctors, lawyers, and journalists for answers. We must send letters and emails, make phone calls, demonstrate, boycott, and write online posts.

We must strive to educate others in a loving manner and to assist our fellow man. We must let our voices be heard, no matter what.

It is our time to call out the shots.

BIBLIOGRAPHY

SO YOU'VE TAKEN THE SHOT, NOW WHAT?

1. https://www.campaignlive.co.uk/article/govt-spent-184m-covid-comms-2020/1708695
2. https://newspunch.com/bidens-hhs-and-cdc-paid-screen-writers-and-comedians-to-mock-the-unvaccinated/
3. https://www.healthline.com/health-news/why-unvaccinated-people-are-being-denied-organ-transplants
4. https://api.politifact.com/factchecks/2021/jul/22/joe-biden/biden-exaggerates-efficacy-covid-19-vaccines/

WHAT HAVE YOU INJECTED INSIDE OF YOURSELF?

1. https://www.miamiherald.com/news/coronavirus/article254111268.html
2. https://www.frontiersin.org/files/Articles/589959/fchem-08-589959-HTML/image_m/fchem-08-589959-g001.jpg
3. https://www.nytimes.com/interactive/2020/health/johnson-johnson-covid-19-vaccine.html
4. https://www.nytimes.com/interactive/2020/health/oxford-astrazeneca-covid-19-vaccine.html

ARE THESE 'GENE THERAPIES'?

1. https://www.fda.gov/vaccines-blood-biologics/cellular-gene-therapy-products/what-gene-therapy
2. https://www.ncbi.nlm.nih.gov/pmc/articles/PMC9141755/
3. https://ui.adsabs.harvard.edu/abs/2004Sci...303..537E/abstract
4. https://www.ncbi.nlm.nih.gov/pmc/articles/PMC3690669/
5. https://pubmed.ncbi.nlm.nih.gov/26342664/
6. https://pubmed.ncbi.nlm.nih.gov/33524990/
7. https://www.ncbi.nlm.nih.gov/pmc/articles/PMC7745181/
8. https://pubmed.ncbi.nlm.nih.gov/33958444/
9. https://pubmed.ncbi.nlm.nih.gov/24089548/
10. https://www.ncbi.nlm.nih.gov/pmc/articles/PMC8166107/
11. https://www.mdpi.com/1467-3045/44/3/73/htm

HOW RELIABLE IS THE ORIGINAL STUDY DATA?

1. https://www.nejm.org/doi/full/10.1056/nejmoa2110345

2. https://www.bmj.com/content/375/bmj.n2635
3. https://phmpt.org/pfizers-documents/
4. shorturl.at/vxNY8
5. https://www.wsj.com/articles/rise-in-non-covid-19-deaths-hits-life-insurers-11645576252

ARE THESE SHOTS "95% EFFECTIVE"?

1. https://www.statnews.com/2020/11/18/pfizer-biontech-covid19-vaccine-fda-data/
2. https://www.thelancet.com/journals/lanmic/article/PIIS2666-5247(21)00069-0/fulltext
3. https://www.fda.gov/media/144245/download
4. https://en.wikipedia.org/wiki/Kary_Mullis
5. https://archive.org/details/kary-mullis-speaks-to-misuse-of-pcr-1993
6. https://pubmed.ncbi.nlm.nih.gov/32986798/
7. https://jamanetwork.com/journals/jama/fullarticle/2783644
8. https://www.bmj.com/content/371/bmj.m4037
9. https://blogs.bmj.com/bmj/2021/01/04/peter-doshi-pfizer-and-modernas-95-effective-vaccines-we-need-more-details-and-the-raw-data/
10. https://www.ons.gov.uk/aboutus/transparencyandgovernance/freedomofinformationfoi/covid19deathsandillnessaftervaccine

DOES IT REDUCE SYMPTOM SEVERITY?

1. https://www.thelancet.com/journals/lancet/article/PIIS0140-6736(21)00947-8/fulltext
2. https://web.archive.org/web/20070712033200/http://www.ocf.berkeley.edu/~barneye/kitty.html
3. https://www.webcitation.org/67mDV0UME?url=http://www.straightdope.com/columns/read/1143/do-cats-always-land-unharmed-on-their-feet-no-matter-how-far-they-fall
4. https://www.eurosurveillance.org/content/10.2807/1560-7917.ES.2021.26.39.2100822
5. https://www.clinicalmicrobiologyandinfection.com/article/S1198-743X(21)00367-0/fulltext

WHAT IS IMMUNITY?

1. https://www.ncbi.nlm.nih.gov/pmc/articles/PMC7270427/

WHAT IS THE INNATE IMMUNE SYSTEM?

1. https://www.ncbi.nlm.nih.gov/pmc/articles/PMC2785020/

2. https://www.ncbi.nlm.nih.gov/pmc/articles/PMC5155499/

WHAT WERE MY ANTIBODY RESULTS?

1. https://www.ncbi.nlm.nih.gov/books/NBK546670/
2. https://www.ncbi.nlm.nih.gov/pmc/articles/PMC4159104/
3. https://www.ncbi.nlm.nih.gov/pmc/articles/PMC6963396/
4. https://www.ncbi.nlm.nih.gov/pmc/articles/PMC4202688/
5. https://www.ncbi.nlm.nih.gov/books/NBK555995/
6. https://www.ncbi.nlm.nih.gov/pmc/articles/PMC4835181/
7. http://www.eurekaselect.com/article/57198

CAN YOU BE IMMUNE WITH A NEG ANTIBODY TEST?

1. https://www.biorxiv.org/content/10.1101/2020.06.29.174888v1.full.pdf

WHY WAS NATURAL IMMUNITY IGNORED?

1. https://www.thelancet.com/journals/lancet/article/PIIS0140-6736(20)32153-X/fulltext
2. https://brownstone.org/articles/79-research-studies-affirm-naturally-acquired-immunity-to-covid-19-documented-linked-and-quoted/

WHY IS NATURAL IMMUNITY THE ONLY WAY OUT?

1. https://www.nejm.org/doi/full/10.1056/NEJMc2108120
2. https://www.biorxiv.org/content/10.1101/2021.12.06.471446v1
3. https://www.ncbi.nlm.nih.gov/pmc/articles/PMC9167431/
4. https://pubmed.ncbi.nlm.nih.gov/34873910/
5. https://pubmed.ncbi.nlm.nih.gov/35380632/
6. https://pubmed.ncbi.nlm.nih.gov/36362500/

WHO ARE THE UNSUNG HEROES?

1. https://science.sciencemag.org/content/371/6529/eabf4063
2. https://www.biorxiv.org/content/10.1101/2021.07.14.452381v1
3. https://www.biorxiv.org/content/10.1101/2021.07.14.452381v1
4. https://www.nature.com/articles/s41392-020-0191-1
5. https://www.nature.com/articles/d41586-021-00367-7#ref-CR2
6. https://science.sciencemag.org/content/373/6556/eabh1766.full
7. https://www.nature.com/articles/s41586-020-2550-z
8. https://www.nature.com/articles/s41590-021-00923-3
9. https://www.cell.com/cell-reports-medicine/fulltext/S2666-3791(21)00203-2

10. https://www.thelancet.com/journals/lanmic/article/PIIS2666-5247(22)00036-2/fulltext
11. https://www.biorxiv.org/content/10.1101/2021.08.11.455984v1
12. https://www.jimmunol.org/content/207/5/1344
13. https://www.ncbi.nlm.nih.gov/pmc/articles/PMC7237901/
14. https://science.sciencemag.org/content/370/6512/89
15. https://www.thelancet.com/journals/ebiom/article/PIIS2352-3964(21)00403-5/fulltext
16. https://www.nature.com/articles/s41423-021-00700-0
17. https://www.telegraph.co.uk/news/2022/01/10/common-cold-might-have-given-britons-protection-covid-pandemic/
18. https://jme.bmj.com/content/early/2022/12/05/jme-2022-108449
19. https://twitter.com/dockaurg/status/1547957109983043584?lang=en

WHAT IS THE KEY TO A WELL FUNCTIONING IMMUNE SYSTEM?

1. https://www.nature.com/articles/s41467-021-22036-z#ref-CR2
2. https://pubmed.ncbi.nlm.nih.gov/33412089/
3. https://www.atsjournals.org/doi/10.1164/rccm.202005-1701LE
4. https://www.atsjournals.org/doi/10.1164/rccm.202005-1701LE

WHY ARE SOME PEOPLE AFFECTED WORSE BY THE VIRUS?

1. https://gh.bmj.com/content/6/12/e006434
2. https://coronavirus.jhu.edu/data/mortality
3. https://www.ons.gov.uk/aboutus/transparencyandgovernance/freedomofinformationfoi/averageageofthosewhohaddiedwithcovid19
4. https://www.ons.gov.uk/peoplepopulationandcommunity/birthsdeathsandmarriages/lifeexpectancies/bulletins/nationallifetablesunitedkingdom/2017to2019
5. https://www.nature.com/articles/s41467-022-29801-8
6. https://www.nature.com/articles/s41467-020-19741-6
7. https://nutrition.bmj.com/content/5/1/10
8. https://www.thelancet.com/journals/landia/article/PIIS2213-8587(21)00244-8/fulltext
9. https://pubmed.ncbi.nlm.nih.gov/32647915/
10. https://www.bmj.com/company/newsroom/insomnia-disrupted-sleep-and-burnout-linked-to-higher-odds-of-severe-covid-19/
11. https://onlinelibrary.wiley.com/doi/pdf/10.1111/add.15194
12. https://bmcinfectdis.biomedcentral.com/articles/10.1186/s12879-021-06617-3
13. https://www.ncbi.nlm.nih.gov/pmc/articles/PMC8569840/
14. https://pubmed.ncbi.nlm.nih.gov/32920234/
15. https://gut.bmj.com/content/70/4/698

16. https://www.ncbi.nlm.nih.gov/pmc/articles/PMC7385774/
17. https://pubmed.ncbi.nlm.nih.gov/12696983/
18. https://bjsm.bmj.com/content/55/19/1099
19. https://www.frontiersin.org/articles/10.3389/fpubh.2021.684112/full
20. https://www.frontiersin.org/articles/10.3389/fcimb.2021.767771/full
21. https://onlinelibrary.wiley.com/doi/10.1111/all.15372
22. https://www.nature.com/articles/s41590-021-01094-x
23. https://www.nature.com/articles/s41467-021-27063-4
24. https://www.science.org/doi/10.1126/science.abg3055
25. https://www.medrxiv.org/content/10.1101/2021.05.03.21256520v1
26. https://journals.plos.org/plospathogens/article?id=10.1371/journal.ppat.1010197
27. https://www.cell.com/iscience/fulltext/S2589-0042(22)00277-2

WHY MAY AN INCREASED EXPOSURE TO SARS-COV-2 IMPROVE IMMUNITY?

1. https://www.drkohilathas.co.uk/ruminations/the-vaccinated-getting-infected-marks-the-end-of-the-pandemic
2. https://www.biorxiv.org/content/10.1101/2021.07.14.452381v1
3. https://www.cdc.gov/pcd/issues/2021/21_0123.htm
4. https://www.nature.com/articles/s41598-021-84092-1
5. https://www.fhi.no/globalassets/dokumenterfiler/rapporter/2020/should-individuals-in-the-community-without-respiratory-symptoms-wear-facemasks-to-reduce-the-spread-of-covid-19-report-2020.pdf
6. https://www.biorxiv.org/content/10.1101/2022.04.30.489997v1
7. https://www.ncbi.nlm.nih.gov/pmc/articles/PMC5278669/
8. https://www.frontiersin.org/articles/10.3389/fimmu.2020.611337/
9. https://www.nature.com/articles/s41385-021-00461-z
10. https://www.nature.com/articles/s41385-020-0309-3
11. https://www.nature.com/articles/s41577-021-00638-4
12. https://www.nature.com/articles/s41467-021-23333-3
13. https://www.scientificamerican.com/article/viruses-can-help-us-as-well-as-harm-us/
14. https://www.ncbi.nlm.nih.gov/pmc/articles/PMC8669911/
15. https://www.ncbi.nlm.nih.gov/pmc/articles/PMC4515362/
16. https://en.m.wikipedia.org/wiki/Marine_viruses
17. https://www.nature.com/articles/s41396-017-0042-4
18. https://pubmed.ncbi.nlm.nih.gov/30734920
19. https://jamanetwork.com/journals/jamanetworkopen/fullarticle/2778936
20. https://journals.plos.org/plosbiology/article?id=10.1371/journal.pbio.1002198
21. https://zenodo.org/record/6904363#.Yx8gvuzMKrw
22. https://www.ncbi.nlm.nih.gov/pmc/articles/PMC2720273/
23. https://www.frontiersin.org/articles/10.3389/fimmu.2020.611337/full

24. https://www.biorxiv.org/content/10.1101/2022.05.16.492138v1
25. https://www.science.org/doi/full/10.1126/scitranslmed.abn6150

WHAT IS THE DIFFERENCE BETWEEN A TH1 AND TH2 RESPONSE?

1. https://www.ncbi.nlm.nih.gov/pmc/articles/PMC2433332/
2. https://www.ncbi.nlm.nih.gov/pmc/articles/PMC8140108/
3. https://pubmed.ncbi.nlm.nih.gov/32669297/
4. https://www.ncbi.nlm.nih.gov/pmc/articles/PMC7108125/
5. https://www.ncbi.nlm.nih.gov/pmc/articles/PMC7190990/
6. https://www.frontiersin.org/articles/10.3389/fimmu.2021.735125/full
7. https://www.ncbi.nlm.nih.gov/pmc/articles/PMC7837114/
8. https://www.ncbi.nlm.nih.gov/pmc/articles/PMC8869678/
9. https://www.nature.com/articles/s41577-020-0402-6
10. https://pubmed.ncbi.nlm.nih.gov/33718270/
11. https://www.frontiersin.org/articles/10.3389/fgene.2021.706902/full
12. https://www.ncbi.nlm.nih.gov/pmc/articles/PMC3917935/
13. https://www.nature.com/articles/nri3536
14. https://www.frontiersin.org/articles/10.3389/fcimb.2020.00317/full
15. https://www.jimmunol.org/content/207/9/2205
16. https://pubmed.ncbi.nlm.nih.gov/15233728/

DO THE JABS INCREASE OUR RISK OF INFECTION?

1. https://www.bmj.com/content/378/bmj-2022-070344
2. https://www.england.nhs.uk/2021/09/nhs-begins-covid-19-booster-vaccination-campaign/
3. https://www.thelancet.com/journals/lanres/article/PIIS2213-2600(22)00010-8/fulltext
4. https://www.ons.gov.uk/aboutus/transparencyandgovernance/freedomofinformationfoi/covid19deathsandillnessaftervaccine
5. https://www.health.govt.nz/covid-19-novel-coronavirus/covid-19-data-and-statistics/covid-19-case-demographics
6. https://www.researchgate.net/publication/343607804_Phase_12_study_of_COVID-19_RNA_vaccine_BNT162b1_in_adults
7. https://www.tandfonline.com/doi/full/10.1080/21645515.2020.1750249
8. https://phmpt.org/wp-content/uploads/2022/03/125742_S1_M1_priority-review-request-1.pdf
9. https://www.sciencedirect.com/science/article/pii/S1201971220302794
10. https://pubmed.ncbi.nlm.nih.gov/34719084/
11. https://www.science.org/doi/full/10.1126/scitranslmed.abn6150
12. https://www.medrxiv.org/content/10.1101/2021.08.24.21262415v1
13. https://www.medrxiv.org/content/10.1101/2022.12.17.22283625v1.full.pdf

WHAT MAY BE SOME LONGER TERM IMMUNOLOGICAL IMPLICATIONS OF TAKING THE SHOT?

1. https://www.sciencedirect.com/science/article/pii/S027869152200206X#bib119
2. https://journals.plos.org/plosone/article?id=10.1371/journal.pone.0249499
3. https://www.science.org/doi/10.1126/scitranslmed.abd2223
4. https://www.nature.com/articles/s41586-020-2639-4
5. https://linkinghub.elsevier.com/retrieve/pii/S0092867422000769
6. https://osf.io/bcsa6/
7. https://linkinghub.elsevier.com/retrieve/pii/S1931524421001225
8. https://www.nature.com/articles/s41421-021-00329-3
9. https://www.medrxiv.org/content/10.1101/2021.04.20.21255677v2.full.pdf
10. https://www.nature.com/articles/s41586-021-03412-7
11. https://www.mdpi.com/2079-9721/9/3/57
12. https://linkinghub.elsevier.com/retrieve/pii/S1525001616454560
13. https://www.jimmunol.org/content/207/10/2405
14. https://phmpt.org/wp-content/uploads/2022/03/125742_S1_M1_priority-review-request-1.pdf
15. https://www.ncbi.nlm.nih.gov/pmc/articles/PMC7123835/
16. https://www.ncbi.nlm.nih.gov/pmc/articles/PMC2846036/
17. https://journals.plos.org/plosone/article?id=10.1371/journal.pone.0070458
18. https://www.ncbi.nlm.nih.gov/pmc/articles/PMC7446632/
19. https://hh-publisher.com/ojs321/index.php/pmmb/article/view/338
20. https://pubmed.ncbi.nlm.nih.gov/30358186/
21. https://www.nature.com/articles/s41577-019-0221-9
22. https://www.ncbi.nlm.nih.gov/pmc/articles/PMC4889009/
23. https://www.voanews.com/a/eu-drug-regulator-warns-against-overuse-of-covid-booster-shots/6395174.html
24. https://www.reuters.com/business/healthcare-pharmaceuticals/eu-drug-regulator-says-more-data-needed-impact-omicron-vaccines-2022-01-11/
25. https://www.nature.com/articles/s41423-020-0401-3
26. https://www.nature.com/articles/s41423-021-00750-4
27. https://www.ncbi.nlm.nih.gov/pmc/articles/PMC7286441/
28. https://www.ncbi.nlm.nih.gov/pmc/articles/PMC7286441/
29. https://www.ncbi.nlm.nih.gov/pmc/articles/PMC4253638/
30. https://molecular-cancer.biomedcentral.com/articles/10.1186/s12943-021-01328-4
31. https://www.ncbi.nlm.nih.gov/pmc/articles/PMC8136783/
32. https://www.frontiersin.org/articles/10.3389/fendo.2018.00402/

33. https://www.ncbi.nlm.nih.gov/pmc/articles/PMC3048316/
34. https://www.ncbi.nlm.nih.gov/pmc/articles/PMC5343750/
35. https://www.jidonline.org/article/S0022-202X(21)02479-9/fulltext
36. https://www.nature.com/articles/ncomms9516
37. https://journals.plos.org/plospathogens/article?id=10.1371/journal.ppat.1009759
38. https://www.frontiersin.org/articles/10.3389/fimmu.2021.656700/full
39. https://www.jcancer.org/v07p1233.htm
40. https://www.sciencedirect.com/science/article/pii/S2542364917301115
41. https://www.mdpi.com/2079-9721/9/3/57/htm
42. https://twitter.com/P_McCulloughMD/status/1514210721122377729

WHY THE SPIKE PROTEIN?

1. https://www.frontiersin.org/articles/10.3389/fimmu.2021.701501/full
2. https://pubmed.ncbi.nlm.nih.gov/35090596/
3. https://www.nature.com/articles/s41423-021-00779-5
4. https://www.politifact.com/factchecks/2021/jun/16/youtube-videos/no-sign-covid-19-vaccines-spike-protein-toxic-or-c/
5. https://www.nature.com/articles/s41593-020-00771-8
6. https://www.frontiersin.org/articles/10.3389/fncel.2021.777738/full
7. https://portlandpress.com/clinsci/article/136/6/431/231092/SARS-CoV-2-spike-protein-causes-cardiovascular
8. https://faseb.onlinelibrary.wiley.com/doi/full/10.1096/fj.202002742RR
9. https://www.ncbi.nlm.nih.gov/pmc/articles/PMC7758180/
10. https://www.mdpi.com/1999-4915/13/10/2056/htm
11. https://www.nature.com/articles/d41586-021-01529-3
12. https://www.science.org/content/article/pandemic-start-anywhere-but-here-argue-papers-chinese-scientists-echoing-party-line#.Yv5P8FFAqPY.twitter
13. https://www.biorxiv.org/content/10.1101/2020.01.30.927871v1
14. https://www.pnas.org/doi/10.1073/pnas.2010722117
15. https://pubmed.ncbi.nlm.nih.gov/20088758/
16. https://www.liebertpub.com/doi/pdfplus/10.1177/153567600601100303
17. https://www.frontiersin.org/articles/10.3389/fimmu.2022.941009/full
18. https://pubmed.ncbi.nlm.nih.gov/34426024/
19. https://www.ncbi.nlm.nih.gov/pmc/articles/PMC8227405/
20. https://onlinelibrary.wiley.com/doi/full/10.1002/jcla.24479
21. https://www.ncbi.nlm.nih.gov/pmc/articles/PMC7237901/
22. https://www.ncbi.nlm.nih.gov/pmc/articles/PMC8463655/

HOW LONG DO SPIKE PROTEINS STAY IN THE BODY?

1. https://www.medrxiv.org/content/10.1101/2022.03.01.22271618v1.full

2. https://linkinghub.elsevier.com/retrieve/pii/S0092867422000769
3. https://www.frontiersin.org/articles/10.3389/fimmu.2021.746021/full
4. https://www.nature.com/articles/s41586-021-03738-2
5. https://www.sciencedaily.com/releases/2021/06/210628170542.htm
6. https://www.nejm.org/doi/full/10.1056/NEJMoa2118946
7. https://www.mdpi.com/2227-9059/10/7/1538/htm
8. https://pubmed.ncbi.nlm.nih.gov/35148837/
9. https://www.ncbi.nlm.nih.gov/pmc/articles/PMC8241425/
10. https://www.ema.europa.eu/en/documents/assessment-report/comirnaty-epar-public-assessment-report_en.pdf
11. https://www.jimmunol.org/content/early/2021/10/11/jimmunol.2100637
12. https://pubmed.ncbi.nlm.nih.gov/23683467/
13. https://jamanetwork.com/journals/jamapediatrics/fullarticle/2796427

WHAT IS THE "HOOK EFFECT"?

1. https://pubmed.ncbi.nlm.nih.gov/34659235/
2. https://www.frontiersin.org/articles/10.3389/fimmu.2021.808932/full
3. https://pubmed.ncbi.nlm.nih.gov/33412089/
4. https://www.nature.com/articles/s41366-021-01016-9

WHAT HAPPENED TO ANTIBODY-DEPENDENT ENHANCEMENT?

1. https://www.nature.com/articles/s41586-020-2538-8
2. https://pubmed.ncbi.nlm.nih.gov/4305197/
3. https://pubmed.ncbi.nlm.nih.gov/12925847/
4. https://pubmed.ncbi.nlm.nih.gov/29097492/
5. https://pubmed.ncbi.nlm.nih.gov/19122397/
6. https://www.nature.com/articles/s41564-020-00789-5/figures/1
7. https://pubmed.ncbi.nlm.nih.gov/25073113/
8. https://pubmed.ncbi.nlm.nih.gov/34193869/
9. https://www.ncbi.nlm.nih.gov/pmc/articles/PMC4018502/
10. https://www.medrxiv.org/content/10.1101/2020.10.08.20209114v1.full
11. https://www.ncbi.nlm.nih.gov/pmc/articles/PMC8351274/
12. https://pubmed.ncbi.nlm.nih.gov/32861333/
13. https://www.nature.com/articles/s41379-022-01069-9

WHAT IS ORIGINAL ANTIGENIC SIN?

1. https://www.jimmunol.org/content/202/2/335
2. https://www.ncbi.nlm.nih.gov/pmc/articles/PMC3165229/
3. https://pubmed.ncbi.nlm.nih.gov/26046565/
4. https://www.mdpi.com/2076-393X/7/3/107\

5. https://www.sciencedirect.com/science/article/pii/S2772613421000068#bib0004
6. https://www.jci.org/articles/view/150613
7. https://www.biorxiv.org/content/10.1101/2021.09.14.460338v1
8. https://www.nature.com/articles/s41586-021-04060-7
9. https://assets.publishing.service.gov.uk/government/uploads/system/uploads/attachment_data/file/1027511/Vaccine-surveillance-report-week-42.pdf
10. https://www.nature.com/articles/28738
11. https://www.cell.com/trends/immunology/fulltext/S1471-4906(21)00177-0
12. https://www.nature.com/articles/s41586-022-05053-w_reference.pdf
13. https://www.sciencedirect.com/science/article/pii/S2772613421000068#bib0004

CAN THESE SHOTS CAUSE AUTOIMMUNE DISEASES?

1. https://zenodo.org/record/1233257#.Ys1e9OzMJQI
2. https://pubmed.ncbi.nlm.nih.gov/24395337/
3. https://www.frontiersin.org/articles/10.3389/fimmu.2019.00043/full
4. https://www.cell.com/cell-systems/fulltext/S2405-4712(20)30363-X
5. https://pubmed.ncbi.nlm.nih.gov/6300911/
6. https://www.science.org/doi/10.1126/scitranslmed.aab2354
7. https://doi.org/10.1111/j.1365-2249.2008.03831.x
8. https://www.sciencedirect.com/science/article/pii/S0896841118305365
9. https://pubmed.ncbi.nlm.nih.gov/15365133/
10. https://pubmed.ncbi.nlm.nih.gov/21699023/
11. https://www.nature.com/articles/s41590-021-00949-7#Fig1
12. https://onlinelibrary.wiley.com/doi/10.1111/sji.13160
13. https://www.cancer.gov/news-events/cancer-currents-blog/2022/mrna-vaccines-to-treat-cancer
14. https://www.frontiersin.org/articles/10.3389/fimmu.2020.617089/full
15. https://www.biorxiv.org/content/10.1101/2021.08.10.455737v1
16. https://www.nature.com/articles/s41420-020-00321-y
17. https://elifesciences.org/articles/58603
18. https://www.cell.com/cell-systems/fulltext/S2405-4712(20)30363-X
19. https://www.medrxiv.org/content/10.1101/2021.02.12.21251298v1
20. https://pubmed.ncbi.nlm.nih.gov/33688651/
21. https://www.frontiersin.org/articles/10.3389/fimmu.2021.705772/full
22. https://www.cell.com/cell-reports-medicine/fulltext/S2666-3791(21)00116-6
23. https://www.medrxiv.org/content/10.1101/2021.02.17.21251953v1?rss=1%22
24. https://www.nature.com/articles/s41366-021-01016-9

25. https://pubmed.ncbi.nlm.nih.gov/33139519/
26. https://www.nejm.org/doi/full/10.1056/NEJMoa2105385
27. https://linkinghub.elsevier.com/retrieve/pii/S1473309920300864
28. https://pubmed.ncbi.nlm.nih.gov/33478949/
29. https://www.ncbi.nlm.nih.gov/pmc/articles/PMC8460308/
30. https://onlinelibrary.wiley.com/doi/10.1111/imm.13443
31. https://www.ncbi.nlm.nih.gov/pmc/articles/PMC9060731/
32. https://pubmed.ncbi.nlm.nih.gov/33861525/
33. https://www.ncbi.nlm.nih.gov/pmc/articles/PMC8239819/figure/bjh17508-fig-0001/
34. https://pubmed.ncbi.nlm.nih.gov/25427992/
35. https://pubmed.ncbi.nlm.nih.gov/33498655/
36. https://www.ncbi.nlm.nih.gov/pmc/articles/PMC6180207/
37. https://www.ncbi.nlm.nih.gov/pmc/articles/PMC4322037
38. https://www.ncbi.nlm.nih.gov/pmc/articles/PMC2716291/

WHAT IS LONG COVID?

1. https://www.ncbi.nlm.nih.gov/pmc/articles/PMC6596083
2. https://pubmed.ncbi.nlm.nih.gov/33206133/
3. https://www.nice.org.uk/guidance/ng188
4. https://www.bmj.com/content/374/bmj.n1648
5. https://physoc.onlinelibrary.wiley.com/doi/full/10.14814/phy2.14726
6. https://www.nature.com/articles/s41591-021-01283-z
7. https://www.science.org/doi/pdf/10.1126/sciimmunol.abm7996
8. https://www.researchsquare.com/article/rs-1844677/v1
9. https://www.nature.com/articles/s41591-022-01840-0
10. https://onlinelibrary.wiley.com/doi/10.1111/all.15372
11. https://translational-medicine.biomedcentral.com/articles/10.1186/s12967-022-03328-4
12. https://www.frontiersin.org/articles/10.3389/fcimb.2022.861703/full
13. https://www.ncbi.nlm.nih.gov/pmc/articles/PMC8699232/
14. https://pubmed.ncbi.nlm.nih.gov/34917659/
15. https://www.ncbi.nlm.nih.gov/pmc/articles/PMC9057012/
16. https://assets.publishing.service.gov.uk/government/uploads/system/uploads/attachment_data/file/1027511/Vaccine-surveillance-report-week-42.pdf
17. https://pubmed.ncbi.nlm.nih.gov/34358460/
18. https://gut.bmj.com/content/early/2022/08/08/gutjnl-2022-328319
19. https://www.medrxiv.org/content/10.1101/2022.08.09.22278592v1
20. https://twitter.com/VirusesImmunity/status/1557391752889307138
21. https://onlinelibrary.wiley.com/doi/10.1111/j.1365-3083.1982.tb00618.x
22. https://www.ncbi.nlm.nih.gov/pmc/articles/PMC1809301/
23. https://www.ncbi.nlm.nih.gov/pmc/articles/PMC4082590/

24. https://www.ncbi.nlm.nih.gov/pmc/articles/PMC9030771/
25. https://pubmed.ncbi.nlm.nih.gov/3428294/
26. https://onlinelibrary.wiley.com/doi/full/10.1046/j.1365-2796.2000.00695.x
27. https://pubmed.ncbi.nlm.nih.gov/22873615/
28. https://www.ncbi.nlm.nih.gov/pmc/articles/PMC5425935
29. https://pubmed.ncbi.nlm.nih.gov/16968806/
30. https://pubmed.ncbi.nlm.nih.gov/23384710/
31. https://www.ncbi.nlm.nih.gov/pmc/articles/PMC7503862/
32. https://www.ncbi.nlm.nih.gov/pmc/articles/PMC7091858/
33. https://www.nature.com/articles/s41591-022-01909-w
34. https://jamanetwork.com/journals/jamapsychiatry/fullarticle/2796097
35. https://www.thelancet.com/journals/lancet/article/PIIS0140-6736(22)02370-4/fulltext#%20

WHAT DOES IMMUNE DYSFUNCTION MEAN FOR HUMANITY?

1. https://dpbh.nv.gov/uploadedFiles/dpbhnvgov/content/Boards/BOH/Meetings/2021/SENEFF~1.PDF
2. https://www.nejm.org/doi/full/10.1056/NEJMoa2203965
3. https://journals.plos.org/plosbiology/article?id=10.1371/journal.pbio.1002198
4. https://www.medrxiv.org/content/10.1101/2022.01.13.22269257v2
5. https://www.rivm.nl/covid-19-vaccinatie/bescherming-coronavaccins-tegen-ziekenhuisopname/booster-en-herhaalprik-bij-ouderen-nodig-om-bescherming-op-peil-te-brengen
6. https://www.gov.mb.ca/health/publichealth/surveillance/covid-19/index.html
7. https://www.news.com.au/world/coronavirus/health/new-zealand-to-add-further-covid-restrictions-as-cases-soar/news-story/535d9a26e3f0df64804c389ee0f6b813
8. https://www.medrxiv.org/content/10.1101/2021.07.28.21261159v1
9. https://www.medrxiv.org/content/10.1101/2021.07.06.21260038v1.full
10. https://pubmed.ncbi.nlm.nih.gov/35131043/
11. https://www.ecdc.europa.eu/en/publications-data/covid-19-public-health-considerations-additional-vaccine-doses
12. https://www.sciencedirect.com/science/article/pii/S2589004222002413
13. https://pubmed.ncbi.nlm.nih.gov/28803888/
14. https://www.nature.com/articles/s41392-022-01100-0

HOW MANY PEOPLE HAVE BEEN INJURED?

1. https://www.nature.com/articles/s41586-022-05028-x
2. https://bnf.nice.org.uk/

3. https://virologytruth.s3.us-east-2.amazonaws.com/vaccines/vaers-reporting.pdf
4. https://www.gov.uk/drug-safety-update/yellow-card-please-help-to-reverse-the-decline-in-reporting-of-suspected-adverse-drug-reactions
5. https://www.ncbi.nlm.nih.gov/pmc/articles/PMC4632204/
6. https://www.sciencedirect.com/science/article/pii/S027869152200206X#bib139
7. https://vaersanalysis.info/2022/08/05/vaers-summary-for-covid-19-vaccines-through-7-29-2022/
8. https://www.gov.uk/government/publications/coronavirus-covid-19-vaccine-adverse-reactions/coronavirus-vaccine-summary-of-yellow-card-reporting
9. https://www.fda.gov/media/144246/download#page=87
10. https://www.cebm.net/covid-19/public-health-england-death-data-revised/
11. https://www.ons.gov.uk/aboutus/transparencyandgovernance/freedomofinformationfoi/covid19deathsandillnessaftervaccine

CAN WE TRUST THE PHARMACEUTICAL INDUSTRY?

1. https://www.ajmc.com/view/fda-recalls-all-ranitidine-products-zantac-citing-increased-risk-of-cancer
2. https://www.sciencemuseum.org.uk/objects-and-stories/medicine/thalidomide
3. https://www.oncozine.com/reversal-of-fortune-how-a-vilified-drug-became-a-life-saving-agent-in-the-war-against-cancer/
4. https://permanent.access.gpo.gov/lps1609/www.fda.gov/fdac/features/2001/201_kelsey.html
5. https://bnf.nice.org.uk/drugs/thalidomide/#pregnancy
6. https://www.theguardian.com/business/2017/sep/15/his-death-still-hurts-the-pfizer-anti-smoking-drug-ruled-to-have-contributed-to-suicide
7. https://www.drugdangers.com/manufacturers/pfizer/
8. https://www.gov.uk/drug-device-alerts/class-2-medicines-recall-pfizer-ltd-champix-all-strengths-film-coated-tablets-el-21-a-slash-25
9. https://www.bmj.com/content/339/bmj.b3657.full
10. https://www.nytimes.com/2009/09/03/business/03health.html
11. https://www.nytimes.com/2020/10/21/health/purdue-opioids-criminal-charges.html
12. https://www.bmj.com/content/353/bmj.i2139.full
13. https://www.cnbc.com/2018/02/22/medical-errors-third-leading-cause-of-death-in-america.html
14. https://www.statnews.com/2017/01/10/moderna-trouble-mrna/

WHAT IS POLYETHYLENE GLYCOL?

1. https://medicaldialogues.in/partner/jbcpl/laxolite
2. https://www.karger.com/Article/Abstract/233309
3. https://www.nature.com/articles/s41565-021-01001-3
4. https://www.sciencedirect.com/science/article/pii/S2214750020304674
5. https://onlinelibrary.wiley.com/doi/10.1111/all.14711
6. https://jamanetwork.com/journals/jama/article-abstract/2776557
7. https://www.ncbi.nlm.nih.gov/pmc/articles/PMC8650829/
8. https://pubmed.ncbi.nlm.nih.gov/31526095/
9. https://www.mdpi.com/1999-4923/13/7/1029
10. https://www.researchgate.net/publication/361261963_PEGylated_COVID-19_vaccines_and_cell-cell_fusion/link/62a906d0c660ab61f87c80af/download

WHY DO ONLY SOME PEOPLE HAVE SIDE-EFFECTS?

1. https://www.euromomo.eu/
2. https://www.pandata.org/about/
3. https://twitter.com/GirardotMarc/status/1555503998353821696
4. https://onlinelibrary.wiley.com/doi/10.1111/sji.13160
5. https://pubmed.ncbi.nlm.nih.gov/33301246/
6. https://www.pmda.go.jp/drugs/2021/P20210212001/672212000_30300AMX00231_I100_1.pdf
7. https://www.ema.europa.eu/en/documents/assessment-report/comirnaty-epar-public-assessment-report_en.pdf
8. https://covidmythbuster.substack.com/p/accidental-iv-injection-is-real-ever
9. https://www.youtube.com/watch?v=hkopHLQjtVQ&t=609s
10. https://pubmed.ncbi.nlm.nih.gov/34406358/
11. https://www.ncbi.nlm.nih.gov/pmc/articles/PMC9060731/
12. https://covidmythbuster.substack.com/p/vaccine-russian-roulette-why-some
13. https://covidmythbuster.substack.com/p/vaccine-russian-roulette-why-some
14. https://twitter.com/GirardotMarc/status/1555507015794950144
15. https://academic.oup.com/cid/article/74/11/1933/6353927
16. https://covidmythbuster.substack.com/p/poking-holes-in-the-brain-blood-barrier
17. https://www.nature.com/articles/nrneurol.2017.188
18. https://www.jstage.jst.go.jp/article/internalmedicine/61/10/61_9407-22/_article
19. https://www.nature.com/articles/s41593-020-00771-8
20. https://covidmythbuster.substack.com/p/can-vaccines-be-dangerous-to-pregnant

WHAT IS THE "THREE CAUSES THREE EFFECTS" HYPOTHESIS?

1. https://www.ncbi.nlm.nih.gov/pmc/articles/PMC7693988/
2. https://www.ncbi.nlm.nih.gov/pmc/articles/PMC8538996/
3. https://www.ncbi.nlm.nih.gov/pmc/articles/PMC7758180/
4. https://www.ncbi.nlm.nih.gov/pmc/articles/PMC8487226/
5. https://faseb.onlinelibrary.wiley.com/doi/full/10.1096/fj.202002742RR
6. https://www.frontiersin.org/articles/10.3389/fncel.2021.777738/full
7. https://www.authorea.com/doi/full/10.22541/au.166069342.27133443/v1
8. https://www.mdpi.com/1999-4915/13/10/2056/htm
9. https://portlandpress.com/clinsci/article/136/6/431/231092/SARS-CoV-2-spike-protein-causes-cardiovascular
10. https://www.biorxiv.org/content/10.1101/2020.12.21.423721v1.full
11. https://www.ncbi.nlm.nih.gov/pmc/articles/PMC8380922/
12. https://www.ncbi.nlm.nih.gov/pmc/articles/PMC7305763/
13. https://pubmed.ncbi.nlm.nih.gov/35195253/
14. https://www.ncbi.nlm.nih.gov/pmc/articles/PMC8354225/
15. https://www.sciencedirect.com/science/article/pii/S1936523320303065
16. https://www.sciencedirect.com/science/article/pii/S0165247821001097
17. https://www.biorxiv.org/content/10.1101/2021.06.09.447484v1.full
18. https://www.preprints.org/manuscript/202103.0551/v1
19. https://www.nature.com/articles/s41422-021-00523-8
20. https://www.cell.com/iscience/fulltext/S2589-0042(21)01450-4?
21. https://www.biorxiv.org/content/10.1101/2022.03.16.484616v2.full
22. https://www.thelancet.com/journals/lanrhe/article/PIIS2665-9913(21)00309-X/fulltext
23. https://www.ahajournals.org/doi/abs/10.1161/circ.144.suppl_1.10712#
24. https://www.ahajournals.org/doi/10.1161/CIRCRESAHA.121.318902
25. https://www.nature.com/articles/s41440-022-00876-6
26. https://my.clevelandclinic.org/health/diseases/22927-microvascular-ischemic-disease
27. https://www.ncbi.nlm.nih.gov/pmc/articles/PMC9030795/
28. https://pubmed.ncbi.nlm.nih.gov/32074468
29. https://jbiomedsci.biomedcentral.com/articles/10.1186/s12929-019-0580-3
30. https://jamanetwork.com/journals/jamanetworkopen/article-abstract/2794886
31. https://pubs.acs.org/doi/10.1021/acscentsci.1c00197
32. https://pubmed.ncbi.nlm.nih.gov/14315085/
33. https://www.nature.com/articles/s41580-020-00314-w
34. https://www.ncbi.nlm.nih.gov/pmc/articles/PMC4166495/
35. https://www.jvascsurg.org/article/S0741-5214(01)22215-0/fulltext
36. https://www.aging-us.com/article/203560/text
37. https://www.frontiersin.org/articles/10.3389/fragi.2022.900028/full

38. https://www.ncbi.nlm.nih.gov/pmc/articles/PMC7857081/
39. https://www.nature.com/articles/s41418-021-00795-y
40. https://www.ncbi.nlm.nih.gov/pmc/articles/PMC4646249/
41. https://www.embopress.org/doi/full/10.15252/embj.2020106267
42. https://www.nature.com/articles/s41577-021-00524-z
43. https://www.ncbi.nlm.nih.gov/pmc/articles/PMC8670263
44. https://www.frontiersin.org/articles/10.3389/fragi.2022.900028/full
45. https://www.ncbi.nlm.nih.gov/pmc/articles/PMC3353745/
46. https://www.cell.com/trends/biochemical-sciences/fulltext/S0968-0004(06)00023-5
47. https://foundationforhealthresearch.org/review-of-covid-19-vaccines-and-the-risk-of-chronic-adverse-events/
48. https://www.sciencedirect.com/science/article/pii/S0006291X2100499X?via%3Dihub
49. https://pubmed.ncbi.nlm.nih.gov/35208734/
50. https://pubs.acs.org/doi/full/10.1021/jacs.2c03925
51. https://www.documentcloud.org/documents/20516010-ema-assessment-report-12-21-2020#document/p35/a2023027
52. https://dpbh.nv.gov/uploadedFiles/dpbhnvgov/content/Boards/BOH/Meetings/2021/SENEFF~1.PDF
53. ema.europa.eu/en/documents/assessment-report/comirnaty-epar-public-assessment-report_en.pdf
54. https://www.authorea.com/users/455597/articles/582067-sars-cov-2-spike-protein-in-the-pathogenesis-of-prion-like-diseases
55. https://www.ncbi.nlm.nih.gov/pmc/articles/PMC9116920/
56. https://www.ahajournals.org/doi/10.1161/01.res.0000256837.40544.4a
57. https://www.sciencedirect.com/science/article/pii/S2213231719314995

HOW DOES THE SPIKE PREY ON WEAKNESS?

1. https://curiosity.lib.harvard.edu/contagion/feature/germ-theory
2. https://www.popsci.com/health/germ-theory-terrain-theory/
3. https://journals.plos.org/plosone/article?id=10.1371/journal.pone.0244815
4. https://www.logically.ai/factchecks/library/0ef46bee
5. My Book
6. https://www.ncbi.nlm.nih.gov/pmc/articles/PMC6011427/
7. https://www.ncbi.nlm.nih.gov/pmc/articles/PMC3158372/
8. https://www.ncbi.nlm.nih.gov/pmc/articles/PMC8544537/
9. https://www.nejm.org/doi/10.1056/NEJMoa2001017
10. https://www.bmj.com/content/374/bmj.n1648
11. https://pubmed.ncbi.nlm.nih.gov/16759303/
12. https://www.nature.com/articles/s41593-020-00771-8
13. https://www.ncbi.nlm.nih.gov/pmc/articles/PMC8130512/

14. https://www.bmj.com/content/369/bmj.m2042
15. https://www.telegraph.co.uk/global-health/science-and-disease/joints-jabs-washington-state-allows-free-cannabis-covid-19-vaccination/
16. https://www.cbsnews.com/news/covid-vaccine-new-york-shake-shack-fries/
17. https://news.sky.com/story/covid-19-vienna-brothel-offers-customers-30-minutes-with-lady-of-their-choice-in-exchange-for-coronavirus-jab-12464616
18. https://ia802607.us.archive.org/7/items/bechamporpasteur00hume_0/bechamporpasteur00hume_0.pdf

HOW MANY MORE EXCESS DEATHS?

1. https://news.sky.com/story/shane-warne-autopsy-reveals-cricket-legend-died-of-natural-causes-12559829
2. https://www.bbc.co.uk/news/uk-scotland-62657986
3. https://www.ons.gov.uk/aboutus/transparencyandgovernance/freedomofinformationfoi/covid19deathsandillnessaftervaccine
4. https://www.gov.uk/government/publications/coronavirus-covid-19-vaccine-adverse-reactions/coronavirus-vaccine-summary-of-yellow-card-reporting#analysis-of-data
5. https://covid.joinzoe.com/post/vaccine-after-effects-more-common-in-those-who-already-had-covid
6. https://www.ons.gov.uk/peoplepopulationandcommunity/birthsdeathsandmarriages/deaths/bulletins/deathsregisteredweeklyinenglandandwalesprovisional/weekending19august2022
7. https://www.bmj.com/content/374/bmj.n2168
8. https://www.thegatewaypundit.com/2022/04/update-jaw-dropping-769-athletes-collapsed-competing-past-year-avg-age-players-suffering-cardiac-arrest-just-23-video/?utm_source=Twitter&utm_medium=PostTopSharingButtons&utm_campaign=websitesharingbuttons

WHY ARE THERE MORE PEOPLE DYING SUDDENLY?

1. https://www.ons.gov.uk/
2. https://www.hartgroup.org/recent-deaths-in-young-people-in-england-and-wales/
3. https://www.ncbi.nlm.nih.gov/pmc/articles/PMC8251361/
4. https://www.bbc.co.uk/news/uk-57517992
5. https://www.bbc.co.uk/news/uk-58112765
6. https://report24.news/ab-13-jahren-lange-liste-ploetzlich-verstorbener-oder-schwerkranker-sportler/
7. https://www.sciencedirect.com/science/article/pii/S0735109722005782

WHAT IS MYOCARDITIS?

1. https://www.express.co.uk/news/science/1518761/france-moderna-vaccine-advice-under-30-coronavirus-covid-jab-heart-problems
2. https://jamanetwork.com/journals/jamacardiology/fullarticle/2781600
3. https://www.bmj.com/content/373/bmj.n1635/rr-0
4. https://www.nejm.org/doi/full/10.1056/NEJMoa2110475
5. https://jamanetwork.com/journals/jama/fullarticle/2784015
6. https://www.preprints.org/manuscript/202208.0151/v1
7. https://www.ncbi.nlm.nih.gov/pmc/articles/PMC7199677/
8. https://www.ncbi.nlm.nih.gov/pmc/articles/PMC3187504/
9. https://www.ncbi.nlm.nih.gov/pmc/articles/PMC8340726/
10. https://www.ncbi.nlm.nih.gov/pmc/articles/PMC3187504/
11. https://www.ncbi.nlm.nih.gov/pmc/articles/PMC8340726/
12. https://academic.oup.com/hmg/article/19/20/4007/646088
13. https://www.ahajournals.org/doi/10.1161/circulationaha.104.507699
14. https://academic.oup.com/cid/advance-article/doi/10.1093/cid/ciab707/6353927
15. https://www.ahajournals.org/doi/abs/10.1161/circ.144.suppl_1.10712
16. https://www.ncbi.nlm.nih.gov/pmc/articles/PMC9372380/
17. https://pubmed.ncbi.nlm.nih.gov/35157759/
18. https://www.cureus.com/articles/110419-catecholamines-are-the-key-trigger-of-covid-19-mrna-vaccine-induced-myocarditis-a-compelling-hypothesis-supported-by-epidemiological-anatomopathological-molecular-and-physiological-findings
19. https://www.ncbi.nlm.nih.gov/pmc/articles/PMC8677426/
20. https://www.ncbi.nlm.nih.gov/pmc/articles/PMC8340726/
21. https://www.biorxiv.org/content/10.1101/2021.09.18.460895v1.full
22. https://www.reuters.com/world/us/us-probing-moderna-vaccine-increased-heart-inflammation-risk-washington-post-2021-08-20/
23. https://www1.racgp.org.au/newsgp/clinical/four-things-about-mrna-covid-vaccines-researchers%5C
24. https://www.ncbi.nlm.nih.gov/pmc/articles/PMC7766481
25. https://ehjournal.biomedcentral.com/articles/10.1186/s12940-015-0022-y
26. https://www.sciencedirect.com/science/article/abs/pii/S134462232100119X
27. https://www.theepochtimes.com/mkt_app/unusual-toxic-components-found-in-covid-vaccines-without-exception-german-scientists_4673873.html
28. https://www.ncbi.nlm.nih.gov/pmc/articles/PMC4768311/
29. https://academic.oup.com/cardiovascres/article/117/3/727/5952673
30. https://pubmed.ncbi.nlm.nih.gov/35934244/

WHAT IS THE RISK OF A DAMAGED HEART?

1. https://www.jpeds.com/article/S0022-3476(22)00282-7/fulltext#tbl1
2. https://onlinelibrary.wiley.com/doi/10.1002/jmri.27036
3. https://www.thelancet.com/journals/lanchi/article/PIIS2352-4642(22)00244-9/fulltext
4. https://pubmed.ncbi.nlm.nih.gov/35660931/
5. https://content.govdelivery.com/accounts/FLDOH/bulletins/3312697

CAN THE SHOTS CAUSE BRAIN DAMAGE?

1. https://www.riotimesonline.com/brazil-news/modern-day-censorship/pfizer-covid-vaccine-has-1291-side-effects-reveals-official-documents/
2. https://childrenshealthdefense.org/defender/pfizer-hired-600-people-vaccine-injury-reports/
3. https://pubmed.ncbi.nlm.nih.gov/35408993/
4. https://www.nature.com/articles/s41593-020-00771-8
5. https://pubmed.ncbi.nlm.nih.gov/35208734/
6. https://www.frontiersin.org/articles/10.3389/fnins.2022.1002770/
7. https://www.ncbi.nlm.nih.gov/pmc/articles/PMC7362815/
8. https://scholarlycommons.hcahealthcare.com/cgi/viewcontent.cgi?article=1420&context=internal-medicine
9. https://www.ons.gov.uk/peoplepopulationandcommunity/birthsdeathsandmarriages/deaths/articles/excessdeathsinenglandandwalesmarch2020tojune2022/2022-09-20#excess-deaths-by-leading-causes

WHY IS JABBING CHILDREN ALL RISK AND NO BENEFIT?

1. https://www.gmc-uk.org/ethical-guidance/ethical-guidance-for-doctors/good-medical-practice/duties-of-a-doctor
2. https://www.standard.co.uk/news/uk/sajid-javid-children-pfizer-health-secretary-england-b955125.html
3. https://www.fda.gov/media/144416/download
4. https://www.wsj.com/articles/cdc-covid-19-coronavirus-vaccine-side-effects-hospitalization-kids-11626706868
5. https://adc.bmj.com/content/105/12/1180
6. https://www.telegraph.co.uk/politics/2020/06/09/school-age-children-likely-hit-lightning-die-coronavirus-oxbridge
7. https://safertowait.com/95-effective/
8. https://www.ndm.ox.ac.uk/covid-19/covid-19-infection-survey/results/new-studies
9. https://www.biorxiv.org/content/10.1101/2020.06.29.174888v1.full.pdf
10. https://www.bmj.com/content/370/bmj.m3563

11. https://pubmed.ncbi.nlm.nih.gov/32668444/
12. https://www.cell.com/cell/fulltext/S0092-8674(20)30610-3
13. https://onlinelibrary.wiley.com/doi/full/10.1111/jpc.14937
14. https://www.thelancet.com/journals/lanchi/article/PIIS2352-4642(20)30251-0/fulltext
15. https://pediatrics.aappublications.org/content/pediatrics/early/2021/01/06/peds.2020-048090.full.pdf
16. https://www.eurosurveillance.org/content/10.2807/1560-7917.ES.2020.26.1.2002011
17. https://www.bbc.co.uk/news/health-55795608
18. https://www.medrxiv.org/content/10.1101/2021.07.28.21261159v1.full
19. https://www.gov.uk/government/publications/coronavirus-covid-19-vaccine-adverse-reactions/coronavirus-vaccine-summary-of-yellow-card-reporting
20. https://www.openvaers.com/covid-data/mortality
21. https://www.medrxiv.org/content/10.1101/2021.08.30.21262866v1.full-text
22. https://www.nejm.org/doi/full/10.1056/nejmoa2110475
23. https://pubmed.ncbi.nlm.nih.gov/30863755/
24. https://www.bbc.co.uk/news/health-58547659
25. https://www.nhs.uk/conditions/vaccinations/nhs-vaccinations-and-when-to-have-them/

CAN THESE SHOTS MAKE ME INFERTILE?

1. https://www.ncbi.nlm.nih.gov/pmc/articles/PMC3885174/
2. https://pubmed.ncbi.nlm.nih.gov/24112745/
3. https://www.forbes.com/sites/matthewherper/2011/11/02/the-second-coming-of-bill-gates/
4. https://www.gov.uk/government/publications/regulatory-approval-of-pfizer-biontech-vaccine-for-covid-19/summary-public-assessment-report-for-pfizerbiontech-covid-19-vaccine
5. https://www.gov.uk/government/publications/covid-19-vaccination-women-of-childbearing-age-currently-pregnant-planning-a-pregnancy-or-breastfeeding/covid-19-vaccination-a-guide-for-women-of-childbearing-age-pregnant-planning-a-pregnancy-or-breastfeeding
6. https://www.science.org/doi/10.1126/sciadv.abm7201
7. https://www.ncbi.nlm.nih.gov/pmc/articles/PMC9087667/
8. https://www.pmda.go.jp/drugs/2021/P20210212001/672212000_30300AMX00231_I100_1.pdf
9. https://www.ema.europa.eu/en/documents/assessment-report/comirnaty-epar-public-assessment-report_en.pdf
10. https://www.ncbi.nlm.nih.gov/pmc/articles/PMC6294055/
11. https://academic.oup.com/aje/article/143/7/707/58332

12. https://academic.oup.com/aje/advance-article/doi/10.1093/aje/kwac011/6511811
13. https://www.sciencedirect.com/science/article/abs/pii/S0890623820302719
14. https://onlinelibrary.wiley.com/doi/10.1111/andr.13209
15. https://www.phmpt.org/wp-content/uploads/2022/03/125742_S1_M2_24_nonclinical-overview.pdf#page=30
16. https://www.ncbi.nlm.nih.gov/pmc/articles/PMC8163337/
17. https://www.ksh.hu/stadat_files/nep/en/nep0067.html,
18. https://www-genesis.destatis.de/genesis/online?operation=abruftabelleBearbeiten&levelindex=1&levelid=1658052524163&auswahloperation=abruftabelleAuspraegungAuswaehlen&auswahlverzeichnis=ordnungsstruktur&auswahlziel=werteabruf&code=12612-0002&auswahltext=&werteabruf=Value+retrieval#abreadcrumb
19. https://www.health.nd.gov/vital/vr-publications
20. https://www.ica.gov.sg/news-and-publications/statistics
21. https://www.ris.gov.tw/app/en/2121?sn=22161405
22. https://www.cdc.gov.tw/Category/Page/9jFXNbCe-sFK9EImRRi2Og
23. https://www.ncbi.nlm.nih.gov/pmc/articles/PMC9047154/
24. https://pubmed.ncbi.nlm.nih.gov/35005663/
25. https://www.nejm.org/doi/full/10.1056/nejmoa2104983
26. https://www.cdc.gov/coronavirus/2019-ncov/vaccines/recommendations/pregnancy.html
27. https://cf5e727d-d02d-4d71-89ff-9fe2d3ad957f.filesusr.com/ugd/adf864_2bd97450072f4364a65e5cf1d7384dd4.pdf
28. https://www.fda.gov/media/152256/download
29. https://www.thelancet.com/journals/laninf/article/PIIS1473-3099(22)00054-8/fulltext
30. https://jamanetwork.com/journals/jama/fullarticle/2781360
31. https://www.ncbi.nlm.nih.gov/pmc/articles/PMC8116639/
32. https://www.medrxiv.org/content/10.1101/2021.04.30.21255690v1.full.pdf
33. https://www.sciencedirect.com/science/article/pii/S1472648321004806?via%3Dihub
34. https://www.nature.com/articles/s41379-022-01061-3
35. https://www.nature.com/articles/s41467-022-30052-w
36. https://www.sciencedirect.com/science/article/pii/S2666776222001041
37. https://www.nejm.org/doi/full/10.1056/NEJMc2114466
38. https://www.medrxiv.org/content/10.1101/2022.07.07.22277371v1
39. https://journals.lww.com/greenjournal/Fulltext/9900/Association_Between_Menstrual_Cycle_Length_and.357.aspx
40. https://www.frontiersin.org/articles/10.3389/frph.2022.952976/full
41. https://www.ncbi.nlm.nih.gov/pmc/articles/PMC8116639/
42. https://www.ncbi.nlm.nih.gov/pmc/articles/PMC9076211/

43. https://www.ncbi.nlm.nih.gov/pmc/articles/PMC8689912/
44. https://www.bmj.com/company/newsroom/new-studies-provide-reassuring-data-on-menstrual-changes-after-covid-19-vaccination/
45. https://thebms.org.uk/2016/07/breast-cancer-mortality-use-hrt/
46. https://www.intechopen.com/chapters/59074
47. https://www.ncbi.nlm.nih.gov/pmc/articles/PMC7730072/
48. https://journals.plos.org/plosmedicine/article?id=10.1371/journal.pmed.1001356
49. https://scotland.shinyapps.io/phs-covid-wider-impact/
50. https://www.heraldscotland.com/news/23028843.covid-scotland-vaccines-ruled-cause-neonatal-deaths-spike/
51. https://bnf.nice.org.uk/drugs/paracetamol/#pregnancy
52. https://pubmed.ncbi.nlm.nih.gov/34681816/
53. https://pharmaceutical-journal.com/article/news/prenatal-exposure-to-paracetamol-linked-with-increased-risk-of-autism-and-adhd

HOW CAN WE TREAT THOSE INJURED?

1. https://www.singlecare.com/blog/news/prescription-drug-statistics/#:~:text=More%20than%20131%20million%20Americans%20take%20at%20least%20one%20prescription%20medication.
2. https://blogs.bmj.com/bmj/2016/06/16/peter-c-gotzsche-prescription-drugs-are-the-third-leading-cause-of-death

WHAT DO WE NEED TO DO BEFORE USING SUPPLEMENTS?

1. https://www.nejm.org/doi/full/10.1056/NEJMc2209371
2. https://pubmed.ncbi.nlm.nih.gov/15617990/
3. https://pubmed.ncbi.nlm.nih.gov/21054335/
4. https://pubmed.ncbi.nlm.nih.gov/15748642/
5. https://pubmed.ncbi.nlm.nih.gov/24770340/
6. https://academic.oup.com/ije/article/37/3/654/743622
7. https://pubmed.ncbi.nlm.nih.gov/10350434/
8. https://pubmed.ncbi.nlm.nih.gov/8922297/
9. https://pubmed.ncbi.nlm.nih.gov/11384870/
10. https://pubmed.ncbi.nlm.nih.gov/15386383/
11. https://pubmed.ncbi.nlm.nih.gov/12907484/
12. https://pubmed.ncbi.nlm.nih.gov/11705562/
13. https://onlinelibrary.wiley.com/doi/10.1111/joim.12496
14. https://pubmed.ncbi.nlm.nih.gov/27876126/
15. https://pubmed.ncbi.nlm.nih.gov/15687362/
16. https://www.ncbi.nlm.nih.gov/pmc/articles/PMC5187459/
17. https://pubmed.ncbi.nlm.nih.gov/24770340/
18. https://pubmed.ncbi.nlm.nih.gov/19626036/

19. https://www.jidonline.org/article/S0022-202X(15)32515-X/fulltext#relatedArticles
20. https://www.nature.com/articles/srep39479
21. https://www.ncbi.nlm.nih.gov/pmc/articles/PMC9349414/
22. https://pubmed.ncbi.nlm.nih.gov/25022687/
23. https://www.ncbi.nlm.nih.gov/pmc/articles/PMC3626364/
24. https://www.ncbi.nlm.nih.gov/pmc/articles/PMC3183972/
25. https://www.ncbi.nlm.nih.gov/pmc/articles/PMC2150773/
26. https://www.ncbi.nlm.nih.gov/pmc/articles/PMC3684798/
27. https://www.ncbi.nlm.nih.gov/pmc/articles/PMC7019735/
28. https://www.ncbi.nlm.nih.gov/pmc/articles/PMC2821804/
29. https://www.ncbi.nlm.nih.gov/pmc/articles/PMC5179549/
30. https://pubmed.ncbi.nlm.nih.gov/20208539/
31. https://pubmed.ncbi.nlm.nih.gov/30697214
32. https://www.ncbi.nlm.nih.gov/pmc/articles/PMC3194221/
33. https://www.ncbi.nlm.nih.gov/pmc/articles/PMC4425186/
34. https://pubmed.ncbi.nlm.nih.gov/25022687/
35. https://pubmed.ncbi.nlm.nih.gov/33065275/
36. https://pubmed.ncbi.nlm.nih.gov/33146028/
37. https://www.nature.com/articles/s41598-022-24053-4
38. https://www.ncbi.nlm.nih.gov/pmc/articles/PMC8899722/
39. https://pubmed.ncbi.nlm.nih.gov/8390483/
40. https://pubmed.ncbi.nlm.nih.gov/18400738/
41. https://www.mayoclinicproceedings.org/article/S0025-6196(11)61465-1/fulltext#secd10773573e1879
42. https://pubmed.ncbi.nlm.nih.gov/32620963/
43. https://www.ncbi.nlm.nih.gov/pmc/articles/PMC6388383/#app1-ijerph-16-00383
44. https://www.ncbi.nlm.nih.gov/books/NBK56078/
45. https://pubmed.ncbi.nlm.nih.gov/7472801/
46. https://www.ncbi.nlm.nih.gov/pmc/articles/PMC8917232/
47. https://pubmed.ncbi.nlm.nih.gov/29902071/
48. https://onlinelibrary.wiley.com/doi/full/10.1111/exd.12715
49. https://www.ncbi.nlm.nih.gov/pmc/articles/PMC5037798/
50. https://pubmed.ncbi.nlm.nih.gov/12771037/
51. https://www.researchgate.net/publication/268032282_Personenbezogene_Messung_der_UV-Exposition_von_Arbeitnehmern_im_Freien
52. https://pubmed.ncbi.nlm.nih.gov/18321444/
53. https://journals.sagepub.com/doi/full/10.1177/1073858413518152
54. https://www.ncbi.nlm.nih.gov/pmc/articles/PMC2824213/
55. https://pubmed.ncbi.nlm.nih.gov/7056735/
56. https://pubmed.ncbi.nlm.nih.gov/16337444/
57. https://journals.physiology.org/doi/full/10.1152/ajpregu.2000.279.3.R786
58. https://pubmed.ncbi.nlm.nih.gov/16102986/

59. https://www.ncbi.nlm.nih.gov/pmc/articles/PMC6689741/
60. https://www.ncbi.nlm.nih.gov/pmc/articles/PMC7195843/
61. https://pubmed.ncbi.nlm.nih.gov/20398008/
62. https://pubmed.ncbi.nlm.nih.gov/10198397/
63. https://pubmed.ncbi.nlm.nih.gov/25535859/
64. https://pubmed.ncbi.nlm.nih.gov/5284360/
65. https://pubmed.ncbi.nlm.nih.gov/17129762/
66. https://pubmed.ncbi.nlm.nih.gov/22024172/
67. https://www.ncbi.nlm.nih.gov/pmc/articles/PMC45363/
68. https://pubmed.ncbi.nlm.nih.gov/12623776/
69. https://pubmed.ncbi.nlm.nih.gov/8047572/
70. https://pubmed.ncbi.nlm.nih.gov/6158420/
71. https://pubmed.ncbi.nlm.nih.gov/7819749/
72. https://www.ncbi.nlm.nih.gov/pmc/articles/PMC2839418/
73. https://pubmed.ncbi.nlm.nih.gov/8502660/
74. https://pubmed.ncbi.nlm.nih.gov/25117535/
75. https://www.ncbi.nlm.nih.gov/pmc/articles/PMC2864873/
76. https://www.ncbi.nlm.nih.gov/pmc/articles/PMC3242694/
77. https://www.ncbi.nlm.nih.gov/pmc/articles/PMC2629403/
78. https://www.ncbi.nlm.nih.gov/pmc/articles/PMC4115328/
79. https://www.nature.com/articles/srep21480/
80. https://www.ncbi.nlm.nih.gov/pmc/articles/PMC3859577/
81. https://pubmed.ncbi.nlm.nih.gov/21632713/
82. https://pubmed.ncbi.nlm.nih.gov/25061767/
83. https://nutrition.bmj.com/content/early/2021/03/03/bmjnph-2021-000228
84. https://pubmed.ncbi.nlm.nih.gov/12218374/
85. https://pubmed.ncbi.nlm.nih.gov/16940468/
86. https://pubmed.ncbi.nlm.nih.gov/21446352/
87. https://books.google.co.uk/books?hl=en&lr=&id=OENyNqxkZ6AC&oi=fnd&pg=PA64&ots=R-u5FoLvc5&sig=U0L1yRibCbjoWRgz4u4e2ZkYkKs&redir_esc=y#v=onepage&q&f=false
88. https://pubmed.ncbi.nlm.nih.gov/26477922/
89. https://onlinelibrary.wiley.com/doi/10.1002/ajh.2830240107
90. https://www.sciencedirect.com/science/article/abs/pii/S0889159109000725
91. https://www.karger.com/Article/Fulltext/430391
92. https://www.ncbi.nlm.nih.gov/pmc/articles/PMC7176256/
93. http://refhub.elsevier.com/S1877-1173(15)00184-2/rf0095
94. https://www.ncbi.nlm.nih.gov/pmc/articles/PMC6523821/
95. https://pubmed.ncbi.nlm.nih.gov/20581713/
96. https://www.ncbi.nlm.nih.gov/pmc/articles/PMC4234964/
97. https://www.frontiersin.org/articles/10.3389/fimmu.2018.00648/

98. https://journals.lww.com/acsm-msse/Abstract/1994/02000/NK_cell_response_to_physical_activity__possible.3.aspx
99. https://pubmed.ncbi.nlm.nih.gov/2266764/
100. https://pubmed.ncbi.nlm.nih.gov/29056598/
101. https://pubmed.ncbi.nlm.nih.gov/10910297/
102. https://www.ncbi.nlm.nih.gov/pmc/articles/PMC5013087/
103. https://pubmed.ncbi.nlm.nih.gov/24798553/
104. https://pubmed.ncbi.nlm.nih.gov/17910910/
105. https://pubmed.ncbi.nlm.nih.gov/26895752/
106. https://journals.lww.com/acsm-msse/Fulltext/2007/04000/Incidence,_Etiology,_and_Symptomatology_of_Upper.1.aspx
107. https://bjsm.bmj.com/content/55/19/1099
108. https://www.who.int/news/item/05-09-2018-launch-of-new-global-estimates-on-levels-of-physical-activity-in-adults
109. https://www.jle.com/fr/revues/mrh/e-docs/exercise_magnesium_and_immune_function_278044/article.phtml
110. https://www.jle.com/fr/revues/mrh/e-docs/exercise_magnesium_and_immune_function_278044/article.phtml
111. https://pubmed.ncbi.nlm.nih.gov/14717743/
112. https://www.ncbi.nlm.nih.gov/pmc/articles/PMC2811891/
113. https://www.sciencedirect.com/science/article/pii/S0168822718302031
114. https://www.ncbi.nlm.nih.gov/pmc/articles/PMC6943267/
115. https://pubmed.ncbi.nlm.nih.gov/34205044/
116. https://pubmed.ncbi.nlm.nih.gov/32647915/
117. https://jamanetwork.com/journals/jamainternalmedicine/fullarticle/216997
118. https://www.frontiersin.org/articles/10.3389/fpubh.2021.695139/full
119. https://assets.publishing.service.gov.uk/government/uploads/system/uploads/attachment_data/file/338934/Adult_obesity_and_type_2_diabetes_.pdf
120. https://www.frontiersin.org/articles/10.3389/fnagi.2019.00127/full
121. https://www.nature.com/articles/s41598-021-91758-3
122. https://pubmed.ncbi.nlm.nih.gov/23298210/
123. https://pubmed.ncbi.nlm.nih.gov/23415911/
124. https://www.jci.org/articles/view/108565
125. https://www.cell.com/cell-metabolism/pdfExtended/S1550-4131(18)30504-7
126. https://www.hindawi.com/journals/iji/2018/2157434/
127. https://www.ncbi.nlm.nih.gov/pmc/articles/PMC7475801/
128. https://translational-medicine.biomedcentral.com/articles/10.1186/s12967-020-02600-9
129. https://pubmed.ncbi.nlm.nih.gov/31485454/
130. https://www.ncbi.nlm.nih.gov/pmc/articles/PMC5452247/
131. https://pubmed.ncbi.nlm.nih.gov/15767618/

132. https://www.ncbi.nlm.nih.gov/pmc/articles/PMC7132133/
133. https://translational-medicine.biomedcentral.com/articles/10.1186/s12967-020-02277-0
134. https://www.ncbi.nlm.nih.gov/pmc/articles/PMC6286979/
135. https://pubmed.ncbi.nlm.nih.gov/11918434/
136. https://translational-medicine.biomedcentral.com/articles/10.1186/s12967-020-02600-9
137. https://www.ncbi.nlm.nih.gov/pmc/articles/PMC7362813/
138. https://pubmed.ncbi.nlm.nih.gov/32765945/
139. https://www.ncbi.nlm.nih.gov/pmc/articles/PMC4352123/
140. https://www.ncbi.nlm.nih.gov/pmc/articles/PMC7189564/
141. https://www.ncbi.nlm.nih.gov/pmc/articles/PMC6402511/
142. https://www.ncbi.nlm.nih.gov/pmc/articles/PMC8250295/
143. https://www.ncbi.nlm.nih.gov/pmc/articles/PMC5012517/
144. https://www.ncbi.nlm.nih.gov/pmc/articles/PMC8250295/
145. https://www.ncbi.nlm.nih.gov/pmc/articles/PMC5313038/
146. https://www.sciencedirect.com/science/article/pii/S0899900721000988
147. https://bmcendocrdisord.biomedcentral.com/articles/10.1186/s12902-020-00558-9
148. https://www.nature.com/articles/d41586-022-00912-y
149. https://www.ncbi.nlm.nih.gov/pmc/articles/PMC8031259/
150. https://pubmed.ncbi.nlm.nih.gov/34151532/
151. https://archive.org/details/1932FishbeinFadsAndQuackeryInHealing/page/n261/mode/2up
152. https://www.britannica.com/topic/fasting
153. https://www.britannica.com/science/starvation
154. https://www.ncbi.nlm.nih.gov/pmc/articles/PMC5411330/
155. https://www.ncbi.nlm.nih.gov/pmc/articles/PMC8744103/
156. https://www.ncbi.nlm.nih.gov/pmc/articles/PMC8102292/
157. https://www.ncbi.nlm.nih.gov/pmc/articles/PMC5857384/
158. https://pubmed.ncbi.nlm.nih.gov/35310455/
159. https://pubmed.ncbi.nlm.nih.gov/16126250/
160. https://www.researchgate.net/figure/Effect-of-a-24h-fast-on-the-TNF-a-IL-1b-IL-6-and-IL-10-response-to-10-or-100-acute_fig1_312374496
161. https://www.ncbi.nlm.nih.gov/pmc/articles/PMC8744103/
162. https://www.ncbi.nlm.nih.gov/pmc/articles/PMC7429999/
163. https://www.ncbi.nlm.nih.gov/pmc/articles/PMC2990190/
164. https://www.ncbi.nlm.nih.gov/pmc/articles/PMC4500936/
165. https://pubmed.ncbi.nlm.nih.gov/30172870
166. https://www.frontiersin.org/articles/10.3389/fbioe.2020.00975/full
167. https://www.ahajournals.org/doi/10.1161/JAHA.118.011863
168. https://pubmed.ncbi.nlm.nih.gov/33770194/
169. https://www.ncbi.nlm.nih.gov/pmc/articles/PMC7275989/
170. https://www.ncbi.nlm.nih.gov/pmc/articles/PMC7415631/

171. https://www.ncbi.nlm.nih.gov/pmc/articles/PMC3676888
172. https://www.frontiersin.org/articles/10.3389/fimmu.2022.816282/full
173. https://www.ncbi.nlm.nih.gov/pmc/articles/PMC9169953/
174. https://www.ncbi.nlm.nih.gov/pmc/articles/PMC7306200/
175. https://pubmed.ncbi.nlm.nih.gov/33806756/
176. https://www.ncbi.nlm.nih.gov/pmc/articles/PMC7232436/
177. https://www.ncbi.nlm.nih.gov/pmc/articles/PMC6414192/
178. https://pubmed.ncbi.nlm.nih.gov/17897073/
179. https://www.ncbi.nlm.nih.gov/pmc/articles/PMC8268053/
180. https://www.ncbi.nlm.nih.gov/pmc/articles/PMC7366458/
181. https://pubmed.ncbi.nlm.nih.gov/28175954/
182. https://www.ncbi.nlm.nih.gov/pmc/articles/PMC3121004/
183. https://www.ncbi.nlm.nih.gov/pmc/articles/PMC8075256/
184. https://pubmed.ncbi.nlm.nih.gov/12360104/
185. https://www.ncbi.nlm.nih.gov/pmc/articles/PMC4691246/
186. https://pubs.acs.org/doi/10.1021/acs.molpharmaceut.9b00459
187. https://pubmed.ncbi.nlm.nih.gov/12512040/
188. https://pubmed.ncbi.nlm.nih.gov/22391012/
189. https://www.ncbi.nlm.nih.gov/pmc/articles/PMC7474734/
190. https://pubmed.ncbi.nlm.nih.gov/27411588
191. https://www.ncbi.nlm.nih.gov/pmc/articles/PMC4102383/
192. https://www.cell.com/cell-stem-cell/fulltext/S1934-5909(14)00151-9
193. https://www.ncbi.nlm.nih.gov/pmc/articles/PMC6460288/
194. https://www.ncbi.nlm.nih.gov/pmc/articles/PMC6818271/
195. https://pubmed.ncbi.nlm.nih.gov/19543266/
196. https://www.nature.com/articles/s41586-022-05128-8
197. https://www.sciencedirect.com/science/article/pii/S1074761321005483
198. https://nutrition.bmj.com/content/early/2022/06/30/bmjnph-2022-000462
199. https://www.sciencedirect.com/science/article/pii/S2589936821000864
200. https://pubmed.ncbi.nlm.nih.gov/30840892/
201. https://www.ncbi.nlm.nih.gov/pmc/articles/PMC6818271/
202. https://www.ncbi.nlm.nih.gov/pmc/articles/PMC8237994/
203. https://lpi.oregonstate.edu/mic/micronutrient-inadequacies/overview
204. https://cir.nii.ac.jp/crid/1571135650174433408
205. https://www.joghr.org/article/17603-micro-nutrient-related-malnutrition-and-obesity-in-a-university-undergraduate-population-and-implications-for-non-communicable-diseases
206. https://pubmed.ncbi.nlm.nih.gov/29980762/
207. https://www.ncbi.nlm.nih.gov/pmc/articles/PMC7352522/
208. https://www.ncbi.nlm.nih.gov/pmc/articles/PMC7193396/
209. https://www.jstor.org/stable/pdf/resrep35660.9.pdf
210. https://www.mdpi.com/1660-4601/19/3/1125
211. https://pubmed.ncbi.nlm.nih.gov/18400738/

212. https://www.ncbi.nlm.nih.gov/pmc/articles/PMC6775441/
213. https://www.ncbi.nlm.nih.gov/pmc/articles/PMC8912822/
214. https://www.who.int/publications/i/item/9789241598019
215. https://www.ncbi.nlm.nih.gov/pmc/articles/PMC7352522/
216. https://www.ncbi.nlm.nih.gov/pmc/articles/PMC2456524/
217. https://www.ncbi.nlm.nih.gov/pmc/articles/PMC4511719/
218. https://cabidigitallibrary.org/doi/10.1079/PAVSNNR20083098
219. https://www.ncbi.nlm.nih.gov/pmc/articles/PMC6162863/
220. https://www.ncbi.nlm.nih.gov/pmc/articles/PMC7019735/
221. https://pubmed.ncbi.nlm.nih.gov/14704330/
222. https://pubmed.ncbi.nlm.nih.gov/16020684/
223. https://www.ncbi.nlm.nih.gov/pmc/articles/PMC4973288/
224. https://pubmed.ncbi.nlm.nih.gov/23688939/
225. https://lpi.oregonstate.edu/mic/health-disease/immunity
226. https://pubmed.ncbi.nlm.nih.gov/34202697/
227. https://pubmed.ncbi.nlm.nih.gov/22113863/
228. https://www.ncbi.nlm.nih.gov/books/NBK109829/
229. https://ods.od.nih.gov/factsheets/VitaminB6-HealthProfessional/
230. https://lpi.oregonstate.edu/mic/vitamins/vitamin-B6
231. https://lpi.oregonstate.edu/mic/glossary#homocysteine
232. https://pubmed.ncbi.nlm.nih.gov/25489409/
233. https://www.cdc.gov/nutritionreport/
234. https://pubmed.ncbi.nlm.nih.gov/8037789/
235. https://pubmed.ncbi.nlm.nih.gov/10434845/
236. https://scholars.direct/Articles/human-nutrition/jhn-2-008.php?jid=human-nutrition
237. https://www.ncbi.nlm.nih.gov/pmc/articles/PMC6478888/
238. https://pdfs.semanticscholar.org/d556/ee510dae113e1505ec788143c3bb7c81f2bf.pdf
239. https://eprints.soton.ac.uk/152657/
240. https://www.hilarispublisher.com/open-access/increased-micronutrient-requirements-during-physiologically-demanding-situations-review-of-the-current-evidence-2376-1318-1000166.pdf
241. https://rupress.org/jem/article/89/2/175/5206/THE-EFFECT-OF-DIET-ON-THE-SUSCEPTIBILITY-OF-THE
242. https://www.frontiersin.org/articles/10.3389/fnut.2020.562051/fu
243. https://pubmed.ncbi.nlm.nih.gov/22116704/
244. https://pubmed.ncbi.nlm.nih.gov/22116703
245. https://pubmed.ncbi.nlm.nih.gov/14584010/
246. https://ebm.bmj.com/content/4/6/182
247. https://pubmed.ncbi.nlm.nih.gov/2047064/
248. https://www.ncbi.nlm.nih.gov/pmc/articles/PMC8495119/
249. https://lpi.oregonstate.edu/mic/vitamins/vitamin-B12
250. https://www.ncbi.nlm.nih.gov/pmc/articles/PMC8226782/

251. https://ods.od.nih.gov/factsheets/VitaminB12-HealthProfessional/
252. https://pubmed.ncbi.nlm.nih.gov/28041597/
253. https://www.ncbi.nlm.nih.gov/pmc/articles/PMC1905232/
254. https://www.ncbi.nlm.nih.gov/pmc/articles/PMC4260394/
255. https://www.ncbi.nlm.nih.gov/pmc/articles/PMC6478888/
256. https://pubmed.ncbi.nlm.nih.gov/17922955/
257. https://www.ncbi.nlm.nih.gov/pmc/articles/PMC7194560/
258. https://assets.researchsquare.com/files/rs-1425014/v1_covered.pdf?c=1646775740
259. https://www.nmcd-journal.com/article/S0939-4753(20)30514-7/fulltext
260. https://www.mountsinai.org/health-library/tests/vitamin-b12-level
261. https://www.ncbi.nlm.nih.gov/pmc/articles/PMC8689946/
262. https://www.ncbi.nlm.nih.gov/books/NBK114302/
263. https://nap.nationalacademies.org/catalog/9810/dietary-reference-intakes-for-vitamin-c-vitamin-e-selenium-and-carotenoids
264. https://ods.od.nih.gov/factsheets/VitaminC-HealthProfessional/
265. https://www.ncbi.nlm.nih.gov/pubmed/12771534%20?dopt=Abstract
266. https://www.ncbi.nlm.nih.gov/pmc/articles/PMC1448351/
267. https://pubmed.ncbi.nlm.nih.gov/4941984/
268. https://www.ncbi.nlm.nih.gov/pmc/articles/PMC5707683/
269. https://pubmed.ncbi.nlm.nih.gov/28353648/
270. https://www.ncbi.nlm.nih.gov/pmc/articles/PMC8078152/
271. https://pubmed.ncbi.nlm.nih.gov/25608928/
272. https://www.ncbi.nlm.nih.gov/pmc/articles/PMC8552785/
273. https://ods.od.nih.gov/factsheets/VitaminC-HealthProfessional/#en8
274. https://pubmed.ncbi.nlm.nih.gov/22698272/
275. https://pubmed.ncbi.nlm.nih.gov/16118484/
276. https://pubmed.ncbi.nlm.nih.gov/9550452/
277. https://ods.od.nih.gov/factsheets/VitaminE-HealthProfessional/
278. https://www.ncbi.nlm.nih.gov/pmc/articles/PMC3997530/
279. https://www.ncbi.nlm.nih.gov/pmc/articles/PMC7352522/
280. https://pubmed.ncbi.nlm.nih.gov/490041/
281. https://doi.org/10.1079%2FPAVSNNR20083098
282. https://www.ncbi.nlm.nih.gov/pmc/articles/PMC6266234/
283. https://pubmed.ncbi.nlm.nih.gov/30697214/
284. https://pubmed.ncbi.nlm.nih.gov/15753137/
285. https://www.tandfonline.com/doi/full/10.1080/09540105.2015.1079600
286. https://www.ncbi.nlm.nih.gov/pmc/articles/PMC6340979/
287. https://scholar.google.com/scholar_lookup?journal=N+Engl+J+Med&title=Azidothymidine+in+the+treatment+of+ATDS&author=A+Ganser&author=J+Greher&author=B+Volkers&author=A+Staszewski&author=D+Hoelzer&volume=318&publication_year=1988&pages=250-1&pmid=3422108&
288. https://www.ncbi.nlm.nih.gov/pmc/articles/PMC1914075/

289. https://ods.od.nih.gov/factsheets/COVID19-HealthProfessional/#h15
290. https://pubmed.ncbi.nlm.nih.gov/33680348/?dopt=Abstract
291. https://pubmed.ncbi.nlm.nih.gov/10684543/
292. https://nap.nationalacademies.org/catalog/9810/dietary-reference-intakes-for-vitamin-c-vitamin-e-selenium-and-carotenoids
293. https://www.ncbi.nlm.nih.gov/pmc/articles/PMC5320409/
294. https://www.ncbi.nlm.nih.gov/pmc/articles/PMC7185114/
295. https://pubmed.ncbi.nlm.nih.gov/16943450/
296. https://pubmed.ncbi.nlm.nih.gov/30914769/
297. https://pubmed.ncbi.nlm.nih.gov/25722698/
298. https://pubmed.ncbi.nlm.nih.gov/28122452/
299. https://pubmed.ncbi.nlm.nih.gov/30107519/
300. https://ods.od.nih.gov/factsheets/Copper-HealthProfessional/#en1
301. https://jhu.pure.elsevier.com/en/publications/modern-nutrition-in-health-and-disease-eleventh-edition
302. https://pubmed.ncbi.nlm.nih.gov/12055353/
303. https://www.ncbi.nlm.nih.gov/pubmed/15559027?dopt=Abstract
304. https://www.sciencedirect.com/science/article/abs/pii/S0946672X11002355
305. https://journals.physiology.org/doi/abs/10.1152/physrev.1985.65.2.238
306. https://www.ncbi.nlm.nih.gov/pmc/articles/PMC6266129/
307. https://pubmed.ncbi.nlm.nih.gov/2082222/
308. https://pubmed.ncbi.nlm.nih.gov/7429759/
309. https://obgyn.onlinelibrary.wiley.com/doi/abs/10.3109/00016349309021153
310. https://pubmed.ncbi.nlm.nih.gov/17989919/
311. https://www.ncbi.nlm.nih.gov/pmc/articles/PMC7850398
312. https://insulinresistance.org/index.php/jir/article/view/43/142
313. https://www.ncbi.nlm.nih.gov/pmc/articles/PMC5535265/
314. https://pubmed.ncbi.nlm.nih.gov/4220265/
315. https://www.ncbi.nlm.nih.gov/pmc/articles/PMC7212532/
316. https://pubmed.ncbi.nlm.nih.gov/34592694/
317. https://www.frontiersin.org/articles/10.3389/fmed.2021.620175/full
318. https://pubmed.ncbi.nlm.nih.gov/26091384/
319. https://pubmed.ncbi.nlm.nih.gov/25844615/
320. https://www.ncbi.nlm.nih.gov/books/NBK557456/
321. https://www.nature.com/articles/7500462
322. https://academic.oup.com/ajcn/article/63/5/846S/4651508
323. https://www.webmd.com/diet/liver-good-for-you
324. https://ods.od.nih.gov/factsheets/Iron-HealthProfessional/
325. https://www.ncbi.nlm.nih.gov/pmc/articles/PMC3676888/
326. http://apps.who.int/iris/bitstream/handle/10665/43894/9789241596657_eng.pdf;jsessionid=FBCFE14C019F698E21F20FD262315654?sequence=1

327. https://pubmed.ncbi.nlm.nih.gov/9091669/
328. https://pubmed.ncbi.nlm.nih.gov/18498447/?dopt=Abstract
329. https://www.ncbi.nlm.nih.gov/pubmed/25668261?dopt=Abstract
330. https://pubmed.ncbi.nlm.nih.gov/22575608/
331. https://pubmed.ncbi.nlm.nih.gov/20533591/?dopt=Abstract
332. https://www.ncbi.nlm.nih.gov/pubmed/18755344?dopt=Abstract
333. https://academic.oup.com/jn/article/131/2/616S/4686847
334. https://www.frontiersin.org/articles/10.3389/fimmu.2022.816282/full
335. https://www.cell.com/med/fulltext/S2666-6340(20)30021-0
336. https://pubmed.ncbi.nlm.nih.gov/20522542/
337. https://www.annualreviews.org/doi/10.1146/annurev-pathol-012513-104651
338. https://pubmed.ncbi.nlm.nih.gov/28974951/
339. https://my.clevelandclinic.org/health/diseases/14477-anemia-of-chronic-disease
340. https://www.ncbi.nlm.nih.gov/pmc/articles/PMC7461220/
341. https://pubmed.ncbi.nlm.nih.gov/33417082/
342. https://pubmed.ncbi.nlm.nih.gov/34593305/
343. https://casereports.bmj.com/content/14/8/e242639
344. https://www.aging-us.com/article/203612/text
345. https://pubmed.ncbi.nlm.nih.gov/26098293/
346. https://ods.od.nih.gov/factsheets/Iodine-HealthProfessional/#h13
347. https://www.sciencedirect.com/science/article/pii/S2376060520303680
348. https://pubmed.ncbi.nlm.nih.gov/18947032/
349. https://www.ncbi.nlm.nih.gov/pmc/articles/PMC7914421/
350. https://www.ingentaconnect.com/content/ben/ccb/2011/00000005/00000003/art00002
351. https://journals.sagepub.com/doi/abs/10.1177/026010600902000204
352. https://pubmed.ncbi.nlm.nih.gov/25018052/
353. https://www.mdpi.com/1422-0067/22/3/1228/htm
354. https://www.sciencedirect.com/science/article/abs/pii/S0891584917312583?via%3Dihub
355. https://europepmc.org/article/med/1972841
356. https://www.frontiersin.org/articles/10.3389/fimmu.2017.01573/full
357. https://pubmed.ncbi.nlm.nih.gov/6858554/
358. https://www.ncbi.nlm.nih.gov/pmc/articles/PMC8552616/
359. https://journals.plos.org/plosone/article?id=10.1371/journal.pone.0254341
360. https://www.liebertpub.com/doi/abs/10.1089/thy.2007.0379?journalCode=thy
361. https://www.oatext.com/iodine-an-effective-substance-against-the-covid-19-pandemic.php
362. https://pubmed.ncbi.nlm.nih.gov/16682732/
363. https://europepmc.org/article/med/8221402/reload=0

364. https://nap.nationalacademies.org/read/10026/chapter/2#1
365. https://www.hindawi.com/journals/scientifica/2017/4179326/
366. https://www.ncbi.nlm.nih.gov/pmc/articles/PMC4455825/
367. https://pubmed.ncbi.nlm.nih.gov/28140318/
368. https://www.ncbi.nlm.nih.gov/pmc/articles/PMC5786912/
369. https://pubmed.ncbi.nlm.nih.gov/11794636/
370. https://pubmed.ncbi.nlm.nih.gov/7327911/
371. https://pubmed.ncbi.nlm.nih.gov/3965244/
372. https://pubmed.ncbi.nlm.nih.gov/16808892/
373. https://pubmed.ncbi.nlm.nih.gov/1489003/
374. https://pubmed.ncbi.nlm.nih.gov/9675754/
375. https://www.ncbi.nlm.nih.gov/pmc/articles/PMC4455825/
376. https://diabetesjournals.org/diabetes/article/65/1/3/34908/Hypomagnesemia-in-Type-2-Diabetes-A-Vicious-Circle
377. https://europepmc.org/article/med/7836621
378. https://pubmed.ncbi.nlm.nih.gov/29480918/
379. https://pubmed.ncbi.nlm.nih.gov/27042258/
380. https://pubmed.ncbi.nlm.nih.gov/12030423/
381. https://www.ncbi.nlm.nih.gov/pmc/articles/PMC5821731/
382. https://pubmed.ncbi.nlm.nih.gov/35051368/
383. https://pubmed.ncbi.nlm.nih.gov/18705536/
384. https://www.sciencedirect.com/science/article/abs/pii/S0092867421015610?dgcid=author
385. https://pubmed.ncbi.nlm.nih.gov/17172008/
386. https://fqresearch.org/pdf_files/Exercise-magnesium-and-immune-function.pdf
387. https://pubmed.ncbi.nlm.nih.gov/17172008/
388. https://www.sciencedirect.com/science/article/pii/B9780128021682000269
389. https://www.frontiersin.org/articles/10.3389/fendo.2022.843152/
390. https://www.frontiersin.org/articles/10.3389/fnut.2022.873162/full
391. https://ods.od.nih.gov/factsheets/Magnesium-HealthProfessional/
392. https://pubmed.ncbi.nlm.nih.gov/14653505/
393. https://www.ncbi.nlm.nih.gov/books/NBK507265/
394. https://link.springer.com/article/10.1111/j.1479-8425.2006.00193.x
395. https://link.springer.com/article/10.1111/j.1479-8425.2007.00262.x
396. https://pubmed.ncbi.nlm.nih.gov/12323090/
397. http://www.ncbi.nlm.nih.gov/entrez/query.fcgi?cmd=Retrieve&db=PubMed&dopt=Abstract&list_uids=15075703
398. https://www.ncbi.nlm.nih.gov/pmc/articles/PMC3262608/#:~:text=Studies%20have%20shown%20that%20EPA,major%20coronary%20events%2C%20and%20anticoagulation.
399. https://www.ncbi.nlm.nih.gov/pmc/articles/PMC4808858/

400. https://www.researchgate.net/figure/Strong-association-of-o-6-in-HUFA-with-CHD-mortality-Heart-attack-death-rates-per_fig4_26756981
401. https://pubmed.ncbi.nlm.nih.gov/21663641/
402. https://www.ncbi.nlm.nih.gov/pmc/articles/PMC7900446/
403. https://pubmed.ncbi.nlm.nih.gov/21816146/
404. https://www.ncbi.nlm.nih.gov/pmc/articles/PMC6834330/
405. https://www.ncbi.nlm.nih.gov/pmc/articles/PMC9012318/
406. https://www.hindawi.com/journals/bmri/2013/464921/
407. https://www.ncbi.nlm.nih.gov/pubmed/24679797
408. https://ods.od.nih.gov/factsheets/Omega3FattyAcids-HealthProfessional/
409. https://www.ncbi.nlm.nih.gov/pmc/articles/PMC8151284/
410. https://www.ncbi.nlm.nih.gov/books/NBK482260/
411. https://www.ncbi.nlm.nih.gov/pmc/articles/PMC2792354/
412. https://www.ajog.org/article/S0002-9378(11)00951-3/fulltext
413. https://www.ncbi.nlm.nih.gov/pmc/articles/PMC3723386/
414. https://www.ncbi.nlm.nih.gov/pmc/articles/PMC5307254/
415. https://pubmed.ncbi.nlm.nih.gov/21318622/
416. https://www.ncbi.nlm.nih.gov/pmc/articles/PMC6480557/
417. https://www.ncbi.nlm.nih.gov/pmc/articles/PMC8033553/#CR49
418. https://www.ncbi.nlm.nih.gov/pmc/articles/PMC7464599/
419. https://www.ncbi.nlm.nih.gov/pmc/articles/PMC344014/
420. https://ods.od.nih.gov/factsheets/Selenium-HealthProfessional/
421. https://www.ncbi.nlm.nih.gov/pmc/articles/PMC4728638/
422. https://onlinelibrary.wiley.com/doi/abs/10.1111/eci.13538
423. https://www.pnas.org/doi/full/10.1073/pnas.1611576114
424. https://pubmed.ncbi.nlm.nih.gov/22705420/?dopt=Abstract
425. https://www.ncbi.nlm.nih.gov/pmc/articles/PMC5659335/
426. https://www.ncbi.nlm.nih.gov/pmc/articles/PMC3048346/
427. https://pubmed.ncbi.nlm.nih.gov/20462857/
428. https://www.ncbi.nlm.nih.gov/pmc/articles/PMC6315874/
429. https://www.ncbi.nlm.nih.gov/pmc/articles/PMC5307254/
430. https://academic.oup.com/jn/article/127/6/1214/4728903
431. https://pubmed.ncbi.nlm.nih.gov/31325027/
432. https://pubmed.ncbi.nlm.nih.gov/21955027/
433. https://www.ncbi.nlm.nih.gov/pmc/articles/PMC7019735/#B109-nutrients-12-00236
434. https://journals.sagepub.com/doi/10.1177/1084822317713300
435. https://pubmed.ncbi.nlm.nih.gov/17242315/
436. https://www.ncbi.nlm.nih.gov/pmc/articles/PMC8569840/
437. https://pubmed.ncbi.nlm.nih.gov/32795605/
438. https://bmcinfectdis.biomedcentral.com/articles/10.1186/s12879-021-06167-8
439. https://pubmed.ncbi.nlm.nih.gov/21318622/

440. https://link.springer.com/article/10.1007/s13668-021-00354-4
441. https://www.nature.com/articles/ijo201081
442. https://pubmed.ncbi.nlm.nih.gov/26646455/
443. https://pubmed.ncbi.nlm.nih.gov/27182867/
444. https://ods.od.nih.gov/factsheets/Zinc-HealthProfessional/
445. https://journals.plos.org/plosone/article?id=10.1371/journal.pone.0270971
446. https://www.ncbi.nlm.nih.gov/pmc/articles/PMC3510072/
447. https://www.ncbi.nlm.nih.gov/pmc/articles/PMC7352522/
448. https://pubmed.ncbi.nlm.nih.gov/29260510/?dopt=Abstract
449. https://pubmed.ncbi.nlm.nih.gov/17682990/?dopt=Abstract
450. https://www.medrxiv.org/content/10.1101/2020.06.14.20131128v1
451. https://www.ncbi.nlm.nih.gov/pubmed/11073753?dopt=Abstract
452. https://pubmed.ncbi.nlm.nih.gov/27915460/?dopt=Abstract
453. https://pubmed.ncbi.nlm.nih.gov/30888253/?dopt=Abstract
454. https://pubmed.ncbi.nlm.nih.gov/30517196/
455. https://pubmed.ncbi.nlm.nih.gov/11594942/?dopt=Abstract
456. https://www.ncbi.nlm.nih.gov/pmc/articles/PMC5793244/
457. https://pubmed.ncbi.nlm.nih.gov/16373990/
458. https://pubmed.ncbi.nlm.nih.gov/17726308/
459. https://pubmed.ncbi.nlm.nih.gov/12730441/
460. https://pubmed.ncbi.nlm.nih.gov/25462582
461. https://pubmed.ncbi.nlm.nih.gov/8075746/
462. https://pubmed.ncbi.nlm.nih.gov/20860857/
463. https://pubmed.ncbi.nlm.nih.gov/11739864/
464. https://pubmed.ncbi.nlm.nih.gov/35599332/
465. https://pubmed.ncbi.nlm.nih.gov/34180610/
466. https://ods.od.nih.gov/factsheets/Zinc-HealthProfessional/#en56
467. https://www.frontiersin.org/articles/10.3389/fnut.2022.806566/full
468. https://www.nature.com/articles/nature.2016.19136
469. https://www.ncbi.nlm.nih.gov/pmc/articles/PMC1959459/
470. https://www.ncbi.nlm.nih.gov/pmc/articles/PMC3027896/
471. https://www.ncbi.nlm.nih.gov/pmc/articles/PMC4854945/
472. https://www.mdpi.com/2072-6643/14/3/466
473. https://gut.bmj.com/content/70/4/698
474. https://pubmed.ncbi.nlm.nih.gov/30144260/
475. http://www.ncbi.nlm.nih.gov/pubmed/30787928
476. http://www.ncbi.nlm.nih.gov/pubmed/27776263
477. http://www.ncbi.nlm.nih.gov/pubmed/16773690
478. http://www.ncbi.nlm.nih.gov/pubmed/29183332
479. http://www.ncbi.nlm.nih.gov/pubmed/25420450
480. http://www.ncbi.nlm.nih.gov/pubmed/25540641
481. https://www.ncbi.nlm.nih.gov/pmc/articles/PMC9051551/
482. https://pubmed.ncbi.nlm.nih.gov/24314205/

483. https://pubmed.ncbi.nlm.nih.gov/21133840/
484. https://www.ncbi.nlm.nih.gov/pmc/articles/PMC7544950/
485. https://pubmed.ncbi.nlm.nih.gov/29255450/
486. https://pubmed.ncbi.nlm.nih.gov/28123052/
487. https://nutritionandmetabolism.biomedcentral.com/articles/10.1186/s12986-021-00635-3
488. https://pubmed.ncbi.nlm.nih.gov/22224928/
489. https://pubmed.ncbi.nlm.nih.gov/24667318/
490. https://www.frontiersin.org/articles/10.3389/fmicb.2015.01177/full#B9
491. https://www.ncbi.nlm.nih.gov/pmc/articles/PMC7655491/
492. https://pubmed.ncbi.nlm.nih.gov/10066652/
493. https://pubmed.ncbi.nlm.nih.gov/11720814/
494. https://pubmed.ncbi.nlm.nih.gov/20803023/
495. https://pubmed.ncbi.nlm.nih.gov/28668682/
496. https://academicjournals.org/journal/AJMR/article-abstract/DC192D160105
497. https://pubmed.ncbi.nlm.nih.gov/22642647/
498. https://pubmed.ncbi.nlm.nih.gov/30886158/
499. https://pubmed.ncbi.nlm.nih.gov/15030604/
500. https://journals.plos.org/plosone/article?id=10.1371/journal.pone.0052132
501. https://www.cell.com/cell/fulltext/S0092-8674(22)00992-8
502. https://pubmed.ncbi.nlm.nih.gov/15738954/
503. https://www.ncbi.nlm.nih.gov/pmc/articles/PMC1361287/
504. https://pubmed.ncbi.nlm.nih.gov/9512816/
505. https://www.ncbi.nlm.nih.gov/pmc/articles/PMC39758/
506. https://pubmed.ncbi.nlm.nih.gov/8416086/
507. https://pubmed.ncbi.nlm.nih.gov/11211068/
508. https://pubmed.ncbi.nlm.nih.gov/8024167/
509. https://www.ncbi.nlm.nih.gov/pmc/articles/PMC4082590/
510. https://pubmed.ncbi.nlm.nih.gov/10080859/
511. https://pubmed.ncbi.nlm.nih.gov/3390497/
512. https://pubmed.ncbi.nlm.nih.gov/8227313/
513. https://pubmed.ncbi.nlm.nih.gov/10461128/
514. https://pubmed.ncbi.nlm.nih.gov/18023961/
515. https://pubmed.ncbi.nlm.nih.gov/26589222/
516. https://www.ncbi.nlm.nih.gov/pmc/articles/PMC3337124/
517. https://pubmed.ncbi.nlm.nih.gov/19686881/?dopt=Abstract
518. https://link.springer.com/chapter/10.1007/978-3-030-16996-1_19
519. https://pubmed.ncbi.nlm.nih.gov/20024706/
520. https://pubmed.ncbi.nlm.nih.gov/28676747/
521. https://pubmed.ncbi.nlm.nih.gov/23510906/?dopt=Abstract
522. https://www.ncbi.nlm.nih.gov/pmc/articles/PMC6458519/
523. https://pubmed.ncbi.nlm.nih.gov/3052653/

524. https://www.nature.com/articles/s41586-022-04890-z
525. https://www.frontiersin.org/articles/10.3389/fpubh.2021.684112/full
526. https://www.medrxiv.org/content/10.1101/2021.12.03.21266946v2.full-text
527. https://pubmed.ncbi.nlm.nih.gov/29262731/
528. https://pubmed.ncbi.nlm.nih.gov/9129266/
529. https://pubmed.ncbi.nlm.nih.gov/36167192/
530. https://pubmed.ncbi.nlm.nih.gov/3003360/
531. https://www.ncbi.nlm.nih.gov/pmc/articles/PMC5143500/
532. https://www.ncbi.nlm.nih.gov/pmc/articles/PMC3944636/
533. https://www.ncbi.nlm.nih.gov/pmc/articles/PMC3687513/
534. https://www.ncbi.nlm.nih.gov/pmc/articles/PMC4945988/
535. https://www.ncbi.nlm.nih.gov/pmc/articles/PMC4214967/
536. https://ehp.niehs.nih.gov/doi/10.1289/EHP9889
537. https://jamanetwork.com/journals/jamanetworkopen/fullarticle/2764067
538. https://pubmed.ncbi.nlm.nih.gov/10696119/
539. https://news.northwestern.edu/stories/2019/07/us-packaged-food-supply-is-ultra-processed/
540. https://bmjopen.bmj.com/content/6/3/e009892
541. https://gh.bmj.com/content/7/3/e008269
542. https://www.bmj.com/content/360/bmj.k322
543. https://www.bmj.com/content/365/bmj.l1451
544. https://pubmed.ncbi.nlm.nih.gov/34348832/
545. https://pubmed.ncbi.nlm.nih.gov/35972529/
546. https://www.ncbi.nlm.nih.gov/pmc/articles/PMC8137628/
547. https://www.ncbi.nlm.nih.gov/pmc/articles/PMC9228591/
548. https://www.sciencedirect.com/science/article/abs/pii/S0899900721002811?via%3Dihub
549. https://www.ncbi.nlm.nih.gov/pmc/articles/PMC8011970/
550. https://www.ncbi.nlm.nih.gov/pmc/articles/PMC7490768/
551. https://pubmed.ncbi.nlm.nih.gov/30945554/
552. https://pubmed.ncbi.nlm.nih.gov/29679410/
553. https://pubmed.ncbi.nlm.nih.gov/29679410/
554. https://www.ncbi.nlm.nih.gov/pmc/articles/PMC9228591/
555. https://www.ncbi.nlm.nih.gov/pmc/articles/PMC7068600/
556. https://www.pnas.org/doi/10.1073/pnas.2111530118
557. https://www.sciencedaily.com/releases/2021/05/210504112637.htm
558. https://www.bbc.co.uk/news/uk-england-hampshire-59622307
559. https://www.sciencedirect.com/science/article/pii/S0048969722020009
560. https://www.sciencedirect.com/science/article/abs/pii/S0048969720374039
561. https://pubmed.ncbi.nlm.nih.gov/33310568/
562. https://www.sciencedirect.com/science/article/pii/S0045653521023705
563. https://www.nature.com/articles/s41598-019-52292-5

564. https://pubmed.ncbi.nlm.nih.gov/32767490/
565. https://www.sciencedirect.com/science/article/abs/pii/S0048969719328384
566. https://www.biorxiv.org/content/10.1101/2022.11.04.515261v1
567. https://www.fda.gov/food/food-additives-petitions/bisphenol-bpa-use-food-contact-application
568. https://pubmed.ncbi.nlm.nih.gov/32380592/
569. https://pubmed.ncbi.nlm.nih.gov/21605673/
570. https://ehjournal.biomedcentral.com/articles/10.1186/1476-069X-14-13
571. https://ift.onlinelibrary.wiley.com/doi/abs/10.1111/1541-4337.12388
572. https://www.ncbi.nlm.nih.gov/pmc/articles/PMC8910940/
573. https://pubmed.ncbi.nlm.nih.gov/12573906/
574. https://pubmed.ncbi.nlm.nih.gov/21987463/
575. https://pubmed.ncbi.nlm.nih.gov/19590677/
576. https://www.ncbi.nlm.nih.gov/pmc/articles/PMC3984226/
577. https://pubmed.ncbi.nlm.nih.gov/22690096/
578. https://journals.plos.org/plosone/article?id=10.1371/journal.pone.0038448
579. https://www.ncbi.nlm.nih.gov/pmc/articles/PMC6477692/
580. https://www.ncbi.nlm.nih.gov/pmc/articles/PMC3997912/
581. https://www.ncbi.nlm.nih.gov/pmc/articles/PMC7906952/
582. https://www.theguardian.com/us-news/2019/may/23/pfas-everyday-products-toxics-guide#:~:text=What%20can%20PFAS%20be%20found,People%20around%20the%20world.
583. https://pubmed.ncbi.nlm.nih.gov/30213782/
584. https://pubmed.ncbi.nlm.nih.gov/28443254/
585. https://www.ncbi.nlm.nih.gov/pmc/articles/PMC7906952/
586. https://journals.plos.org/plosone/article?id=10.1371/journal.pone.0244815
587. https://pubmed.ncbi.nlm.nih.gov/22274686/
588. https://www.sciencedirect.com/science/article/pii/S2405844021022635
589. https://pubmed.ncbi.nlm.nih.gov/29106950/
590. https://pubmed.ncbi.nlm.nih.gov/25601914/
591. https://www.nature.com/articles/s41370-018-0097-y
592. https://pubmed.ncbi.nlm.nih.gov/27003842/
593. https://www.ncbi.nlm.nih.gov/pmc/articles/PMC9103108/
594. https://bmcoralhealth.biomedcentral.com/articles/10.1186/s12903-015-0153-0
595. https://www.ncbi.nlm.nih.gov/pmc/articles/PMC6195894/
596. https://www.fluorideresearch.org/483/files/FJ2015_v48_n3_p195-204_pq.pdf
597. https://www.ncbi.nlm.nih.gov/pmc/articles/PMC6923889/
598. https://fluorideresearch.org/332/files/FJ2000_v33_n2_p74-78.pdf

599. https://www.researchgate.net/publication/292716556_The_influence_of_fluoride_andor_aluminium_on_free_radical_toxicity_in_the_brain_of_female_mice_and_beneficial_effects_of_some_antidotes
600. https://www.researchgate.net/publication/311349663_Fluoride_induced_oxidative_stress_immune_system_and_apoptosis_in_animals_a_review
601. https://pubmed.ncbi.nlm.nih.gov/3328040/
602. https://pubmed.ncbi.nlm.nih.gov/19387566/
603. https://pubmed.ncbi.nlm.nih.gov/20390376/
604. https://pubmed.ncbi.nlm.nih.gov/1921770/
605. https://www.theguardian.com/society/2021/sep/23/fluoride-will-be-added-to-uk-drinking-water-to-cut-tooth-decay
606. https://pubmed.ncbi.nlm.nih.gov/21255877/
607. https://www.ncbi.nlm.nih.gov/pmc/articles/PMC7598058/
608. https://www.thelancet.com/journals/lancet/article/PIIS0140-6736(16)31679-8/fulltext
609. https://books.google.co.uk/books?hl=en&lr=&id=-A4LDgAAQBAJ&oi=fnd&pg=PP1&ots=dcnh1U7lyD&sig=Fx3aWVWXz1efiZrm_OZNkKRo4UY&redir_esc=y#v=onepage&q&f=false
610. https://www.mdpi.com/1660-4601/15/7/1380
611. https://www.frontiersin.org/articles/10.3389/fcell.2020.00091/full#B21
612. https://www.sciencedirect.com/science/article/abs/pii/S0048969719307545?via%3Dihub
613. https://www.mdpi.com/1660-4601/14/9/950
614. https://www.atsjournals.org/doi/10.1164/rccm.201709-1883OC
615. https://www.nature.com/articles/s41598-021-83577-3
616. https://www.frontiersin.org/articles/10.3389/fcell.2020.00091/full#B21
617. https://europepmc.org/article/med/24507396
618. https://linkinghub.elsevier.com/retrieve/pii/S0091674910018609
619. https://www.sciencedirect.com/science/article/abs/pii/S0300483X14001826?via%3Dihub
620. https://www.tandfonline.com/doi/abs/10.3109/08958378.2012.731093?journalCode=iiht20
621. https://pubmed.ncbi.nlm.nih.gov/23322918/
622. https://www.sciencedirect.com/science/article/pii/S0161589020304065
623. https://particleandfibretoxicology.biomedcentral.com/articles/10.1186/s12989-020-00362-2
624. https://particleandfibretoxicology.biomedcentral.com/articles/10.1186/s12989-020-00362-2
625. https://www.researchgate.net/publication/320349175_PM25_Meets_Blood_in_vivo_Damages_and_Immune_Defense
626. https://www.ncbi.nlm.nih.gov/pmc/articles/PMC7598058/#B3

627. https://pubs.acs.org/doi/10.1021/acs.est.1c05383
628. https://aqli.epic.uchicago.edu/reports/
629. https://www.theguardian.com/environment/2022/jun/14/air-pollution-got-worse-during-lockdown-in-many-countries-study-finds
630. https://link.springer.com/article/10.1007/s11869-020-00963-y
631. https://www.nature.com/articles/s41598-021-81935-9
632. https://ehjournal.biomedcentral.com/articles/10.1186/s12940-021-00784-1
633. https://link.springer.com/article/10.1007/s10640-020-00486-1
634. https://pubmed.ncbi.nlm.nih.gov/21247619/
635. https://atm.amegroups.com/article/view/72939/
636. https://corporatewatch.org/monsanto-company-profile/
637. https://www.corp-research.org/e-letter/monsanto-and-genetically-engineering-crops
638. https://enveurope.springeropen.com/articles/10.1186/s12302-016-0070-0
639. https://www.iarc.who.int/featured-news/media-centre-iarc-news-glyphosate
640. https://pubmed.ncbi.nlm.nih.gov/29843257/
641. https://pubmed.ncbi.nlm.nih.gov/10854122/
642. https://pubmed.ncbi.nlm.nih.gov/32897110/
643. https://www.sciencedirect.com/science/article/abs/pii/S0300483X21001748
644. https://pubmed.ncbi.nlm.nih.gov/25434756/
645. https://pubmed.ncbi.nlm.nih.gov/20685618/
646. https://pubmed.ncbi.nlm.nih.gov/9536512/
647. https://www.frontiersin.org/articles/10.3389/fimmu.2022.854837/full
648. https://pubmed.ncbi.nlm.nih.gov/35629374/
649. https://www.oatext.com/Endocrine-disruption-and-cytotoxicity-of-Glyphosate-and-Roundup-in-human-JAr-cells-in-vitro.php
650. https://animalmicrobiome.biomedcentral.com/articles/10.1186/s42523-022-00165-0
651. https://www.ncbi.nlm.nih.gov/pmc/articles/PMC4169648/
652. https://pubmed.ncbi.nlm.nih.gov/35773603/
653. https://www.researchgate.net/publication/291057194_Effect_of_quercetin_against_roundupR_andor_fluoride_induced_biochemical_alterations_and_lipid_peroxidation_in_rats
654. https://pubmed.ncbi.nlm.nih.gov/21859351/
655. https://www.sciencedirect.com/science/article/pii/S0304389422009876
656. https://stacks.cdc.gov/view/cdc/109265
657. https://www.science.org/doi/10.1126/science.aba1510
658. https://pubmed.ncbi.nlm.nih.gov/3556209/
659. https://linkinghub.elsevier.com/retrieve/pii/S0013935117305790

660. https://www.sciencedirect.com/science/article/abs/pii/S0048969721026267?via%3Dihub
661. https://www.mdpi.com/2571-8789/6/1/30
662. https://pmj.bmj.com/content/79/933/391
663. https://www.tandfonline.com/doi/abs/10.1081/CLT-100102447?journalCode=ictx19
664. https://pubmed.ncbi.nlm.nih.gov/9486671/
665. https://www.sciencedirect.com/science/article/abs/pii/S2468202017300955
666. https://pubmed.ncbi.nlm.nih.gov/12928151/
667. https://pubmed.ncbi.nlm.nih.gov/23164666/
668. https://pubmed.ncbi.nlm.nih.gov/22617429/
669. https://www.ncbi.nlm.nih.gov/pmc/articles/PMC4063836/
670. https://pubmed.ncbi.nlm.nih.gov/27289040/
671. https://www.ncbi.nlm.nih.gov/pmc/articles/PMC3855504/
672. https://pubmed.ncbi.nlm.nih.gov/21147604/
673. https://pubmed.ncbi.nlm.nih.gov/21190988/
674. https://journals.plos.org/plosntds/article?id=10.1371/journal.pntd.0003518
675. https://www.ncbi.nlm.nih.gov/pmc/articles/PMC2737023/
676. http://ncbi.nlm.nih.gov/pmc/articles/PMC3727341/
677. https://www.ncbi.nlm.nih.gov/pmc/articles/PMC7563920/
678. https://www.ncbi.nlm.nih.gov/pmc/articles/PMC3783787/
679. https://www.ncbi.nlm.nih.gov/pmc/articles/PMC5580875/
680. https://pubmed.ncbi.nlm.nih.gov/26992476/
681. https://jamanetwork.com/journals/jamapediatrics/fullarticle/2796427
682. https://www.mdpi.com/2073-4360/14/13/2700
683. https://www.ncbi.nlm.nih.gov/pmc/articles/PMC4244211/
684. https://books.google.co.uk/books?id=DT4uDwAAQBAJ&pg=PT878&lpg=PT878&dq=4000+years+to+describe+this+fungal+diversity+based+on+present+discovery+rate+of+about+1200+new+species+per+year&source=bl&ots=8nDYCxo8Jr&sig=ACfU3U3aWQpzIRy4ideOxCu3_uNuVlc1Ew&hl=en&sa=X&ved=2ahUKEwjMuNmlt936AhUzoVwKHbX9B84Q6AF6BAgGEAM#v=snippet&q=4000%20years&f=false
685. https://www.nrcs.usda.gov/wps/portal/nrcs/detail-full/soils/health/biology/?cid=nrcs142p2_053864
686. https://www.sciencedirect.com/science/article/pii/S2215017X19307003
687. https://returntonow.net/2018/06/04/mushroom-based-pesticide-could-make-chemical-pesticides-obsolete/
688. https://www.nature.com/articles/s41598-018-32194-8
689. https://www.wbur.org/hereandnow/2019/01/28/mushrooms-fungi-disease-bees
690. https://www.ncbi.nlm.nih.gov/pmc/articles/PMC7826851/
691. https://www.sciencedirect.com/science/article/pii/S2772753X22000120

692. https://www.ncbi.nlm.nih.gov/pmc/articles/PMC8998036/
693. https://www.researchgate.net/publication/297751864_A_safety_assessment_of_Coriolus_versicolor_biomass_as_a_food_supplement
694. https://pubmed.ncbi.nlm.nih.gov/33058392/
695. https://www.sciencedirect.com/topics/medicine-and-dentistry/krestin
696. https://pubmed.ncbi.nlm.nih.gov/15183073/
697. https://sciendo.com/pdf/10.2478/acph-2021-0007
698. https://www.ncbi.nlm.nih.gov/labs/pmc/articles/PMC5929448/
699. https://www.ncbi.nlm.nih.gov/labs/pmc/articles/PMC6010034/
700. https://www.ncbi.nlm.nih.gov/books/NBK92757/#ch9_sec1
701. https://pubmed.ncbi.nlm.nih.gov/17182202/
702. https://pubmed.ncbi.nlm.nih.gov/16169168/\
703. https://pubmed.ncbi.nlm.nih.gov/9096652/
704. https://pubmed.ncbi.nlm.nih.gov/12916709/
705. https://www.ncbi.nlm.nih.gov/pmc/articles/PMC4684114/
706. https://www.ncbi.nlm.nih.gov/pmc/articles/PMC2841828/
707. https://www.frontiersin.org/articles/10.3389/fimmu.2019.00388/full
708. https://www.ncbi.nlm.nih.gov/pmc/articles/PMC8007786/
709. https://pubmed.ncbi.nlm.nih.gov/16630939/
710. https://pubmed.ncbi.nlm.nih.gov/19969338/
711. https://www.frontiersin.org/articles/10.3389/fimmu.2020.624411/full
712. https://www.biorxiv.org/content/10.1101/2022.04.30.489997v1
713. https://pubmed.ncbi.nlm.nih.gov/32473127/
714. https://insight.jci.org/articles/view/146316
715. https://www.nature.com/articles/s41586-020-2550-z
716. https://www.nature.com/articles/s41598-021-92521-4
717. https://www.jimmunol.org/content/early/2021/10/01/jimmunol.2100606
718. https://www.science.org/doi/10.1126/sciimmunol.abn3127
719. https://www.ncbi.nlm.nih.gov/pmc/articles/PMC4049052/
720. https://pubmed.ncbi.nlm.nih.gov/10444630/
721. https://www.ncbi.nlm.nih.gov/pmc/articles/PMC2856774/

OTHER SUPPLEMENTS

1. https://www.ncbi.nlm.nih.gov/pmc/articles/PMC5876976/
2. https://www.nature.com/articles/d41586-021-02978-6
3. https://www.medrxiv.org/content/10.1101/2022.04.08.22273614v1.full
4. https://www.mdpi.com/2072-6643/13/6/1963/pdf
5. https://www.frontiersin.org/articles/10.3389/fcimb.2020.00096/full
6. https://www.ncbi.nlm.nih.gov/pmc/articles/PMC8564795/
7. https://www.ncbi.nlm.nih.gov/pmc/articles/PMC3389160/
8. https://www.sciencedirect.com/science/article/abs/pii/S0031942213004536?via%3Dihub

9. https://www.ncbi.nlm.nih.gov/pmc/articles/PMC3770732/
10. https://www.ncbi.nlm.nih.gov/pmc/articles/PMC3150605/
11. https://www.ncbi.nlm.nih.gov/pmc/articles/PMC3948846/
12. https://www.sciencedirect.com/science/article/abs/pii/S0091305714000835?via%3Dihub
13. https://www.ncbi.nlm.nih.gov/pmc/articles/PMC4240709/
14. https://pubmed.ncbi.nlm.nih.gov/24043773/
15. https://pubmed.ncbi.nlm.nih.gov/26715291/
16. https://pubmed.ncbi.nlm.nih.gov/24535427/
17. https://pubmed.ncbi.nlm.nih.gov/28295316/
18. https://examine.com/supplements/7-8-dihydroxyflavone/
19. https://pubmed.ncbi.nlm.nih.gov/15363636/
20. https://www.sciencedirect.com/science/article/abs/pii/S0304394017306353
21. https://pubmed.ncbi.nlm.nih.gov/25463525/
22. https://www.pnas.org/doi/10.1073/pnas.1801609115
23. https://pubmed.ncbi.nlm.nih.gov/29076953/
24. https://linkinghub.elsevier.com/retrieve/pii/S105913111600042X
25. https://pubmed.ncbi.nlm.nih.gov/23614584/
26. https://pubmed.ncbi.nlm.nih.gov/23563705/
27. https://www.webmd.com/vitamins/ai/ingredientmono-834/acetyl-l-carnitine
28. https://www.ncbi.nlm.nih.gov/pmc/articles/PMC4595381/
29. https://www.ncbi.nlm.nih.gov/pmc/articles/PMC2789318/
30. https://pubmed.ncbi.nlm.nih.gov/1428296/
31. https://www.ncbi.nlm.nih.gov/pmc/articles/PMC8775685/
32. https://pubmed.ncbi.nlm.nih.gov/12637119/
33. https://pubmed.ncbi.nlm.nih.gov/24156263/
34. https://pubmed.ncbi.nlm.nih.gov/29042830/
35. https://examine.com/supplements/alpha-gpc/#references
36. https://pubmed.ncbi.nlm.nih.gov/32587943/
37. https://pubmed.ncbi.nlm.nih.gov/34817582/
38. https://pubmed.ncbi.nlm.nih.gov/21414376/
39. https://www.ncbi.nlm.nih.gov/labs/pmc/articles/PMC5613902/
40. https://www.ncbi.nlm.nih.gov/pmc/articles/PMC7504512/
41. https://www.ncbi.nlm.nih.gov/pmc/articles/PMC5613902/
42. https://pubmed.ncbi.nlm.nih.gov/22906565/
43. https://pubmed.ncbi.nlm.nih.gov/26482148/
44. https://www.thelancet.com/journals/ebiom/article/PIIS2352-3964(21)00326-1/fulltext
45. https://pubmed.ncbi.nlm.nih.gov/32278858/
46. https://www.ncbi.nlm.nih.gov/pmc/articles/PMC7504512/#B116-molecules-25-03809
47. https://bnrc.springeropen.com/articles/10.1186/s42269-022-00786-0

48. https://pubmed.ncbi.nlm.nih.gov/26374184/
49. https://pubmed.ncbi.nlm.nih.gov/25709796/
50. https://pubmed.ncbi.nlm.nih.gov/8957153/
51. https://www.sciencedirect.com/science/article/pii/S2095809918305423
52. https://draxe.com/nutrition/artemisia-annua-benefits/
53. https://www.ncbi.nlm.nih.gov/pmc/articles/PMC2758403/
54. https://www.ncbi.nlm.nih.gov/pmc/articles/PMC4297758/
55. https://pubmed.ncbi.nlm.nih.gov/33141328/
56. https://pubmed.ncbi.nlm.nih.gov/32405226/
57. https://pubmed.ncbi.nlm.nih.gov/34465091/
58. https://www.ncbi.nlm.nih.gov/pmc/articles/PMC6557089/
59. https://draxe.com/health/artemisinin/
60. https://www.drugs.com/npp/sweet-wormwood.html
61. https://www.sciencedirect.com/science/article/pii/S1756464620305636
62. https://link.springer.com/article/10.1007/s11655-019-3039-1
63. https://www.sciencedirect.com/science/article/pii/S1756464620305636#b0280
64. https://www.spandidos-publications.com/10.3892/etm.2018.6501
65. https://www.hindawi.com/journals/ecam/2013/654643/
66. https://www.sciencedirect.com/science/article/abs/pii/S0141813016330707?via%3Dihub
67. https://www.sciencedirect.com/science/article/pii/S1567576916304477?via%3Dihub
68. https://www.mdpi.com/1420-3049/24/2/373
69. https://www.spandidos-publications.com/10.3892/etm.2018.6501
70. https://www.dovepress.com/astragaloside-iv-an-effective-drug-for-the-treatment-of-cardiovascular-peer-reviewed-fulltext-article-DDDT
71. https://pubmed.ncbi.nlm.nih.gov/28303172/
72. https://pubmed.ncbi.nlm.nih.gov/27034688/
73. https://pubmed.ncbi.nlm.nih.gov/32682983/
74. https://www.ncbi.nlm.nih.gov/pmc/articles/PMC3968031
75. https://www.ncbi.nlm.nih.gov/pmc/articles/PMC4936768/
76. https://pubmed.ncbi.nlm.nih.gov/1471613/i
77. https://examine.com/supplements/astragalus/
78. https://pubmed.ncbi.nlm.nih.gov/15898709/
79. https://pubmed.ncbi.nlm.nih.gov/31126578/
80. https://pubmed.ncbi.nlm.nih.gov/27365272/
81. https://www.ncbi.nlm.nih.gov/pmc/articles/PMC4564636/
82. https://www.sciencedirect.com/science/article/abs/pii/S0306452209001833?via%3Dihub
83. https://www.ncbi.nlm.nih.gov/pmc/articles/PMC7803732/
84. https://pubmed.ncbi.nlm.nih.gov/11498727/
85. https://pubmed.ncbi.nlm.nih.gov/23320031/
86. https://examine.com/supplements/bacopa-monnieri/

87. https://pubmed.ncbi.nlm.nih.gov/28588366/
88. https://www.ncbi.nlm.nih.gov/pmc/articles/PMC8493948/
89. https://www.ncbi.nlm.nih.gov/pmc/articles/PMC6025220/
90. https://pubmed.ncbi.nlm.nih.gov/24849036/
91. https://pubmed.ncbi.nlm.nih.gov/25435015/
92. https://pubmed.ncbi.nlm.nih.gov/21920425/
93. https://pubmed.ncbi.nlm.nih.gov/15853750/
94. https://pubmed.ncbi.nlm.nih.gov/34666140/
95. https://pubmed.ncbi.nlm.nih.gov/36051349/
96. https://pubmed.ncbi.nlm.nih.gov/30668313/
97. https://www.ncbi.nlm.nih.gov/pmc/articles/PMC8493948/
98. https://ovarianresearch.biomedcentral.com/articles/10.1186/s13048-022-00965-7
99. https://www.sciencedirect.com/science/article/pii/S0014579315002495
100. https://www.ncbi.nlm.nih.gov/pmc/articles/PMC6535191/
101. https://pubmed.ncbi.nlm.nih.gov/27352310/
102. https://pubmed.ncbi.nlm.nih.gov/33753147/
103. https://www.researchsquare.com/article/rs-1844677/v1
104. https://linkinghub.elsevier.com/retrieve/pii/S1471490600018123
105. https://www.ncbi.nlm.nih.gov/pmc/articles/PMC7407580/
106. https://assets.researchsquare.com/files/rs-1344323/v1/aaf12e39-aadd-4283-be20-c0396f4143c5.pdf?c=1644516561
107. https://pubs.acs.org/doi/10.1021/ol070748n
108. https://pubmed.ncbi.nlm.nih.gov/21820898/
109. https://pubs.acs.org/doi/10.1021/acs.jnatprod.9b00724
110. https://pubchem.ncbi.nlm.nih.gov/compound/Shikonin#section=Non-Human-Toxicity-Excerpts
111. https://www.ncbi.nlm.nih.gov/pmc/articles/PMC182643/
112. https://www.ncbi.nlm.nih.gov/pmc/articles/PMC9383814/
113. https://www.ncbi.nlm.nih.gov/pmc/articles/PMC8240111/
114. https://pubmed.ncbi.nlm.nih.gov/23679238/
115. https://www.ncbi.nlm.nih.gov/pmc/articles/PMC8124789/
116. https://scholar.google.com/scholar_lookup?journal=Edible+Fungi+China&title=Extraction+of+Inonotus+obliquus+polysaccharide+and+the+effect+of+anti-proliferation+on+SMMC7721+cells+of+lung+cancer&author=Z.+Huili&author=Y.+Song&author=L.+Yu&volume=25&publication_year=2006&pages=31-33&
117. https://pubmed.ncbi.nlm.nih.gov/25270791/
118. https://pubmed.ncbi.nlm.nih.gov/33610845/
119. https://www.ncbi.nlm.nih.gov/pmc/articles/PMC8124789/
120. https://pubmed.ncbi.nlm.nih.gov/28954386/
121. https://www.ncbi.nlm.nih.gov/pmc/articles/PMC4100277/
122. https://www.tandfonline.com/doi/full/10.1080/21691401.2019.1577877

123. https://www.sciencedirect.com/science/article/pii/S1567576917304459?via%3Dihub
124. https://www.nutraingredients-usa.com/Article/2012/06/13/ORAC-has-ongoing-value-says-expert-as-USDA-removes-online-database
125. https://www.sciencedirect.com/science/article/abs/pii/000989819506133X?via%3Dihub
126. https://examine.com/supplements/chaga/
127. https://pubmed.ncbi.nlm.nih.gov/32419395/
128. https://pubmed.ncbi.nlm.nih.gov/30276648/
129. https://www.ncbi.nlm.nih.gov/pmc/articles/PMC5807419/
130. https://pubmed.ncbi.nlm.nih.gov/20193705/
131. https://pubmed.ncbi.nlm.nih.gov/17482527/
132. https://ift.onlinelibrary.wiley.com/doi/abs/10.1111/1541-4337.12539
133. https://pubmed.ncbi.nlm.nih.gov/19960455/
134. https://pubmed.ncbi.nlm.nih.gov/24124769/
135. https://pubmed.ncbi.nlm.nih.gov/16621054/
136. https://pubmed.ncbi.nlm.nih.gov/18579827/
137. https://pubmed.ncbi.nlm.nih.gov/24384733/
138. https://www.immunologyresearchjournal.com/articles/coenzyme-q10-and-vitamin-d-interventions-could-ameliorate-covid-19-related-cellular-bioenergetic-dysfunction-and-cytokine-storms.pdf
139. https://www.embopress.org/doi/full/10.15252/emmm.202013001
140. https://pubmed.ncbi.nlm.nih.gov/34967652/
141. https://www.mdpi.com/1422-0067/23/20/12345
142. https://pubmed.ncbi.nlm.nih.gov/25810566/
143. https://pubmed.ncbi.nlm.nih.gov/25308577/
144. https://pubmed.ncbi.nlm.nih.gov/22704112/
145. https://pubmed.ncbi.nlm.nih.gov/24704922/
146. https://www.ncbi.nlm.nih.gov/pmc/articles/PMC4568976/
147. https://www.ncbi.nlm.nih.gov/pmc/articles/PMC5870379/
148. https://examine.com/supplements/coenzyme-q10/
149. http://diposit.ub.edu/dspace/bitstream/2445/181270/3/701264.pdf
150. https://www.ncbi.nlm.nih.gov/pmc/articles/PMC8950003/
151. https://www.ncbi.nlm.nih.gov/pmc/articles/PMC5812812/
152. https://www.sciencedirect.com/science/article/abs/pii/S0953620521003320
153. https://pubmed.ncbi.nlm.nih.gov/21193035/
154. https://www.jimmunol.org/content/174/8/4584
155. https://www.ncbi.nlm.nih.gov/pmc/articles/PMC4684410/
156. https://www.ncbi.nlm.nih.gov/pmc/articles/PMC5058879/
157. https://pubmed.ncbi.nlm.nih.gov/35787150/
158. https://www.ncbi.nlm.nih.gov/pmc/articles/PMC5049504/
159. https://pubmed.ncbi.nlm.nih.gov/35381033/
160. https://pubmed.ncbi.nlm.nih.gov/35833737/

161. https://www.ncbi.nlm.nih.gov/pmc/articles/PMC8078534/
162. https://www.ncbi.nlm.nih.gov/pmc/articles/PMC9136918/
163. https://pubmed.ncbi.nlm.nih.gov/34657777/
164. https://pubmed.ncbi.nlm.nih.gov/33002524/
165. https://www.ncbi.nlm.nih.gov/pmc/articles/PMC3257684/
166. https://www.ncbi.nlm.nih.gov/pmc/articles/PMC8308243/
167. https://pubmed.ncbi.nlm.nih.gov/24571383/
168. https://pubmed.ncbi.nlm.nih.gov/25781716/
169. https://www.ncbi.nlm.nih.gov/pmc/articles/PMC4302452/
170. https://www.ncbi.nlm.nih.gov/pmc/articles/PMC8307123/
171. https://www.tandfonline.com/doi/full/10.1080/09540105.2021.1892594
172. https://pesquisa.bvsalud.org/global-literature-on-novel-coronavirus-2019-ncov/resource/pt/covidwho-1202490
173. https://journals.plos.org/plosone/article?id=10.1371/journal.pone.0268806
174. https://www.ncbi.nlm.nih.gov/pmc/articles/PMC8469309/
175. https://www.frontiersin.org/articles/10.3389/fphar.2021.666600/full
176. https://academic.oup.com/ae/article/40/4/235/2389394
177. https://www.ncbi.nlm.nih.gov/books/NBK92758/
178. https://pubmed.ncbi.nlm.nih.gov/16873101/
179. https://pubmed.ncbi.nlm.nih.gov/19350364/
180. https://www.ncbi.nlm.nih.gov/pmc/articles/PMC7356751/
181. https://pubmed.ncbi.nlm.nih.gov/25704018/
182. https://pubmed.ncbi.nlm.nih.gov/15506292/
183. https://pubmed.ncbi.nlm.nih.gov/12165189/
184. https://pubmed.ncbi.nlm.nih.gov/10755473/
185. https://www.ncbi.nlm.nih.gov/pmc/articles/PMC7898063/#B42
186. https://www.ncbi.nlm.nih.gov/pmc/articles/PMC7754931/
187. https://pubmed.ncbi.nlm.nih.gov/27315037/
188. https://examine.com/supplements/cordyceps/
189. https://www.ncbi.nlm.nih.gov/pmc/articles/PMC8072387/
190. https://pubmed.ncbi.nlm.nih.gov/21476212/
191. https://pubmed.ncbi.nlm.nih.gov/18570234/
192. https://pubmed.ncbi.nlm.nih.gov/22745069/
193. https://pubmed.ncbi.nlm.nih.gov/31255730/
194. https://www.ncbi.nlm.nih.gov/pmc/articles/PMC8072387/
195. https://pubmed.ncbi.nlm.nih.gov/21982433/
196. https://www.ncbi.nlm.nih.gov/pmc/articles/PMC7023136/
197. https://pubmed.ncbi.nlm.nih.gov/9358903/
198. https://pubmed.ncbi.nlm.nih.gov/27989876/
199. https://pubmed.ncbi.nlm.nih.gov/24794906/
200. https://pubmed.ncbi.nlm.nih.gov/12553052/
201. https://www.ncbi.nlm.nih.gov/pmc/articles/PMC3883055/
202. https://www.ncbi.nlm.nih.gov/pmc/articles/PMC2637808/

203. https://pubmed.ncbi.nlm.nih.gov/27470399/
204. https://www.ncbi.nlm.nih.gov/pmc/articles/PMC3964021/
205. https://www.ncbi.nlm.nih.gov/pmc/articles/PMC2964958/
206. https://www.ncbi.nlm.nih.gov/pmc/articles/PMC3814973/
207. https://linkinghub.elsevier.com/retrieve/pii/S1756464615000092
208. https://pubmed.ncbi.nlm.nih.gov/17569207/
209. https://pubmed.ncbi.nlm.nih.gov/17545551/
210. https://www.ncbi.nlm.nih.gov/pmc/articles/PMC5664031/
211. https://pubmed.ncbi.nlm.nih.gov/14994335/
212. https://pubmed.ncbi.nlm.nih.gov/30145851/
213. https://www.nature.com/articles/s41420-019-0234-y
214. https://pubmed.ncbi.nlm.nih.gov/17569217/
215. https://www.sciencedirect.com/science/article/abs/pii/S0304389420311493
216. https://www.ncbi.nlm.nih.gov/pmc/articles/PMC8170768/
217. https://www.ncbi.nlm.nih.gov/pmc/articles/PMC7551052/
218. https://pubmed.ncbi.nlm.nih.gov/25277322/
219. https://pubmed.ncbi.nlm.nih.gov/24982601/
220. https://pubmed.ncbi.nlm.nih.gov/19589293/
221. https://www.ncbi.nlm.nih.gov/pmc/articles/PMC8268053/
222. https://www.nature.com/articles/s41598-021-81462-7
223. https://pubs.rsc.org/en/content/articlelanding/2020/ra/d0ra03167d
224. https://www.ncbi.nlm.nih.gov/pmc/articles/PMC9044632/
225. https://pubmed.ncbi.nlm.nih.gov/35057437/
226. https://trialsjournal.biomedcentral.com/articles/10.1186/s13063-022-06375-w
227. https://pubmed.ncbi.nlm.nih.gov/26528921/
228. https://examine.com/supplements/curcumin/
229. https://pubmed.ncbi.nlm.nih.gov/29480523/
230. https://pubmed.ncbi.nlm.nih.gov/17044766/
231. https://www.ncbi.nlm.nih.gov/pmc/articles/PMC6414192/
232. https://pubmed.ncbi.nlm.nih.gov/11857414/
233. https://www.ncbi.nlm.nih.gov/pmc/articles/PMC8754353/
234. https://www.ncbi.nlm.nih.gov/pmc/articles/PMC3535405/
235. https://pubmed.ncbi.nlm.nih.gov/11348657/
236. https://www.nature.com/articles/s41569-021-00536-1
237. https://www.ncbi.nlm.nih.gov/pmc/articles/PMC5929433/
238. https://www.frontiersin.org/articles/10.3389/fneur.2020.00437/full
239. https://pubmed.ncbi.nlm.nih.gov/8530509/
240. https://pubmed.ncbi.nlm.nih.gov/15888438/
241. https://www.mdpi.com/2077-0383/11/19/5882
242. https://pubmed.ncbi.nlm.nih.gov/20502000/
243. https://ascpt.onlinelibrary.wiley.com/doi/10.1002/cpt.2317
244. https://pubmed.ncbi.nlm.nih.gov/16501251/

245. https://www.nature.com/articles/s41598-022-11219-3
246. https://pubmed.ncbi.nlm.nih.gov/9782673/
247. https://www.ncbi.nlm.nih.gov/pmc/articles/PMC3689181/
248. https://pubmed.ncbi.nlm.nih.gov/25272572/
249. https://pubmed.ncbi.nlm.nih.gov/33187049/
250. https://pubmed.ncbi.nlm.nih.gov/8298183/
251. https://pubmed.ncbi.nlm.nih.gov/11351248/
252. https://www.ncbi.nlm.nih.gov/pmc/articles/PMC3220618/
253. https://pubmed.ncbi.nlm.nih.gov/22524676/
254. https://www.ncbi.nlm.nih.gov/pmc/articles/PMC2765609/
255. https://www.ncbi.nlm.nih.gov/pmc/articles/PMC8839434/
256. https://www.ncbi.nlm.nih.gov/pmc/articles/PMC5527824/
257. https://www.preprints.org/manuscript/202209.0440/v1
258. https://www.nature.com/articles/s41598-020-59894-4
259. https://pubmed.ncbi.nlm.nih.gov/30312797/
260. https://www.aging-us.com/article/203560/text
261. https://www.ncbi.nlm.nih.gov/pmc/articles/PMC6197652/
262. https://pubmed.ncbi.nlm.nih.gov/29317180/
263. https://nootropicsexpert.com/fisetin/#fisetin-recommended-dosage
264. https://koreascience.kr/article/JAKO201025665646491.page
265. https://www.kew.org/read-and-watch/ginkgo-biloba-maidenhair-tree-kew-gardens
266. https://examine.com/supplements/ginkgo-biloba/
267. https://www.ncbi.nlm.nih.gov/pmc/articles/PMC7047126/
268. https://www.ncbi.nlm.nih.gov/pmc/articles/PMC8944638/
269. https://www.ncbi.nlm.nih.gov/pmc/articles/PMC8944638/
270. https://pubmed.ncbi.nlm.nih.gov/25446810/
271. https://www.researchgate.net/publication/348552634_Ginkgo_biloba_modulates_hippocampal_BDNF_expression_in_a_rat_model_of_chronic_restraint_stress-induced_depression
272. https://journals.plos.org/plosone/article?id=10.1371/journal.pone.0225761
273. https://www.ncbi.nlm.nih.gov/pmc/articles/PMC3157487/
274. https://www.karger.com/Article/Fulltext/381744
275. https://pubmed.ncbi.nlm.nih.gov/16801106/#:~:text=It%20is%20effective%20in%20the,oral%20anti%2Dplatelet%20therapeutic%20agent.
276. https://www.ncbi.nlm.nih.gov/pmc/articles/PMC8375244/
277. https://examine.com/supplements/ginkgo-biloba/
278. https://pubmed.ncbi.nlm.nih.gov/25046825/
279. https://www.ncbi.nlm.nih.gov/pmc/articles/PMC7993717/
280. https://pubmed.ncbi.nlm.nih.gov/27876669/
281. https://www.mdpi.com/2073-4409/9/5/1107/htm
282. https://pubmed.ncbi.nlm.nih.gov/25850282/

283. http://www.chinadoi.cn/portal/mr.action?doi=10.3969/j.issn.1005-4561.2017.08.003
284. https://pubmed.ncbi.nlm.nih.gov/27082952/
285. https://pubmed.ncbi.nlm.nih.gov/24502632/
286. https://pubmed.ncbi.nlm.nih.gov/24873669/
287. https://www.ncbi.nlm.nih.gov/pmc/articles/PMC2893180/
288. https://www.ncbi.nlm.nih.gov/pmc/articles/PMC7930927/
289. https://www.ncbi.nlm.nih.gov/pmc/articles/PMC5648830/
290. https://pubmed.ncbi.nlm.nih.gov/29036812/
291. https://pubmed.ncbi.nlm.nih.gov/17183312/
292. https://pubmed.ncbi.nlm.nih.gov/32066253/
293. https://www.alzdiscovery.org/uploads/cognitive_vitality_media/Ginsenoside-Rg1-Cognitive-Vitality-For-Researchers.pdf
294. https://examine.com/supplements/panax-ginseng/
295. https://www.ncbi.nlm.nih.gov/pmc/articles/PMC3116297/
296. https://pubmed.ncbi.nlm.nih.gov/26602573/
297. https://pubmed.ncbi.nlm.nih.gov/11081995/
298. https://pubmed.ncbi.nlm.nih.gov/10518115/
299. https://pubmed.ncbi.nlm.nih.gov/31998466/
300. https://pubmed.ncbi.nlm.nih.gov/16105244/
301. https://pubmed.ncbi.nlm.nih.gov/20144879/
302. https://pubmed.ncbi.nlm.nih.gov/18191355/
303. https://www.ncbi.nlm.nih.gov/pmc/articles/PMC4908235/
304. https://pubmed.ncbi.nlm.nih.gov/27279066/
305. https://www.ncbi.nlm.nih.gov/pmc/articles/PMC3834700/
306. https://www.ncbi.nlm.nih.gov/pmc/articles/PMC3594936/
307. https://pubmed.ncbi.nlm.nih.gov/6238770/
308. https://www.ncbi.nlm.nih.gov/pmc/articles/PMC6755196/
309. https://www.webmd.com/vitamins/ai/ingredientmono-753/gotu-kola
310. https://www.healthline.com/health/gotu-kola-benefits
311. https://www.fao.org/3/i4480e/i4480e.pdf
312. https://pubmed.ncbi.nlm.nih.gov/21466438/
313. https://pubmed.ncbi.nlm.nih.gov/27338088
314. https://pubmed.ncbi.nlm.nih.gov/27073430/
315. https://www.ncbi.nlm.nih.gov/pmc/articles/PMC6149506/
316. https://pubmed.ncbi.nlm.nih.gov/28864169/
317. https://www.ncbi.nlm.nih.gov/pmc/articles/PMC4675646/
318. https://www.frontiersin.org/articles/10.3389/fnins.2021.718188/full
319. https://pubmed.ncbi.nlm.nih.gov/25991666/
320. https://www.ncbi.nlm.nih.gov/pmc/articles/PMC5831959/
321. https://cellandbioscience.biomedcentral.com/articles/10.1186/s13578-021-00680-8
322. https://www.ncbi.nlm.nih.gov/books/NBK299060/
323. https://www.sciencedirect.com/science/article/pii/S0273230018300928

324. https://efsa.onlinelibrary.wiley.com/doi/epdf/10.2903/j.efsa.2018.5239
325. https://pubmed.ncbi.nlm.nih.gov/22641606/
326. https://www.ncbi.nlm.nih.gov/pmc/articles/PMC8540791/
327. https://www.healthline.com/health/is-jiaogulan-the-new-ginseng
328. https://link.springer.com/article/10.1007/s11101-005-3754-4
329. https://www.ncbi.nlm.nih.gov/pmc/articles/PMC5037898/
330. https://pubmed.ncbi.nlm.nih.gov/33556477/
331. https://pubmed.ncbi.nlm.nih.gov/24752286/
332. https://pubmed.ncbi.nlm.nih.gov/31499195/
333. https://www.ncbi.nlm.nih.gov/pmc/articles/PMC6271118/
334. https://pubmed.ncbi.nlm.nih.gov/21897202/
335. https://pubmed.ncbi.nlm.nih.gov/25371572/
336. https://europepmc.org/article/cba/352403
337. https://www.ncbi.nlm.nih.gov/pmc/articles/PMC3572697/
338. https://www.ncbi.nlm.nih.gov/pmc/articles/PMC3484409/
339. https://onlinelibrary.wiley.com/doi/full/10.1111/jhn.12936
340. https://onlinelibrary.wiley.com/doi/full/10.1002/oby.20539
341. https://examine.com/supplements/jiaogulan/
342. https://www.ncbi.nlm.nih.gov/pmc/articles/PMC7194064/
343. https://pubmed.ncbi.nlm.nih.gov/34207199/
344. https://pubmed.ncbi.nlm.nih.gov/22000769/
345. https://pubmed.ncbi.nlm.nih.gov/25207357/
346. https://www.sciencedirect.com/science/article/pii/S1568163720302245
347. https://www.ncbi.nlm.nih.gov/pmc/articles/PMC5505738/
348. https://www.sciencedirect.com/science/article/pii/S2214647416300381
349. https://www.ncbi.nlm.nih.gov/pmc/articles/PMC5215870/
350. https://www.ncbi.nlm.nih.gov/pmc/articles/PMC8233727/
351. https://pubmed.ncbi.nlm.nih.gov/30889017/
352. https://pubmed.ncbi.nlm.nih.gov/31585673/
353. https://pubmed.ncbi.nlm.nih.gov/24486607/
354. https://www.frontiersin.org/articles/10.3389/fneur.2020.00952/full
355. https://pubmed.ncbi.nlm.nih.gov/28593105/
356. https://pubmed.ncbi.nlm.nih.gov/15914953/
357. https://www.ncbi.nlm.nih.gov/pmc/articles/PMC1554554/
358. https://pubmed.ncbi.nlm.nih.gov/30074108/
359. http://monomed.pl/img/lampy/t2.pdf
360. https://pleijsalon.com/the-definitive-guide-to-choosing-a-red-light-therapy-device/
361. https://redlightman.com/blog/complete-guide-light-therapy-dosing/
362. https://pubmed.ncbi.nlm.nih.gov/6308762/
363. https://covid19criticalcare.com/wp-content/uploads/2020/11/FLCCC-Ivermectin-in-the-prophylaxis-and-treatment-of-COVID-19.pdf
364. https://www.nature.com/articles/ja201711
365. https://www.ncbi.nlm.nih.gov/pmc/articles/PMC7129059/

366. https://europepmc.org/article/ppr/ppr243457#S7
367. https://pubmed.ncbi.nlm.nih.gov/32871846/
368. https://pubmed.ncbi.nlm.nih.gov/19109745/
369. https://www.ncbi.nlm.nih.gov/pmc/articles/PMC8088823/
370. https://www.ncbi.nlm.nih.gov/pmc/articles/PMC7550891/
371. https://www.ncbi.nlm.nih.gov/pmc/articles/PMC8248252/
372. https://www.ncbi.nlm.nih.gov/pmc/articles/PMC9215332/
373. https://www.ncbi.nlm.nih.gov/pmc/articles/PMC9308124/
374. https://www.theguardian.com/world/2021/sep/20/ivermectin-shortage-horse-owners-covid
375. https://twitter.com/US_FDA/status/1429050070243192839?s=20
376. https://fullfact.org/health/coronavirus-vaccine-pfizer-transmission-test/
377. https://www.covid19treatmentguidelines.nih.gov/therapies/antiviral-therapy/
378. https://www.researchgate.net/publication/344318845_POST-ACUTE_OR_PROLONGED_COVID-19_IVERMECTIN_TREATMENT_FOR_PATIENTS_WITH_PERSISTENT_SYMPTOMS_OR_POST-ACUTE
379. https://pubmed.ncbi.nlm.nih.gov/28087447/
380. https://agris.fao.org/agris-search/search.do?request_locale=fr&recordID=US201301489412&countryResource=
381. https://pubmed.ncbi.nlm.nih.gov/25288148/
382. https://www.jstage.jst.go.jp/article/biomedres/32/1/32_1_67/_pdf/-char/en
383. https://pubmed.ncbi.nlm.nih.gov/20834180/
384. https://pubmed.ncbi.nlm.nih.gov/18844328/
385. https://pubmed.ncbi.nlm.nih.gov/23668749/
386. https://en.cnki.com.cn/Article_en/CJFDTOTAL-LYLC201401002.htm
387. https://pubmed.ncbi.nlm.nih.gov/11842649/
388. https://www.sciencedirect.com/science/article/abs/pii/S1359511313002821
389. https://pubmed.ncbi.nlm.nih.gov/20637576/
390. https://pubmed.ncbi.nlm.nih.gov/29801717/
391. https://pubmed.ncbi.nlm.nih.gov/32402583/
392. https://pubmed.ncbi.nlm.nih.gov/19149659/
393. https://pubmed.ncbi.nlm.nih.gov/16688936/
394. https://pubmed.ncbi.nlm.nih.gov/30319424/
395. https://www.ncbi.nlm.nih.gov/pmc/articles/PMC8478534/
396. https://pubmed.ncbi.nlm.nih.gov/19610032/
397. https://www.ncbi.nlm.nih.gov/pmc/articles/PMC5470611/
398. https://pubmed.ncbi.nlm.nih.gov/29595544/
399. https://www.ncbi.nlm.nih.gov/pmc/articles/PMC7422625/
400. https://pubmed.ncbi.nlm.nih.gov/34717250/
401. https://pubs.acs.org/doi/10.1021/jp509752s
402. https://www.tandfonline.com/doi/full/10.1080/13880200601113057

403. https://pubmed.ncbi.nlm.nih.gov/31362009/
404. https://pubmed.ncbi.nlm.nih.gov/32208856/
405. https://www.ncbi.nlm.nih.gov/pmc/articles/PMC7138288/
406. https://www.ncbi.nlm.nih.gov/pmc/articles/PMC2937579/
407. https://journals.sagepub.com/doi/10.1177/039463201202500201
408. https://www.sciencedirect.com/science/article/abs/pii/S0149291813001781
409. https://pubmed.ncbi.nlm.nih.gov/21193035/
410. https://www.nature.com/articles/tp2015142
411. https://pubmed.ncbi.nlm.nih.gov/32013309
412. https://pubmed.ncbi.nlm.nih.gov/18937165/
413. https://www.ncbi.nlm.nih.gov/pmc/articles/PMC7267424/
414. https://www.nature.com/articles/s41598-022-14664-2
415. https://pubs.rsc.org/en/content/articlelanding/2022/me/d1me00119a
416. https://www.frontiersin.org/articles/10.3389/fimmu.2021.769011/full
417. https://doi.org/10.26434%2Fchemrxiv.11871402.v3
418. https://pubmed.ncbi.nlm.nih.gov/12055336
419. https://pubmed.ncbi.nlm.nih.gov/31951246/
420. https://pubmed.ncbi.nlm.nih.gov/11890390/
421. https://www.sciencedirect.com/science/article/abs/pii/S0963996920308449
422. https://www.ncbi.nlm.nih.gov/pmc/articles/PMC3096456/
423. https://www.ncbi.nlm.nih.gov/pmc/articles/PMC5018343/
424. https://pubmed.ncbi.nlm.nih.gov/12472620/
425. https://pubmed.ncbi.nlm.nih.gov/29359412/
426. https://pubmed.ncbi.nlm.nih.gov/11753476/
427. https://examine.com/supplements/maca/#dosage-information
428. https://www.frontiersin.org/articles/10.3389/fendo.2019.00249/full
429. https://www.mdpi.com/2076-3921/9/11/1088/htm
430. https://pubmed.ncbi.nlm.nih.gov/12204540/
431. https://pubmed.ncbi.nlm.nih.gov/63506/
432. https://pubmed.ncbi.nlm.nih.gov/18316227/
433. https://pubmed.ncbi.nlm.nih.gov/10739303/
434. https://www.ncbi.nlm.nih.gov/books/NBK550972/
435. https://pubmed.ncbi.nlm.nih.gov/11721091/
436. https://pubmed.ncbi.nlm.nih.gov/7350183/
437. https://www.nature.com/articles/s41398-021-01464-x
438. https://pubmed.ncbi.nlm.nih.gov/22850476/
439. https://www.ncbi.nlm.nih.gov/pmc/articles/PMC7767214
440. https://www.sleep.theclinics.com/article/S1556-407X(08)00012-X/fulltext
441. https://www.sciencedirect.com/science/article/abs/pii/030645309390025G?via%3Dihub
442. https://bnf.nice.org.uk/drugs/melatonin/
443. https://ojs.ptbioch.edu.pl/index.php/abp/article/view/3264

444. https://onlinelibrary.wiley.com/doi/10.1111/j.1600-079X.2007.00529.x
445. https://pubmed.ncbi.nlm.nih.gov/31679041/
446. https://academic.oup.com/carcin/article/34/5/1051/2463212
447. https://www.oncotarget.com/article/16379/text/
448. https://onlinelibrary.wiley.com/doi/10.1002/jcp.29036
449. https://anatomypubs.onlinelibrary.wiley.com/doi/full/10.1002/ar.21361
450. https://linkinghub.elsevier.com/retrieve/pii/S1040842817300884
451. https://doi.org/10.1152/ajpheart.00163.2009
452. https://onlinelibrary.wiley.com/doi/10.1111/jpi.12299
453. https://doi.org/10.1007/978-3-319-63245-2_10
454. https://link.springer.com/article/10.1007/s10557-020-07052-3
455. https://www.spandidos-publications.com/10.3892/mmr.2014.2753
456. https://onlinelibrary.wiley.com/doi/10.1111/j.1600-079X.2008.00643.x
457. https://journals.sagepub.com/doi/10.3727/000000003108746786
458. https://linkinghub.elsevier.com/retrieve/pii/S0024320514002276
459. http://www.eurekaselect.com/article/82252
460. https://onlinelibrary.wiley.com/doi/10.1002/jbt.22430
461. https://www.ncbi.nlm.nih.gov/pmc/articles/PMC7346071/
462. https://academic.oup.com/jpp/article/70/1/70/6121796
463. https://www.ncbi.nlm.nih.gov/pmc/articles/PMC7233010/
464. https://linkinghub.elsevier.com/retrieve/pii/S0303846720302213
465. https://pubmed.ncbi.nlm.nih.gov/15119946/
466. https://www.mdpi.com/1422-0067/19/9/2802
467. https://rbej.biomedcentral.com/articles/10.1186/1477-7827-9-108
468. https://linkinghub.elsevier.com/retrieve/pii/S1043661819302889
469. https://link.springer.com/article/10.1177/1933719117711262
470. https://doi.org/10.3389/fendo.2019.00273
471. https://www.sciencedirect.com/science/article/abs/pii/S0165032718328210?via%3Dihub
472. https://www.hindawi.com/journals/omcl/2019/8218650/
473. https://linkinghub.elsevier.com/retrieve/pii/S0301211511004593
474. https://pubmed.ncbi.nlm.nih.gov/29462985/
475. https://www.advbiores.net/article.asp?issn=2277-9175;year=2016;volume=5;issue=1;spage=174;epage=174;aulast=Javanmard
476. https://www.sciencedirect.com/science/article/abs/pii/S0011224017303498?via%3Dihub
477. https://onlinelibrary.wiley.com/doi/abs/10.1111/j.1600-079X.2010.00822.x
478. https://www.ejog.org/article/S0301-2115(11)00459-3/fulltext
479. https://onlinelibrary.wiley.com/doi/10.1111/jpi.12172
480. https://www.mdpi.com/1422-0067/14/4/8638
481. https://www.ncbi.nlm.nih.gov/pubmed/32314850
482. https://link.springer.com/article/10.1007/s00018-021-04102-3

483. https://www.sciencedirect.com/science/article/pii/S0026286221000583?via%3Dihub
484. https://www.mdpi.com/1422-0067/22/2/764
485. https://www.ncbi.nlm.nih.gov/pmc/articles/PMC5187924/
486. https://pubmed.ncbi.nlm.nih.gov/33477032/
487. https://www.ncbi.nlm.nih.gov/pmc/articles/PMC9157541/
488. https://www.ncbi.nlm.nih.gov/pmc/articles/PMC9368024/
489. https://www.ncbi.nlm.nih.gov/pmc/articles/PMC7670925/
490. https://www.ncbi.nlm.nih.gov/pmc/articles/PMC7367032/
491. https://www.ncbi.nlm.nih.gov/pmc/articles/PMC9088601/
492. https://academic.oup.com/biomedgerontology/article/73/10/1330/4942467
493. https://www.ncbi.nlm.nih.gov/pmc/articles/PMC8465482/
494. https://www.ncbi.nlm.nih.gov/pmc/articles/PMC7959850/
495. https://www.ncbi.nlm.nih.gov/pmc/articles/PMC6449196/
496. https://www.ncbi.nlm.nih.gov/pmc/articles/PMC7426637/
497. https://www.ncbi.nlm.nih.gov/pmc/articles/PMC6177209/
498. https://openheart.bmj.com/content/8/1/e001568
499. https://www.ncbi.nlm.nih.gov/pmc/articles/PMC8506572/
500. https://www.mdpi.com/1420-3049/27/3/705
501. https://pubmed.ncbi.nlm.nih.gov/18289163/
502. https://www.mdpi.com/2076-3921/10/9/1483/htm
503. http://www.melatonin-research.net/index.php/MR/article/view/86
504. https://onlinelibrary.wiley.com/doi/abs/10.1111/j.1600-079X.2010.00762.x
505. https://www.sciencedirect.com/science/article/abs/pii/S0887233321001168
506. https://www.sciencedirect.com/science/article/abs/pii/S0531556501002297
507. https://www.nature.com/articles/s41419-019-1556-7
508. https://pubmed.ncbi.nlm.nih.gov/25010497/
509. https://pubmed.ncbi.nlm.nih.gov/28089603/
510. https://journals.plos.org/plosone/article?id=10.1371/journal.pone.0099943
511. https://pubmed.ncbi.nlm.nih.gov/32474586/
512. https://www.ncbi.nlm.nih.gov/pmc/articles/PMC5768956/
513. https://pubmed.ncbi.nlm.nih.gov/27500468/
514. https://doris-loh.com/home
515. https://www.ncbi.nlm.nih.gov/pmc/articles/PMC3334267/
516. https://www.ncbi.nlm.nih.gov/pmc/articles/PMC7893939/
517. https://bnf.nice.org.uk/drugs/melatonin/#indications-and-dose
518. https://www.ncbi.nlm.nih.gov/pubmed/9378688
519. https://www.ncbi.nlm.nih.gov/pubmed/31722088
520. https://ncbi.nlm.nih.gov/pubmed/30663964

521. https://pubmed.ncbi.nlm.nih.gov/27576224/
522. https://pubmed.ncbi.nlm.nih.gov/19082413/
523. https://www.ncbi.nlm.nih.gov/pmc/articles/PMC3087269/
524. https://www.ncbi.nlm.nih.gov/pmc/articles/PMC6147575/
525. https://pubmed.ncbi.nlm.nih.gov/10646879/
526. https://pubmed.ncbi.nlm.nih.gov/27699422/
527. https://pubmed.ncbi.nlm.nih.gov/23022479/
528. https://pubmed.ncbi.nlm.nih.gov/15115294/
529. https://pubmed.ncbi.nlm.nih.gov/14724055/
530. https://pubmed.ncbi.nlm.nih.gov/33669457/
531. https://www.ncbi.nlm.nih.gov/pmc/articles/PMC8699482/
532. https://pubmed.ncbi.nlm.nih.gov/16464752/
533. https://www.ncbi.nlm.nih.gov/pmc/articles/PMC4686104/
534. https://www.researchgate.net/publication/264390565_Therapeutic_Benefits_of_Methylene_Blue_on_Cognitive_Impairment_during_Chronic_Cerebral_Hypoperfusion
535. https://www.frontiersin.org/articles/10.3389/fncel.2020.00130/full
536. https://www.ncbi.nlm.nih.gov/pmc/articles/PMC3265679/
537. https://pubmed.ncbi.nlm.nih.gov/12384216/
538. https://www.ncbi.nlm.nih.gov/pmc/articles/PMC3836814/
539. https://pubmed.ncbi.nlm.nih.gov/25018057/
540. https://www.ncbi.nlm.nih.gov/pmc/articles/PMC5018244/
541. https://pubmed.ncbi.nlm.nih.gov/31144270/
542. https://pubmed.ncbi.nlm.nih.gov/24316434/
543. https://www.ncbi.nlm.nih.gov/pmc/articles/PMC5018244/#R1
544. https://www.nature.com/articles/s41598-021-92481-9
545. https://pubmed.ncbi.nlm.nih.gov/34019535/
546. https://www.sciencedirect.com/science/article/abs/pii/S1572100021003653
547. https://jamanetwork.com/journals/jamadermatology/article-abstract/534807
548. https://bmccancer.biomedcentral.com/articles/10.1186/s12885-017-3179-7
549. https://clinicaltrials.gov/ct2/show/NCT04933864
550. https://www.ncbi.nlm.nih.gov/pmc/articles/PMC4312803/
551. https://www.ncbi.nlm.nih.gov/pmc/articles/PMC7440159/
552. https://pubmed.ncbi.nlm.nih.gov/33010384/
553. https://link.springer.com/book/10.1007/0-387-27600-9
554. https://pubmed.ncbi.nlm.nih.gov/19010359/
555. https://pubmed.ncbi.nlm.nih.gov/10720331/
556. https://pubmed.ncbi.nlm.nih.gov/10390371/
557. https://pubmed.ncbi.nlm.nih.gov/15024000/
558. https://pubmed.ncbi.nlm.nih.gov/7416064/
559. https://pubmed.ncbi.nlm.nih.gov/27882052/

560. https://openheart.bmj.com/content/9/1/e001989
561. https://pubmed.ncbi.nlm.nih.gov/22724555/
562. https://pubmed.ncbi.nlm.nih.gov/13143077/
563. https://pubmed.ncbi.nlm.nih.gov/9130398/
564. https://www.ncbi.nlm.nih.gov/pmc/articles/PMC6798087/
565. https://pubmed.ncbi.nlm.nih.gov/4479416/
566. https://pubmed.ncbi.nlm.nih.gov/21285318/?dopt=Abstract
567. https://pubmed.ncbi.nlm.nih.gov/2370888/
568. https://pubmed.ncbi.nlm.nih.gov/21414183/
569. https://pubmed.ncbi.nlm.nih.gov/23764390/
570. https://www.ncbi.nlm.nih.gov/pmc/articles/PMC5078644/
571. https://pubmed.ncbi.nlm.nih.gov/10625935/
572. https://pubmed.ncbi.nlm.nih.gov/14608114/
573. https://pubmed.ncbi.nlm.nih.gov/10850638/
574. https://pubmed.ncbi.nlm.nih.gov/24424706/
575. https://pubmed.ncbi.nlm.nih.gov/15654927/
576. https://pubmed.ncbi.nlm.nih.gov/10219066/
577. https://openheart.bmj.com/lookup/external-ref?access_num=http://www.n&link_type=MED&atom=%2Fopenhrt%2F9%2F1%2Fe001989.atom
578. https://pubmed.ncbi.nlm.nih.gov/22296306/
579. https://pubmed.ncbi.nlm.nih.gov/25259724/
580. https://pubmed.ncbi.nlm.nih.gov/23336594/
581. https://www.hindawi.com/journals/ije/2020/6461254/
582. https://www.ncbi.nlm.nih.gov/pmc/articles/PMC8227031/
583. https://www.ncbi.nlm.nih.gov/pmc/articles/PMC5728865/
584. https://www.ncbi.nlm.nih.gov/pmc/articles/PMC5056296/
585. https://www.ncbi.nlm.nih.gov/pmc/articles/PMC6844281/
586. https://www.frontiersin.org/articles/10.3389/fimmu.2013.00047/full
587. https://pubmed.ncbi.nlm.nih.gov/27315814/
588. https://www.ncbi.nlm.nih.gov/pmc/articles/PMC5331475/
589. https://www.ncbi.nlm.nih.gov/pmc/articles/PMC7833496/
590. https://examine.com/supplements/inositol/\
591. https://www.sciencedirect.com/topics/neuroscience/acetylcysteine
592. https://www.ncbi.nlm.nih.gov/pmc/articles/PMC3254057/
593. https://pubmed.ncbi.nlm.nih.gov/10440166/
594. https://www.ncbi.nlm.nih.gov/pmc/articles/PMC7649937/
595. https://pubmed.ncbi.nlm.nih.gov/19732754/
596. https://www.nature.com/articles/1209954
597. https://link.springer.com/article/10.1385%2FCT%3A6%3A2%3A111
598. https://www.ncbi.nlm.nih.gov/pmc/articles/PMC5570602/
599. https://www.ncbi.nlm.nih.gov/pmc/articles/PMC397455/
600. https://www.ncbi.nlm.nih.gov/pmc/articles/PMC3664242/
601. https://pubmed.ncbi.nlm.nih.gov/16531564/

602. https://www.ncbi.nlm.nih.gov/pmc/articles/PMC4688235/
603. https://pubmed.ncbi.nlm.nih.gov/16175180/
604. https://www.frontiersin.org/articles/10.3389/fimmu.2020.598444/full
605. https://pubmed.ncbi.nlm.nih.gov/1520537/
606. https://pubmed.ncbi.nlm.nih.gov/23118923/
607. https://pubmed.ncbi.nlm.nih.gov/32198291/
608. https://journals.plos.org/plosone/article?id=10.1371/journal.pone.0087229
609. https://pubmed.ncbi.nlm.nih.gov/12404881/]
610. https://pubmed.ncbi.nlm.nih.gov/19732754/
611. https://www.ncbi.nlm.nih.gov/pmc/articles/PMC6250560/
612. https://pubmed.ncbi.nlm.nih.gov/15944340/
613. https://www.ncbi.nlm.nih.gov/pmc/articles/PMC8234027/
614. https://www.ncbi.nlm.nih.gov/pmc/articles/PMC8211525/
615. https://pubmed.ncbi.nlm.nih.gov/31826654/
616. https://pubmed.ncbi.nlm.nih.gov/28617566/
617. https://pubmed.ncbi.nlm.nih.gov/18534556/
618. https://pubmed.ncbi.nlm.nih.gov/23131885/
619. https://www.ncbi.nlm.nih.gov/pmc/articles/PMC5993450/
620. https://www.ncbi.nlm.nih.gov/pmc/articles/PMC2826714/
621. https://pubmed.ncbi.nlm.nih.gov/21606648/
622. https://pubmed.ncbi.nlm.nih.gov/19428083/
623. https://pubmed.ncbi.nlm.nih.gov/19091331/
624. https://pubmed.ncbi.nlm.nih.gov/24577230/
625. https://www.ncbi.nlm.nih.gov/pmc/articles/PMC3783787/
626. https://www.ncbi.nlm.nih.gov/pmc/articles/PMC6599212/
627. https://www.webmd.com/vitamins/ai/ingredientmono-1018/n-acetyl-cysteine-nac
628. https://www.sciencedaily.com/releases/2007/09/070904175353.htm
629. https://pubmed.ncbi.nlm.nih.gov/27927636/
630. https://pubmed.ncbi.nlm.nih.gov/3478223/
631. https://www.nature.com/articles/srep11601
632. https://www.ncbi.nlm.nih.gov/pmc/articles/PMC5372539/
633. https://pubmed.ncbi.nlm.nih.gov/8593442/
634. https://www.ncbi.nlm.nih.gov/pmc/articles/PMC6043915/
635. https://www.ncbi.nlm.nih.gov/pmc/articles/PMC3879341/
636. https://pubmed.ncbi.nlm.nih.gov/22040882/
637. https://pubmed.ncbi.nlm.nih.gov/28763875/
638. https://pubmed.ncbi.nlm.nih.gov/19786378/
639. https://pubmed.ncbi.nlm.nih.gov/23821590/
640. https://www.researchgate.net/publication/293056528_An_open_clinical_pilot_study_to_evaluate_the_safety_and_efficacy_of_natto_kinaseas_an_add-

on_oral_fibrinolytic_agent_tolow_molecular_weight_heparin_anti-plateletsin_acute_ischeamic_stroke
641. https://www.ncbi.nlm.nih.gov/pmc/articles/PMC9441630/
642. https://pubmed.ncbi.nlm.nih.gov/26740078/
643. https://pubmed.ncbi.nlm.nih.gov/18310985/
644. https://www.ncbi.nlm.nih.gov/pmc/articles/PMC4264722/
645. https://pubmed.ncbi.nlm.nih.gov/36080170/
646. https://www.ncbi.nlm.nih.gov/pmc/articles/PMC8648369/
647. https://www.ncbi.nlm.nih.gov/pmc/articles/PMC8380922/
648. https://jhoonline.biomedcentral.com/articles/10.1186/s13045-020-00954-7
649. https://www.drugs.com/npp/nattokinase.html
650. https://pubmed.ncbi.nlm.nih.gov/36312453/
651. https://www.ncbi.nlm.nih.gov/pmc/articles/PMC4523006/
652. https://www.ncbi.nlm.nih.gov/pmc/articles/PMC2779993/
653. https://www.ncbi.nlm.nih.gov/pmc/articles/PMC3724370/
654. https://onlinelibrary.wiley.com/doi/10.1111/exd.13819
655. https://www.ncbi.nlm.nih.gov/pmc/articles/PMC7275989/
656. https://www.ncbi.nlm.nih.gov/pmc/articles/PMC7428453/
657. https://www.ons.gov.uk/aboutus/transparencyandgovernance/freedomofinformationfoi/averageageofthosewhohaddiedwithcovid19
658. https://www.ncbi.nlm.nih.gov/pmc/articles/PMC5291468/
659. https://pubmed.ncbi.nlm.nih.gov/28522577/
660. https://www.ncbi.nlm.nih.gov/pmc/articles/PMC7275989/
661. https://www.frontiersin.org/articles/10.3389/fimmu.2020.01708/full
662. https://www.researchgate.net/publication/47544942_Niacin_attenuates_lung_inflammation_and_improves_survival_during_sepsis_by_downregulating_the_nuclear_factor-B_pathway
663. https://pubmed.ncbi.nlm.nih.gov/19382275/
664. https://pubmed.ncbi.nlm.nih.gov/7527336/
665. https://www.nature.com/articles/s41418-020-0530-3#ref-CR7
666. https://www.hindawi.com/journals/jna/2010/157591/
667. https://pubmed.ncbi.nlm.nih.gov/10616035/
668. https://pubmed.ncbi.nlm.nih.gov/32386566/
669. https://pubmed.ncbi.nlm.nih.gov/30813414/
670. https://www.ncbi.nlm.nih.gov/pmc/articles/PMC4840455/
671. https://jamanetwork.com/journals/jamapsychiatry/article-abstract/490850
672. https://www.ncbi.nlm.nih.gov/pmc/articles/PMC6007359/
673. https://clinmedjournals.org/articles/jide/journal-of-infectious-diseases-and-epidemiology-jide-7-195.php?jid=jide
674. https://academic.oup.com/bib/article/22/2/1279/5964187?login=true
675. https://pubmed.ncbi.nlm.nih.gov/35457123/
676. https://www.mdpi.com/2073-4409/11/4/710/htm

677. https://www.ncbi.nlm.nih.gov/pmc/articles/PMC6577427/
678. https://examine.com/supplements/vitamin-b3/
679. https://www.ncbi.nlm.nih.gov/pmc/articles/PMC8510689/
680. https://www.ncbi.nlm.nih.gov/pmc/articles/PMC4752613/
681. https://www.ncbi.nlm.nih.gov/pmc/articles/PMC8225153/
682. https://linkinghub.elsevier.com/retrieve/pii/B9780081026595000136
683. https://www.academia.edu/4003248/Imtiaz_Ahmad_Preliminary_Phytochemical_Studies_of_the_Miracle_Herb_of_the_Century_Nigella_sativa_L_Black_Seed_
684. https://sunnah.com/bukhari/76
685. https://www.ncbi.nlm.nih.gov/pmc/articles/PMC2702918/
686. https://www.ncbi.nlm.nih.gov/pmc/articles/PMC6535880/
687. https://academic.oup.com/fqs/article/2/1/1/4823052
688. https://pubmed.ncbi.nlm.nih.gov/27394440/
689. https://pubmed.ncbi.nlm.nih.gov/28236403/
690. https://www.ncbi.nlm.nih.gov/pmc/articles/PMC3933240/
691. https://www.ncbi.nlm.nih.gov/pmc/articles/PMC7225850/
692. https://www.ncbi.nlm.nih.gov/pmc/articles/PMC6406245/
693. https://www.derpharmachemica.com/abstract/characterization-of-antiradical-and-antiinflammatory-activities-of-some-coldrnpressed-oils-in-carrageenaninduced-rat-mod-4555.html
694. https://pubmed.ncbi.nlm.nih.gov/28216638/
695. https://www.ncbi.nlm.nih.gov/pmc/articles/PMC5116410/
696. https://www.ncbi.nlm.nih.gov/pmc/articles/PMC6317145/
697. https://pubmed.ncbi.nlm.nih.gov/28892789/
698. https://pubmed.ncbi.nlm.nih.gov/29405769/
699. https://pubmed.ncbi.nlm.nih.gov/29405769/
700. https://www.sciencedirect.com/science/article/pii/S2468227618301650?via%3Dihub
701. https://pubmed.ncbi.nlm.nih.gov/30091737/
702. https://pubmed.ncbi.nlm.nih.gov/31728856/
703. https://pubmed.ncbi.nlm.nih.gov/30668372/
704. https://www.mdpi.com/2227-9717/8/4/388
705. https://pubmed.ncbi.nlm.nih.gov/30259603/
706. https://pubmed.ncbi.nlm.nih.gov/26500095/
707. https://www.ncbi.nlm.nih.gov/pmc/articles/PMC4946859/
708. https://pubmed.ncbi.nlm.nih.gov/28552110/
709. https://www.ncbi.nlm.nih.gov/pmc/articles/PMC5620515/
710. https://www.ijper.org/article/460
711. https://www.researchgate.net/publication/321324359_The_efficacy_of_black_cumin_seed_Nigella_sativa_oil_and_hypoglycemic_drug_combination_to_reduce_HbA1c_level_in_patients_with_metabolic_syndrome_risk
712. https://pubmed.ncbi.nlm.nih.gov/28098097/

713. https://pubmed.ncbi.nlm.nih.gov/32510754/
714. https://www.sciencedirect.com/science/article/pii/S2221169117300382?via%3Dihub
715. https://pubmed.ncbi.nlm.nih.gov/31286398/
716. https://www.aloki.hu/pdf/1504_031048.pdf
717. https://www.ncbi.nlm.nih.gov/pmc/articles/PMC5292131/
718. https://pubmed.ncbi.nlm.nih.gov/32035219/
719. https://pubmed.ncbi.nlm.nih.gov/32053036/
720. https://pubmed.ncbi.nlm.nih.gov/30575005/
721. https://pubmed.ncbi.nlm.nih.gov/27696167/
722. https://www.ncbi.nlm.nih.gov/pmc/articles/PMC6111118/
723. https://pubmed.ncbi.nlm.nih.gov/28669218/
724. https://pubmed.ncbi.nlm.nih.gov/24680621/
725. https://www.ncbi.nlm.nih.gov/pmc/articles/PMC4387233/
726. http://eprints.mums.ac.ir/10195/
727. https://pubmed.ncbi.nlm.nih.gov/26510692/
728. http://ams.uokerbala.edu.iq/wp/wp-content/uploads/sites/7/2018/07/Study-the-effect-of-Nigella-Sativa-on-thyroid-function.pdf
729. https://pubmed.ncbi.nlm.nih.gov/30020313/
730. https://pubmed.ncbi.nlm.nih.gov/32548864/
731. https://www.tandfonline.com/doi/full/10.1080/13102818.2016.1257925
732. https://www.ncbi.nlm.nih.gov/pmc/articles/PMC5412196/
733. https://pubmed.ncbi.nlm.nih.gov/26826815/
734. https://pubmed.ncbi.nlm.nih.gov/31847893/
735. https://www.innovareacademics.in/journals/index.php/ajpcr/article/view/16227
736. https://www.cabdirect.org/globalhealth/abstract/20203092873
737. https://pubmed.ncbi.nlm.nih.gov/31300109/
738. https://www.sciencedirect.com/science/article/abs/pii/S2210803318300563?via%3Dihub
739. https://www.ncbi.nlm.nih.gov/pmc/articles/PMC3847425/
740. https://www.ajol.info/index.php/ajid/article/view/116542
741. https://c19early.org/nsmeta.html#fig_fp
742. https://onlinelibrary.wiley.com/doi/10.1002/ptr.7277
743. https://www.researchgate.net/publication/352134969_Clinical_Trial_of_Black_Seeds_Against_COVID_-19_in_Kirkuk_City_Iraq
744. https://pjmhsonline.com/2021/jan/384.pdf
745. https://www.medrxiv.org/content/10.1101/2020.10.30.20217364v2
746. https://examine.com/supplements/black-seed/#dosage-information
747. https://pubmed.ncbi.nlm.nih.gov/29705470/
748. https://covid19criticalcare.com/wp-content/uploads/2020/11/FLCCC-Alliance-I-MASKplus-Protocol-ENGLISH.pdf
749. https://www.ncbi.nlm.nih.gov/pmc/articles/PMC5392257/
750. https://www.ncbi.nlm.nih.gov/pmc/articles/PMC3002804/

751. https://www.seriouseats.com/guide-to-olive-varieties
752. https://pubmed.ncbi.nlm.nih.gov/24843404/
753. https://pubmed.ncbi.nlm.nih.gov/27847271/
754. https://pubmed.ncbi.nlm.nih.gov/11746176/
755. https://pubmed.ncbi.nlm.nih.gov/9464466/
756. https://pubmed.ncbi.nlm.nih.gov/12615669/
757. https://www.ncbi.nlm.nih.gov/pmc/articles/PMC9409738/
758. https://pubmed.ncbi.nlm.nih.gov/11905662
759. https://pubmed.ncbi.nlm.nih.gov/19079898/
760. https://pubmed.ncbi.nlm.nih.gov/15869811/
761. https://www.ncbi.nlm.nih.gov/pmc/articles/PMC3892135/
762. https://pubmed.ncbi.nlm.nih.gov/24211687/
763. https://pubmed.ncbi.nlm.nih.gov/21333710/
764. https://pubmed.ncbi.nlm.nih.gov/26873189/
765. https://www.ncbi.nlm.nih.gov/pmc/articles/PMC1878493/
766. https://www.ncbi.nlm.nih.gov/pmc/articles/PMC2626601/
767. https://www.ncbi.nlm.nih.gov/pmc/articles/PMC9319675/
768. https://linkinghub.elsevier.com/retrieve/pii/S0006291X07000812
769. https://www.frontiersin.org/articles/10.3389/fphar.2022.879118/full
770. https://pubmed.ncbi.nlm.nih.gov/22713943/
771. https://onlinelibrary.wiley.com/doi/10.1002/mnfr.201601066
772. https://pubmed.ncbi.nlm.nih.gov/25988120/
773. https://pubmed.ncbi.nlm.nih.gov/32356316/
774. https://examine.com/supplements/olive-leaf-extract/
775. https://www.ncbi.nlm.nih.gov/pmc/articles/PMC9496116/
776. https://pubmed.ncbi.nlm.nih.gov/35985182/
777. https://pubmed.ncbi.nlm.nih.gov/31236960/
778. https://pubmed.ncbi.nlm.nih.gov/33217688/
779. https://www.ncbi.nlm.nih.gov/pmc/articles/PMC4859791/
780. https://www.ncbi.nlm.nih.gov/pmc/articles/PMC3842302/
781. https://pubmed.ncbi.nlm.nih.gov/29091888/
782. https://pubmed.ncbi.nlm.nih.gov/29476730/
783. https://pubmed.ncbi.nlm.nih.gov/22526619/
784. https://www.ncbi.nlm.nih.gov/pmc/articles/PMC3792198/
785. https://pubmed.ncbi.nlm.nih.gov/24995563/
786. https://www.ncbi.nlm.nih.gov/pmc/articles/PMC4650553/
787. https://pubmed.ncbi.nlm.nih.gov/19135124/
788. https://pubmed.ncbi.nlm.nih.gov/22607196/
789. https://pubmed.ncbi.nlm.nih.gov/27533597/
790. https://pubmed.ncbi.nlm.nih.gov/25213258/
791. https://pubmed.ncbi.nlm.nih.gov/19585117/
792. https://www.ncbi.nlm.nih.gov/pmc/articles/PMC5564777/
793. https://pubmed.ncbi.nlm.nih.gov/31927505/
794. https://pubmed.ncbi.nlm.nih.gov/34204966/

795. https://pubmed.ncbi.nlm.nih.gov/26895180/
796. https://pubmed.ncbi.nlm.nih.gov/20680459/
797. https://www.ncbi.nlm.nih.gov/pmc/articles/PMC8013958/
798. https://neuropedia.com/oroxylin-a/
799. https://examine.com/supplements/baikal-skullcap/
800. https://eu.usatoday.com/story/news/factcheck/2021/06/15/fact-check-white-pine-tea-likely-not-helpful-against-covid-19/7651765002/
801. https://www.jimmunol.org/content/early/2021/10/11/jimmunol.2100637
802. https://pubmed.ncbi.nlm.nih.gov/23683467/
803. https://pubmed.ncbi.nlm.nih.gov/33911876/
804. https://www.medrxiv.org/content/10.1101/2022.04.28.22274443v1
805. https://www.ncbi.nlm.nih.gov/pmc/articles/PMC7038244/
806. https://siberiangreen.com/blogs/news/sources-of-natural-suramin-in-siberian-trees-and-its-health-benefits
807. https://pubmed.ncbi.nlm.nih.gov/13543900/
808. https://pubmed.ncbi.nlm.nih.gov/22069350/
809. https://www.ncbi.nlm.nih.gov/pmc/articles/PMC4576071/
810. https://pubmed.ncbi.nlm.nih.gov/15869993/
811. https://pubmed.ncbi.nlm.nih.gov/22248627/
812. https://pubmed.ncbi.nlm.nih.gov/26457430/
813. https://pubmed.ncbi.nlm.nih.gov/23474269/
814. https://pubmed.ncbi.nlm.nih.gov/7043783/
815. https://pubmed.ncbi.nlm.nih.gov/15203120/
816. https://pubmed.ncbi.nlm.nih.gov/15961104/
817. https://pubmed.ncbi.nlm.nih.gov/1313577/
818. https://www.nature.com/articles/s41594-021-00570-0
819. https://www.immunology.ox.ac.uk/covid-19/covid-19-immunology-literature-reviews/suramin-inhibits-sars-cov-2-infection-in-cell-culture-by-interfering-with-early-steps-of-the-replication-cycle
820. https://pubmed.ncbi.nlm.nih.gov/13435962/
821. https://www.ncbi.nlm.nih.gov/pmc/articles/PMC5497533/
822. https://pubmed.ncbi.nlm.nih.gov/21243780/
823. https://www.sciencedirect.com/topics/chemistry/shikimic-acid#:~:text=Shikimic%20acid%2C%20obtained%20from%20s-tar,a%20cyclohexene%2C%20and%20a%20cyclitol.
824. https://pubmed.ncbi.nlm.nih.gov/23553030/
825. https://www.ncbi.nlm.nih.gov/pmc/articles/PMC7153330
826. https://www.magonlinelibrary.com/doi/full/10.12968/hmed.2020.0580
827. https://www.ncbi.nlm.nih.gov/pmc/articles/PMC8992306/
828. https://www.ncbi.nlm.nih.gov/pmc/articles/PMC7730152/
829. https://pubmed.ncbi.nlm.nih.gov/26580596/
830. https://pubmed.ncbi.nlm.nih.gov/33825313/
831. http://www.surgicalcosmetic.org.br/details/342/en-US/shikimic-acid--a-potential-active-principle-for-skin-exfoliation

832. https://www.ncbi.nlm.nih.gov/pmc/articles/PMC7301717/
833. https://www.ncbi.nlm.nih.gov/pmc/articles/PMC6057698/
834. https://www.ncbi.nlm.nih.gov/pmc/articles/PMC6353859/
835. https://pubmed.ncbi.nlm.nih.gov/28478071/
836. https://pubmed.ncbi.nlm.nih.gov/28478071/
837. https://pubmed.ncbi.nlm.nih.gov/30733674/
838. https://pubmed.ncbi.nlm.nih.gov/23499702/
839. https://pubmed.ncbi.nlm.nih.gov/16273023
840. https://pubmed.ncbi.nlm.nih.gov/19429065/
841. https://pubmed.ncbi.nlm.nih.gov/19699261/
842. https://examine.com/supplements/polygala-tenuifolia/
843. https://pubmed.ncbi.nlm.nih.gov/15669543/
844. https://pubmed.ncbi.nlm.nih.gov/33245776/
845. https://pubmed.ncbi.nlm.nih.gov/35163255/
846. https://pubmed.ncbi.nlm.nih.gov/17217322/
847. https://pubmed.ncbi.nlm.nih.gov/12788891/
848. https://pubmed.ncbi.nlm.nih.gov/22649404/
849. https://pubmed.ncbi.nlm.nih.gov/22281161/
850. https://pubmed.ncbi.nlm.nih.gov/27631986/
851. https://austinpublishinggroup.com/womens-health/fulltext/ajwh-v6-id1032.pdf
852. https://pubmed.ncbi.nlm.nih.gov/32142651/
853. https://www.ncbi.nlm.nih.gov/pmc/articles/PMC8349425/
854. https://pubmed.ncbi.nlm.nih.gov/27307386/
855. https://www.ncbi.nlm.nih.gov/pmc/articles/PMC3043630/
856. https://pubmed.ncbi.nlm.nih.gov/32353859/
857. https://www.ncbi.nlm.nih.gov/pmc/articles/PMC7201103/
858. https://pubmed.ncbi.nlm.nih.gov/2899776/
859. https://www.ncbi.nlm.nih.gov/pmc/articles/PMC4823480/
860. https://pubmed.ncbi.nlm.nih.gov/23357432/
861. https://pubmed.ncbi.nlm.nih.gov/11208769/
862. https://www.ncbi.nlm.nih.gov/pmc/articles/PMC4849272/
863. https://pubmed.ncbi.nlm.nih.gov/23458628/
864. https://www.ncbi.nlm.nih.gov/pmc/articles/PMC4794096/
865. https://pubmed.ncbi.nlm.nih.gov/10969178/
866. https://www.ncbi.nlm.nih.gov/pmc/articles/PMC7896492/
867. https://www.ncbi.nlm.nih.gov/pmc/articles/PMC9032170/
868. https://www.ncbi.nlm.nih.gov/pmc/articles/PMC6273625/
869. https://www.ncbi.nlm.nih.gov/pmc/articles/PMC4808895/
870. https://www.ncbi.nlm.nih.gov/pmc/articles/PMC7425105/
871. https://pubmed.ncbi.nlm.nih.gov/18417116/
872. https://www.ncbi.nlm.nih.gov/pmc/articles/PMC6651418/
873. https://pubmed.ncbi.nlm.nih.gov/33906539/
874. https://www.ncbi.nlm.nih.gov/pmc/articles/PMC2816429/

875. https://pubmed.ncbi.nlm.nih.gov/30551359/
876. https://www.ncbi.nlm.nih.gov/pmc/articles/PMC8249127/
877. https://www.ncbi.nlm.nih.gov/pmc/articles/PMC3085798/
878. https://pubmed.ncbi.nlm.nih.gov/29132096/
879. https://pubmed.ncbi.nlm.nih.gov/23211366/
880. https://pubmed.ncbi.nlm.nih.gov/23376836/
881. http://article.sapub.org/10.5923.j.diabetes.20120103.01.html
882. https://www.sid.ir/paper/344066/en
883. https://pubmed.ncbi.nlm.nih.gov/14581383/
884. https://pubmed.ncbi.nlm.nih.gov/24039778/
885. https://pubmed.ncbi.nlm.nih.gov/12198000/
886. https://pubmed.ncbi.nlm.nih.gov/30392493/
887. https://www.ncbi.nlm.nih.gov/pmc/articles/PMC7254783/
888. https://pubmed.ncbi.nlm.nih.gov/27694000/
889. https://pubmed.ncbi.nlm.nih.gov/27756054/
890. https://pubmed.ncbi.nlm.nih.gov/30016632/
891. https://pubmed.ncbi.nlm.nih.gov/30639267/
892. https://www.ncbi.nlm.nih.gov/pmc/articles/PMC5936869/
893. https://pubmed.ncbi.nlm.nih.gov/29355544/
894. https://pubmed.ncbi.nlm.nih.gov/23000251/
895. https://pubmed.ncbi.nlm.nih.gov/30142541/
896. https://pubmed.ncbi.nlm.nih.gov/30978523/
897. https://pubmed.ncbi.nlm.nih.gov/19440933/
898. https://pubmed.ncbi.nlm.nih.gov/30599890/
899. https://pubmed.ncbi.nlm.nih.gov/25774442/
900. https://pubmed.ncbi.nlm.nih.gov/23000494/
901. https://pubmed.ncbi.nlm.nih.gov/26754609/
902. https://pubmed.ncbi.nlm.nih.gov/26864337/
903. https://chemrxiv.org/engage/chemrxiv/article-details/60c74980f96a00352b28727c
904. https://www.ncbi.nlm.nih.gov/pmc/articles/PMC8662201/
905. https://www.ncbi.nlm.nih.gov/pmc/articles/PMC9137692/\
906. https://www.ncbi.nlm.nih.gov/pmc/articles/PMC8573830
907. https://www.ncbi.nlm.nih.gov/pmc/articles/PMC8238537/
908. https://www.frontiersin.org/articles/10.3389/fphar.2022.898062
909. https://pubmed.ncbi.nlm.nih.gov/26992476/
910. https://www.researchgate.net/publication/291057194_Effect_of_quercetin_against_roundupR_andor_fluoride_induced_biochemical_alterations_and_lipid_peroxidation_in_rats
911. https://www.ncbi.nlm.nih.gov/pmc/articles/PMC7176256/
912. https://pubmed.ncbi.nlm.nih.gov/30668339/
913. https://pubmed.ncbi.nlm.nih.gov/16910729/
914. https://pubmed.ncbi.nlm.nih.gov/33187342/
915. https://www.sciencedirect.com/science/article/pii/S0753332222005662#

916. https://www.nature.com/articles/s41598-021-02544-0
917. https://pubmed.ncbi.nlm.nih.gov/25050823/
918. https://pubmed.ncbi.nlm.nih.gov/25669932/
919. https://examine.com/supplements/quercetin/#dosage-information
920. https://pubmed.ncbi.nlm.nih.gov/1102509/
921. https://pubmed.ncbi.nlm.nih.gov/30425336/
922. https://www.nature.com/articles/nature08221
923. https://pubmed.ncbi.nlm.nih.gov/34089901
924. https://www.nature.com/articles/s41586-018-0162-7
925. https://www.ncbi.nlm.nih.gov/pmc/articles/PMC3972801/
926. https://www.sciencedirect.com/science/article/pii/S2211124713003926
927. https://www.tandfonline.com/doi/abs/10.4161/auto.8824
928. https://www.oncotarget.com/article/1272/text/
929. https://onlinelibrary.wiley.com/doi/10.1111/acel.12194
930. https://link.springer.com/article/10.1007/s12035-016-0129-3
931. https://pubmed.ncbi.nlm.nih.gov/29943667/
932. https://www.ncbi.nlm.nih.gov/pmc/articles/PMC4571606/
933. https://www.nature.com/articles/cddis2016491
934. https://pubmed.ncbi.nlm.nih.gov/19183256/
935. https://pubmed.ncbi.nlm.nih.gov/22417271/
936. https://link.springer.com/article/10.1007/s11357-019-00087-x
937. https://onlinelibrary.wiley.com/doi/10.1111/j.1474-9726.2012.00832.x
938. https://onlinelibrary.wiley.com/doi/10.1111/acel.12109
939. https://www.ahajournals.org/doi/full/10.1161/JAHA.116.004106
940. https://pubmed.ncbi.nlm.nih.gov/31801138/
941. https://pubmed.ncbi.nlm.nih.gov/16043946/
942. https://pubmed.ncbi.nlm.nih.gov/30259816/
943. https://www.ahajournals.org/doi/10.1161/CIRCRESAHA.119.315185
944. https://www.sciencedirect.com/science/article/pii/S0006497120342798
945. https://www.ncbi.nlm.nih.gov/pmc/articles/PMC4166495/
946. https://www.ncbi.nlm.nih.gov/pmc/articles/PMC7857081/
947. https://sljch.sljol.info/articles/abstract/10.4038/sljch.v45i3.8132/
948. https://www.ncbi.nlm.nih.gov/pmc/articles/PMC5418203/
949. https://www.nature.com/articles/nature08155
950. https://www.science.org/doi/abs/10.1126/scitranslmed.aaq1564
951. https://www.ncbi.nlm.nih.gov/pmc/articles/PMC6021456/
952. https://www.ncbi.nlm.nih.gov/pmc/articles/PMC8001969/
953. https://www.sciencedirect.com/science/article/pii/S2211124719306990
954. https://www.nature.com/articles/s41591-018-0092-9
955. https://journals.lww.com/drug-monitoring/Abstract/2000/10000/Pharmacokinetics_and_Safety_of_Single_Oral_Doses.6.aspx
956. https://pubmed.ncbi.nlm.nih.gov/22461615/
957. https://www.nature.com/articles/s41419-019-1822-8
958. https://www.ncbi.nlm.nih.gov/pmc/articles/PMC6814615/

959. https://pubmed.ncbi.nlm.nih.gov/26020944/
960. https://www.rapamycin.news/t/what-is-the-rapamycin-dose-dosage-for-anti-aging-or-longevity/102
961. https://pubmed.ncbi.nlm.nih.gov/29408453/
962. https://www.ncbi.nlm.nih.gov/pmc/articles/PMC4942868/#b9
963. https://pubmed.ncbi.nlm.nih.gov/9395251/
964. https://www.ncbi.nlm.nih.gov/pmc/articles/PMC7143620/
965. https://pubmed.ncbi.nlm.nih.gov/8985016/
966. https://pubmed.ncbi.nlm.nih.gov/22465220/
967. https://www.ncbi.nlm.nih.gov/pmc/articles/PMC8289612/
968. https://www.ncbi.nlm.nih.gov/pmc/articles/PMC8542789/
969. https://pubmed.ncbi.nlm.nih.gov/29951747/
970. https://pubmed.ncbi.nlm.nih.gov/29407880/
971. https://pubmed.ncbi.nlm.nih.gov/30570816/
972. https://pubmed.ncbi.nlm.nih.gov/24150206/
973. https://www.ncbi.nlm.nih.gov/pmc/articles/PMC4068748/
974. https://pubmed.ncbi.nlm.nih.gov/25851110/
975. https://pubmed.ncbi.nlm.nih.gov/26440667/
976. https://pubmed.ncbi.nlm.nih.gov/25627672/
977. https://www.ncbi.nlm.nih.gov/pmc/articles/PMC4404420/
978. https://pubmed.ncbi.nlm.nih.gov/25061707/
979. https://pubmed.ncbi.nlm.nih.gov/24478430/
980. https://www.ncbi.nlm.nih.gov/pmc/articles/PMC4333343/
981. https://pubmed.ncbi.nlm.nih.gov/26854575/
982. https://pubmed.ncbi.nlm.nih.gov/31102993/
983. https://pubmed.ncbi.nlm.nih.gov/32985211/
984. https://www.nature.com/articles/s41598-022-13920-9
985. https://www.ncbi.nlm.nih.gov/pmc/articles/PMC713894
986. https://www.ncbi.nlm.nih.gov/pmc/articles/PMC7763587
987. https://pubmed.ncbi.nlm.nih.gov/30894514/
988. https://www.ncbi.nlm.nih.gov/pmc/articles/PMC8123193
989. https://www.ncbi.nlm.nih.gov/pmc/articles/PMC6608268/
990. https://pubmed.ncbi.nlm.nih.gov/22648627/
991. https://www.ncbi.nlm.nih.gov/pmc/articles/PMC6147949/
992. https://www.ncbi.nlm.nih.gov/pmc/articles/PMC3810808/
993. https://pubmed.ncbi.nlm.nih.gov/17956300/
994. https://www.ncbi.nlm.nih.gov/pmc/articles/PMC7139620/#B65-ijms-21-02084
995. https://pubmed.ncbi.nlm.nih.gov/28668442/
996. https://www.ncbi.nlm.nih.gov/pmc/articles/PMC6164842/
997. https://pubmed.ncbi.nlm.nih.gov/11205889/
998. https://pubmed.ncbi.nlm.nih.gov/17583542/
999. https://pubmed.ncbi.nlm.nih.gov/17392095/
1000. https://pubmed.ncbi.nlm.nih.gov/19695122/

1001. https://pubmed.ncbi.nlm.nih.gov/23793060/
1002. https://examine.com/supplements/resveratrol/#dosage-information
1003. https://pubmed.ncbi.nlm.nih.gov/20378318/
1004. https://www.ncbi.nlm.nih.gov/pmc/articles/PMC3541197/
1005. https://scholar.google.com/scholar_lookup?title=Medicinal+plants+in+Mongolian+medicine&author=Z+Khaidaev&author=TA+Menshikova&publication_year=1978&
1006. https://www.ncbi.nlm.nih.gov/pmc/articles/PMC9228580/
1007. https://pubmed.ncbi.nlm.nih.gov/11410073/
1008. https://pubmed.ncbi.nlm.nih.gov/17990971/
1009. https://www.sciencedirect.com/science/article/pii/S0753332219329671#:~:text=Rhodiola%20rosea%20L.%2C%20a%20-worldwide,diabetes%2C%20sepsis%2C%20and%20cancer.
1010. https://pubmed.ncbi.nlm.nih.gov/27013349/
1011. https://www.ncbi.nlm.nih.gov/pmc/articles/PMC3541197/
1012. https://pubmed.ncbi.nlm.nih.gov/20308973/
1013. https://pubmed.ncbi.nlm.nih.gov/28073099/
1014. https://pubmed.ncbi.nlm.nih.gov/22427203/
1015. https://www.ncbi.nlm.nih.gov/pmc/articles/PMC4070792/
1016. https://pubmed.ncbi.nlm.nih.gov/26548654/
1017. https://pubmed.ncbi.nlm.nih.gov/16401550
1018. https://www.ncbi.nlm.nih.gov/pmc/articles/PMC3538178
1019. https://www.ncbi.nlm.nih.gov/pmc/articles/PMC5901654/
1020. https://pubmed.ncbi.nlm.nih.gov/32461080/
1021. https://pubmed.ncbi.nlm.nih.gov/24818779/
1022. https://www.ncbi.nlm.nih.gov/pmc/articles/PMC4727095/
1023. https://pubmed.ncbi.nlm.nih.gov/26497336/
1024. https://pubmed.ncbi.nlm.nih.gov/11081987/
1025. https://pubmed.ncbi.nlm.nih.gov/22228617/
1026. https://pubmed.ncbi.nlm.nih.gov/19016404/
1027. https://pubmed.ncbi.nlm.nih.gov/28219059/
1028. https://pubmed.ncbi.nlm.nih.gov/18307390/
1029. https://pubmed.ncbi.nlm.nih.gov/17990195/
1030. https://pubmed.ncbi.nlm.nih.gov/34209617/
1031. https://pubmed.ncbi.nlm.nih.gov/23443221/
1032. https://pubmed.ncbi.nlm.nih.gov/25146085/
1033. https://www.ncbi.nlm.nih.gov/pmc/articles/PMC7281162/
1034. https://pubmed.ncbi.nlm.nih.gov/26063084/
1035. https://pubmed.ncbi.nlm.nih.gov/24188805/
1036. https://pubmed.ncbi.nlm.nih.gov/35337143/
1037. https://examine.com/supplements/rhodiola-rosea/#dosage-information
1038. https://www.ncbi.nlm.nih.gov/pmc/articles/PMC7601550/
1039. https://www.ncbi.nlm.nih.gov/pmc/articles/PMC6802361/
1040. https://www.ncbi.nlm.nih.gov/pmc/articles/PMC7601109/

1041. https://pubmed.ncbi.nlm.nih.gov/17625346/
1042. https://www.ncbi.nlm.nih.gov/pmc/articles/PMC5793241/
1043. https://www.ncbi.nlm.nih.gov/pmc/articles/PMC6305251/
1044. https://pubmed.ncbi.nlm.nih.gov/30711561/
1045. https://journals.sagepub.com/doi/abs/10.3181/00379727-99-24442
1046. https://pubmed.ncbi.nlm.nih.gov/18856648/
1047. https://www.cnki.net/kcms/doi/10.16429/j.1009-7848.2016.01.003.html
1048. https://www.thieme-connect.de/products/ejournals/abstract/10.1055/s-0032-1321154
1049. https://pubmed.ncbi.nlm.nih.gov/30933519/
1050. https://www.ncbi.nlm.nih.gov/pmc/articles/PMC6470943/
1051. https://pubmed.ncbi.nlm.nih.gov/31820078/
1052. https://pubmed.ncbi.nlm.nih.gov/31529692/
1053. https://pubmed.ncbi.nlm.nih.gov/31622731/
1054. https://pubmed.ncbi.nlm.nih.gov/26190785/
1055. https://pubmed.ncbi.nlm.nih.gov/19376837/
1056. https://www.ncbi.nlm.nih.gov/pmc/articles/PMC4350847/
1057. https://www.ncbi.nlm.nih.gov/pmc/articles/PMC5124115/
1058. https://www.ncbi.nlm.nih.gov/pmc/articles/PMC7014095/
1059. https://pubmed.ncbi.nlm.nih.gov/18075862/
1060. https://linkinghub.elsevier.com/retrieve/pii/S030881461001602X
1061. https://pubmed.ncbi.nlm.nih.gov/17213647/
1062. https://www.sciencedirect.com/science/article/pii/B9780323854009000034
1063. https://www.ncbi.nlm.nih.gov/pmc/articles/PMC4103725/
1064. https://www.ncbi.nlm.nih.gov/pmc/articles/PMC7397171/
1065. https://examine.com/supplements/royal-jelly/
1066. https://www.ncbi.nlm.nih.gov/pmc/articles/PMC3988729/
1067. https://pubmed.ncbi.nlm.nih.gov/9257239/
1068. https://pubmed.ncbi.nlm.nih.gov/18419679/
1069. https://pubmed.ncbi.nlm.nih.gov/16553520/
1070. https://www.ncbi.nlm.nih.gov/pmc/articles/PMC7533016/
1071. https://www.ncbi.nlm.nih.gov/pmc/articles/PMC6391314/
1072. https://www.ncbi.nlm.nih.gov/pmc/articles/PMC1804380/
1073. https://thorax.bmj.com/content/76/12/1242
1074. https://pubmed.ncbi.nlm.nih.gov/34451904/
1075. https://pubmed.ncbi.nlm.nih.gov/34745111/
1076. https://pubmed.ncbi.nlm.nih.gov/34241597/
1077. https://pubmed.ncbi.nlm.nih.gov/12173712/
1078. https://pubmed.ncbi.nlm.nih.gov/20238162/
1079. https://pubmed.ncbi.nlm.nih.gov/19793165/
1080. https://pubmed.ncbi.nlm.nih.gov/25102244/
1081. https://pubmed.ncbi.nlm.nih.gov/26523510/
1082. https://www.ncbi.nlm.nih.gov/pmc/articles/PMC4954764/

1083. https://www.ncbi.nlm.nih.gov/pmc/articles/PMC6215385/
1084. https://www.ncbi.nlm.nih.gov/pmc/articles/PMC3606118/
1085. https://www.ncbi.nlm.nih.gov/pmc/articles/PMC7533016/
1086. https://pubmed.ncbi.nlm.nih.gov/28396195/
1087. https://pubmed.ncbi.nlm.nih.gov/25077998/
1088. https://pubmed.ncbi.nlm.nih.gov/25419632/
1089. https://pubmed.ncbi.nlm.nih.gov/20501859/
1090. https://pubmed.ncbi.nlm.nih.gov/24916702/
1091. https://pubmed.ncbi.nlm.nih.gov/16286460/
1092. https://pubmed.ncbi.nlm.nih.gov/22773971/
1093. https://pubmed.ncbi.nlm.nih.gov/29787004/
1094. https://pubmed.ncbi.nlm.nih.gov/20621088/
1095. https://www.ncbi.nlm.nih.gov/pmc/articles/PMC6072146/
1096. https://pubmed.ncbi.nlm.nih.gov/19793165/
1097. https://examine.com/supplements/danshen/
1098. https://pubmed.ncbi.nlm.nih.gov/24899780/
1099. https://pubmed.ncbi.nlm.nih.gov/3218894/
1100. https://pubmed.ncbi.nlm.nih.gov/11165553/
1101. https://www.ncbi.nlm.nih.gov/pmc/articles/PMC2718593/
1102. https://pubmed.ncbi.nlm.nih.gov/28053227/
1103. https://pubmed.ncbi.nlm.nih.gov/2759081/
1104. https://link.springer.com/article/10.1007/BF02172188
1105. https://doi.org/10.1152%2Fajpregu.1995.269.1.R38
1106. https://link.springer.com/article/10.1007/s004240050905
1107. https://journals.sagepub.com/doi/10.1177/002215549804601109
1108. https://www.frontiersin.org/articles/10.3389/fnagi.2020.581374/full
1109. https://www.authorea.com/users/455597/articles/582067-sars-cov-2-spike-protein-in-the-pathogenesis-of-prion-like-diseases
1110. https://www.ncbi.nlm.nih.gov/pmc/articles/PMC5941775/
1111. https://pubmed.ncbi.nlm.nih.gov/11583886/
1112. https://pubmed.ncbi.nlm.nih.gov/15564698/
1113. https://pubmed.ncbi.nlm.nih.gov/16105634/
1114. https://pubmed.ncbi.nlm.nih.gov/20682487/
1115. https://www.ncbi.nlm.nih.gov/pmc/articles/PMC2248601/
1116. https://www.ncbi.nlm.nih.gov/pmc/articles/PMC5941775/
1117. https://pubmed.ncbi.nlm.nih.gov/23411620/
1118. https://www.sciencedirect.com/science/article/pii/S0531556521002916
1119. https://pubmed.ncbi.nlm.nih.gov/23844383/
1120. https://www.ncbi.nlm.nih.gov/pmc/articles/PMC3312275/
1121. https://www.ncbi.nlm.nih.gov/pmc/articles/PMC5069380/
1122. https://pubmed.ncbi.nlm.nih.gov/22253637/
1123. https://pubmed.ncbi.nlm.nih.gov/23213291/
1124. https://pubmed.ncbi.nlm.nih.gov/30486813/
1125. https://pubmed.ncbi.nlm.nih.gov/25705824/

1126. https://pubmed.ncbi.nlm.nih.gov/27001189/
1127. https://pubmed.ncbi.nlm.nih.gov/12842264/
1128. https://pubmed.ncbi.nlm.nih.gov/25748743/
1129. https://pubmed.ncbi.nlm.nih.gov/27932366/
1130. https://pubmed.ncbi.nlm.nih.gov/16871826/
1131. https://www.ncbi.nlm.nih.gov/pmc/articles/PMC7908414/
1132. https://antiquitynow.org/2014/11/12/bon-appetit-wednesday-seaweed-for-thanksgiving/
1133. https://pubmed.ncbi.nlm.nih.gov/25744337/
1134. https://pubmed.ncbi.nlm.nih.gov/22683660/
1135. https://www.ncbi.nlm.nih.gov/pmc/articles/PMC7345263/
1136. https://www.ncbi.nlm.nih.gov/pmc/articles/PMC5706049/
1137. https://linkinghub.elsevier.com/retrieve/pii/S004484860800820X
1138. https://www.ncbi.nlm.nih.gov/pmc/articles/PMC8232781/
1139. https://pubmed.ncbi.nlm.nih.gov/10227153/
1140. https://pubmed.ncbi.nlm.nih.gov/15896707/
1141. https://pubmed.ncbi.nlm.nih.gov/15056863/
1142. https://pubmed.ncbi.nlm.nih.gov/18616277/
1143. https://www.ncbi.nlm.nih.gov/pmc/articles/PMC5859842/
1144. https://pubmed.ncbi.nlm.nih.gov/7539671/
1145. https://pubmed.ncbi.nlm.nih.gov/17067880/
1146. https://pubmed.ncbi.nlm.nih.gov/17296677/
1147. https://pubmed.ncbi.nlm.nih.gov/27346541/
1148. https://pubmed.ncbi.nlm.nih.gov/18789961/
1149. https://pubmed.ncbi.nlm.nih.gov/24285223/
1150. https://linkinghub.elsevier.com/retrieve/pii/S0040402005017576
1151. https://pubmed.ncbi.nlm.nih.gov/32747241/
1152. https://pubmed.ncbi.nlm.nih.gov/30840077/
1153. https://pubmed.ncbi.nlm.nih.gov/23634989/
1154. https://pubmed.ncbi.nlm.nih.gov/31730947/
1155. https://www.ncbi.nlm.nih.gov/pmc/articles/PMC5405917/
1156. https://www.ncbi.nlm.nih.gov/pmc/articles/PMC5918985/
1157. https://pubmed.ncbi.nlm.nih.gov/8128484/
1158. https://pubmed.ncbi.nlm.nih.gov/29954354/
1159. https://www.nature.com/articles/s41421-020-00192-8
1160. https://www.mdpi.com/1422-0067/22/24/13202
1161. https://www.ncbi.nlm.nih.gov/pmc/articles/PMC7798825
1162. https://bpspubs.onlinelibrary.wiley.com/doi/10.1002/prp2.810
1163. https://journals.physiology.org/doi/full/10.1152/ajplung.00552.2020
1164. https://www.ncbi.nlm.nih.gov/pmc/articles/PMC6551690/
1165. https://nap.nationalacademies.org/read/10026/chapter/2#1
1166. https://pubmed.ncbi.nlm.nih.gov/22414981/
1167. https://pubmed.ncbi.nlm.nih.gov/26011104/
1168. https://pubmed.ncbi.nlm.nih.gov/9876004/

1169. https://pubmed.ncbi.nlm.nih.gov/8106628/
1170. https://pubmed.ncbi.nlm.nih.gov/15220938/
1171. https://pubmed.ncbi.nlm.nih.gov/25749125/
1172. https://examine.com/articles/how-can-i-safely-consume-seaweed/
1173. https://pubmed.ncbi.nlm.nih.gov/26817952/
1174. https://pubmed.ncbi.nlm.nih.gov/27517127/
1175. https://examine.com/supplements/brown-seaweed-extract/#dosage-information
1176. https://www.ncbi.nlm.nih.gov/pmc/articles/PMC7585045/
1177. https://pubmed.ncbi.nlm.nih.gov/11273304/
1178. https://pubmed.ncbi.nlm.nih.gov/12911824/
1179. https://pubmed.ncbi.nlm.nih.gov/450050/
1180. https://pubmed.ncbi.nlm.nih.gov/18272344/
1181. https://pubmed.ncbi.nlm.nih.gov/2688125/
1182. https://www.ncbi.nlm.nih.gov/pmc/articles/PMC7032259/
1183. https://pubmed.ncbi.nlm.nih.gov/7694216/
1184. https://www.ncbi.nlm.nih.gov/pmc/articles/PMC7167820/
1185. https://pubmed.ncbi.nlm.nih.gov/23811076/
1186. https://journals.sagepub.com/doi/abs/10.1177/1721727X1201000322
1187. https://www.ncbi.nlm.nih.gov/pmc/articles/PMC4149131/
1188. https://www.ncbi.nlm.nih.gov/pmc/articles/PMC5028551/
1189. https://www.frontiersin.org/articles/10.3389/fphar.2021.603997/full
1190. https://www.ncbi.nlm.nih.gov/pmc/articles/PMC2876922/
1191. https://pubmed.ncbi.nlm.nih.gov/21785188/
1192. https://www.ncbi.nlm.nih.gov/pmc/articles/PMC3296184/
1193. https://www.sciencedirect.com/science/article/abs/pii/S0146638008002647
1194. https://onlinelibrary.wiley.com/doi/abs/10.1002/ptr.2650090113
1195. https://onlinelibrary.wiley.com/doi/abs/10.1002/ptr.2650050505
1196. https://onlinelibrary.wiley.com/doi/abs/10.1002/ptr.2650030606
1197. https://www.ncbi.nlm.nih.gov/pmc/articles/PMC6364418/
1198. https://pubmed.ncbi.nlm.nih.gov/26395129/
1199. https://pubmed.ncbi.nlm.nih.gov/27414521/
1200. https://www.biorxiv.org/content/10.1101/2021.08.11.456012v2.full
1201. https://www.serravit.com.tr/wp-content/uploads/2020/08/Medical-aspects-of-Humic-Acid.pdf
1202. https://www.researchgate.net/publication/270097258_Fulvic_Acids_and_Viral_Infections
1203. https://www.ncbi.nlm.nih.gov/pmc/articles/PMC7554000/
1204. https://pubs.acs.org/doi/10.1021/am301358b
1205. https://www.sciencedirect.com/science/article/abs/pii/S1385894717310525
1206. https://cdn.shopify.com/s/files/1/0575/6574/1236/files/ION_White_Paper_Clinical_Trial.pdf

1207. https://www.ncbi.nlm.nih.gov/pmc/articles/PMC7640951/
1208. https://www.mdpi.com/2304-8158/11/5/694
1209. https://pubmed.ncbi.nlm.nih.gov/1245381/
1210. https://www.ncbi.nlm.nih.gov/pmc/articles/PMC3501277/
1211. https://www.ncbi.nlm.nih.gov/pmc/articles/PMC3929995/
1212. https://pubmed.ncbi.nlm.nih.gov/17053427/
1213. https://cdnsciencepub.com/doi/10.1139/cjpp-2019-0313
1214. https://pubmed.ncbi.nlm.nih.gov/23170060/
1215. https://www.biomolther.org/journal/view.html?volume=26&number=3&spage=225&year=2018
1216. https://pubmed.ncbi.nlm.nih.gov/1509945/
1217. https://www.ncbi.nlm.nih.gov/pmc/articles/PMC5933890/
1218. https://www.pnas.org/doi/full/10.1073/pnas.1809045115
1219. https://pubmed.ncbi.nlm.nih.gov/25833532/
1220. https://pubmed.ncbi.nlm.nih.gov/15649278/
1221. https://pubmed.ncbi.nlm.nih.gov/24065043/
1222. https://www.mdpi.com/2072-6643/9/8/795
1223. https://www.ncbi.nlm.nih.gov/pmc/articles/PMC3894431/
1224. https://pubmed.ncbi.nlm.nih.gov/23933994/
1225. https://pubmed.ncbi.nlm.nih.gov/23179085/
1226. https://www.ncbi.nlm.nih.gov/pmc/articles/PMC5097872/
1227. https://pubmed.ncbi.nlm.nih.gov/22936072/
1228. https://pubmed.ncbi.nlm.nih.gov/23257519/
1229. https://pubmed.ncbi.nlm.nih.gov/19234572/
1230. https://pubmed.ncbi.nlm.nih.gov/12075268/
1231. https://pubmed.ncbi.nlm.nih.gov/22718614/
1232. https://pubmed.ncbi.nlm.nih.gov/25833520/
1233. https://pubmed.ncbi.nlm.nih.gov/23392923/
1234. https://www.ncbi.nlm.nih.gov/pmc/articles/PMC4061860/
1235. https://www.ncbi.nlm.nih.gov/pmc/articles/PMC4630664/
1236. https://pubmed.ncbi.nlm.nih.gov/25894843/
1237. https://pubmed.ncbi.nlm.nih.gov/7403183/
1238. https://pubmed.ncbi.nlm.nih.gov/27444300/
1239. https://pubmed.ncbi.nlm.nih.gov/28118062/
1240. https://pubmed.ncbi.nlm.nih.gov/26781281
1241. https://pubmed.ncbi.nlm.nih.gov/27412799/
1242. https://pubmed.ncbi.nlm.nih.gov/16797868/
1243. https://pubmed.ncbi.nlm.nih.gov/27875962/
1244. https://pubmed.ncbi.nlm.nih.gov/12490622/
1245. https://www.ncbi.nlm.nih.gov/pmc/articles/PMC7889472/
1246. https://pubmed.ncbi.nlm.nih.gov/10516137/
1247. https://www.explorationpub.com/uploads/Article/A100188/100188.pdf
1248. https://www.medrxiv.org/content/10.1101/2021.07.07.21260092v1.full.pdf

1249. https://examine.com/supplements/taurine/#dosage-information
1250. https://www.ncbi.nlm.nih.gov/pmc/articles/PMC3910118/
1251. https://www.ncbi.nlm.nih.gov/pmc/articles/PMC4296439/
1252. https://link.springer.com/article/10.1007/s13596-012-0061-7
1253. https://pubmed.ncbi.nlm.nih.gov/15553132
1254. https://www.thieme-connect.de/products/ejournals/abstract/10.1055/s-0035-1565644
1255. https://www.ncbi.nlm.nih.gov/pmc/articles/PMC5376420/
1256. https://pubmed.ncbi.nlm.nih.gov/26899341/
1257. https://www.ncbi.nlm.nih.gov/pmc/articles/PMC4774317/
1258. https://pubmed.ncbi.nlm.nih.gov/3253489/
1259. https://pubmed.ncbi.nlm.nih.gov/24871663/
1260. https://www.ncbi.nlm.nih.gov/pmc/articles/PMC2816535/
1261. https://pubmed.ncbi.nlm.nih.gov/10782484/
1262. https://pubmed.ncbi.nlm.nih.gov/24621337/
1263. https://pubmed.ncbi.nlm.nih.gov/9973087/
1264. https://pubmed.ncbi.nlm.nih.gov/10464416/
1265. https://pubmed.ncbi.nlm.nih.gov/9198110/
1266. https://pubmed.ncbi.nlm.nih.gov/17887944/
1267. https://www.tandfonline.com/doi/abs/10.1080/10496475.2012.712939
1268. https://pubmed.ncbi.nlm.nih.gov/18277466/
1269. https://pubmed.ncbi.nlm.nih.gov/18946617/
1270. https://www.semanticscholar.org/paper/Ethanolic-Extracts-of-Ocimum-sanctum%2C-Azadirachta-Jha-Jha/91ae5d5c28990a9aee7eb61ff16049ce86b72935
1271. https://pubmed.ncbi.nlm.nih.gov/17669454/
1272. https://pubmed.ncbi.nlm.nih.gov/23061282/
1273. https://www.researchgate.net/publication/291296699_A_study_of_hepatoprotective_activity_of_Ocimum_sanctum_Krishna_tulas_extracts_in_chemically_induced_liver_damage_in_albino_mice
1274. https://www.jstage.jst.go.jp/article/jcbn1986/20/2/20_2_113/_pdf
1275. https://www.researchgate.net/publication/264037368_Protective_Effect_of_Ocimum_sanctum_on_Ethanol-induced_Oxidative_Stress_in_Swiss_Albino_Mice_Brain
1276. https://www.researchgate.net/profile/Dilip-Kedia/publication/288420493_Protective_effect_of_Ocimum_sanctum_leaf_extracts_against_rogor_induced_ovarian_toxicity_in_Clarias_batrachus_Linn/links/58b5376345851503bea1adcb/Protective-effect-of-Ocimum-sanctum-leaf-extracts-against-rogor-induced-ovarian-toxicity-in-Clarias-batrachus-Linn.pdf
1277. https://pubmed.ncbi.nlm.nih.gov/21430913/

1278. http://www.veterinaryworld.org/Vol.4/January%20-%202011/Imuuno%20modulatory%20effect%20of%20Ocimum%20sanctum%20against%20endosulfan%20induced%20immunotoxicity.pdf
1279. https://pubmed.ncbi.nlm.nih.gov/19130861/
1280. https://pubmed.ncbi.nlm.nih.gov/21976818/
1281. https://www.ncbi.nlm.nih.gov/pmc/articles/PMC3119265/
1282. https://ijp-online.com/article.asp?issn=0253-7613;year=2007;volume=39;issue=2;spage=87;epage=89;aulast=pemminati
1283. https://pubmed.ncbi.nlm.nih.gov/15266961/
1284. http://veterinaryworld.org/Vol.4/June%20-%202011/Hematobiochemical%20changes%20of%20lead%20Poisoning%20and%20amelioration%20with%20Ocimum%20sanctum%20in%20wistar%20albino%20rats.pdf
1285. https://pubmed.ncbi.nlm.nih.gov/19111884/
1286. https://pubmed.ncbi.nlm.nih.gov/16924835/
1287. https://pubmed.ncbi.nlm.nih.gov/12587743/
1288. https://pubmed.ncbi.nlm.nih.gov/22087607/
1289. https://pubmed.ncbi.nlm.nih.gov/7275241/
1290. https://pubmed.ncbi.nlm.nih.gov/2329804/
1291. https://www.researchgate.net/publication/263448784_Aqueous_Tulsi_leaf_Ocimum_sanctum_extract_possesses_antioxidant_properties_and_protects_against_cadmium-induced_oxidative_stress_in_rat_heart
1292. https://pubmed.ncbi.nlm.nih.gov/16965878/
1293. https://pubmed.ncbi.nlm.nih.gov/27093754/
1294. https://pubmed.ncbi.nlm.nih.gov/17379314/
1295. https://pubmed.ncbi.nlm.nih.gov/15619567/
1296. https://pubmed.ncbi.nlm.nih.gov/21812651/
1297. https://www.ijpsonline.com/articles/cholinergic-basis-of-memory-improving-effect-of-ocimum-tenuiflorum-linn.html?view=mobile&crsi=6624964158&cicada_org_src=healthwebmagazine.com&cicada_org_mdm=direct
1298. https://pubmed.ncbi.nlm.nih.gov/19253862/
1299. https://pubmed.ncbi.nlm.nih.gov/21977056/
1300. https://pubmed.ncbi.nlm.nih.gov/21106356/
1301. https://www.amrita.edu/publication/hypolipidemic-efficacy-of-ocimum-sanctum-in-the-prevention-of-atherogenesis-in-male-albino-rabbits/
1302. https://www.ncbi.nlm.nih.gov/pmc/articles/PMC4296439/#ref48
1303. https://www.ncbi.nlm.nih.gov/pmc/articles/PMC3178181/
1304. https://www.karger.com/Article/Abstract/497569
1305. https://pubmed.ncbi.nlm.nih.gov/18085503/
1306. https://pubmed.ncbi.nlm.nih.gov/8880292/
1307. https://www.researchgate.net/profile/Kartik-Salwe/publication/266885994_EVALUATION_OF_THE_ANTIDIABETIC_EFFECT_OF_OCIMUM_SANCTUM_IN_TYPE_2_DIABETIC_PATIENTS/links/

548bb0880cf225bf669f8b0f/EVALUATION-OF-THE-ANTIDIABETIC-EFFECT-OF-OCIMUM-SANCTUM-IN-TYPE-2-DIABETIC-PATIENTS.pdf

1308. https://www.ncbi.nlm.nih.gov/pmc/articles/PMC5539010/
1309. https://www.tandfonline.com/doi/abs/10.1080/09735070.2009.11886330
1310. https://shodhganga.inflibnet.ac.in/handle/10603/76115
1311. https://pubmed.ncbi.nlm.nih.gov/21619917/
1312. https://www.sciencedirect.com/science/article/abs/pii/S2222180812601893
1313. https://pubmed.ncbi.nlm.nih.gov/21914546/
1314. https://www.tandfonline.com/doi/abs/10.1080/0972060X.2008.10643611
1315. https://www.ajol.info/index.php/ajb/article/view/92439
1316. https://www.cabdirect.org/cabdirect/abstract/20093343446
1317. https://pubmed.ncbi.nlm.nih.gov/19909781/
1318. https://www.researchgate.net/publication/280004308_Antibacterial_Activity_of_Ocimum_sanctum_Linn_and_its_application_in_Water_Purification
1319. https://www.cabdirect.org/globalhealth/abstract/20133079769
1320. https://www.semanticscholar.org/paper/Antifatigue-and-neuroprotective-properties-of-of-L-Prasad/e8deb24d8bea4b29ded5f3e11f3dcb5e8f325ec3
1321. http://repository.ias.ac.in/76148/
1322. https://www.ncbi.nlm.nih.gov/pmc/articles/PMC8531902/
1323. https://www.ncbi.nlm.nih.gov/pmc/articles/PMC8357497/
1324. https://www.ncbi.nlm.nih.gov/pmc/articles/PMC6268661/
1325. https://pubmed.ncbi.nlm.nih.gov/21455446/
1326. https://academic.oup.com/qjmed/article/111/suppl_1/hcy200.188/5244568
1327. https://pubmed.ncbi.nlm.nih.gov/33109038/
1328. https://www.ncbi.nlm.nih.gov/pmc/articles/PMC5376420/
1329. https://www.ncbi.nlm.nih.gov/pmc/articles/PMC5494092/
1330. https://pubmed.ncbi.nlm.nih.gov/9230919/
1331. https://www.ncbi.nlm.nih.gov/pmc/articles/PMC9611527/
1332. https://pubmed.ncbi.nlm.nih.gov/17158229/
1333. https://pubmed.ncbi.nlm.nih.gov/5027768/
1334. https://pubmed.ncbi.nlm.nih.gov/22154083/
1335. https://pubmed.ncbi.nlm.nih.gov/24668744/
1336. https://www.ncbi.nlm.nih.gov/pmc/articles/PMC4670816/
1337. https://www.ncbi.nlm.nih.gov/pmc/articles/PMC3511118/
1338. https://www.ncbi.nlm.nih.gov/pmc/articles/PMC7590292/
1339. https://pubmed.ncbi.nlm.nih.gov/8684484/
1340. https://www.ncbi.nlm.nih.gov/pmc/articles/PMC3052787/
1341. https://www.ncbi.nlm.nih.gov/pmc/articles/PMC3864001/
1342. https://www.ncbi.nlm.nih.gov/pmc/articles/PMC3668813/
1343. https://www.ncbi.nlm.nih.gov/pmc/articles/PMC3735704/

1344. https://pubmed.ncbi.nlm.nih.gov/23407450/
1345. https://www.nature.com/articles/s41598-020-63013-8
1346. https://www.nature.com/articles/386078a0
1347. https://www.ncbi.nlm.nih.gov/pmc/articles/PMC7578635/
1348. https://www.ncbi.nlm.nih.gov/pmc/articles/PMC6413124/
1349. https://www.ncbi.nlm.nih.gov/pmc/articles/PMC7601762/
1350. https://www.ncbi.nlm.nih.gov/pmc/articles/PMC9312339/
1351. https://pubmed.ncbi.nlm.nih.gov/8323961/
1352. https://pubmed.ncbi.nlm.nih.gov/9354587/
1353. https://pubmed.ncbi.nlm.nih.gov/15450084/
1354. https://pubmed.ncbi.nlm.nih.gov/22582012/
1355. https://www.ncbi.nlm.nih.gov/pmc/articles/PMC5831512/
1356. https://www.ncbi.nlm.nih.gov/pmc/articles/PMC3138866/
1357. https://pubmed.ncbi.nlm.nih.gov/10580503/
1358. https://pubmed.ncbi.nlm.nih.gov/25694037/
1359. https://pubmed.ncbi.nlm.nih.gov/23525894/
1360. https://pubmed.ncbi.nlm.nih.gov/19179058/
1361. https://pubmed.ncbi.nlm.nih.gov/15514282/
1362. https://pubmed.ncbi.nlm.nih.gov/28345303/
1363. https://pubmed.ncbi.nlm.nih.gov/21403017/
1364. https://pubmed.ncbi.nlm.nih.gov/19410972/
1365. https://www.ncbi.nlm.nih.gov/pmc/articles/PMC2909045/
1366. https://pubmed.ncbi.nlm.nih.gov/27100101/
1367. https://www.frontiersin.org/articles/10.3389/fmed.2020.00154/full
1368. https://www.ncbi.nlm.nih.gov/pmc/articles/PMC7504709/
1369. https://pubmed.ncbi.nlm.nih.gov/24285428/
1370. https://pubmed.ncbi.nlm.nih.gov/22475810/
1371. https://pubmed.ncbi.nlm.nih.gov/17982686/
1372. https://pubmed.ncbi.nlm.nih.gov/19929921/
1373. https://pubmed.ncbi.nlm.nih.gov/11861756/
1374. https://pubmed.ncbi.nlm.nih.gov/17404108/
1375. https://pubmed.ncbi.nlm.nih.gov/20676681/
1376. https://pubmed.ncbi.nlm.nih.gov/16400650/
1377. https://www.ncbi.nlm.nih.gov/pmc/articles/PMC3591458/
1378. https://pubmed.ncbi.nlm.nih.gov/17445536/
1379. https://www.ncbi.nlm.nih.gov/pmc/articles/PMC9312339/]
1380. https://www.ncbi.nlm.nih.gov/pmc/articles/PMC7499546/
1381. https://journals.sagepub.com/doi/full/10.1177/00033197221121007
1382. https://pubmed.ncbi.nlm.nih.gov/33601125/
1383. https://www.ncbi.nlm.nih.gov/pmc/articles/PMC7406600/
1384. https://pubmed.ncbi.nlm.nih.gov/24089220/
1385. https://pubmed.ncbi.nlm.nih.gov/17012108
1386. https://pubmed.ncbi.nlm.nih.gov/9349732/
1387. https://www.ncbi.nlm.nih.gov/pmc/articles/PMC5613455

1388. https://www.ncbi.nlm.nih.gov/pmc/articles/PMC6413124/#B13-ijms-20-00896
1389. https://examine.com/supplements/vitamin-k/
1390. https://www.ncbi.nlm.nih.gov/pmc/articles/PMC4458242/
1391. https://pubmed.ncbi.nlm.nih.gov/31857587/
1392. https://pubmed.ncbi.nlm.nih.gov/34497484/
1393. https://link.springer.com/article/10.1007/s13311-015-0417-z
1394. https://pubmed.ncbi.nlm.nih.gov/30355189/
1395. https://pubmed.ncbi.nlm.nih.gov/26058501/
1396. https://www.ncbi.nlm.nih.gov/labs/pmc/articles/PMC3295231/
1397. https://pubmed.ncbi.nlm.nih.gov/25689839/
1398. https://www.nature.com/articles/nn0199_94
1399. https://pubmed.ncbi.nlm.nih.gov/23245749/
1400. https://www.ncbi.nlm.nih.gov/labs/pmc/articles/PMC3679540/
1401. https://www.ncbi.nlm.nih.gov/pmc/articles/PMC5928377/
1402. https://pubmed.ncbi.nlm.nih.gov/25164906/
1403. https://www.ncbi.nlm.nih.gov/pmc/articles/PMC7100921/
1404. https://pubmed.ncbi.nlm.nih.gov/28862330/
1405. https://www.seizure-journal.com/article/S1059-1311(18)30011-6/fulltext
1406. https://www.ncbi.nlm.nih.gov/pmc/articles/PMC4666924/
1407. https://physoc.onlinelibrary.wiley.com/doi/full/10.1113/EP087351
1408. https://www.frontiersin.org/articles/10.3389/fcvm.2021.766676/full
1409. https://www.ncbi.nlm.nih.gov/pmc/articles/PMC4082307/
1410. https://pubmed.ncbi.nlm.nih.gov/10839541/
1411. https://pubmed.ncbi.nlm.nih.gov/11247812/
1412. https://www.ncbi.nlm.nih.gov/pmc/articles/PMC3715840/
1413. https://www.frontiersin.org/articles/10.3389/fnins.2019.00877/full
1414. https://www.ncbi.nlm.nih.gov/pmc/articles/PMC9028764/
1415. https://www.ncbi.nlm.nih.gov/pmc/articles/PMC7850225/
1416. https://pubmed.ncbi.nlm.nih.gov/36353127/
1417. https://www.researchsquare.com/article/rs-1716096/v1
1418. https://pubmed.ncbi.nlm.nih.gov/30328647/
1419. https://www.ncbi.nlm.nih.gov/pmc/articles/PMC8313807/
1420. https://www.ncbi.nlm.nih.gov/labs/pmc/articles/PMC4543605/
1421. https://www.ncbi.nlm.nih.gov/pmc/articles/PMC1919431/
1422. https://www.nature.com/articles/aps2016149
1423. https://www.pnas.org/doi/10.1073/pnas.0409888102
1424. https://www.sciencedirect.com/science/article/pii/S0753332221004248
1425. https://www.frontiersin.org/articles/10.3389/fphar.2021.590201/full
1426. https://www.pnas.org/doi/full/10.1073/pnas.0803601105
1427. https://www.sciencedirect.com/science/article/pii/S0002944012008905
1428. https://pubmed.ncbi.nlm.nih.gov/22717234/
1429. https://www.sciencedirect.com/science/article/pii/S000294401000177X
1430. https://pubmed.ncbi.nlm.nih.gov/32560286/

1431. https://pubmed.ncbi.nlm.nih.gov/31841509/
1432. https://pubmed.ncbi.nlm.nih.gov/31711937/
1433. https://pubmed.ncbi.nlm.nih.gov/30469079/
1434. https://pubmed.ncbi.nlm.nih.gov/30343038/
1435. https://pubmed.ncbi.nlm.nih.gov/26748309/
1436. https://pubmed.ncbi.nlm.nih.gov/28729222/
1437. https://pubmed.ncbi.nlm.nih.gov/28624443/
1438. https://pubmed.ncbi.nlm.nih.gov/30836069/
1439. https://pubmed.ncbi.nlm.nih.gov/28026135/
1440. https://pubmed.ncbi.nlm.nih.gov/27379721/
1441. https://pubmed.ncbi.nlm.nih.gov/21356367/
1442. https://pubmed.ncbi.nlm.nih.gov/31109132/
1443. https://pubmed.ncbi.nlm.nih.gov/22326488/
1444. https://www.sciencedirect.com/science/article/abs/pii/S0091305714001956
1445. https://pubmed.ncbi.nlm.nih.gov/27077495/
1446. https://www.ncbi.nlm.nih.gov/pmc/articles/PMC3255347/
1447. https://pubmed.ncbi.nlm.nih.gov/23747418/
1448. https://pubmed.ncbi.nlm.nih.gov/32365556/
1449. https://pubmed.ncbi.nlm.nih.gov/28545573/
1450. https://pubmed.ncbi.nlm.nih.gov/26408161/
1451. https://pubmed.ncbi.nlm.nih.gov/30799631/
1452. https://pubmed.ncbi.nlm.nih.gov/19457575/
1453. https://pubmed.ncbi.nlm.nih.gov/21789506/
1454. https://pubmed.ncbi.nlm.nih.gov/28992427/
1455. https://pubmed.ncbi.nlm.nih.gov/22448282/
1456. https://pubmed.ncbi.nlm.nih.gov/25171128/
1457. https://www.sciencedirect.com/science/article/abs/pii/S0009279718316284
1458. https://www.sciencedirect.com/science/article/abs/pii/S0031938414003400
1459. https://www.ncbi.nlm.nih.gov/pmc/articles/PMC9208571/
1460. https://www.ncbi.nlm.nih.gov/pmc/articles/PMC7410791/
1461. https://pubmed.ncbi.nlm.nih.gov/32557405/

THIS IS ALL THAT WE'VE GOT

1. https://pubmed.ncbi.nlm.nih.gov/23985420/
2. https://pubmed.ncbi.nlm.nih.gov/21811020/
3. https://pubmed.ncbi.nlm.nih.gov/22914588/
4. https://pubmed.ncbi.nlm.nih.gov/27884585/
5. https://www.ncbi.nlm.nih.gov/pmc/articles/PMC2574024/
6. https://pubmed.ncbi.nlm.nih.gov/24280255/
7. https://pubmed.ncbi.nlm.nih.gov/20129316/

8. https://pubmed.ncbi.nlm.nih.gov/22766770/
9. https://pubmed.ncbi.nlm.nih.gov/7256279/
10. https://pubmed.ncbi.nlm.nih.gov/12370853/
11. https://pubmed.ncbi.nlm.nih.gov/24918436/
12. https://journals.lww.com/pancreasjournal/Abstract/2013/05000/Uridine_Triphosphate_Increases_Proliferation_of.17.aspx
13. https://pubmed.ncbi.nlm.nih.gov/25972546/
14. https://www.ncbi.nlm.nih.gov/pmc/articles/PMC6105847/
15. https://www.bmj.com/content/370/bmj.m3489/rr-3
16. https://www.ncbi.nlm.nih.gov/pmc/articles/PMC9250701/
17. https://www.ncbi.nlm.nih.gov/pmc/articles/PM-C7553911/pdf/41598_2020_Article_73864.pdf
18. https://pubmed.ncbi.nlm.nih.gov/29442306/
19. https://pubmed.ncbi.nlm.nih.gov/25495394/
20. https://pubmed.ncbi.nlm.nih.gov/10687868/
21. https://pubmed.ncbi.nlm.nih.gov/33091497/
22. https://www.ncbi.nlm.nih.gov/pmc/articles/PMC6365538/
23. https://pubmed.ncbi.nlm.nih.gov/24477002/
24. https://www.sciencedirect.com/science/article/abs/pii/S0956566322008661?via%3Dihub
25. https://pubmed.ncbi.nlm.nih.gov/26466563/
26. https://www.bmj.com/content/376/bmj.o102
27. https://pubmed.ncbi.nlm.nih.gov/35821373/
28. https://www.ncbi.nlm.nih.gov/pmc/articles/PMC1182327/
29. https://blogs.bmj.com/bmj/2017/06/05/paul-glasziou-and-iain-chalmers-can-it-really-be-true-that-50-of-research-is-unpublished/
30. https://fortune.com/well/2022/10/26/omicron-booster-new-may-not-work-better-than-original-covid-shot-vaccine-jab-wuhan-strain-ba4-ba5-original-pandemic-endemic/

WHAT WILL OUR FUTURE LOOK LIKE?

1. https://www.ncbi.nlm.nih.gov/pmc/articles/PMC7375349/
2. https://www.mdpi.com/1660-4601/19/15/9295
3. https://brownstone.org/articles/more-than-400-studies-on-the-failure-of-compulsory-covid-interventions/
4. https://pubmed.ncbi.nlm.nih.gov/33301246/
5. https://www.nature.com/articles/d41586-020-03441-8
6. https://depts.washington.edu/bhdept/ethics-medicine/bioethics-topics/detail/67
7. https://systematicreviewsjournal.biomedcentral.com/articles/10.1186/s13643-019-1034-4
8. https://www.nejm.org/doi/full/10.1056/nejm199711133372006

MASKING DEATH

1. 1. https://fullfact.org/health/coronavirus-vaccine-pfizer-transmission-test/
2. https://www.sciencedirect.com/science/article/pii/S2589537022000359
3. https://www.mdpi.com/1660-4601/19/15/9295
4. https://www.mdpi.com/1660-4601/18/8/4344
5. https://www.acpjournals.org/doi/10.7326/M20-6817
6. https://www.telegraph.co.uk/politics/2021/06/10/face-masks-should-continue-forever-says-sagescientist/
7. https://www.sciencedirect.com/science/article/pii/S004896972204712X

WHY DID WE HAVE A PANDEMIC?

1. https://www.youtube.com/watch?v=6Af6b_wyiwl
2. https://www.nature.com/articles/S41591-020-0820-9
3. https://www.thelancet.com/journals/lancet/article/PIIS0140-6736(22)01585-9/fulltext
4. https://www.jeffsachs.org/interviewsandmedia/64rtmykxdl56ehbjwy37m5hfahwnm5
5. https://www.help.senate.gov/imo/media/doc/report_an_analysis_of_the_origins_of_covid-19_102722.pdf
6. https://observer.com/2020/12/how-bill-gates-helped-make-the-covid-19-vaccine-possible/
7. https://www.biometricupdate.com/202206/fortify-rights-links-personal-id-documents-listing-ethnicity-with-repression-genocides
8. https://web.kominfo.go.id/sites/default/files/G20%20Bali%20Leaders%27%20Declaration%2C%2015-16%20November%202022%2C%20incl%20Annex.pdf
9. https://www.darpa.mil/
10. https://www.darpa.mil/attachments/ADEPTVignetteFINAL.pdf
11. https://www.gao.gov/products/gao-21-319
12. https://www.goodreads.com/book/show/82256.The_Sovereign_Individual

WWW.CALLINGOUTTHESHOTS.XZY

Made in the USA
Monee, IL
03 May 2023

32903760R10297